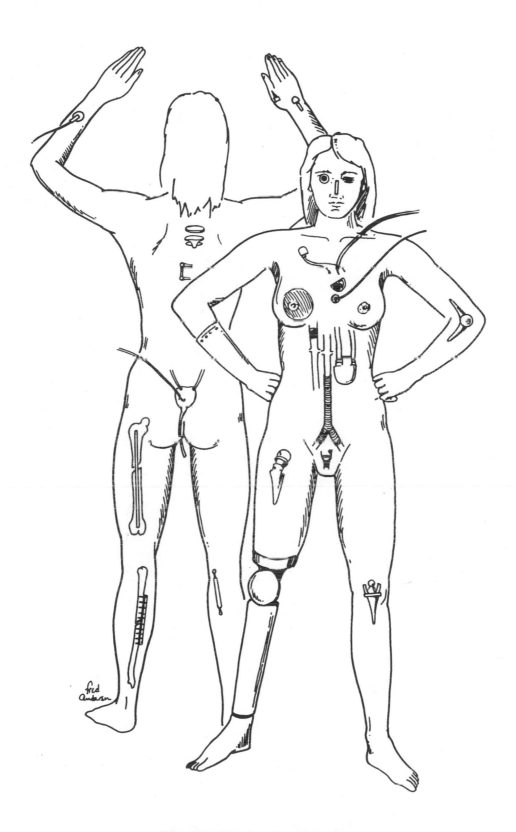

The BioMechanical Woman

Radiologic Guide to Medical Devices and Foreign Bodies

Radiologic Guide to Medical Devices and Foreign Bodies

EDITED BY

Tim B. Hunter, M.D., F.A.C.R.
Professor, Department of Radiology,
University of Arizona;
Chief of Diagnostic Radiology,
Arizona Health Sciences Center,
Tucson, Arizona;

David G. Bragg, M.D.
Professor and Chairman,
Department of Radiology,
University of Utah,
Salt Lake City, Utah

with **1269** illustrations

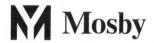

M Mosby

St. Louis Baltimore Boston Chicago London Madrid Philadelphia Sydney Toronto

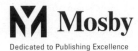

Editor: Anne S. Patterson
Managing editor: Elaine Steinborn
Project manager: Mark Spann
Production editor: Carl Masthay
Book and cover designer: David Zielinski
Production: Celeste Clingan

Printed in the United States of America.

Mosby–Year Book, Inc.
11830 Westline Industrial Drive
St. Louis, Missouri 63146

Library of Congress Cataloging-in-Publication Data
Radiologic guide to medical devices and foreign bodies / edited by Tim
   B. Hunter, David G. Bragg.
      p.   cm.
   Includes bibliographical references and index.
   ISBN 0-8016-6574-4
   1. Radiography, Medical—Complications.   2. Implants, Artificial.
3. Foreign bodies (Surgery)   I. Hunter, Tim B.   II. Bragg, David
G., 1933-
   [DNLM: 1. Diagnostic Imaging.   2. Implants, Artificial.
3. Foreign Bodies.   4. Artifacts.   WN 210 R128 1993]
RC78.3.R36   1994
616.07'54—dc20
DNLM/DLC   93-1357
for Library of Congress   CIP

94 95 96 97 98 CL/MY 9 8 7 6 5 4 3 2 1

Contributors

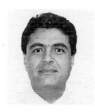 **Nicholas A. Awad, M.D.**
Radiologist,
Kingman, Arizona

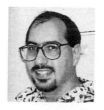 **Ammar Darkazanli, M.Sc.**
Research Lecturer,
Department of Radiology,
University of Arizona,
Tucson, Arizona

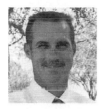 **James B. Benjamin, M.D.**
Associate Professor,
Department of Surgery,
University of Arizona,
Tucson, Arizona

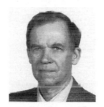 **Martin L. Fackler, M.D.**
President,
International Wound Ballistics
    Association,
Hawthorne, Florida

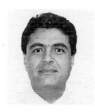 **David G. Bragg, M.D.**
Professor and Chairman,
Department of Radiology,
University of Utah,
Salt Lake City, Utah

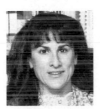 **Laurie L. Fajardo, M.D.**
Associate Professor,
Head, Section of Mammography
    and Breast Imaging,
Department of Radiology,
University of Arizona,
Tucson, Arizona

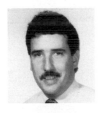 **Luis Cueva, D.D.S., P.T.**
Dentist,
Tucson, Arizona

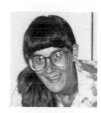 **Linda J. Goodwill**
Photographer and Research Assistant,
Department of Radiology,
University of Arizona,
Tucson, Arizona

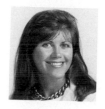 **Julie S. Curtis, M.D.**
Pueblo Radiology Medical Group,
Santa Barbara, California

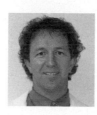 **Stephen Harkins, D.D.S.**
Dentist, Specializing in
    TMJ Dysfunction and
    Craniofacial Pain,
Tucson, Arizona

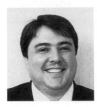

Jeremy J. Hollerman, M.D.

Assistant Professor,
Department of Radiology,
University of Minnesota,
Assistant Chief,
Department of Medical Imaging,
Hennepin County Medical Center,
Minneapolis, Minnesota

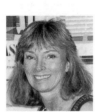

K. Rebecca Hunt, M.D.

Clinical Associate Professor and
  Director Residency Training,
Department of Radiology,
University of Arizona,
Tucson, Arizona

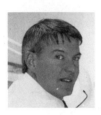

Tim B. Hunter, M.D., F.A.C.R.

Professor, Department of Radiology
University of Arizona;
Chief of Diagnostic Radiology,
Arizona Health Sciences Center,
Tucson, Arizona

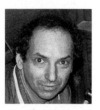

David H. Levy, M.A.

Amateur Astronomer,
Astronomical Writer
University of Arizona,
Tucson, Arizona

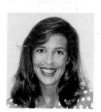

Pamela J. Lund, M.D.

Assistant Professor,
Head, Section of Diagnostic
  Ultrasound,
Department of Radiology,
University of Arizona,
Tucson, Arizona

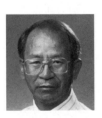

Joon B. Park, Ph.D.

Department of Biomedical
  Engineering,
The University of Iowa,
Iowa City, Iowa

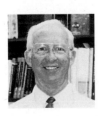

Dennis D. Patton, M.D.

Professor and Chief,
Division of Nuclear Medicine,
Department of Radiology,
University of Arizona,
Tucson, Arizona

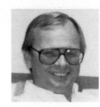

Gerald D. Pond, M.D.

Professor
Head, Section of Vascular and
  Interventional Radiology
Department of Radiology
University of Arizona,
Tucson, Arizona

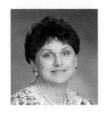

Eve Saenz, R.N.

Risk Manager,
Legal Risk Management,
The University Physicians, Inc.,
Tucson, Arizona

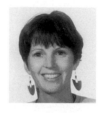

Kathleen A. Scanlan, M.D.

Associate Professor,
Chief of Diagnostic Ultrasound,
Department of Diagnostic Radiology,
University of Wisconsin,
Madison, Wisconsin

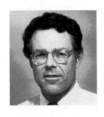

William W. Scott, Jr., M.D.

Associate Professor, Department of
  Radiology,
School of Medicine,
The Johns Hopkins Medical
  Institutions,
Baltimore, Maryland

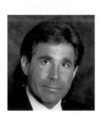

**Frank G. Shellock, Ph.D.,
  F.A.C.S.M., F.A.C.C.**

Director of Research and
  Development and
  Advanced Applications,
Tower Imaging;
Assistant Professor of Radiological
  Sciences,
University of California–Los Angeles
  School of Medicine,
Los Angeles, California

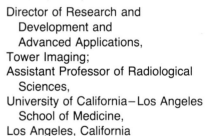

Welland O. Short, M.D.

Radiologist,
Albuquerque, New Mexico;
Formerly Clinical Assistant Professor,
Department of Radiology,
University of Arizona,
Tucson, Arizona

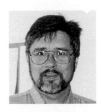

Stephen H. Smyth, M.D.
Clinical Assistant Professor,
Department of Radiology,
University of Arizona;
Clinical Director,
VAMC Radiology,
Tucson, Arizona

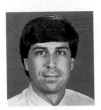

Steven L. Solomon, M.D.
Radiological Associates, P.C.;
Formerly Assistant Professor,
Mallinckrodt Institute of Radiology
Washington University Medical
    Center,
St. Louis, Missouri

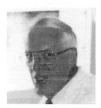

James R. Standen, M.D.
Clinical Professor,
Head, Section of Thoracic Radiology,
Department of Radiology,
University of Arizona,
Tucson, Arizona

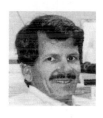

Evan Charles Unger, M.D.
Director,
Computed Tomography and Magnetic
    Resonance Imaging,
Associate Professor,
    Department of Radiology,
University of Arizona,
Tucson, Arizona

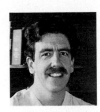

James A. Warneke, M.D.
Assistant Professor,
Department of Surgery,
University of Arizona,
Tucson, Arizona

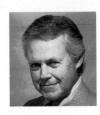

Paul S. Wheeler, M.D.
Associate Professor,
    Department of Radiology,
The Johns Hopkins Medical
    Institutions,
Baltimore, Maryland

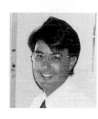

Mark T. Yoshino, M.D.
Radiologist;
Formerly Assistant Professor,
Section of Neuroradiology,
Department of Radiology,
University of Arizona,
Tucson, Arizona

Wizard of Id   By Brant Parker & Johnny Hart

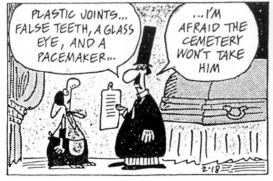
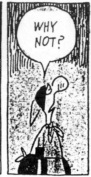
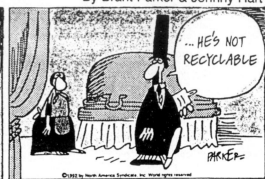

Foreword

Radiologists are avid writers and readers of books devoted to their field. Most of these books are dedicated to descriptions of disease states imaged by various modalities. In the midst of this plethora, it is rewarding to find one that deviates from this pattern, finds a vacuum, and successfully fills it. Drs. Hunter and Bragg have done just that in their book.

Progress in medicine has introduced a host of devices and appliances. These are recognizable as such radiographically, but their proper identification and an understanding of their function and adequacy is not always a simple process for the radiologist, who is often not versed in all the nuances of medical hardware. Providing a ready reference source for this kind of information applicable to the entire body represents a valuable contribution.

The mark of a radiologist's expertise is often his or her ability to sort out what is important or real from what is not. To help in this, the authors have included chapters on artifacts to aid in avoiding error of commission. They have also included comprehensive discussions of foreign bodies. The identification of foreign bodies is frequently of as much clinical importance as their localization, and this too has been treated only superficially in the literature. The authors and their contributors have culled and documented a wide spectrum of foreign materials in all parts of the body to help in identification.

I am delighted to see this volume of new material. It will prove a useful reading bench companion. I congratulate the authors for a job well done.

Theodore E. Keats, M.D.
Charlottesville, Virginia

Preface

· ·

A number of years ago I suggested to the Year Book Medical Publishers that it would be very useful to have a book available to illustrate the various devices that can be found in the human body, both operatively placed and traumatically induced. My inertia and other priorities delayed this project from being realized until Mosby–Year Book, Inc., was approached by Tim Hunter with a similar idea. With a clever concept and unlimited energies, Tim completed this book with the help of a distinguished group of contributing authors in short order. I believe this text, *Radiologic Guide to Medical Devices and Foreign Bodies,* will be an extremely useful companion to our daily professional lives, and I am pleased to have played the parental role as I have stated above.

The purpose of our text is to provide an approach to the identification, classification, and understanding of medical devices, foreign bodies, and common artifacts found during radiologic examinations. The text is not intended to be encyclopedic because the field of device development is too vast and rapidly moving to expect such all-inclusive coverage.

The chapters are organized in a logical, user-oriented manner, which we hope will be both instructional and efficient. The initial chapters discuss the general topic of biomaterials, devices, and their visibility. After Tim Hunter's chapter "Foreign Bodies" a general anatomic chapter orientation is presented to allow you to refer to body sites for referencing medical devices. A brief description of the more common surgical procedures seemed appropriate to place a fair number of surgical artifacts and devices in an imaging perspective. The final chapters cover various computed tomographic, ultrasound, magnetic resonance imaging, and nuclear imaging artifacts.

Chapter 19, "Bullets, Pellets, and Wound Ballistics," is an important one for our radiology community to understand. With our increasingly hostile environments, each of our communities seems to form combat zones, requiring our knowledge of weapons and their associated injuries. The final chapter, "How This Book Was Illustrated," is a useful approach to medical photography, as illustrated by this text.

tended it to be. Please help us enlarge and improve upon this effort in future editions, based upon your experiences and observations.

David G. Bragg

Acknowledgments

This large, complex book could not have been completed without the support and encouragement of many persons, including our families and colleagues, who have had to suffer through our single-minded determination to put aside all other obligations while working on the project. The idea for the book is not original with the editors, though each of us had independently thought of it several years ago. Anne S. Patterson, Editor-in-Chief of Medicine for Mosby–Year Book, stimulated us to collaborate and provided support from Mosby–Year Book for the book's eventual completion. Without her encouragement, the project would not have been undertaken because it just seemed too overwhelming.

This book greatly reflects the hard work and dedication of Linda Goodwill, our editorial assistant. She was a godsend who spent endless hours performing difficult, time-consuming tasks that would have defeated us early in the game. Linda literally produced the majority of the illustrations in the book. She set up a studio in her apartment, learned how to photograph devices and radiographs, and coordinated all the manuscript and illustration preparation. At least 25% of the radiographs used as illustrations were personally retrieved from the chapter authors by Linda. In addition, she maintained extensive records of the devices and radiographs photographed. Moreover, Linda even wrote a chapter for the book and produced the list of manufacturers found in the Appendix.

Linda Goodwill was also invaluable in the final manuscript preparation. She and the senior editor (TBH) checked the legends and figure labels on every illustration in the book. For over 1000 prints, she put the needed illustrative arrows on the prints, placed labels on the back of the prints, and mounted the prints in notebooks. To make the book as accurate as possible, Linda personally attempted to look up every single reference in the book! She used the journals and texts in the senior editor's office and the books and journals in the University of Arizona Health Sciences Center

(AHSC) Library to accomplish this task. In this effort, she was greatly helped by the capable assistance of Hannah M. Fisher, reference librarian.

The book contains approximately 900 references. Linda personally found 755 of the references and corrected significant errors in 317 (42%) of them. These errors ranged from incorrect spelling of authors' names to a totally incorrect listing for an article, such that it could not be found at all.

Linda Goodwill worked very closely on a daily basis with Scot Photo (5470 E. Speedway, Tucson, Arizona). Scot Photo performed the majority of the audiovisual work for the book. We could not have found a more accommodating vendor. Every person (Fig. 1) at Scot Photo went out of his or her way to help us. The prices

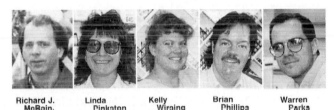

Richard J. MoBain, proprietor   Linda Pinkston   Kelly Wirsing   Brian Phillips   Warren Parks

charged were more than generous, particularly considering all our retakes, rush orders, and special printing requests. We want to particularly thank Richard J. McBain, proprietor, Linda Pinkston, Black & White Lab Technician, Kelly Wirsing, Lab Technician, Warren Parkes, Camera Sales, and Brian Phillips, Camera Sales.

Materials Management at the University Medical Center (UMC), Tucson, Arizona, was invaluable to us. This complex department handles the medical supplies for a busy university medical center. Almost all the devices photographed by Linda Goodwill were lent to us by Materials Management. Not only did this organization provide access to these devices, but its helpful employees (Fig. 2) also provided us with much needed information and advice concerning various devices. The employees' courtesy and respect for our efforts is much ap-

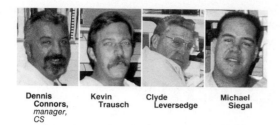

Dennis
Connors,
manager,
CS

Kevin
Trausch

Clyde
Leversedge

Michael
Siegal

preciated. We were also most impressed by their concern for providing the best of professional care for the patients at UMC. We want to particularly thank Dennis R. Connors, Manager, Central Service, Clyde Leversedge, Kevin Trausch, and Mike Siegal.

The University of Arizona College of Medicine Book Store supplied many of the everyday materials used in the book's preparation. Karen Coy and Estelle Bornhurst went out of their way to provide advice and supply hard-to-get items at a moment's notice.

Because this book covers a multitude of disciplines, it was necessary to work with persons from many different medical backgrounds and specialties. The following individuals from UMC or the University of Arizona College of Medicine were especially helpful in providing information and access to various medical devices: Sharon Snyder, Department of Cardiothoracic Surgery, Lloyd Constable, Department of Orthopedic Surgery, and Sheril Howard, Director, Department of Speech Pathology.

We could not have gone very far without the advice and help of numerous manufacturers' sales representatives and representatives from local medical-supply companies. They provided us access to rare and valuable devices, illustrations of devices, package inserts, references, and much helpful advice and encouragement. We want to especially thank Cheryl Wilder (American Medical Systems), Greg Wilson (Biomet, Inc.), Andrew H. Worth (Dow Corning Corp.), Monty Montierth (De Puy), Alan Reid (HowMedica, Inc.), James Dempsey (Inter-Tech Orthopedics, Inc.), Bill Dormandy (Interventional Therapeutics Corp.), Tom Patterson (LifeStyle Hearing, Inc.), Tom Brown (Med-Tech West, Inc.), Alan Nichols (Richards Medical Company), Craig W. Lynn (Synthes Ltd., USA), Dan Johnston (Target Therapeutics), James Davenport, Jane Espinoza, Karen Martin, and Ruth Martin (Tucson Limb & Brace), Daniel E. Donahue (Wilson Cook), and Bob Mieler (Zimmer).

No edited work can be accomplished without the support of the individual chapter authors. Ours all accomplished their assignments in a cheerful, cooperative fashion, usually on time. They remained friendly toward the editors despite periodic badgering by the senior editor for them to turn in their manuscripts. What counts most is the high quality of work that resulted from their efforts. The editors truly believe that much of what is contained in the book is unique and not found elsewhere.

Biomedical Communications, College of Medicine, University of Arizona, Tucson, is an acknowledged leader in providing the state of the art in audiovisual materials. The most difficult photographic and artwork assignments for this book were provided by BioMedical Communications. The senior editor has enjoyed a long, close relationship with Biomedical Communications and greatly appreciates their support for this project. Of particular note are the figures of the BioMechanical Man and Woman and the Trauma Woman drawn by Fred Anderson and the Gallery of Medical Devices drawn by Stacey K. Lane.

Word processors are wonderful tools, and this book could not have been done without one. The book, as submitted to the publisher, consisted of about 1,124,400 bytes in WordPerfect 5.1 files (Word Perfect Corporation, Orem, Utah). The book as the reader now sees it is the work of Elaine Steinborn, Managing Editor, Development, Mosby—Year Book, and her coworkers. The book's WordPerfect files were entered by the individual authors, the senior editor, or the authors' indispensable secretaries, who, though they have not been individually named, deserve mention for their valuable work. Sandra Boltinghouse has worked closely with the senior editor for many years. Her support is much appreciated, not so much for her typing of difficult, complex manuscripts, of which she has done plenty, but for her always remaining encouraging, calm, and collected in many a trying circumstance.

The editors finally want to thank all those whom we may inadvertently have forgotten to mention. Any large project, such as this book, is the product of many individuals, some of whom do not get the recognition they properly deserve. We thank them nonetheless.

Tim B. Hunter

David G. Bragg

Contents

· ·

Gallery of Medical Devices

Tim B. Hunter

Illustrated by
Stacey K. Lane

The following figures illustrate a wide variety of medical devices. These drawings are to be used only for quick reference to identify some of the common devices appearing on everyday radiologic studies. This section is not meant to be encyclopedic and is of necessity incomplete. For information concerning the use and complications of a particular device, please refer to the appropriate chapter.

Knowing the specific name of a device is not usually important, especially the eponyms attached to many devices. These names have often evolved from their original meaning. For example, a slight change in the design of an indwelling central venous catheter or a slight modification in the design of an orthopedic prosthesis may cause it to have a completely different name. However, it continues to have the same basic function. What is important concerning the identification of medical devices is the recognition of their presence and an understanding of their use and their complications.

The following illustrations were drawn on a Slidetek computer system with output to a typeset-quality imagesetter. They were produced in Biomedical Communications, Arizona Health Sciences Center, The University of Arizona, Tucson, Arizona.

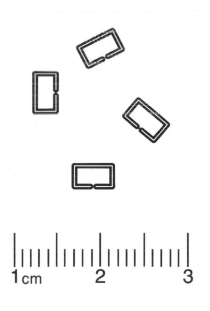

Skin (Scalp) Staple

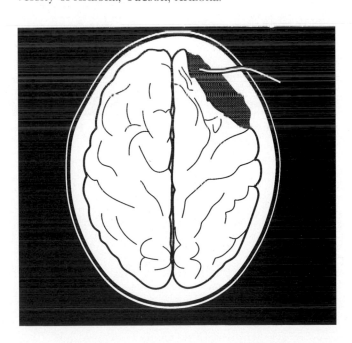

Subdural Drainage Catheter

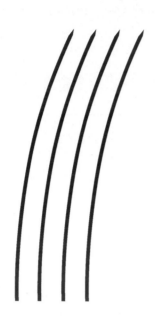

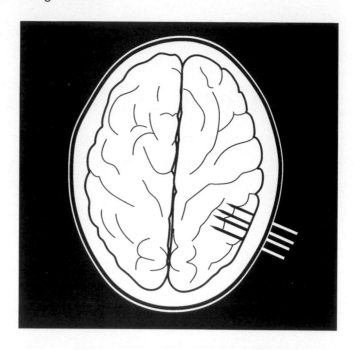

Brachytherapy Catheters

Brachytherapy Catheters

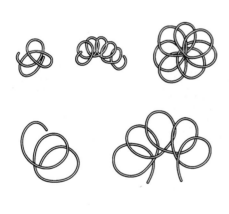

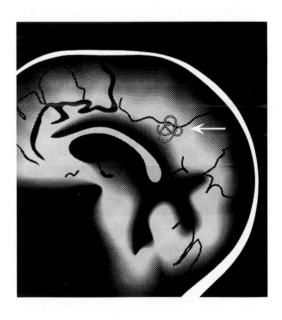

Platinum Coils

Platinum Coils

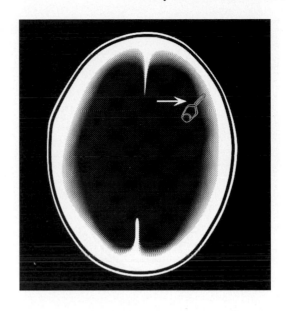

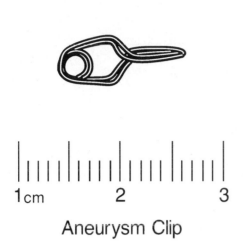

Aneurysm Clip

Aneurysm Clip

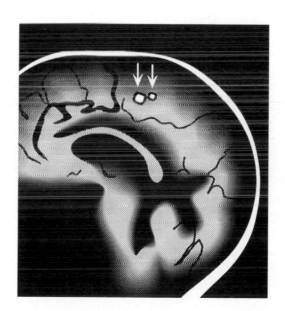

Cerebral Blood Flow Probe

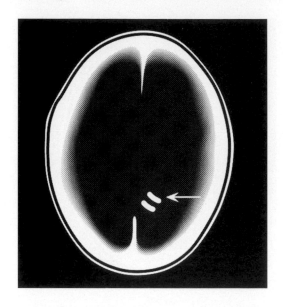

Cerebellar Stimulators

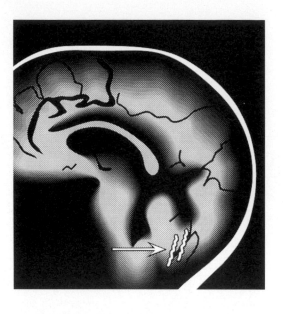

Cerebellar Stimulators

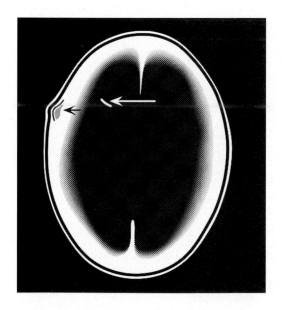

Ventriculoperitoneal Shunt

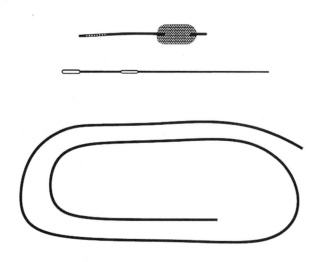

Pudenz VP Shunt

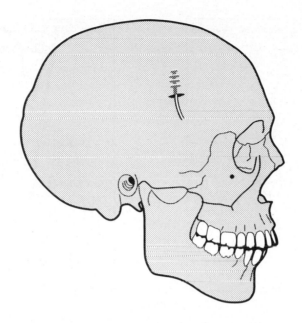

Portnoy Ventriculoperitoneal Shunt

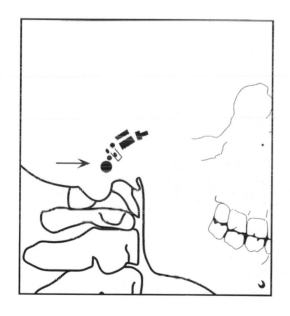

Hearing Aid

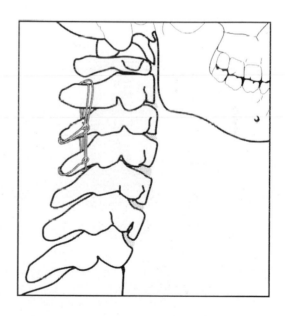

Sublaminar Wires

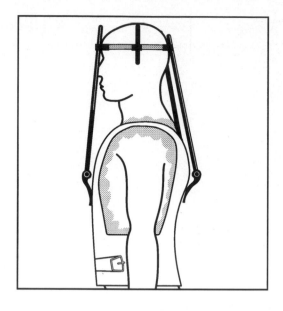

Halo Vest and Brace

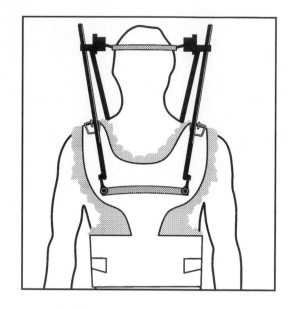

Halo Vest and Brace

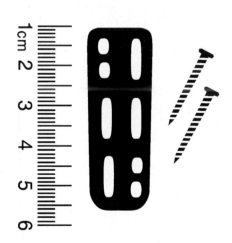

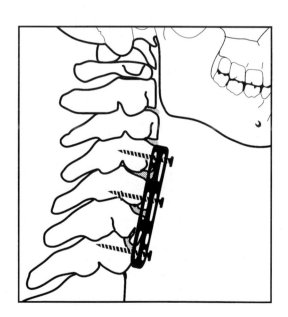

Anterior Cervical Fusion Plate

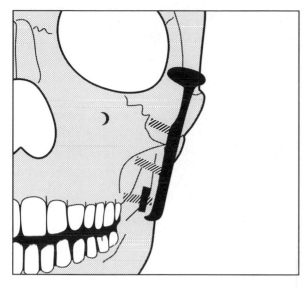

Temporomandibular Joint (TMJ)
Prosthesis

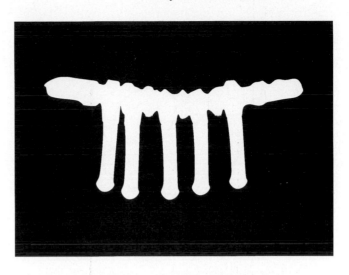

Osseointegrated Dental Implants
with Fixed Dental Bridgework

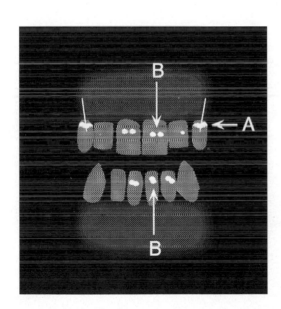

A. Root Canal Fillings with Denture
   Retention Posts
B. Porcelain Denture Teeth with Pins

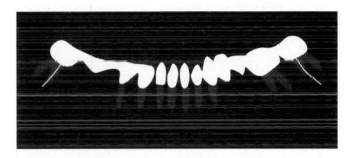

Fixed Dental Bridge with Root Canal Fillings

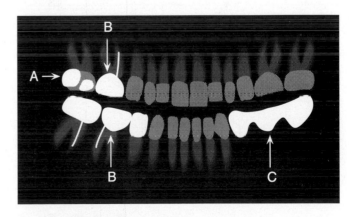

A. Alloy Dental Restoration
B. Root Canal Filling with Porcelain Veneer Crowns
   and Posts
C. Fixed Bridge Pontic with Abutment Crowns

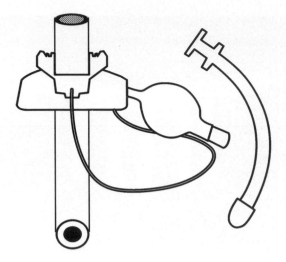

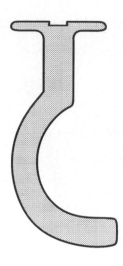

Cuffed Tracheostomy Tube

Oral Airway

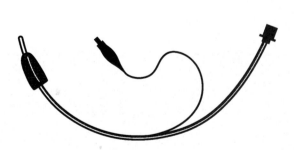

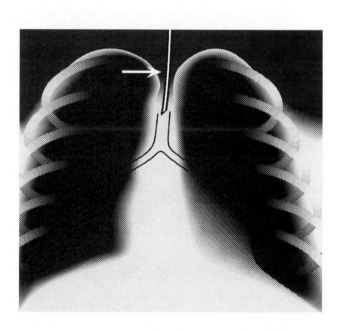

Endotracheal Tube

Endotracheal Tube

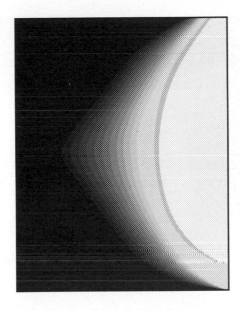

Retropectoral Breast Implant

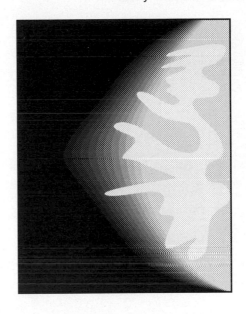

Collapsed Implant

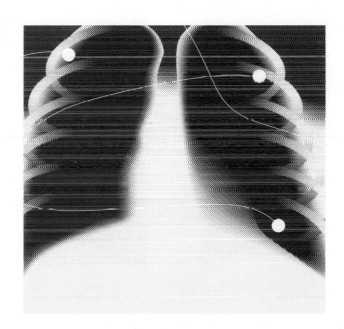

ECG Leads

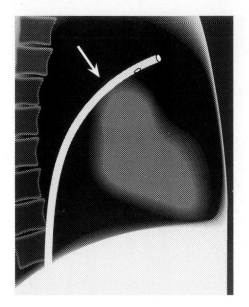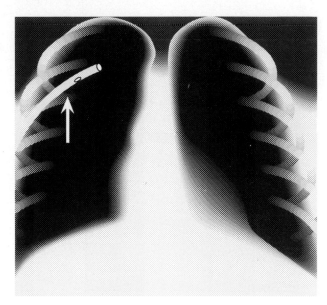

Chest (Thoracostomy) Tube

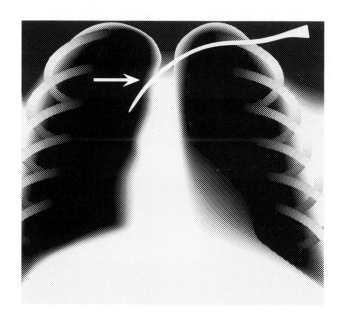

CVP Catheter or
Hemodialysis Catheter

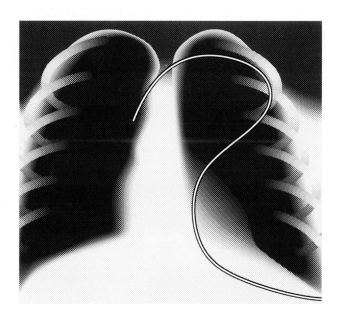

Central Venous Catheter
(Possible Types: Hickman, Hohn,
Cordis, Broviac, Leonard, Groshong)

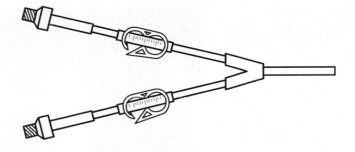

Hickman and Leonard Dual Lumen Catheter

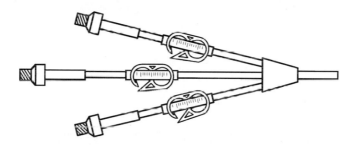

Hickman Triple Lumen Catheter

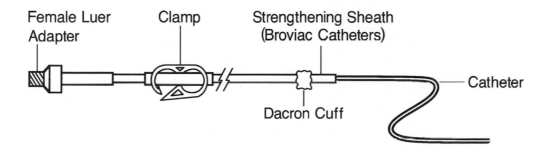

Female Luer Adapter   Clamp   Strengthening Sheath (Broviac Catheters)   Catheter

Dacron Cuff

Hickman and Broviac Single Lumen Catheter

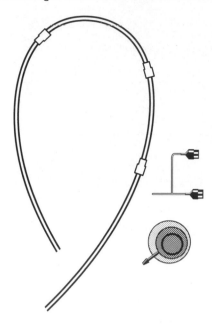

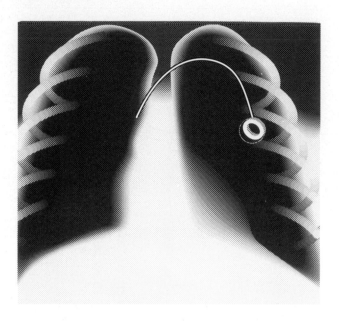

Subcutaneous Access
Port Device

Central Venous Catheter
Attached to Subcutaneous Port

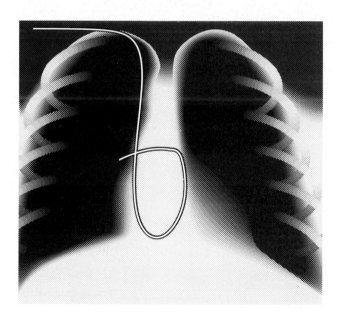

Swan-Ganz Catheter

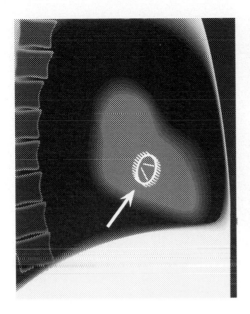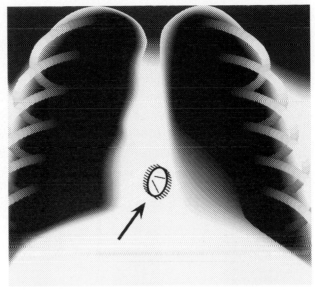

Hemex Tilting Bileaflet
Mechanical Valve (in Mitral Position)

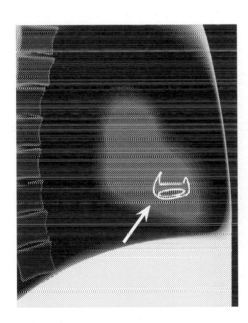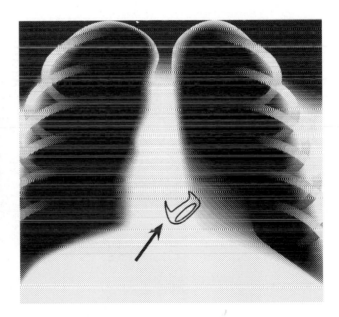

Ionescu–Shiley Valve
Prosthesis in Aortic Position

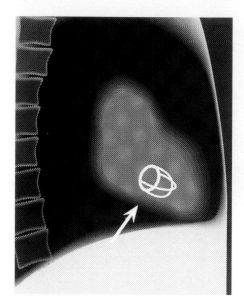
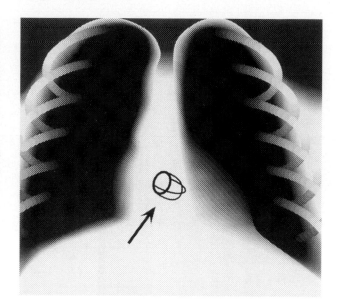

**Starr-Edwards Prosthesis
(in Mitral Valve Position)**

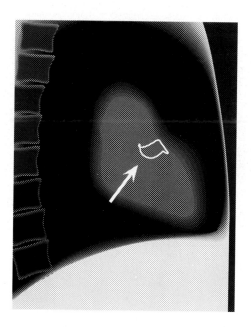

**Ionescu-Shiley Low Profile Pericardial Bovine
Valve Prosthesis (in Aortic Position)**

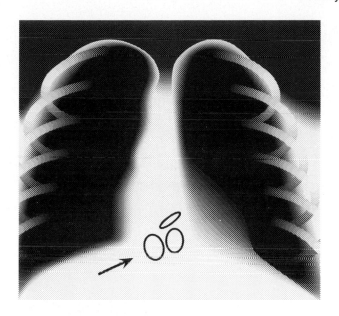

Hancock Porcine Valve Prostheses
(in Tricuspid, Mitral, and
Aortic Positions)

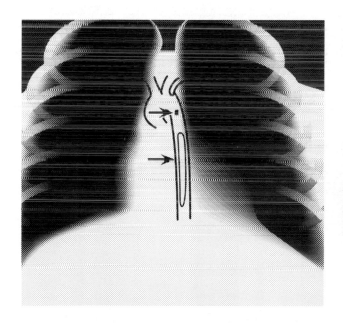

Intra-aortic Balloon Device (IABD)
with Balloon Inflated

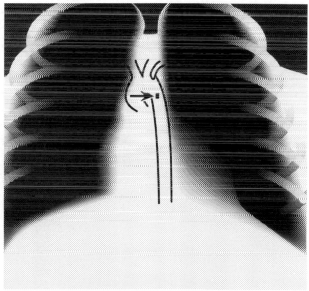

Intra-aortic Balloon Device (IABD)
with Balloon Deflated

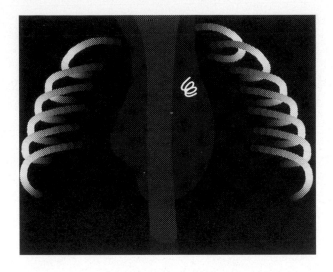

Gianturco Coil for Occlusion of
a Patent Ductus Arteriosus (PDA)

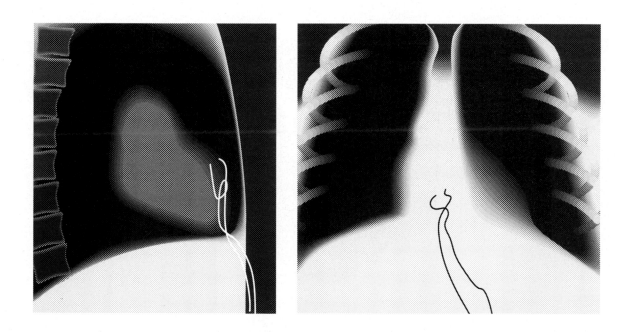

Temporary Epicardial Pacemaker Leads

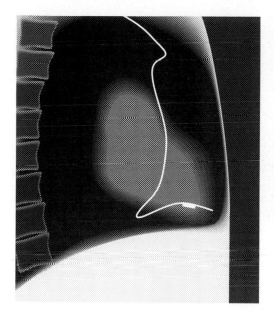
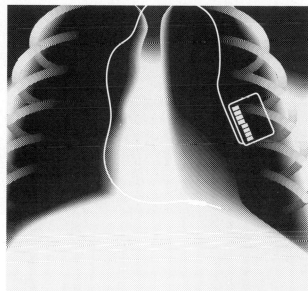

Transvenous Pacemaker

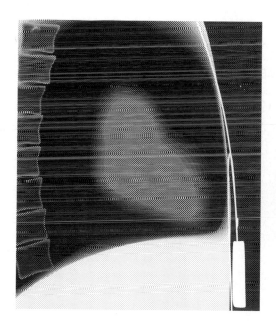
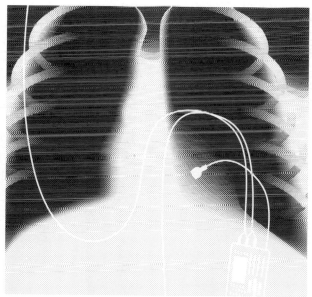

Remote Telemetry Transmitter

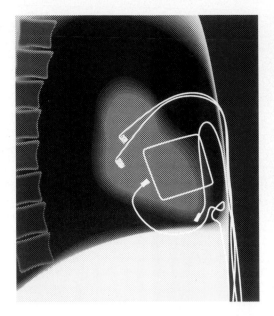
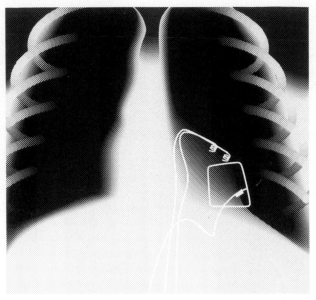

Automatic Implantable Cardioverter
Defibrillator (AICD)

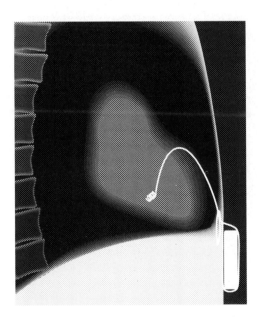
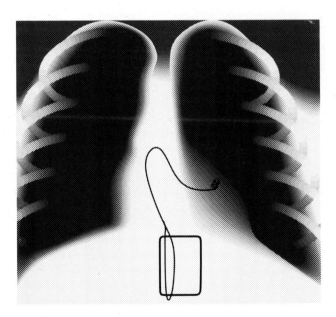

Single Electrode Epicardial
"Corkscrew" Subxiphoid Pacemaker

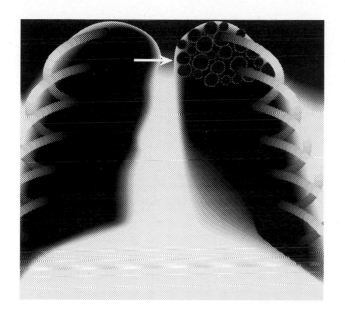

Ping-Pong Ball Plumbage

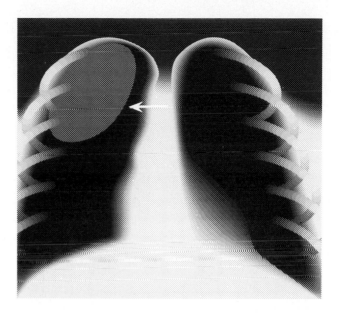

Oleothorax

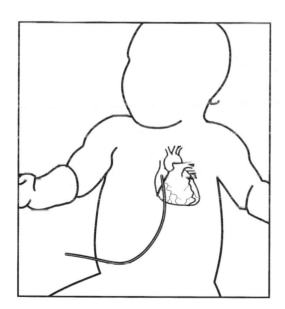

Umbilical Venous Catheter

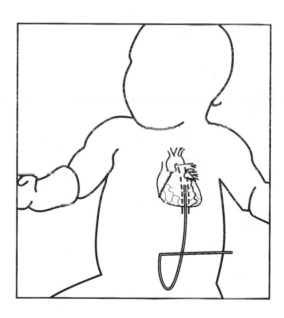

Umbilical Arterial Catheter

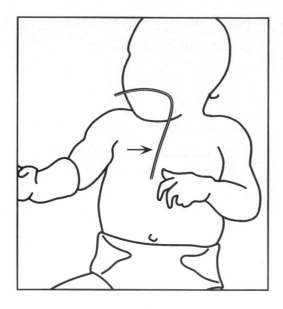

pH Probe

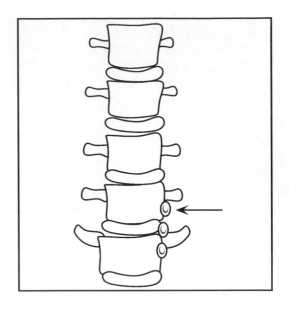

Dorsal Column Stimulator

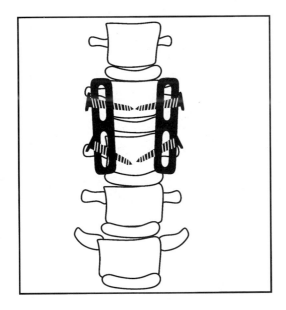

Steffee Plates and Screws

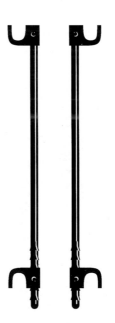

Harrington Rods

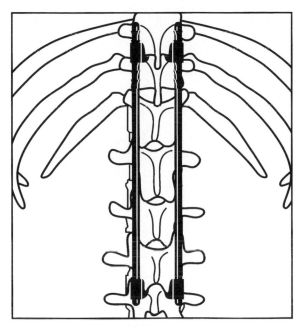

Harrington Rods

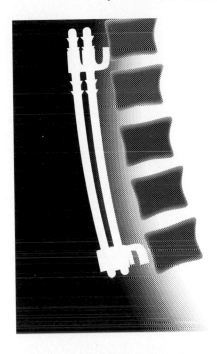

Harrington Rods

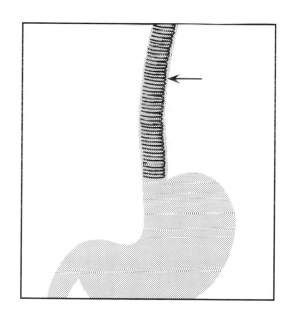

Esophagus Stent

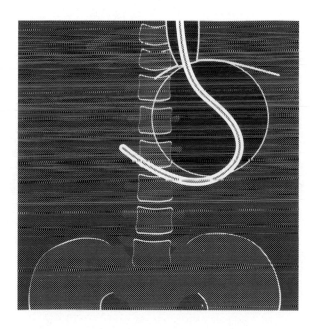

Sangstaken–Blakemore Tube

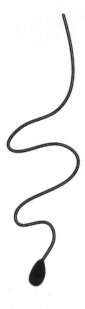

**Mercury-Weighted
Decompression Tube**

(Miller-Abbot, Cantor Tube)

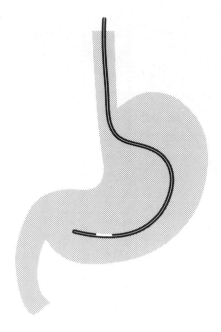

Nasogastric Tube

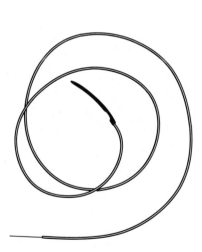

Feeding Tube

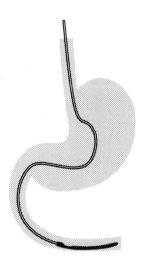

Feeding Tube

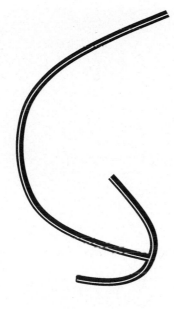

T-tube Drain

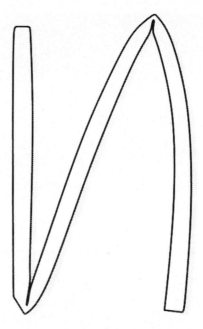

Penrose Tubing

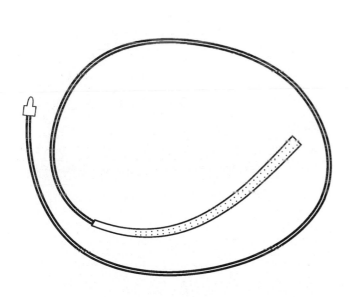

Silicone Flat Drain

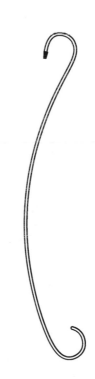

Ureteral Stent

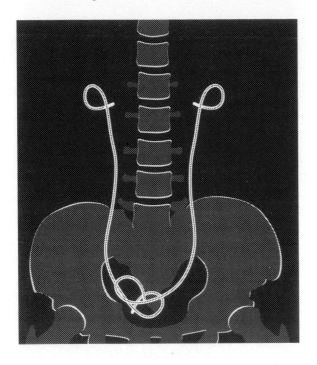

Ureteral Stents

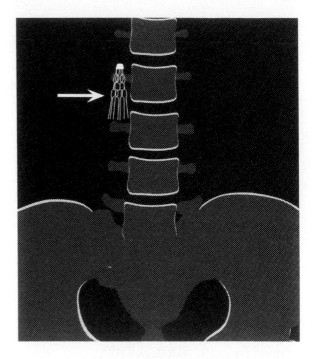

**Inferior Vena Cava Filter
(Greenfield)**

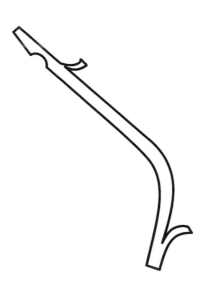

Biliary Stent

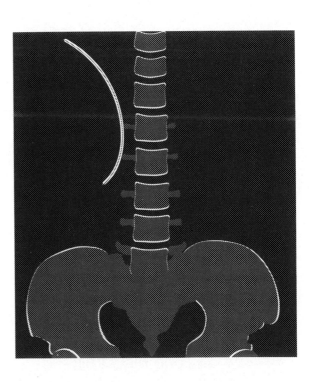

Biliary Drainage Catheter

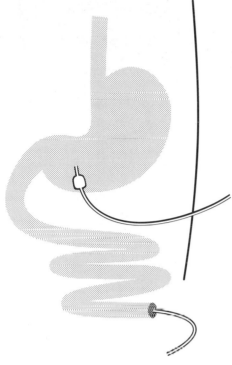

Gastrostomy/Jejunostomy

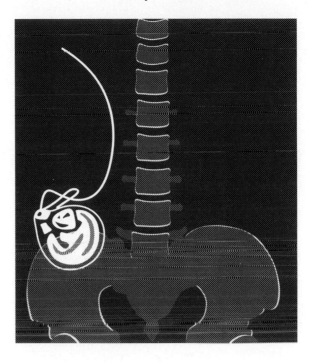

Chemotherapy Infusion Pump

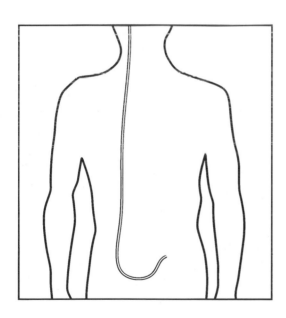

Ventriculoperitoneal Shunt

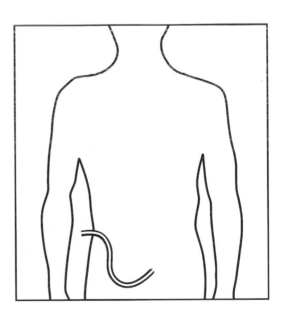

Peritoneal Dialysis Catheter

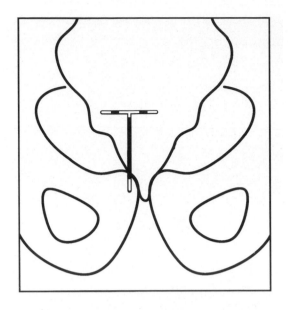

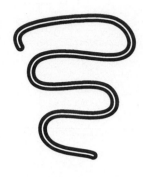

Lippes Loop IUD

IUD (Progestasert or
Copper T)

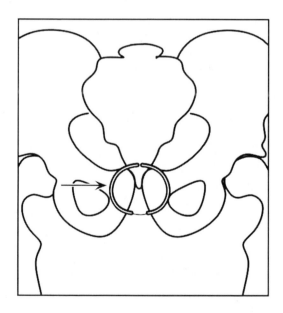

Pessary

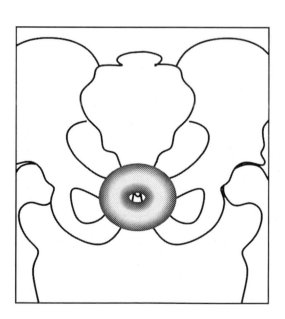

Pessary

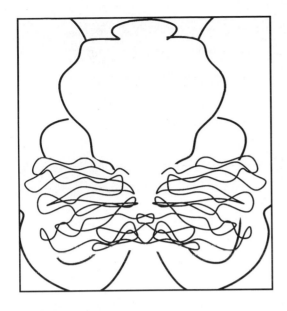

Tantalum Mesh

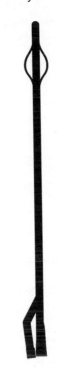

Foley Catheter

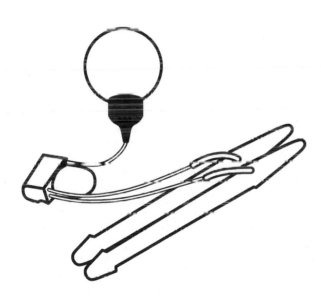

Penile Prosthesis

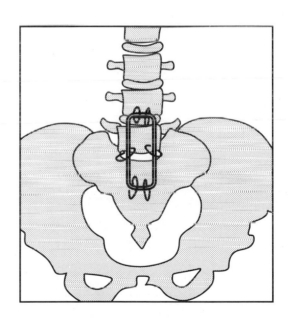

Hartsholl Rectangle

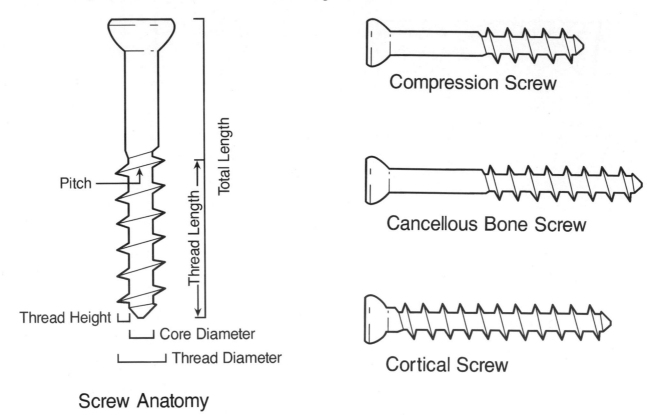

Screw Anatomy

Compression Screw

Cancellous Bone Screw

Cortical Screw

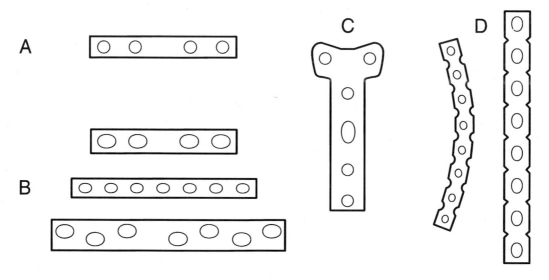

Internal Fixation Plates

A. One Third Tubular Plate
B. Dynamic Compression Plates
C. T-plate
D. Reconstruction Plates

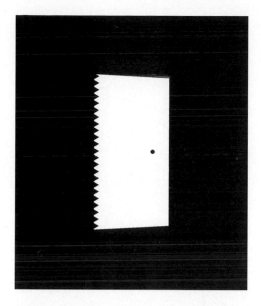

Brown corrugated fasteners

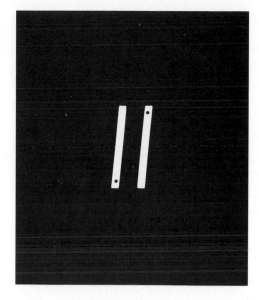

Michel clips

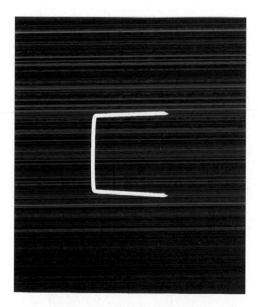

Staple (Downing)

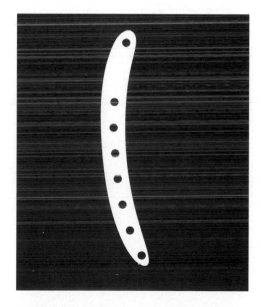

Wilson spinal fusion plate

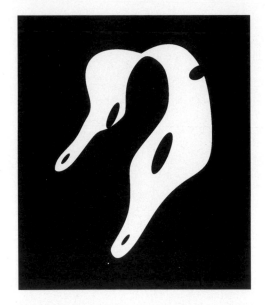

Elbow (Trochlear) prosthesis (Wade)

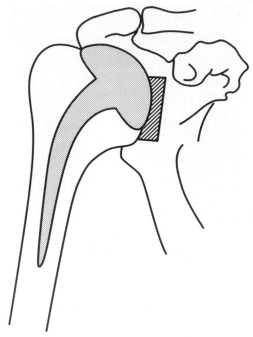

Neer Prosthesis

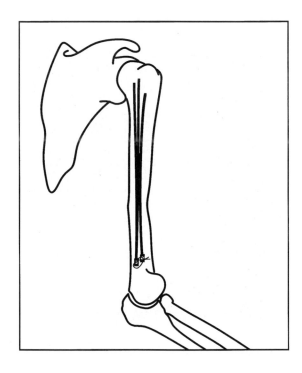

Flexible Intramedullary Rods in Humerus

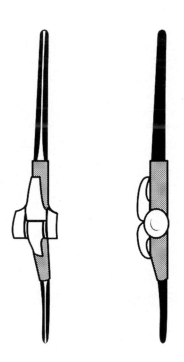

Total Elbow Prosthesis

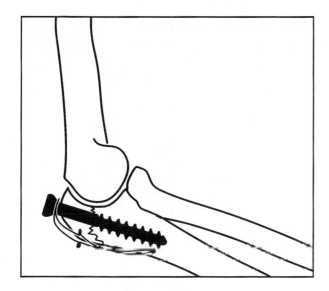

Tension Band Fixation of
Olecranon Fracture Using a
Cancellous Bone Screw

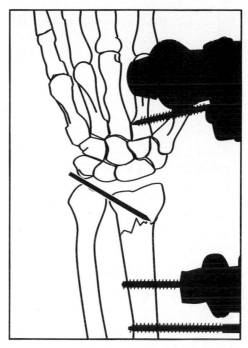

Distal Radius Fracture with
External Fixator Device and
Percutaneous Pin

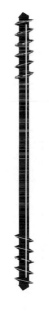

Herbert Screw

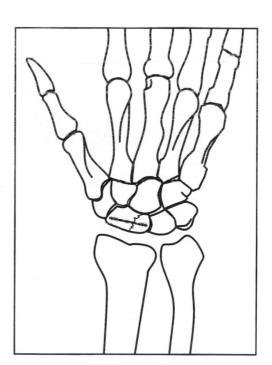

Herbert Screw
Transfixing Scaphoid Fracture

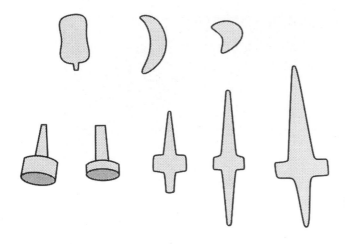

Various Silastic Implants
for Small Joints

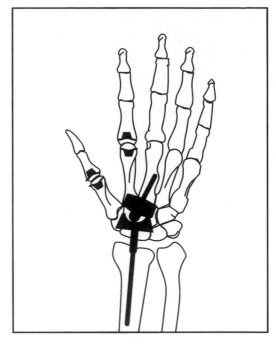

Total Wrist Arthroplasty and
Silastic Metacarpophalangeal Implants

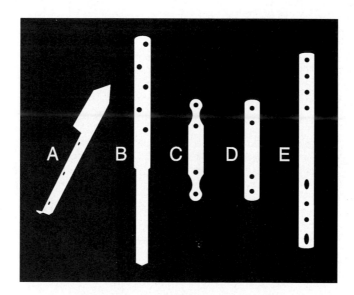

A. Bosworth spline (shoulder)
B. Bosworth spline (femur)
C. Sherman plate
D. Venable plate
E. Venable coaptation splint

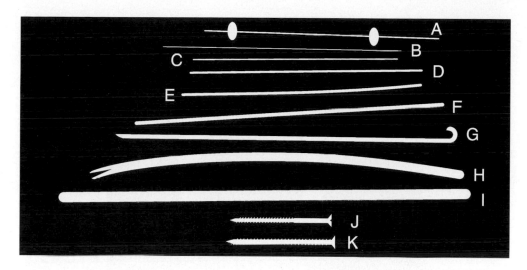

A. Web tibial bolt
B. Kirschner wire
C. Guide wire
D. Steinman pin
E. Küntscher intramedullary nail (forearm)
F. Hanson-Street diamond-shaped nail (intramedullary)

G. Rush intramedullary nail
H. Küntscher nested intramedullary nail (tibia)
I. Küntscher clover-leaf nail (intramedullary) femur
J. Arthrodesis wood screw
K. Arthrodesis full-threaded screw

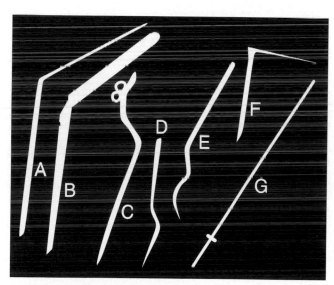

A. Moore blade plate
B. Neufeld nail
C. Moe plate
D. Blount plate
E. Curved Blount plate
F. Wright knee plate
G. Austin-Moore nail (hip)

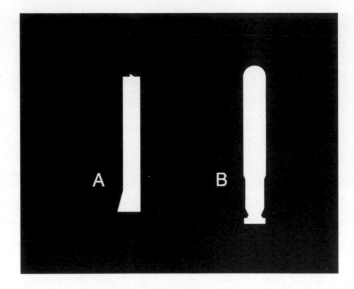

A. Smith–Peterson nail
B. Böhler nail

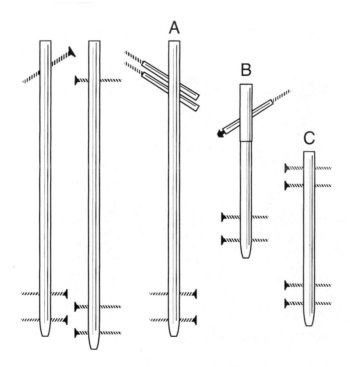

Locking Femoral Intramedullary Rods
A. Reconstruction Rod
B. Intramedullary Hip Screw
C. Supracondylar Rod

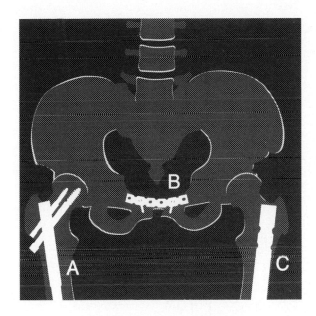

A. Reconstruction Rod
B. Reconstruction Plate
C. Unlocked Intramedullary Rod

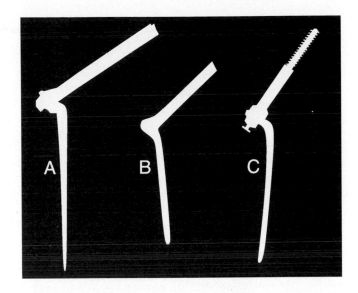

A. Smith-Peterson nail with McLaughlin bar
B. Jewett nail
C. Lorenzo screw and plate

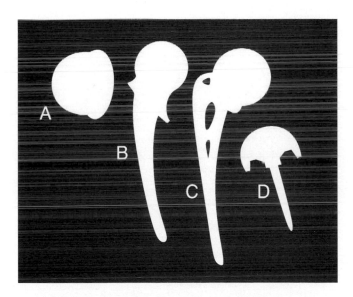

A. Smith-Peterson Vitallium cup
B. Fred Thompson hip prosthesis
C. Austin-Moore hip prosthesis
D. Judet acrylic prosthesis (hip)

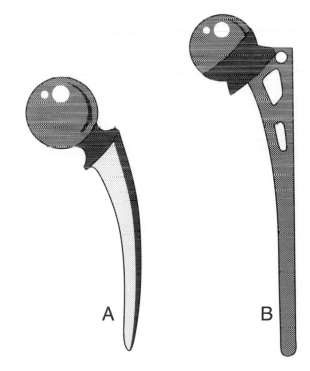

Single Piece Endoprostheses
A. Used with cement   B. Cementless

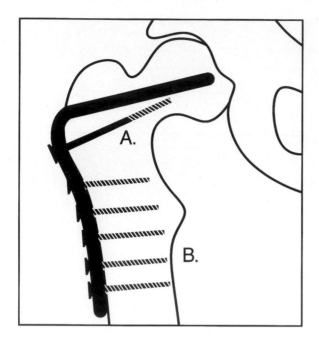

Blade Plate

A. Cancellous Screw
B. Cortical Screws

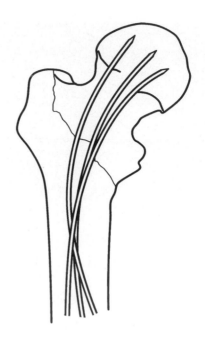

Enders Nails

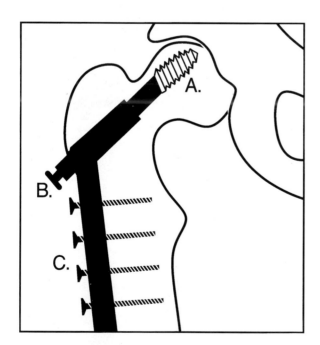

Compression Hip Screw

A. Lag Screw
B. Compression Screw
C. Barrel and Side Plate

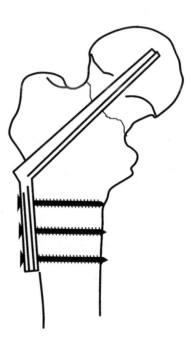

Nail and Side Plate

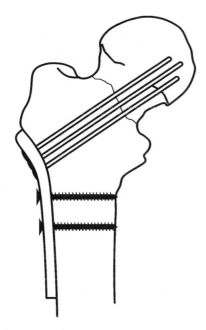

Multiple Pins with Side Plate
(Deyerle Apparatus)

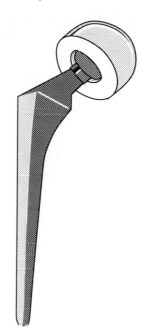

Bipolar Endoprosthesis

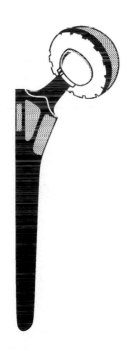

Modular Noncemented
Total Hip Prosthesis

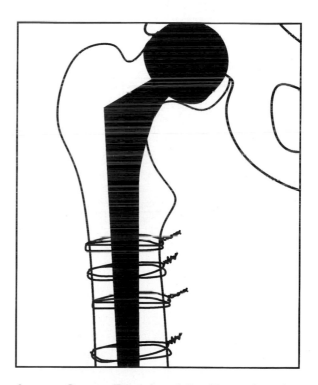

Long Stem Bipolar Hip Prosthesis
with Cerclage Wires

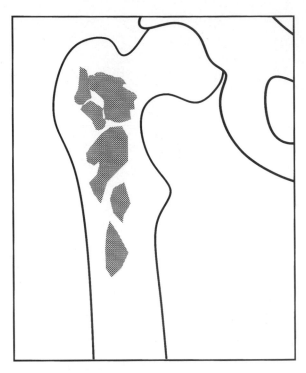

Methyl methacrylate
Antibiotic Beads

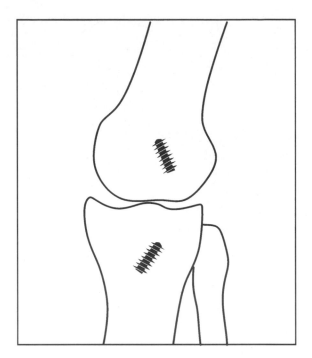

Kurosaka Screws

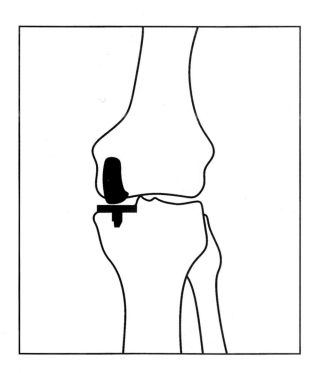

Unicompartmental Knee Prosthesis

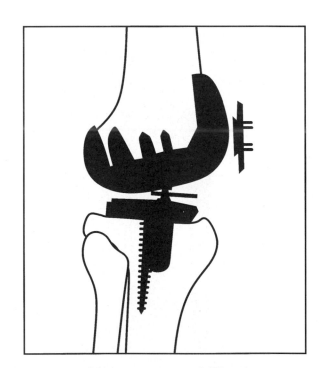

Noncemented Total
Knee Arthroplasty

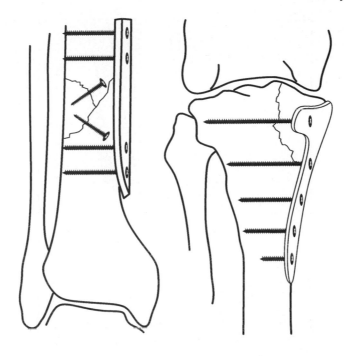

Neutralization Plate   Buttress Plate

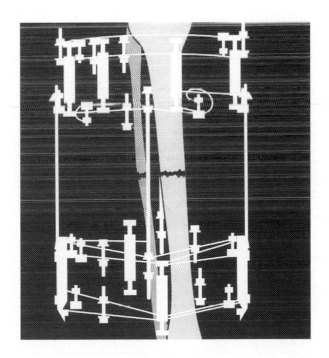

Ilizarov Device

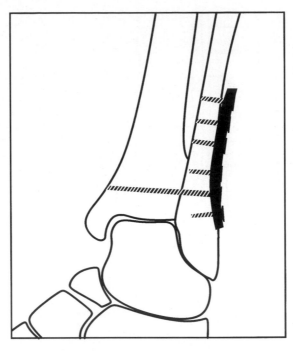

Dynamic Compression Plate
and Syndesmotic Screw

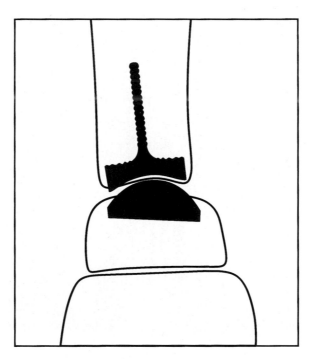

Total Ankle Arthroplasty

What to Do About an Unusual Radiologic Finding

· ·

Tim B. Hunter

Unusual radiologic findings are common. A significant percentage of these findings can be explained by the presence of a medical device, imaging artifact, or, less commonly, a foreign body in or on the patient.

A good education and a large experience are the prime requisites for the interpretation of difficult radiologic studies. There is no substitute for these. Nevertheless, even the most inexperienced observer can often solve the problem of an unusual radiologic finding by taking an ordered approach. The first question to be asked is: Is the finding a film artifact or an artifact of the imaging modality itself (computed radiography, computed tomography, ultrasound, magnetic resonance imaging, nuclear medicine)? If neither of these, does it represent a medical device, or the results of medical treatment (bandages on the arm, pills in the stomach, and so on), or is it truly related to the patient?

FILM ARTIFACTS

Film artifacts should be one of the first considerations when one is working through an unusual radiologic finding. Film artifacts represent those peculiarities that are actually on the film itself and that arise from mistakes in the handling, exposure, and development of the film. Many of them are readily evident to the observer and include large static electricity marks, areas of noticeably uneven development, bent and torn films, chemical stains, film fogging from light leaks, double exposures, film scratches, and so forth (Figs. I-1 to I-5).[1]

Film artifacts are less likely to cause mistakes in diagnosis than artifacts related to an imaging modality because film artifacts are usually readily evident and most observers are more familiar with them. Film artifacts are, nonetheless, very important. Almost all imaging studies are interpreted and archived on film. Therefore film artifacts are a constant threat to any imaging study, in addition to those artifacts inherent with the imaging modality itself. Usually, film artifacts are immediately recognizable and are a minor annoyance. However, they may limit the diagnostic usefulness of an exam or even require a repeat study, adding to patient inconvenience, discomfort, and radiation exposure.

At times, film artifacts may be subtle and lead to diagnostic errors. Foreign material on a cassette screen can simulate a radiopaque foreign body; a tiny static electricity mark may appear to represent a fine, linear fracture line; or emulsion flaking may mimic an area of clustered calcifications on a mammogram. Most physicians and medical personnel, including radiologists, fail to appreciate the amount of quality control that is necessary for the production of artifact-free films. This includes using the proper radiographic exposure with the correct film and screen, having proper processing technique (correct chemicals, temperature, and times), and using careful film handing and storage. Depending on one's definition, mislabeling of films with incorrect patient name, number, date, time, or body side is another film artifact that is common and requires constant vigilance to avoid.

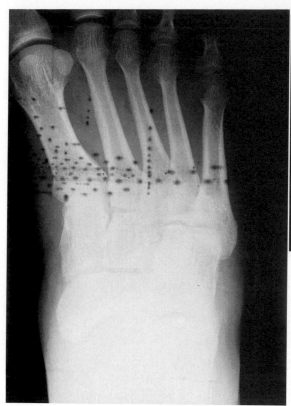

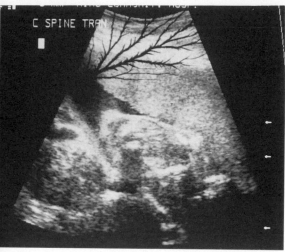

Fig. I-1. Typical static electricity marks. **A,** Plain radiograph of the foot. **B,** Transverse ultrasound image of a fetal neck from an obstetric ultrasound study. Notice how the static electricity marks significantly degrade the image. (Courtesy Bill Quirk and Douglas D. Schroeder, Tucson, Arizona.)

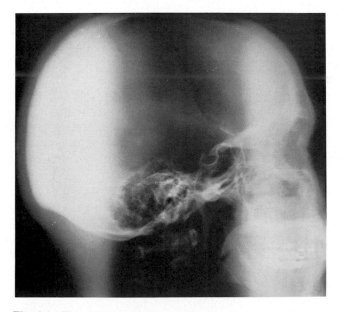

Fig. I-2. This bizarre skull appearance was caused by uneven processor development. (Courtesy Bill Quirk and Douglas D. Schroeder, Tucson.)

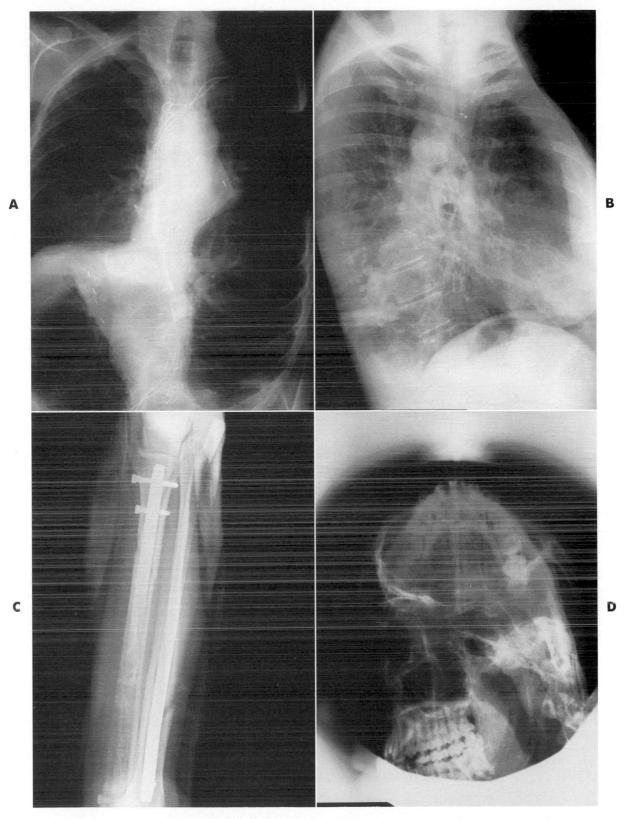

Fig. I-3. A to **D**, Various double exposures. Sometimes, inexperienced radiology residents attempt to interpret such films!   *Continued.*

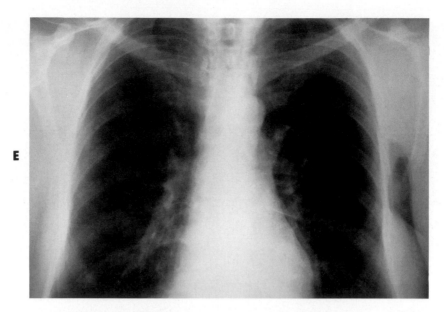

E

Fig. 1-3, cont'd. E, A particularly deceptive double exposure. The patient breathed between the two exposures. Notice the "double" ribs on the right and the double heart border. (Courtesy Bill Quirk and Douglas D. Schroeder, Tucson.)

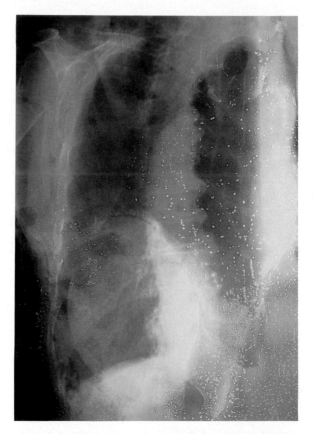

Fig. I-4. This image shows almost all the things that can go wrong with film handling and development, including films sticking together in the processor, double exposures, uneven film development, foreign material on the film and cassettes, and film tearing and bending. (Courtesy Bill Quirk and Douglas D. Schroeder, Tucson.)

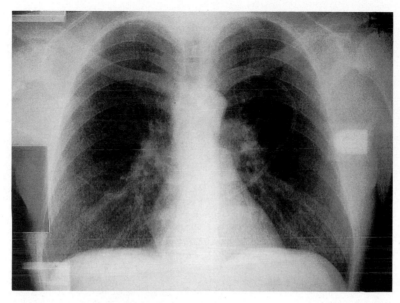

Fig. I-5. Mottled, uneven appearance to this image, as well as the rectangular densities on the right and left side, were caused by the computed radiography cassette being inadvertently turned over and exposed through the back of the cassette. (Courtesy Bill Quirk and Douglas D. Schroeder, Tucson.)

IMAGING MODALITY ARTIFACTS

Artifacts peculiar to the imaging modality itself are a particular problem with computed radiography, ultrasound, CT, MRI, and nuclear medicine studies. These types of artifact are important for several reasons: they can degrade a study or render it useless; they may be difficult to recognize and may lead to mistaken diagnoses; they are often caused or made worse by medical devices. Moreover, medical devices may not only produce severe imaging artifacts, but also their very presence may constitute a risk to the patient and may represent a contraindication for the performance of an exam, particularly MR studies (see Chapters 16, 17, and 19).

MEDICAL DEVICES

The imaging of medical devices is the essence of this book. There are hundreds of them, and they come in all sizes and shapes and have a multitude of uses. The figures of the BioMechanical Man and Woman on the inside front and back covers illustrate the types of devices that may be present in a patient (though not all at the same time!). These include orthopedic implants, heart pacemakers, spinal cord stimulators, peripheral and central venous catheters, intestinal tubes, casts, bandages, plates and screws, ostomy appliances, sutures, staples, skin clips, electrodes, wires, drains, stents, artificial sphincters, and so forth. How many of them can you identify on the figures?

Whenever one is working through the identification of an unusual radiologic finding, a medical device should be considered. The computer-generated drawings in the Gallery of Medical Devices (pp. 1 to 40) have been especially designed for rapid identification of those tubes, catheters, implants, and other devices most likely to be seen. A more detailed description of the devices and others like them are found in the respective chapters.

FOREIGN BODIES

The figure of the Trauma Woman (inside back cover) illustrates the types of objects that can be lying on top of, underneath, or in the clothing of a patient. These items often produce unusual "shadows" and simulate disease. Simple objects, such as bandages, buttons, belt buckles, earrings, pills in a pocket, a locket of hair overlying the apex of the chest, and tattoos (Figs. I-6 to I-10) have been known to cause a misdiagnosis because their true nature was not recognized. On the other hand, significant internal foreign bodies and medical devices have been overlooked because they were assumed to be on the outside of the patient!

Internal foreign bodies are not as common in most situations as external foreign objects, but they are important because they can cause significant symptoms and often go unrecognized. Internal foreign bodies are discussed in Chapters 2, 3, 5, 6, 7, 9, 14, and 17. These may have been inadvertently or deliberately swallowed or inserted into a body orifice. Internal foreign bodies may also result from an external accidental injury or be the unexpected outcome of medical treatment, such as

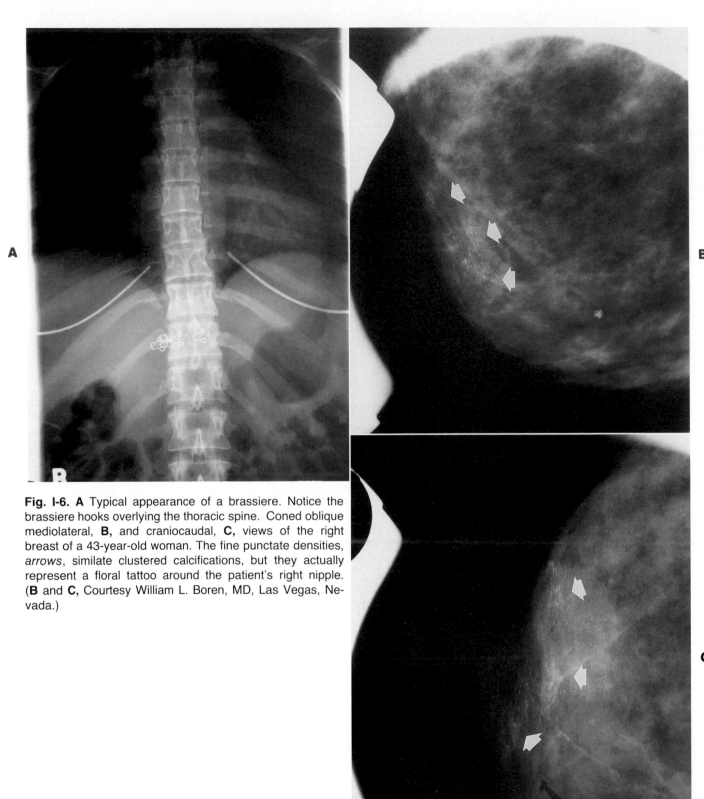

Fig. I-6. A Typical appearance of a brassiere. Notice the brassiere hooks overlying the thoracic spine. Coned oblique mediolateral, **B,** and craniocaudal, **C,** views of the right breast of a 43-year-old woman. The fine punctate densities, *arrows*, simulate clustered calcifications, but they actually represent a floral tattoo around the patient's right nipple. (**B** and **C,** Courtesy William L. Boren, MD, Las Vegas, Nevada.)

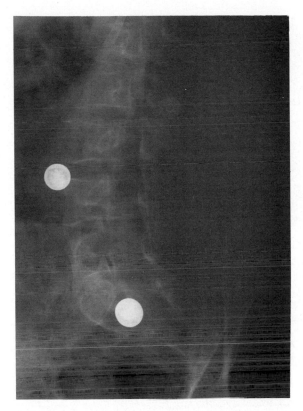

Fig. I-7. The two metallic densities visible on this oblique view of the lumbar spine represent buttons. (Courtesy Bill Quirk and Douglas D. Schroeder, Tucson.)

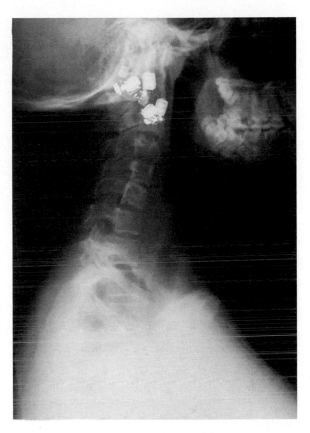

Fig. I-8. This patient's earrings simulate the appearance of a complex electronic device. (Courtesy Bill Quirk and Douglas D. Schroeder, Tucson.)

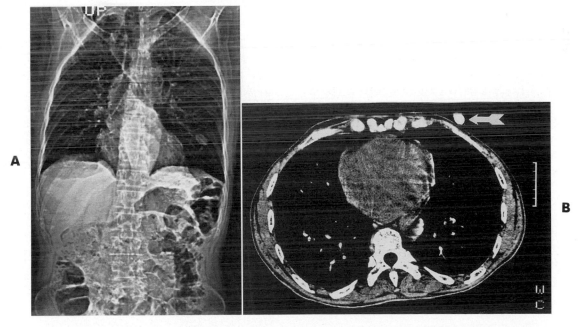

Fig. I-9. Elderly man undergoing chest and abdominal computed tomographic (CT) examinations. **A,** The scout film of the chest showed what appeared to be a mass in his left lung. **B,** It could not be seen on his chest CT slices and was found to be a lemon drop candy, *arrow,* in his shirt pocket.

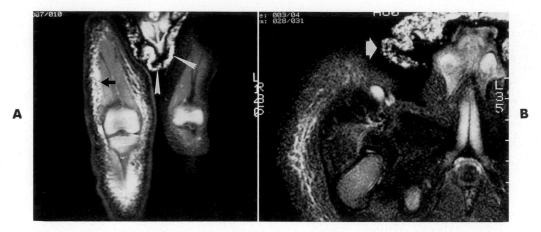

Fig. I-10. Eight-month-old male with unexplained enlargement of the right leg. **A,** STIR (short tau inversion recovery) coronal magnetic resonance image of the legs shows extensive lymphedema of the right leg, *black arrow,* and apparent lymphedema of the scrotum, *white arrowheads.* **B,** Axial fast spin-echo T$_2$ fat saturation magnetic resonance image of the proximal portion of the right thigh again shows the "scrotal edema," *arrow.* It was found to be a urine-soaked diaper. The child had no visible scrotal swelling.

a retained surgical sponge. Bullet wounds and gunshot injuries are a particular problem in our society and are discussed in depth in Chapter 19.

Internal foreign bodies are generally an unusual occurrence. They will not be properly diagnosed unless they are part of one's thought process whenever an unusual radiologic finding is encountered.

NORMAL VARIANTS

If an unusual radiologic finding does not represent an artifact, medical device, or foreign body, it may simply be a normal variant. A fundamental part of diagnostic radiology training is the appreciation for the wide variety of normal anatomy that occurs in humans. This is basic to the interpretation of all imaging studies. Pathologic processes can be properly recognized and diagnosed only when the possibility of normal variation has been excluded.[2] This process of exclusion involves education, experience, periodic reference to anatomic and radiologic texts, and the seeking of advice from other observers.

GOOD HABITS

There are two good habits that all observers of medical imaging studies should develop: the obtaining of prior studies and the reading of the prior radiology reports. These simple measures will often solve the prob-

lem of the unusual radiologic finding. The previous observer may have already noted the finding and reported its nature. If it was not present before, it might now be obvious that the finding is simply an artifact or a recently placed device. Or it might be evident that the finding definitely represents a new pathologic process. Moreover, consistent reviewing of prior examinations and reading of prior reports (not just glancing at the notations on the front of the film jacket) will frequently prevent the embarrassment of missing a finding noted by others, provide consistency in the interpretation of a series of studies, reveal errors made by previous observers, and sometimes even impart new medical knowledge to the reader.[3]

These good habits coupled with an orderly process for considering artifacts, medical devices, foreign bodies, and normal variants will provide a solid starting point for the proper interpretation of an unusual radiologic finding.

REFERENCES

1. Sweeney RJ: *Radiographic artifacts: their cause and control,* Philadelphia, 1983, Lippincott.
2. Keats TE: *Atlas of normal roentgen variants that may simulate disease,* St. Louis, 1992, Mosby.
3. Hunter TB, Boyle RR: The value of reading the previous radiology report, *AJR* 150:697-698, 1988.

1

Biomaterials: An Overview

· ·

Joon B. Park

Any material that is brought into contact with living tissue for the purpose of treating medical and dental problems can be thought of as a biomaterial. Obviously, any substance used as a biomaterial should be compatible with tissues chemically, mechanically, and pharmacologically. Specifically, biomaterials should have adequate strength, resisting fatigue (mechanical compatibility); be chemically inert and stable (chemical compatibility); and should not elicit allergenic, carcinogenic, immunogenic, or toxic reactions (pharmacologic compatibility). Moreover, sound engineering design and cost are also important considerations for a particular application.

Biomaterials can be classified in many ways: according to the source (man-made, or synthetic, versus nature-made, or natural), according to their expected duration inside the body (permanent or transient), according to their tissue types or uses (soft tissue, hard tissue, and blood), and according to the medical discipline involved (cardiovascular, dental, neurosurgical, orthopedic, otolaryngology, pediatrics, and so on).

Other terms are also used to describe biomaterials. Implants generally refer to materials placed in vivo, and prostheses denote artificial substitutes for a missing body part. In many situations, (such as hip implant or total hip prosthesis) these words can have the same meaning.

Development of implants did not progress significantly until Dr. J. Lister's aseptic surgical technique was advanced during the American Civil War. Before the concept of asepsis, various metal wires and pins made of iron, steel, gold, copper, silver, platinum, and so on, could not be evaluated properly because of infection, which masked the true effects of materials on tissues.

Development of noncorrosive metal alloys for the chemical industry in the beginning of the twentieth century together with early understanding of tissue response to foreign materials made possible more applications in medicine and dentistry. One of the early uses of plastics was the Judet femoral head prosthesis made of an acrylic, poly(methyl methacrylate). The same acrylic polymer is also used to fabricate corneal implants and is noted for its reasonable mechanical strength, high refractive index, and good biocompatibility. Open-heart surgical techniques made possible the development of artificial blood vessels in the 1950s and heart valves in the 1960s. The first successful direct pacemaker stimulation of the heart was also done in the late 1950s. By 1982 a total heart implant had been developed and tested in a human patient.

The study of structure-property of human tissues is beyond the scope of this chapter. However, Table 1-1 provides some comparison of the mechanical properties of human tissues and implant materials for a quick reference. As one might expect, metals and ceramics are primarily used for constructing implants that bear a large load, whereas elastomers (rubbers), plastics, and carbons are used largely for soft-tissue replacements and for tubes, drains, and catheters. Recently, composite materials are being considered for fabricating implants. One should be careful not to generalize concerning the use of implant materials because soft materials may also be used for hard-tissue applications, such as silicone rubber for toe and finger joint replacements, and polyethylene for the acetabular cup in hip joint replacement.

Table 1-1   Comparison of Properties of Tissues and Biomaterials

Materials	Young's modulus (MPa)	Fracture strength (MPa)	Fracture strain (%)	Density (g/cm³)
Metals				
316L stainless steel	200,000	540-620	55-60	7.9
Co-Cr alloy (wrought)	230,000	900	60	9.2
Ti-6Al-4 alloy	110,000	900	10	4.5
Polymers				
Silicone rubber	1-10	6-7	350-600	1.12-1.23
Polyamide (nylon 66)	2800	76	90	1.14
Ultrahigh molecular weight (UHMW) polyethylene	1500	34	200-250	0.93-0.94
Acrylic (PMMA)*	3000	60	1-3	1.10-1.23
Ceramics and carbons				
Al_2O_3 (single crystal)	363,000	490	<1	3.9
Hydroxyapatite	120,000	150	<1	3.2
Pyrolytic carbon	280,000	517	<1	1.5-2.0
Composites				
Carbon-fiber reinforced polymer (CFRP)	70,000-200,000	650	<1	2
Tissues				
Skin	0.34/38†	7.6	60	~1.0
Aorta (transverse)	0.1/2†	1.1	77	~1.0
Tendon	200/2500†	60	12	~1.0
Bone (femur)	17,200	121	~1	~2.0
Tooth (dentin)	13,800	138‡	<1	~1.9

*Poly(methyl methacrylate).

†The initial portion and final portions of the stress-strain curve are distinctly different for most soft tissues, and the modulus is expressed for the two portions. All tissues also exhibit anisotropy of properties because of their anisotropy of structure.

‡Compressive strength.

METALS

Metals tend to oxidize or corrode by reacting with oxygen in air or in an aqueous solution. This process poses two problems. One is weakening of the implant itself, and the other is undesirable tissue reaction to the corrosion products locally and systemically. The ban on the use of stainless steels for implant fabrications in Scandinavian countries is attributable to the metal sensitivity (mainly nickel) developed by many patients. These problems limit the number of metallic biomaterials to a few such as 316L stainless steel, Co-Cr alloys, or Ti alloys.

Stainless Steels

The first stainless steel used for implant fabrication was type 18-8 (18% Ni−8% Cr) or type 302 in modern classification of the stainless steels. Later, a small amount of molybdenum (2% to 4%) was added to improve its corrosion resistance in salt water. This allowed for the ultimate development of the type 316L stainless steel, which limits the amount of carbon content to 0.03% instead of 0.08% for type 316, providing for even better corrosion resistance in vivo. Only 316L stainless steel is suitable for making implants. Interestingly, cutting surgical tools are usually made of martensitic stainless steel, such as type 420, which contains no nickel but a higher percentage of carbon than type 316L has.

Cobalt-Chromium Alloys

Cobalt-chromium alloys are manufactured into final products by either a cast or a wrought process. The compositions of these alloys vary considerably. For example, the small amount of molybdenum (Mo) in the cast alloys decreases the grain size during solidification, which increases its strength. The mechanical properties of the cobalt-chromium alloys are better than those of the stainless steels. Furthermore, they have excellent corrosion and fatigue resistance.

The cast alloys are frequently used in dental work for their excellent reproducibility of details. The casting procedure for this alloy is the "lost-wax" investment technique. In this procedure, one has to control the alloy grain size and its distribution by controlling solidi-fication temperature, mold surface, and the presence of other elements (such as molybdenum) to achieve a homogeneous solid solution, which results in superior physical properties.

Titanium and its Alloys

Titanium and its alloys are used as implant materials because of their high corrosion resistance and relatively low density (4.5 g/cm^3 compared with 7.9, 8.3, and 9.2 g/cm^3 for stainless steel and for cast and wrought cobalt-chrome alloys respectively). The excellent corrosion resistance of pure titanium is attributable to the tenacious oxide film (TiO_2) on the surface, as in the case of aluminum oxide (Al_2O_3), which protects the surface from further oxidation. Unlike aluminum, the titanium oxide film is very stable in saline solution at room temperature. Because of the inferior mechanical properties of titanium in its pure form, it is often used for biologic purposes by being alloyed with other elements, such as aluminum, vanadium, manganese, silicon, molybdenum, and tin.

Shape-memory alloys (SMA) are being investigated for making implants. One of the SMA is nitinol (Ti-Ni alloy), which has been tested for implant application since the 1960s and has shown good biocompatibility. This alloy permits one to design an implant that can be changed to its desirable body form by a well-controlled heating process. One may even manipulate the transformation temperatures by controlling the relative amount of titanium in the alloy or by adding small amounts of other metals, such as cobalt. The transformation is attributable to actual structural change taking place (austenite to martensite phase) by deformation, and, importantly, the alloy can be reverted to its original structure by further heating.

Other Metals

Another corrosion-resistant metal used for implant manufacture is tantalum. It forms an oxide film similar to that of titanium. The mechanical properties are similar to those of the stainless steels, but it has a much higher density of 16.6 g/cm^3, making the metal less attractive to use. This metal is mostly used to fabricate sutures for neural and plastic surgery.

Platinum metals (platinum, ruthenium, rhodium, palladium, osmium, and iridium) and their alloys have been utilized from time to time for surgical implants, though high cost combined with relatively poor mechanical properties restricts their use to special cases, including dental bridges and electrodes for special circumstances (such as pacemaker tips).

POLYMERS

Polymers (*poly* = 'many'; *mer* = 'part') are composed of individual molecular units linked together by *pri-*

mary covalent bonding in the main *backbone* chain by means of C, N, O, and Si atoms. The simplest example is polyethylene, which is made from ethylene ($CH_2{=}CH_2$). The carbon atoms share electrons with two other hydrogen and carbon atoms: $-CH_2-(CH_2-CH_2)_n-CH_2-$, where n indicates a number of repeating units in an average length chain. To have a strong solid material, the repeating unit, n, should be well over 1000, making the molecular weight (MW) of the polymer over 28,000 grams per mole. This is the reason that polymers consist of giant molecules. At low molecular weight the material behaves as a wax (such as paraffin wax used for household candles) or at a still lower molecular weight as an oil or as a gas.

The main backbone chain can be of entirely different atoms; for example, the polydimethyl siloxane (silicone rubber) has silicone (Si) and oxygen (O) as its backbone atoms, that is, $-Si(CH_3)_2[O-Si(CH_3)_2]_n-O-$. The side-group atoms can be changed; thus, if we substitute the hydrogen atoms of polyethylene with fluorine (F), the resulting material is well-known Teflon (polytetrafluoroethylene).

To link the small molecules (monomers), one has to force the monomers to lose electrons by the processes of condensation and addition. By controlling the reaction temperature, pressure, and time in the presence of a catalyst or catalysts one can manipulate the degree to which monomers are put together into a chain. In the 1930s this polymerization process was first commercially used to make nylon, a polyamide.

Typical condensation polymers are polyester (Dacron), polyurethane, and polydimethylsiloxane (Silastic elastomer). Natural polymers, polysaccharides and proteins, are also made by condensation polymerization. The condensing molecule of natural polymers is always water (H_2O).

One can achieve "addition polymerization" by rearranging the bond within each monomer. Since each "mer" has to share at least two covalent electrons with other mers, the monomers have to have at least one double or triple bond. For example, in case of vinyl polymers:

$$n\;\overset{\displaystyle H\;\;H}{\underset{\displaystyle H\;\;R}{C{=}C}} \qquad\qquad \left(-\overset{\displaystyle H\;\;H}{\underset{\displaystyle H\;\;R}{C-C}}-\right)_n \tag{1}$$

Some of the commercially important vinyl monomers used for addition polymerization are given in Table 1-2.

Polymeric materials have a wide variety of applications for biomedical use, since they can be easily fabricated into many forms: fibers, textiles, films, gels, sols, and solids. Almost all commercial polymers can be used for making biomedical implants provided that each

Table 1-2 Monomers for Addition Polymerization

Monomer Name	Chemical Formula
Vinyl chloride	$CH_2{=}CHCl$
Vinyl acetate	$CH_3COOCH{=}CH_2$
Styrene	$CH_2{=}CH{-}C_6H_5$
Vinylidene chloride	$CH_2{=}CCl_2$
Methyl acrylate	$CH_2{=}CH{-}COOCH_3$
Methyl methacrylate	$CH_2{=}\underset{\underset{COOCH_3}{\mid}}{\overset{\overset{CH_3}{\mid}}{C}}$
Acrylonitrile	$CH_2{=}CH{-}CN$

polymer has undergone extensive in vitro and in vivo testing, including clinical trials. Because of the cost and time involved, not all the polymers have been tested for possible use. Polymers bear a close resemblance to natural tissue components, such as collagen, which allows direct bonding with other substances, such as heparin coating on the surface of polymers for the prevention of blood clotting. Adhesive polymers can be used to close wounds or glue orthopedic implants in place.

Polyolefins (Polyethylene and Polypropylene)

Polyethylene and polypropylene and their copolymers are called "polyolefins." These are linear thermoplastics that can be remelted and reused. Polyethylene is available commercially in three major grades: low density, high density, and ultrahigh molecular weight (UHMWPE). Polyethylene is one of the vinyl polymers in equation (2) which has the repeating unit structure with R$=$H.

The ultrahigh molecular weight polyethylene (MW $>2 \times 10^6$ g/mol) has been used extensively for orthopedic implant fabrications, especially for load-bearing surfaces such as total hip and knee joints. This material has no known solvent at room temperature; therefore only high temperature and pressure sintering may be used to produce desired products. Conventional extrusion or molding processes are difficult to use.

Polypropylene is another olefin polymer with R$=$CH$_3$. Polypropylene can be synthesized by use of a Ziegler type of stereospecific catalyst, which controls the position of each monomer unit as it is being polymerized to allow the formation of a regular chain structure from the asymmetric repeating unit. Polypropylene has an exceptionally high flex life; hence it is used to make integrally molded hinges for finger-joint prostheses. It also has excellent environmental stress-cracking resistance.

Polyamides (Nylons)

The polyamides are known as nylons and are designated by the number of carbon atoms in the parent diamine and diacid. Nylons can be polymerized by step-reaction or ring-scission polymerization, or both processes. They have excellent fiber-forming abilities because of interchain hydrogen bonding and a high degree of crystallinity, which increases strength in the fiber direction.

The basic chemical structure of the repeating unit of polyamides can be written in two ways:

$$-[NH(CH_2)_xNHCO(CH_2)_yCO]_n-$$

and

$$[NH(CH_2)_xCO]_n$$

The former equation represents polymers made from diamines and diacids such as type 66 and 610. The later polyamides are made from omega (ω)-amino acids and are designated as nylon 6 ($x = 5$), 11 ($x = 10$), and 12 ($x = 11$).

The nylons are hygroscopic (absorb water) and lose their strength in vivo when implanted. Water molecules serve as *plasticizers* and attack the nylons' amorphous region, which is less densely packed than the crystalline region. Proteolytic enzymes may also aid hydrolyzation by attacking the amide groups.

Acrylic Polymers

These polymers are used extensively in medical applications as (hard) contact lenses, implantable ocular lenses, and bone cement for joint fixation. Dentures and maxillofacial prostheses are also made from acrylics because they have excellent physical and coloring properties, and they are easy to fabricate.

The basic chemical structure of repeating units of acrylics can be represented by

$$-(CH_2{-}\underset{\underset{COOR_2}{\mid}}{\overset{\overset{R_1}{\mid}}{C}})_n- \tag{2}$$

The poly(methyl methacrylate), or PMMA, has both R groups CH$_3$. These polymers are addition (or free radical) polymerized. They can be obtained in liquid monomer form or as fully polymerized beads, sheets, and rods.

Because of the bulky side groups, these polymers are usually obtained in clear amorphous state. PMMA has high tensile strength (60 MPa) and softening temperature (125° C). PMMA has an excellent light transparency (92% transmission), a high index of refraction (1.49), and excellent weathering properties. This material can be cast, molded, or machined with conventional tools. It has an excellent chemical resistivity and is highly biocompatible in pure form. The material is brittle in comparison with other polymers.

Recently, bone cement has been used in greater numbers of clinical application to secure a firm fixation of joint prostheses, such as hip and knee joints. Bone cement is primarily made of poly(methyl methacrylate) powder and monomer methyl methacrylate liquid. One commercial product, Surgical Simplex Radiopaque bone cement, is an ampule containing a colorless, flammable liquid monomer that has a sweet, slightly acrid odor and has the following composition:

Methyl methacrylate (monomer)	97.4 vol%
N,N,-dimethyl-p-toluidine	2.6 vol%
Hydroquinone	75 ± 15 ppm

The hydroquinone is added to prevent premature polymerization, which may occur under certain conditions, such as exposure to light, elevated temperatures, or radiation. N,N-dimethyl-p-toluidine is added to promote or accelerate "cold-curing" of the finished compound. (The "cold-curing" is used to describe the manner in which the polymerization process occurs at room temperature as opposed to some acrylics polymerized under high temperature and pressure.) The liquid component is sterilized by membrane filtration.

The other component is a packet of 40 g of finely ground white powder (mixture of poly[methyl methacrylate], methyl methacrylate–styrene copolymer, and barium sulfate, U.S.P.) of the following composition:

Poly(methyl methacrylate)	15.0 weight %
Methyl methacrylate–styrene copolymer	75.0 weight %
Barium sulfate ($BaSO_4$), U.S.P.	10.0 weight %

When the two components are mixed together, the monomer liquid is polymerized by the free radical (addition) polymerization process. A minute amount of an initiator, dibenzoyl peroxide, present in the powder, will react with the monomer to initiate free radical generation. The propagation process will continue until long-chain molecules are produced. The monomer liquid wets the polymer powder particle surfaces and links them together after being polymerized.

Fluorocarbon Polymers

The best known fluorocarbon polymer is polytetrafluoroethylene (PTFE), commonly known as Teflon (du Pont). Other polymers containing fluorine are polytrifluorochloroethylene (PTFCE), polyvinylfluoride (PVF), and fluorinated ethylene propylene (FEP). Only PTFE will be discussed here, since the others have rather inferior chemical and physical properties and are seldom used for implant fabrication.

PTFE is made from tetrafluoroethylene under pressure with a peroxide catalyst in the presence of excess water for removal of heat. The repeating unit is similar to that of polyethylene, except that the hydrogen atoms are replaced fluorine atoms.

The polymer is highly crystalline (over 94% crystallinity) with an average molecular weight of 0.5 ~ 5 × 10^6 g/mol. This polymer has a very high density (2.2 g/cm^3) and a low modulus of elasticity of tensile strength. It also has a very low surface tension (18.5 erg/cm^2) and low friction coefficient (0.1). This material is used to fabricate artificial blood vessels in knitted or (porous) expanded form (Gore-Tex). PTFE cannot be injection molded or melt extruded because of its very high melt viscosity, and it cannot be plasticized. Usually, the powders are sintered to above 327° C under pressure to produce solids.

High-Strength Thermoplastics

Recently, new polymeric materials have been developed to match the properties of light metals. These polymers have excellent mechanical, thermal, and chemical properties because of their stiffened main backbone chains. Polyacetals and polysulfones are being tested as implant materials, whereas polycarbonates have found their applications in the heart/lung assist devices, food packaging, and so on.

These polymers have a reasonably high molecular weight (greater than 20,000 g/mol) and have excellent mechanical and thermal properties. More importantly, they display an excellent resistance to most chemicals and to water over wide temperature ranges.

Rubbers

Three types of rubber, silicone, natural, and synthetic rubbers, have been used to fabricate implants. Rubber is defined by American Standards for Testing and Materials (ASTM) as "a material which at room temperature can be stretched repeatedly to at least twice its original length and upon release of the stress, returns immediately with force to its approximate original length." Rubbers are stretchable because of the kinks of the individual chains. The repeated stretchability is attributable to the cross-links between chains that hold the chains together. The amount of cross-linking for natural rubber controls the flexibility of the rubber: the addition of 2% to 3% sulfur results in a flexible rubber, whereas adding as much as 30% sulfur makes it a hard rubber. Rubbers contain antioxidants to protect them against decomposition by oxidation, hence improving aging properties. Fillers such as carbon black or silica powders are also used to improve their physical properties.

Natural rubber is made mostly from the latex of the *Hevea brasiliensis* tree and the chemical formula is the same as that of polyisoprene. Natural rubber was found to be compatible with blood in its pure form. Also, cross-linking by x rays and organic peroxides produces rubber with superior blood compatibility compared with rubbers made by the conventional sulfur vulcanization.

Synthetic rubbers were developed to substitute for natural rubber. The Natta and Ziegler types of stereospecific polymerization techniques have made this development possible. Synthetic rubbers, however, have rarely been used for biomedical purposes.

Silicone rubber, developed by Dow Corning company, is one of the few polymers developed for medical use. It is used in a wide variety of applications for tubes, catheters, and drains. The repeating unit is dimethyl siloxane

$$-(\underset{\underset{CH_3}{|}}{\overset{\overset{CH_3}{|}}{Si}}-O)_n-$$

which undergoes condensation polymerization. Low molecular weight polymers have low viscosity and can be cross-linked to make a rubberlike material. Medical-grade silicone rubbers use stannous octate as a catalyst and can be mixed with base polymer at the time of implant fabrication.

Silicone rubbers use silica (SiO_2) powder as fillers to improve their mechanical properties. The more fillers that are used, the higher the density and the harder the rubber, since silica has higher density and hardness.

CERAMICS

Ceramics are inorganic compounds that include silicates, metallic oxides, carbides, and various refractory hydrides, sulfides, and nitrides. Oxides such as Al_2O_3, MgO, and SiO_2 contain metallic and nonmetallic elements, whereas other ceramics are ionic salts, NaCl, CsCl, ZnS, and so on. Exceptions to the "inorganic" nature of the ceramics are the "carbons" (diamond and carbonaceous structures like graphite and pyrolized carbons, which are covalently bonded).

Recently, ceramics have been given a lot of attention as candidates for implant materials because they possess highly desirable characteristics for some applications. Ceramics have been used for some time in dentistry as crowns; they are inert to body fluids and have high compressive strength and a good esthetic appearance.

Carbons have found use as artificial heart valve disks, percutaneous buttons, and dental implants. Although their black color can be a drawback in dental application, carbons have such desirable qualities as good biocompatibility and ease of fabrication.

Ceramics are generally hard; in fact the measurement of hardness is calibrated against ceramic materials. Diamond is the hardest with a score of 10 on Mohs' scale and talc ($Mg_3Si_4O_{10}[OH]_2$) is the softest with a score of 1. Others like alumina (Al_2O_3; score 9), quartz (SiO_2; score 8), and apatite ($Ca_5P_3O_{12}F$; score 5) are in between. Another characteristic of ceramic materials is their high melting temperatures because of their high bonding energy.

Unlike metals and polymers, ceramics are difficult to shear because of the ionic nature of their bonding. For shear to take place, planes of atoms must slip past each other. However, in ceramic materials ions with the same electric charge repel each other; hence, moving the planes of atoms is very difficult. This makes the ceramics nonductile, and creep at room temperature is almost nonexistent.

On the other hand, ceramics are very sensitive to notching or microcracks. Instead of undergoing plastic deformation (or yield), they will fracture elastically once a crack propagates. This is also the reason ceramics have low tensile strength compared to their compressive strength. In compression, any cracks or pores tend to be closed, but in tension the opposite is true. In case of compression, the cross-sectional area of the narrowest section does not decrease, whereas in tension it becomes smaller. Since the area is made smaller by the applied force, the actual stress becomes larger, worsening the stress-concentration effect, which is, in fact, a much more important factor than the change in cross-sectional area. If a ceramic is made flawless, it becomes very strong even in tension. Glass fibers made this way have tensile strengths twice that of steel.

Although the use of ceramic materials is well known in dentistry, their use in medicine is relatively new. The main advantage of ceramics over others biomaterials is their "inertness" or "biocompatibility," which is attributable to their low chemical reactivity. However, ceramics sometimes are made reactive to induce direct bonding between an implant and hard tissues.

Aluminum Oxides

The main source of high-purity alumina is bauxite and native corundum. The commonly available (alpha) α-alumina can be prepared by calcination of alumina trihydrate, resulting in calcined alumina. The American Society for Testing and Materials (ASTM) specifies 99.5% pure alumina and less than 0.1% of combined SiO_2 and alkali oxides (mostly Na_2O) for implant use.

The alpha alumina has rhombohedral crystal structure (a = 0.4758 nm and c = 1.2991 nm). The single crystal of alumina known as sapphire and ruby (depending on the types of impurities) has been used successfully to make implants. One can make these large single crystals by feeding fine alumina powders onto the surface of a seed crystal, which is slowly withdrawn from the electric arc or oxy-hydrogen flame as the fused powder builds up. Alumina crystals up to a 10 cm diameter have been grown by this method.

The strength of polycrystalline alumina depends on the porosity and grain sizes. Generally, the smaller the grains and porosity the higher is the resulting strength. Alumina in general is a quite hard material. This high hardness is responsible for using alumina as an abrasive (emery) and bearing for watch movements. The high hardness is accompanied by low friction and wear, which are major advantages of using alumina as a joint replacement material despite its brittleness.

Hydroxyapatite

Hydroxyapatite has been tried many times for use as a form of artificial bone. Recently, this material has been synthesized and used for manufacturing various forms of implants both in a solid and in a porous form and as coating on other implants.

The mineral part of bone and teeth is made of apatite of calcium and phosphate similar to hydroxyapatite crystals, $Ca_{10}(PO_4)_6(OH)_2$. The apatite family of minerals, $A_{10}(BO_4)_6X_2$, crystallize into the hexagonal rhombic prism and have unit-cell dimensions a = 0.0432 nm and c = 0.6881 nm. The ideal Ca/P ratio of hydroxyapatite is 10/6 and the calculated density is 3.219 g/cm^3. It is interesting to note that the substitution of OH with F will give a greater chemical stability. This is probably one of the reasons for the better caries resistance of teeth by fluoridation.

There seems to be a wide variation of the mechanical properties of hydroxyapatite attributable largely to differences in manufacturing methods and testing procedures. The most interesting property of hydroxyapatite is its excellent biocompatibility to the extent that it appears to form a direct chemical bonding with hard tissues.

Glass-Ceramics

Glass-ceramics are polycrystalline ceramics made by controlled crystallization of glasses developed by S.D. Stookey of Corning Glass Works in the early 1960s. They were first utilized in photosensitive glasses in which small amounts of copper, silver, and gold are precipitated by ultraviolet irradiation. These metallic precipitates help to nucleate and crystallize the glass into a fine grained ceramic, which possesses excellent mechanical and thermal properties. Bioglass and Ceravital are two glass ceramics developed for implants.

The main drawback of glass-ceramics is their brittleness similar to other glasses and ceramics. Also, because of restrictions on their composition for them to remain biocompatible (to stimulate osteogenicity), their mechanical strength cannot be substantially improved as for other glass-ceramics. Therefore they cannot be used for making major load-bearing devices, such as joint implants. It is also doubtful that their direct bonding with hard tissues can be maintained for a long time, since old cells are replaced by new ones, constantly destroying the initial bonding. Glass-ceramics can, however, be successfully used as fillers for bone cement, as dental restorative composites, and as coating material.

Other Ceramics

In addition to the ceramic materials mentioned so far, there have been experiments with many other ceramics, notably titanium oxide (TiO_2), barium titanate ($BaTiO_2$), tricalcium phosphate ($Ca_3[PO_4]_2$), and calcium aluminate ($CaO \cdot Al_2O_3$). Their potential applications range from inducing tissue ingrowth to regenerating new bone and stimulating growth in adjacent tissues.

Carbons

Carbons can be made in many forms: allotropic, crystalline diamond and graphite, noncrystalline glassy, and quasicrystalline pyrolytic carbon. Among these, only pyrolytic carbon is widely utilized for implant fabrication.

The mechanical properties of carbons, especially the pyrolytic carbon, are largely dependent on their density. Increased mechanical properties are directly related to an increased density, which indicates that the properties depend mainly on the aggregate structure of the material. Carbons show excellent compatibility with tissues; for example, there is superb compatibility of pyrolytic carbon with blood, and it is used to coat heart valves.

Pyrolytic carbon has been successfully deposited onto the surfaces of blood vessel implants made of polymers. This is called "ultralow temperature isotropic (ULTI) carbon" instead of "low temperature isotropic (LTI) carbon." The deposited carbon is thin enough not to interfere with the flexibility of the grafts, yet it exhibits excellent blood compatibility.

Composites

The rationale for incorporating inclusions in a polymer matrix is to increase its stiffness, strength, fatigue life, and other properties. For that reason, carbon fibers have been incorporated in carbon itself and into plastics (usually epoxy). The ultrahigh molecular weight or high-density polyethylenes have been converted into composites for making implants to improve their wear resistance and increase their longevity. Improvement in the resistance to creep of the polymeric component is also desirable. Excessive creep results in an indentation of the polymeric component after long-term use. Enhancements of various mechanical properties by a factor of 2 are feasible.

Fibers have also been incorporated into poly(methyl methacrylate), or PMMA, bone cement on an experimental basis. Significant improvements in the mechanical properties can be achieved. However, this approach has not found much acceptance because the fibers also increase the viscosity of the unpolymerized material. It is consequently difficult to form and shape the polymerizing cement during the surgical procedure. Metal wires have been used as macroscopic "fibers" to reinforce PMMA cement used in spinal stabilization surgery, but such wires are not useful in joint replacements because of the limited space available.

Particle reinforcement has also been used to improve the properties of bone cement. For example, inclusion of bone particles in PMMA cement somewhat improves its stiffness and considerably improves its fatigue life. Moreover, the bone particles at the interface with the patient's bone are ultimately resorbed and are replaced by ingrowing bone tissue. This approach is currently in the experimental stage.

FURTHER READING

Bechtol CO, Ferguson AB, Laing PG: *Metals and engineering in bone and joint surgery,* London, 1959, Balliere, Tindall & Cox.

Black J: *Biological performance of materials,* New York, 1981, Marcel Dekker.

Bloch B, Hastings GW: *Plastic materials in surgery,* ed 2, Springfield, Ill, 1972, Charles C Thomas.

Bokros JC, Arkins RJ, Shim HS, et al: Carbon in prosthetic devices. In Deviney ML, O'Grady TM, editors: *Petroleum derived carbons,* Am Chem Soc Symp, Series No. 21, Washington, DC, 1976, American Chemical Society.

Bruck SD: *Blood compatible synthetic polymers: an introduction,* Springfield, Ill, 1974, Charles C Thomas.

Bruck SD: *Properties of biomaterials in the physiological environment,* Boca Raton, Fla, 1980, CRC Press.

Charnley J: *Acrylic cement in orthopedic surgery,* Edinburgh & London, 1970, Livingstone.

Dardik H, editor: *Graft materials in vascular surgery,* Chicago, Ill, 1978, Year Book Medical Publishers (Mosby, St. Louis).

Ducheyne P, Van der Perre G, Aubert AE, editors: *Biomaterials and biomechanics,* Amsterdam, 1984, Elsevier Science.

Dumbleton JH, Black J: *An introduction to orthopedic materials,* Springfield, Ill, 1975, Charles C Thomas.

Edwards WS: *Plastic arterial grafts,* Springfield, Ill, 1965, Charles C Thomas.

Guidelines for physiochemical characterization of biomaterials, Report of the National Heart, Lung, and Blood Institute Work Group, Devices and Technology Branch, NHLBI, NIH Pub. No. 80-2186, Sept 1980.

Guidelines for blood-material interactions, Report of the National Heart, Lung, and Blood Institute Work Group, Devices and Technology Branch, NHLBI, NIH Pub. No. 80-2185, Revised Sept 1985.

Hastings GW, Williams DF, editors: *Mechanical properties of biomaterials,* New York, 1980, J Wiley.

Homsy CA, Armeniades CD, editors: *Biomaterials for skeletal and cardiovascular applications,* J Biomed Mater Symp, No. 3, New York, 1972, J Wiley.

Hulbert SF, Young FA, Moyle DD, editors: *J Biomed Mater Res Symp,* No. 2, 1972.

Kronenthal RL, Oser Z, editors: *Polymers in medicine and surgery,* New York, 1975, Plenum Press.

Lee H, Neville K: *Handbook of biomedical plastics,* Pasadena, Calif, 1971, Pasadena Technology Press.

Lee SM, editor: *Advances in biomaterials,* Lancaster, Pa, 1987, Technomic Pub. AG.

Leinninger RI: *Polymers as surgical implants,* CRC Crit Rev Bioeng 2:333-360, 1972.

Levine SN, editor: Polymers and tissue adhesives, *Ann NY Acad Sci,* Part IV, 146, 1968.

Levine SN, editor: Materials in biomedical engineering, *Ann NY Acad Sci,* Part IV, 146, 1968.

Lynch W: *Implants: reconstructing human body,* New York, 1982, Van Nostrand Reinhold.

Mears DC: *Materials and orthopedic surgery,* Baltimore, Md, 1979, Williams & Wilkins.

Park JB: *Biomaterials: an introduction,* New York, London, 1979, Plenum.

Park JB: *Biomaterials science and engineering,* New York, London, 1984, Plenum.

Rubin LR, editor: *Biomaterials in reconstructive surgery,* St. Louis, 1983, Mosby.

Schaldach M, Hohmann D, editors: *Advances in artificial hip and knee joint technology,* Berlin, 1976, Springer-Verlag.

Schnitman PA, Schulman LB, editors: *Dental implants: benefits and risks,* An NIH-Harvard Consensus Development Conference, NIH Pub. No. 81-1531, US Dept of Health and Human Services, Bethesda, Md, 1980.

Sharma CP, Szycher M, editors: *Blood compatible materials and devices,* Lancaster, Pa, 1991, Technomic Pub. AG.

Syrett BC, Acharya A, editors: *Corrosion and degradation of implant materials,* ASTM STP 684, Philadelphia, Pa, 1979, American Society for Testing and Materials.

Szycher M, Robinson WJ, editors: *Synthetic biomedical polymers: concepts and applications,* Westport, Conn, 1980, Technomic Pub.

Transactions of American Society for Artificial Internal Organs, published yearly and contains studies related to this chapter.

Williams DF, editor: *Biocompatibility in clinical practice,* Vol. I and II, Boca Raton, Fla, 1982, CRC Press.

Williams DF, editor: *Systemic aspects of blood compatibility,* Boca Raton, Fla, 1981, CRC Press.

Williams DF, editor: *Compatibility of implant materials,* London, 1976, Sector Pub.

Williams DF, editor: *Fundamental aspects of biocompatibility,* Vol. I and II, Boca Raton, Fla, 1981, CRC Press.

2

Medical Devices and Their Radiologic Visibility

Paul S. Wheeler
William W. Scott, Jr.

Medical devices are a growth industry both in the variety and in the number of devices produced. Medical items placed in humans range from sponges and venous catheters intended for temporary use to prostheses intended to last nearly a lifetime. All medical devices are designed to improve the quality of life and, in many instances, are necessary to prolong or even save a life. However, they are also capable of causing the patient harm; they can give false readings, break, malfunction, or become displaced or infected, and they may require diagnostic imaging and active intervention to reverse their bad effects.

Becoming familiar with the enormous range and function of the medical devices available is a considerable challenge for all physicians. It is also a risk-prevention role for the diagnostic imaging department because there are two important factors that are not controlled or sometimes appreciated by the radiologist and referring physician.[1,2] In many cases, the radiologic visibility of a device has been designed with no input from the radiologic community. Moreover, devices may be purchased by a hospital, clinic, or medical center by administrators looking for the lowest price. Often they fail to seek advice from radiologists and other physicians concerning the radiologic detectability of the devices they purchase.

RADIOPACITY

The simplest design flaw of many medical devices is the failure of the manufacturer to make them ra-

diopaque. For example, a common problem with some large- and small-bore venous catheters is their poor radiopacity. Often, the catheters are not visible on plain films. Yet thrombi and perforation can result from catheter tips lying against vein walls, particularly if the infusate is hypertonic or chemically irritating, as is the case with chemotherapeutic agents and hyperalimentation fluids. In addition, a long venous catheter can form a knot (Fig. 2-1) or reach the right ventricle, causing arrhythmias, pain (Fig. 2-2), or even perforation with cardiac tamponade. Patient coughing can flip a catheter tip into unusual sites (Fig. 2-3), such as the azygous and jugular veins, or it may even break a catheter. For all these reasons, vascular catheters must be visible on plain film radiographs, even in obese patients, so that these dangerous and potentially catastrophic complications can be avoided or at least recognized and corrected as soon as they occur.

Surprisingly, most vascular grafts and several heart valves are not radiopaque. Although it would seem logical to be able to visualize them on radiographs, apparently their designers believe that there are no major consequences if the devices are invisible. However, in at least one instance, poor device radiopacity caused significant patient morbidity. Only the very tip of a ventriculoatrial shunt was visible on posteroanterior and lateral chest radiographs, and it was easily missed and confused with a tiny film artifact (Fig. 2-4). The shunt broke, coiled in the heart, and led to subacute bacterial endocarditis with vegetations on the tubing and tricuspid valve before the problem was recognized. The broken shunt was extracted at fluoroscopy, but the procedure was complicated by the angiographers having to look for movement of the tiny opaque tip to know if

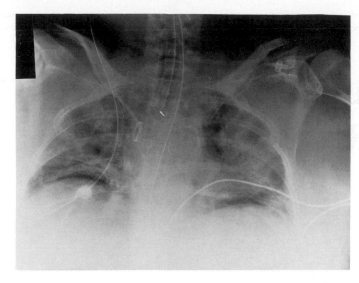

Fig. 2-1. Linear markers and wires abound on portable chest films. Notice knotted portion of Swan-Ganz catheter in superior vena cava.

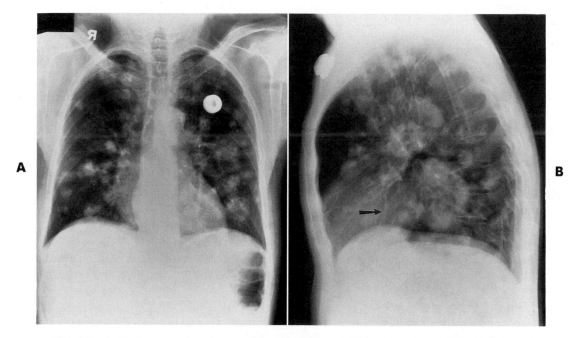

Fig. 2-2. **A,** Posteroanterior chest radiograph shows multiple metastases in the lungs. The patient is being treated with chemotherapy through a central venous catheter. The patient had chest pain and pericardial friction rub. **B,** Lateral view shows the venous catheter in the lower right ventricle, *arrow.*

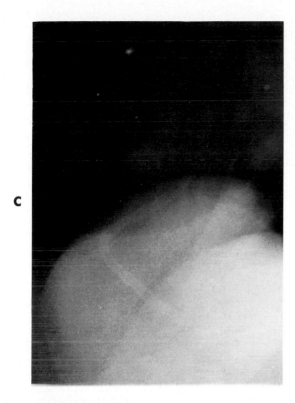

Fig. 2-2, cont'd. C, Close-up view of the catheter on the lateral view. It is deep in the right ventricle.

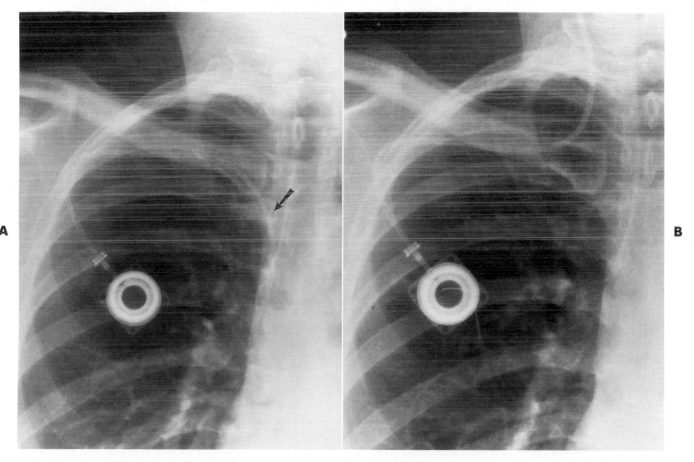

Fig. 2-3. A, Venous catheter for chemotherapy with tip in the superior vena cava, *arrow.*
B, Venous catheter has flipped into the jugular vein on a follow-up film.

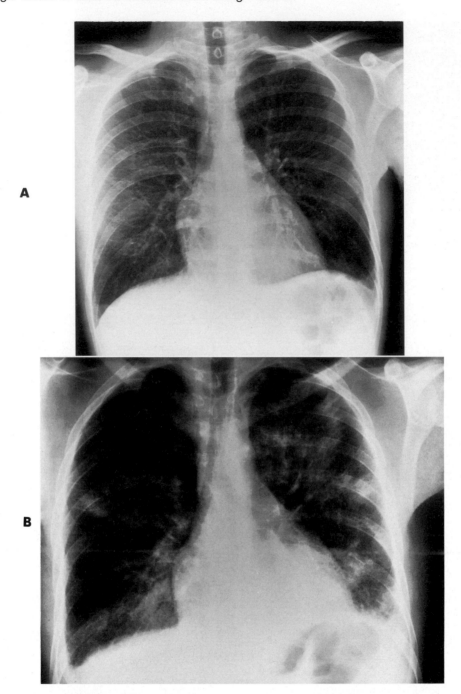

A

B

Fig. 2-4. **A,** Posteroanterior chest radiograph shows a patient with subacute bacterial endocarditis. An invisible ventriculoatrial shunt broke and coiled in the right atrium. It was covered with vegetations. The tiny tip marker is hidden by the spine. **B,** Shower of septic infarcts after removal of the broken, infected ventriculoatrial shunt.

they had proper grasp of the shunt tubing. Furthermore, withdrawal of the shunt from the patient led to a shower of septic emboli.

Another example where there has been inadequate attention toward making a device sufficiently radiopaque for ready visibility concerns a small tube designed to be introduced through an endotracheal tube. It is intended for suctioning secretions from the left main stem and lower lobe bronchus and is meant to be both therapeutic and diagnostic. Unfortunately, the tube is composed entirely of Silastic rubber, which is radiolucent, and is therefore invisible on radiographs. How can one

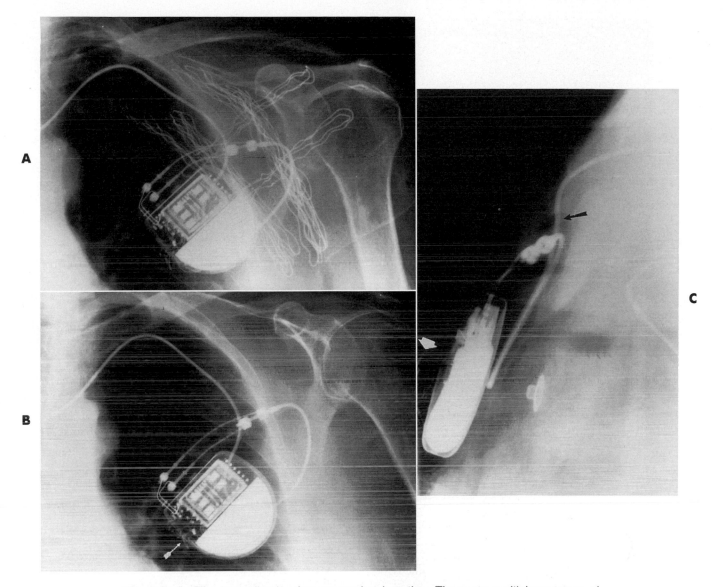

Fig. 2-5. A, Film immediately after pacemaker insertion. There are multiple sponges at the operative site. **B,** Abscess near pacemaker caused by retained sponge whose markers look like tiny circuit wires on inferior medial margin of the pacemaker, *arrow.* **C,** Lateral view showing air-fluid level, *arrow,* in the soft tissues above the pacemaker and sponge markers barely visible at the edge of the film anterior to the pacemaker, *arrowhead.*

actually tell if the tube is in the left main stem bronchus? Consideration is now being given toward using a marker wire within the tube or a small metal tube retrofitted in the tip so it can be seen on chest radiographs. Wouldn't it be better if the radiologic visibility of a device was one of the first considerations in its design rather than a late afterthought?

Manufacturers may have the best intentions for making their products sufficiently radiopaque. Unfortunately, they may then place such small or abstract opaque markers on their devices that the markers are easily overlooked by the uninitiated. Surgical sponges

(see Chapter 9) range from small pledgets used in neurosurgery to large laparotomy pads. They have a diversity of markers.[3] The small markers can easily be mistaken for broken wire sutures, and the large ones may have an appearance similar to a Penrose drain. Some sponges can even look like circuit wires in a pacemaker (Fig. 2-5). Laparotomy sponge markers are slightly denser than most rubber drains, and many are distinguished by a tiny row of stitch holes (Fig. 2-6). Most cases where a sponge has been left in a patient are more embarrassing then life threatening; however, their recognition would be aided if there were a clearly defined

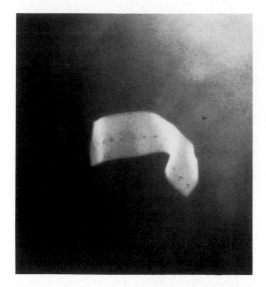

Fig. 2-6. Laparotomy sponge marker within the abdomen. Notice row of tiny stitch holes in its midline.

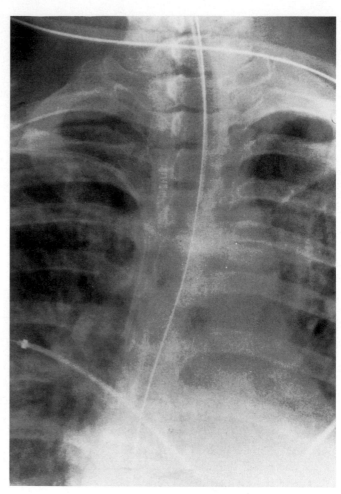

Fig. 2-8. Linear markers of endotracheal tube and nasogastric tube overlying each other and making tip location uncertain.

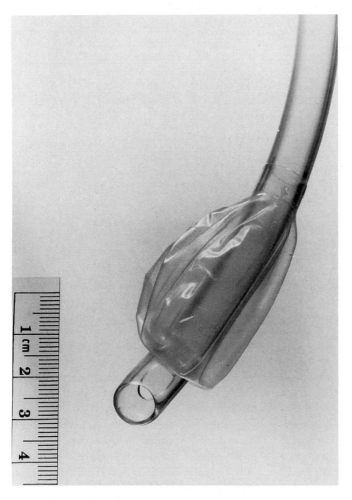

Fig. 2-7. Endotracheal tube has one thin barium stripe. The marker should also be around the lower rim.

and accepted standard for their opaque markers.

Endotracheal tubes are very common, and the location of their tip is quite important (Fig. 2-7). Most are marked with a longitudinal linear barium stripe, which can be mistaken for a similar marking on a nasogastric tube whose tip is in the cervical esophagus. The two linear markers can even be perfectly superimposed on each other, making it impossible to locate the tip of the endotracheal tube (Fig. 2-8). A marker stripe on the entire rim of the endotracheal tube tip is a long overdue improvement. It would be especially useful when the tip is near the carina or at the top edge of the film near or even in or above the larynx (Fig. 2-9).

A problem encountered much less frequently, except for overlying orthopedic casts and braces, is a device being too radiopaque. A device with too much opacity can hide underlying bone and soft-tissue detail. It may also simulate disease. For example, radiopaque ECG patches are notorious for mimicking lung masses and hilar adenopathy.

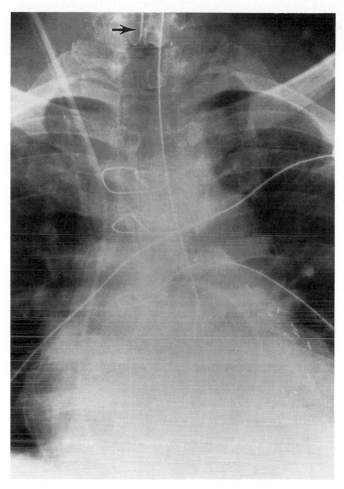

Fig. 2-9. High endotracheal tube with tip, *arrow*, near larynx at the upper edge of the film partly hidden by the spine. Patient in great distress "bucking" the respirator.

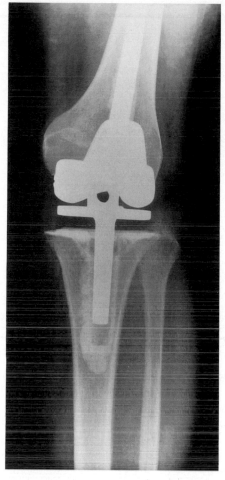

Fig. 2-10. Confusing prosthetic design. The metal tibial component is surrounded by radiolucent plastic. The appearance simulates tibial component loosening.

CONFUSING APPEARANCES

Manufacturers may inadvertently design their equipment in such a manner as to confuse the inexperienced physician because the normal radiographic appearance of the device may actually simulate a pathologic condition. Loosening of orthopedic prostheses is usually detected by visualization of a lucent zone between the prosthesis and surrounding bone (see Chapter 11). One knee joint prosthesis includes a layer of nonopaque plastic, which perfectly mimics loosening. This may indicate an incorrect diagnosis by anyone who is seeing the prosthesis for the first time and is unfamiliar with its expected appearance (Fig. 2-10).

CONCLUSION

Medical devices improve health and save lives. They are a most important part of modern medicine. A broad familiarity with them is a necessity for physicians and health care workers. A small percentage of devices will have complications that harm patients. Medical devices pose a special challenge to those in the imaging field because of the number and variety of devices available and because of the lack of standardization and consistency in their radiologic visibility. The radiologic community should have a more significant input in their design, and device visibility should be an important factor in their purchase and use.

REFERENCES

1. Scott WW Jr, Wheeler PS: Markers for implanted devices: need for standardization, *AJR* 146:387-390, 1986.
2. Wheeler PS: Device identification: deficient marking systems, *AJR* 146:418-419, 1986.
3. Spiegel SM, Palayew MJ: Retained surgical sponges: diagnostic dilemma and an aid to their recognition, *RadioGraphics* 2:53-68, 1982.

3

Foreign Bodies

. . . .

Tim B. Hunter

People are capable of ingesting, inserting, or injecting themselves or others with all manner of foreign bodies. The psychology of these ingestions, insertions, injections, and stabbings is beyond the scope of this book. The present chapter illustrates examples of foreign devices or objects found in or on patients' bodies and illustrates the range of significant, unusual injuries that can be seen from time to time in an average radiologic practice. These cases of foreign-body ingestion or insertion fall into four broad categories of patients:

1. Children
2. Mentally handicapped or retarded persons (Unlike children, these persons frequently are "repeat offenders." They will often be seen many times for unusual injuries and foreign-body insertions or ingestions.)
3. Adults with unusual sexual behavior
4. "Normal" adults and children (These persons are injured while engaging in criminal activities or are those who are subjected to spouse abuse or child abuse.)

FOREIGN-BODY INGESTIONS

Foreign-body ingestion cases range from children swallowing coins to mentally handicapped adults swallowing razor blades and silverware (Figs. 3-1 to 3-27). Most of all the objects swallowed pass through the gastrointestinal tract without consequence (Table 3-1).[1-6] Elongated or sharp objects, such as needles, bobby pins, or razor blades, are more likely to lodge at areas of narrowing (from bowel adhesions or strictures) or impinge at regions of anatomic acute angulation. The duodenal loop, the duodenojejunal junction, the appendix, and the ileocecal valve region seem to be more predisposed to impaction from these types of objects (Fig. 3-21).[1-10]

The occurrence of appendicitis secondary to an impacted foreign body is an interesting problem.[9,10] There are many reports of appendicitis, appendiceal perforation, and appendiceal abscess formation developing months to years after the ingestion of a foreign object.[9] Because appendicitis is a common disease, its association with a foreign body may be coincidental. It is certainly well known that small round objects, such as lead shot, BB's, and barium and mercury globules, can reside in the appendix for years without apparent effect (Figs. 3-5 and 3-6). Probably, sharp objects, such as pins and toothpicks, are somewhat more likely to induce appendiceal inflammation or perforation. On the other hand, small round objects are probably harmless as far as the appendix is concerned. Larger, round objects, such as an airgun pellet, lodged in the appendix may predispose to appendicitis.[10] It remains controversial whether there should be elective surgery in such instances in an asymptomatic patient.[10]

Large round or cylindrical objects may pass through the esophagus only to be unable to pass through the pylorus.[11] Some large, round objects (such as coins and meat) can become impacted at the thoracic inlet or the gastroesophageal junction (Figs. 3-7, 3-12, 3-22, and 3-23).[12-16]

Disk (button) batteries used in watches, calculators, hearing aids, and cameras produce a potentially very dangerous type of foreign-body ingestion (Fig. 3-16).[17-18] Because of their small size and resemblance to a dime, watch batteries are attractive to children and mentally incapacitated persons. They are seemingly harmless, since their small, round contour should per-

Text continued on p. 81.

Table 3-1 Foreign-Body Ingestions

General Principles

1. Most foreign bodies traverse the gastrointestinal tract without problem.
2. Elongated objects (such as needles, bobby pins) may become impacted at a point of narrowing or at a tight bend (such as the duodenal loop, duodenojejunal junction, terminal ileum).
3. Opaque objects:
   a. Glass of all types
   b. Most metallic objects
   c. Some foods and medicines
   d. Most chicken bones; some fish bones
   e. Sand and gravel
   f. Some medications and poisons—*CHIPES* [chloral hydrate, heavy metals, iodides, phenothiazines, enteric coated pills, solvents]
4. Nonopaque objects:
   a. Most food and medicine
   b. Wood of all types
   c. Most fish bones
   d. Most plastics
   e. Most aluminum objects
5. Consider an unexpected esophageal or airway-tract foreign body in children or mentally incapacitated persons with unexplained stridor, drooling, or respiratory symptoms.
6. Always look for second and third foreign bodies. Never rest after finding one.
7. Examine the entire gastrointestinal tract from the nasopharynx to the rectum.

Predisposed Patients

1. Young children
2. Emotionally disturbed persons
3. Persons with decreased palatal sensitivity caused by:
   a. Dentures
   b. Excessive alcohol or drug intake
   c. Ingestion of very cold liquids
4. Persons with poor vision
5. Persons who eat rapidly

Complications

1. Perforation or peritonitis
2. Obstruction
3. Abscess formation

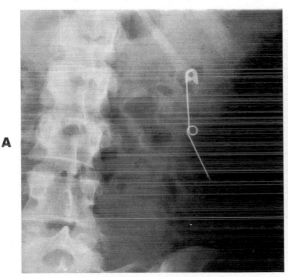
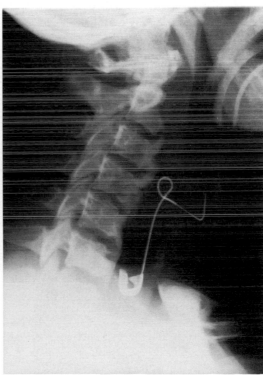

Fig. 3-1. A, A 28-year-old woman who periodically swallowed pins and razor blades. The open safety pin in her descending colon passed without difficulty. **B,** This 37-year-old mentally retarded woman was admitted comatose with a 24-hour history of difficulty in breathing. A safety pin had perforated through the wall of her esophagus and penetrated her larynx. It was extracted at laryngoscopy, and she recovered without sequelae.

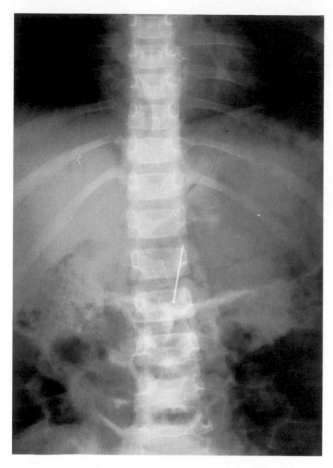

Fig. 3-2. Girl, 5 years of age, who swallowed a pin. It passed without difficulty.

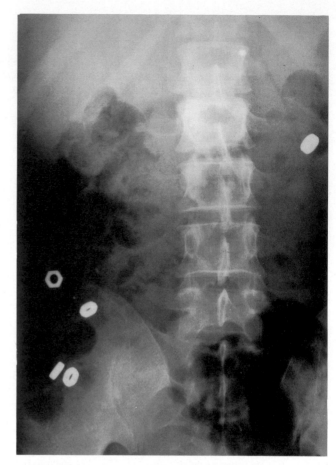

Fig. 3-3. Mentally retarded adult who periodically swallowed foreign objects. Notice the scattered nuts in his bowel. (Courtesy Dr. Brahm B. Hyams, Montreal, Quebec.)

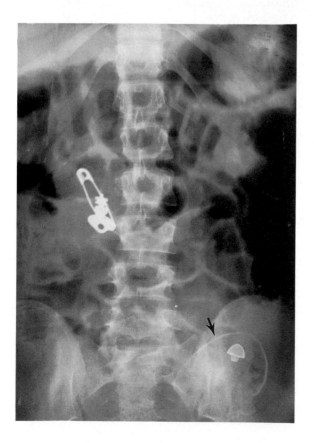

Fig. 3-4. Retarded child, 15 years of age, repeatedly swallowed foreign objects. Notice the safety pin and the key in the jejunum and the flexible rubber Khrushchev doll head, *arrow,* in the descending colon. The objects passed without complications. (Courtesy Dr. George R. Barnes, Jr., Tucson, Arizona.)

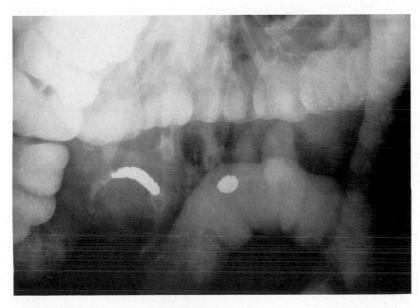

Fig. 3-5. Metallic mercury in the appendix resulting from rupture of the mercury bag on a Miller-Abbott tube. The patient had no symptoms.

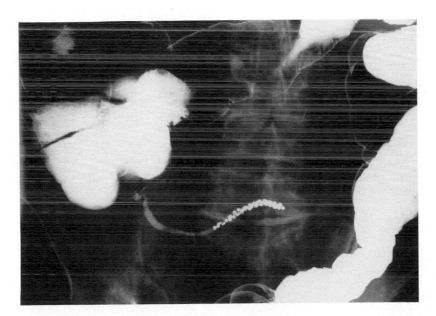

Fig. 3-6. BB's in the appendix. Man, 72 years of age, with no gastrointestinal symptoms. He used to eat BB's as a child.

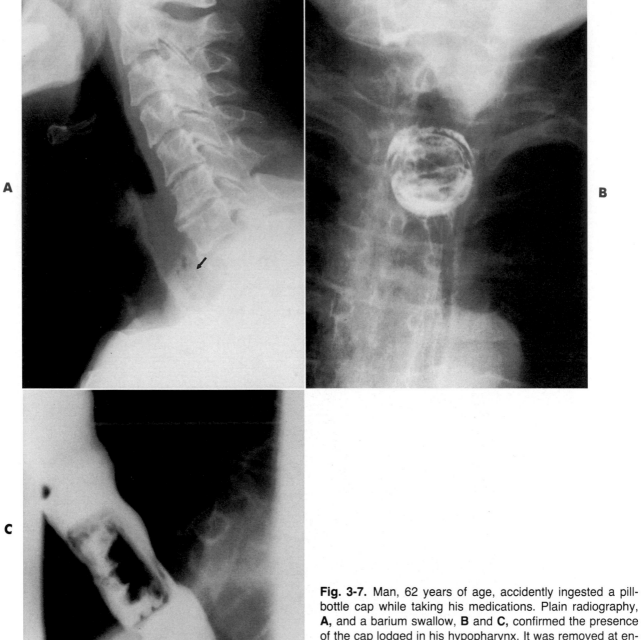

Fig. 3-7. Man, 62 years of age, accidently ingested a pill-bottle cap while taking his medications. Plain radiography, **A,** and a barium swallow, **B** and **C,** confirmed the presence of the cap lodged in his hypopharynx. It was removed at endoscopy. (**B** and **C,** Courtesy Hunter TB: *AJR* 157:411-412, 1991.)

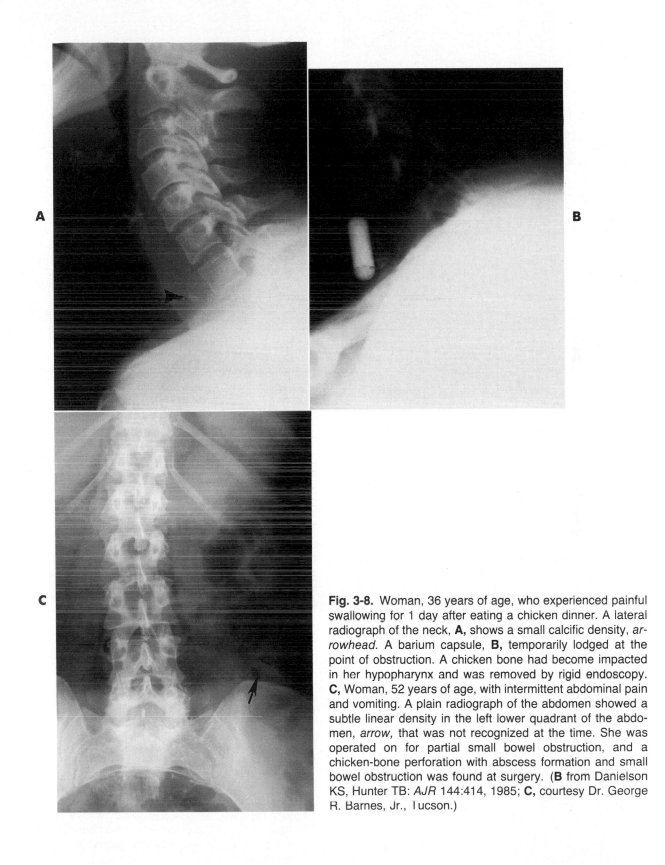

Fig. 3-8. Woman, 36 years of age, who experienced painful swallowing for 1 day after eating a chicken dinner. A lateral radiograph of the neck, **A,** shows a small calcific density, *arrowhead.* A barium capsule, **B,** temporarily lodged at the point of obstruction. A chicken bone had become impacted in her hypopharynx and was removed by rigid endoscopy. **C,** Woman, 52 years of age, with intermittent abdominal pain and vomiting. A plain radiograph of the abdomen showed a subtle linear density in the left lower quadrant of the abdomen, *arrow,* that was not recognized at the time. She was operated on for partial small bowel obstruction, and a chicken-bone perforation with abscess formation and small bowel obstruction was found at surgery. (**B** from Danielson KS, Hunter TB: *AJR* 144:414, 1985; **C,** courtesy Dr. George R. Barnes, Jr., Tucson.)

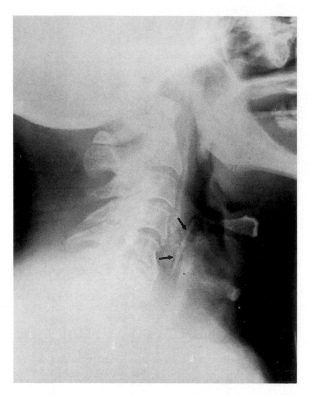

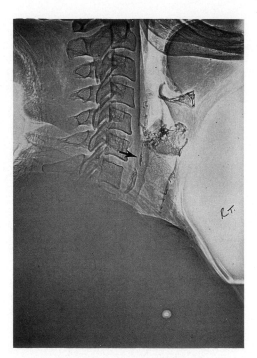

Fig. 3-9. Man, 81 years of age, swallowed a turkey bone. It could not be seen at direct laryngoscopy but was removed at endoscopy. Notice the bone sliver, *arrows,* located just posterior to the calcified thyroid cartilage.

Fig. 3-10. An elderly gentleman experienced painful swallowing after having a bowl of "oxtail" soup. Notice the prominent piece of impacted bone lying anterior to the seventh cervical vertebra. Also notice the prominently calcified posterior margin of the cricoid bone, *arrow.* This normal variant can easily be mistaken for a foreign body. In this patient an impacted bone fragment was removed from the hypopharynx at endoscopy.

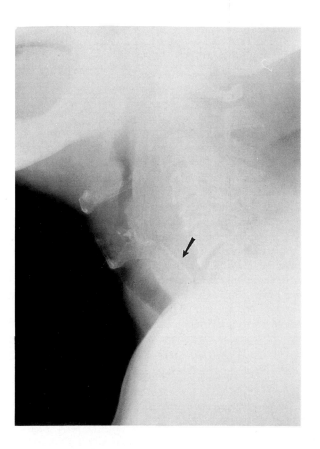

Fig. 3-11. Man, 68 years of age, with 2 days of difficulty swallowing after eating a fish dinner. Indirect laryngoscopy was negative. A fish bone, *arrow,* was removed at surgery after unsuccessful endoscopy. The bone had perforated the hypopharyngeal wall and was lodged in the soft tissues of the neck.

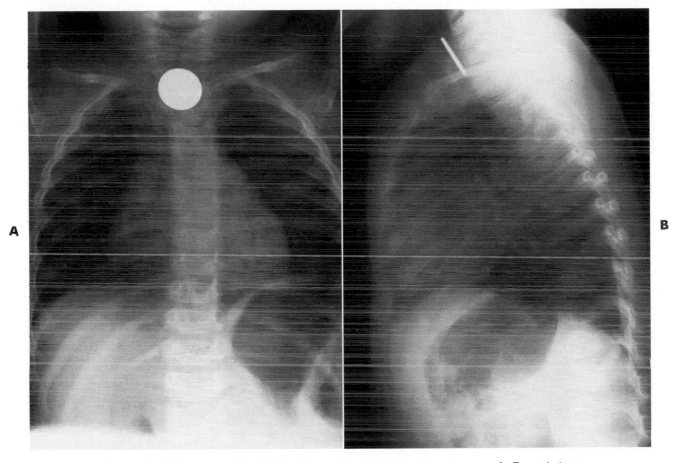

Fig. 3-12. Eighteen-month-old girl with a coin lodged in her hypopharynx. **A,** Frontal view. **B,** Lateral view. (Courtesy Dr. Robert Gatenby, Huntingdon Valley, Pa.)

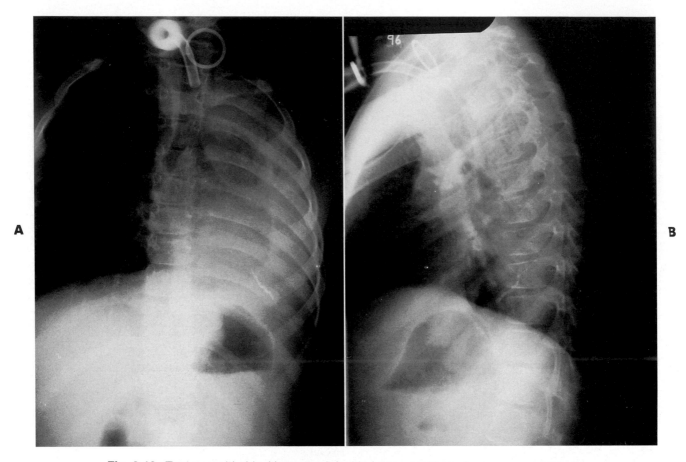

Fig. 3-13. Two-year-old girl with severe left-sided pneumonitis and empyema requiring a tracheostomy. For several days the ringlike metallic density noted on her portable chest radiographs was assumed to be associated with her tracheostomy tube. Finally, standard frontal, **A,** and lateral, **B,** chest radiographs revealed that she had a foreign body in her hypopharynx. A bingo chip was removed at endoscopy.

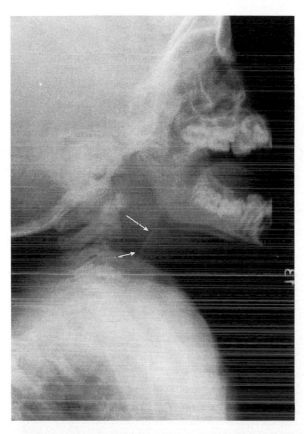

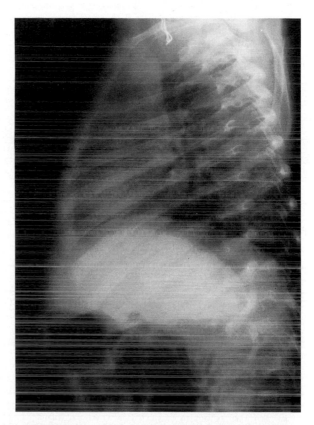

Fig. 3-14. One-year-old girl had coughing after swallowing a red coinlike plastic wafer. A soft-tissue radiograph of the neck shows the object, *arrows,* lodged in her hypopharynx. She coughed it up a few minutes after the radiograph was taken. It is unusual for a plastic object to be opaque on plain film radiography.

Fig. 3-15. Eight-month-old boy with vague respiratory symptoms. A piece of wire was removed from his hypopharynx at endoscopy.

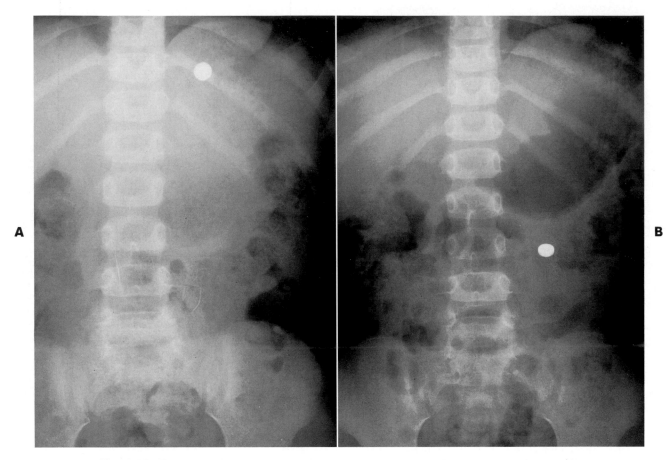

Fig. 3-16. Four-year-old girl ingested a watch battery. **A,** The battery is in the fundus of the stomach. **B,** The battery is now in the transverse colon. It passed without complications.

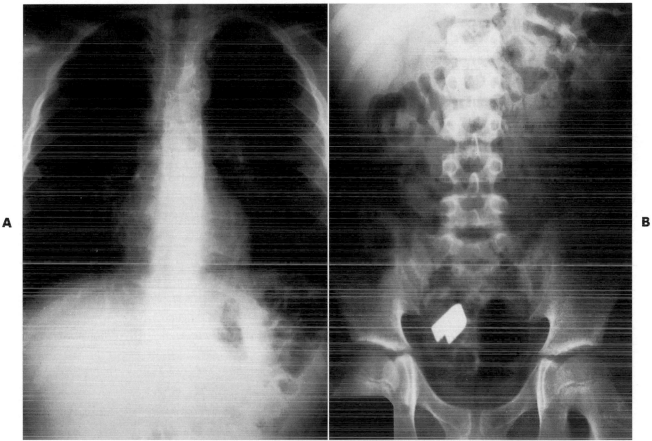

Fig. 3-17. Eight-year-old boy who was said to have swallowed some foreign object. **A,** First film presented to the radiologist shows no opaque object in the chest or stomach. However, the radiologist asked for a repeat film to include all the abdomen and pelvis. **B,** This radiograph shows a metallic object in the distal area of the child's small bowel.

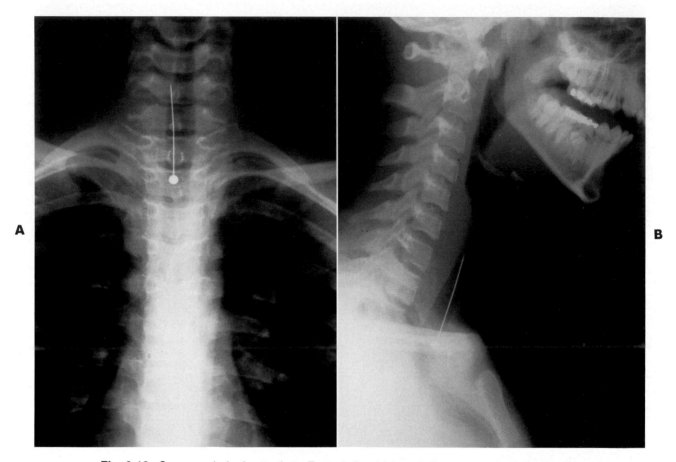

Fig. 3-18. Corsage pin in the trachea. Frontal, **A,** and lateral, **B,** views. A 13-year-old boy was playing with a blowgun and inhaled the pin. It was removed at bronchoscopy. (Courtesy Dr. George R. Barnes, Jr., Tucson.)

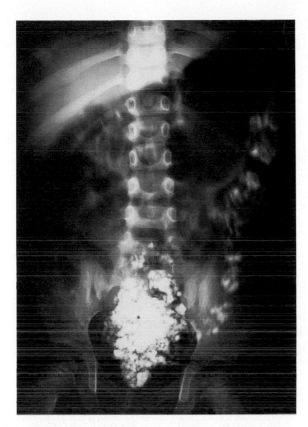

Fig. 3-19. Three-year-old boy with a long history of periodically ingesting gravel, dirt, and small stones. Sometimes he would develop rectal impaction because of the foreign material in his colon.

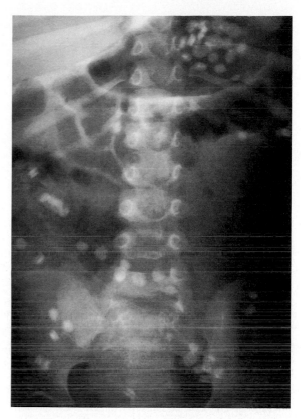

Fig. 3-20. Three-year-old boy ingested multiple iron tablets probably containing ferrous gluconate and ferrous sulfate salts. He recovered without sequelae. (Courtesy Dr. George R. Barnes, Jr., Tucson.)

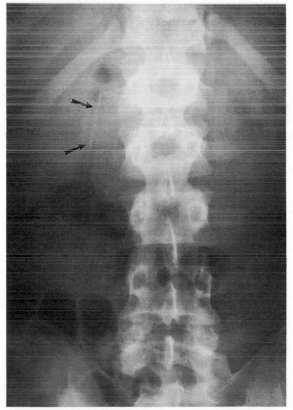

Fig. 3-21. Pencil, *arrows,* lodged in the duodenum. (Courtesy Dr. Charles A. Rohrmann, Jr., Seattle, Wash.)

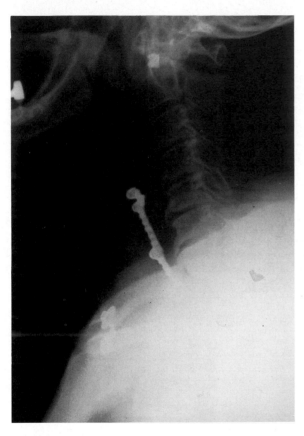

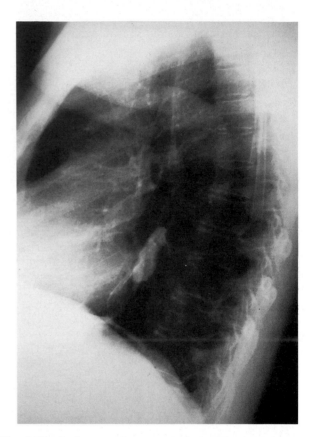

Fig. 3-22. Elderly man who swallowed his upper denture. The back of his lower denture is visible over the mandible. (Courtesy Dr. Brahm B. Hyams, Montreal, Quebec.)

Fig. 3-23. Coffee-cup fragment is lodged in the distal area of the esophagus.

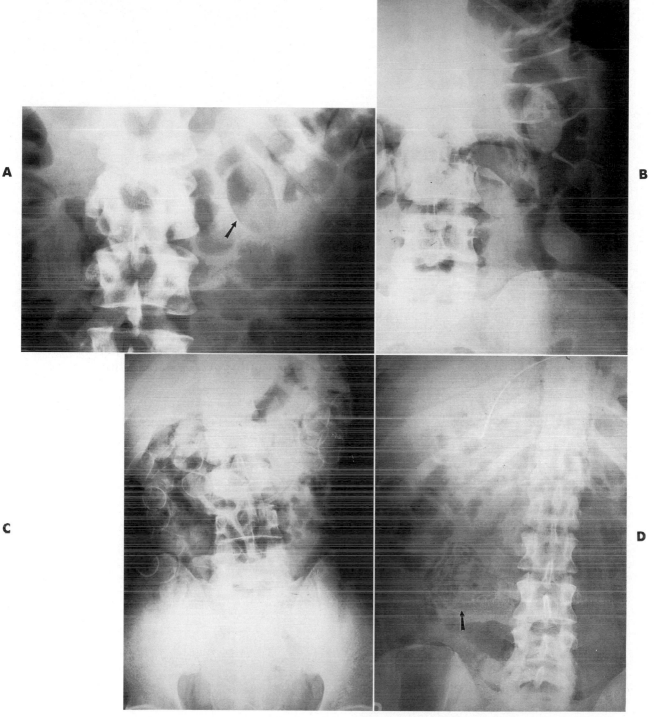

Fig. 3-24. Three examples of adults who were smuggling drugs, **A** to **C,** and an adult who was in the habit of swallowing rubber gloves, **D. A,** Packet, *arrow,* is in the transverse colon. Notice the rim of the lucency. **B** and **C,** Relatively opaque packets in the transverse and descending colon. **D,** The mottled lucency, *arrow,* in the right lower quadrant of the abdomen represents a rolled-up rubber glove in the terminal area of the ileum. It has a similar appearance to swallowed drug packets. (Courtesy Dr. Charles A. Rohrmann, Jr., Seattle.)

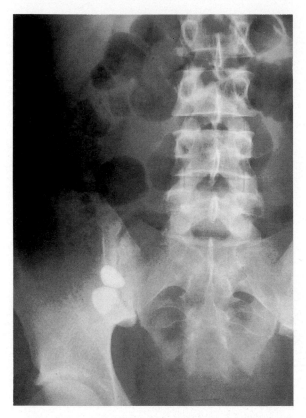

Fig. 3-25. Pepto-Bismol tablets in the right lower quadrant of the abdomen producing "pseudoappendicolith." (Courtesy Dr. Charles A. Rohrmann, Jr., Seattle.)

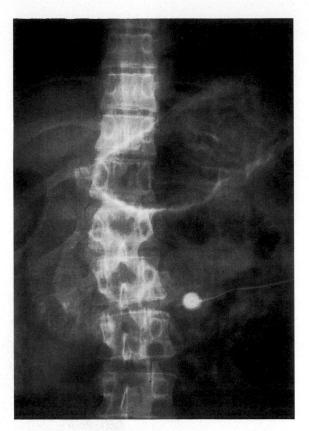

Fig. 3-26. Twenty-five-year-old schizophrenic chemist who ingested lead nitrate. The lead compound produced a mild opacification to the patient's stomach and small intestine. He recovered from the poisoning and was hospitalized for his schizophrenia. (Courtesy Dr. David Vanderkin, Tucson.)

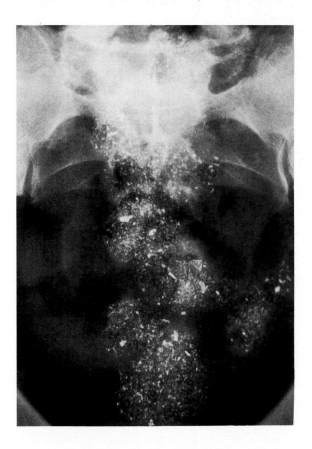

Fig. 3-27. Typesetter who inadvertently ingested high amounts of metallic lead over a period years while eating his lunch at the plant. He had very high blood lead levels, neurologic symptoms, anorexia, and constipation. Notice the opaque lead visible within the rectosigmoid portion of his colon.

mit easy passage through the gastrointestinal tract. In fact, most of them pass without difficulty. However, they can cause grave injury or even death. They contain a variety of alkaline corrosive agents, like aqueous potassium hydroxide, as well as heavy metals, such as mercury and cadmium. If their containers fracture, they can spill their caustic contents, which may lead to perforation and systemic toxicity from heavy metal poisoning.

The treatment for watch-battery ingestion is controversial.[17-19] Most authorities would avoid surgery or endoscopy in routine cases where the battery reaches the stomach. Any evidence for lack of progression through the gastrointestinal tract is a cause for concern and probable intervention. Batteries usually can be removed from the esophagus, stomach, and duodenum by endoscopy- or fluoroscopy-directed interventional techniques with magnets, Foley catheters, forceps, or some type of retrieval basket.[19-21] Watch batteries are magnetic because their case contains nickel. Disk batteries impacted in the esophagus are considered to be especially dangerous and should be removed promptly.

Another seemingly innocuous but potentially extremely dangerous ingested foreign body is the plastic clip used to close plastic bags or bread packages.[22-26] These have been observed to grip various portions of the bowel mucosa, producing inflammation and ulceration, eventually leading to such severe complications as perforation, obstruction, intussusception, fistula formation, abdominal abscess formation, and death. Unfortunately, these objects are not radiopaque on plain radiographs and are difficult to detect. They may become encrusted with mineral or bile salts and thereby be rendered opaque.

Fewer than 1% of ingested foreign bodies cause perforation of the gastrointestinal tract. Sharp, elongated objects are the most likely to penetrate.[3,27-32] Perforations are more common in the ileocecal region, especially in Meckel's diverticulum or the appendix. Foreign-body ingestion should be considered in atypical cases of abdominal pain, peritonitis, abdominal abscess formation, obstruction, and perforation.[26] Metallic objects, fish bones, and chicken bones are the foreign bodies most frequently reported to have caused a perforation.[3] Unusual densities and lucencies or encrustation of objects by bile and mineral salts may be the only clue to an unsuspected foreign-body ingestion.

Plastic objects and thin aluminum objects, such as pull tabs on aluminum cans, are not radiopaque. All chicken and most meat bones are radiopaque on plain films (Figs. 3-8 to 3-11), whereas the majority of fish bones are not, though a minority of them are readily evident (Fig. 3-11).[3,32] Glass is always radiopaque. Its radiopacity does not depend on its lead or other metal content.[33-35]

The relative radiolucency of aluminum is not appreciated by many physicians and radiologists.[36-38] Ingested or inhaled aluminum objects are simply not easily detected on radiographs. The United States Federal Government actually abandoned plans to produce an aluminum penny because many physicians pointed out the very real hazard of a common coin being radiolucent[36-38] because coin ingestions are so common in children. Pop tops and the Italian lira consist of aluminum, are relatively radiolucent, and have caused esophageal perforations.[36]

The diagnosis of an ingested foreign body may be difficult in those patients who cannot furnish an adequate history or who have swallowed objects that are not inherently opaque.[1-2,12-15,39,40] In selected cases, contrast studies with barium tablets, barium capsules (Fig. 3-8), barium-impregnated cotton balls, or barium-coated food may be useful.[41] Computed tomography of the abdomen or chest may even be helpful, particularly if an unusual density or lucency is found and the diagnosis of a perforating foreign body is entertained.[42]

We, unfortunately, live in a world plagued by illicit drug traffic and use. The importation of illegal drugs is a major industry. Some of the more interesting players in this trade are the "mules" or "body packers" who smuggle drugs by ingesting or inserting into their rectum or vagina drug-filled packets. These are usually filled with cocaine, though heroin is also common. The packing material is typically a condom or balloon, and the packets vary in their relative opacities. Some are opaque, whereas others are isodense or hypodense compared to the bowel.[13]

On serial plain abdominal films (Fig. 3-24), these packets may be detected by observation of a definite crescent of air surrounding an ovoid density. This is sometime called the double-condom sign. The packets may also be noted as multiple well-defined densities in the stomach, small intestine, or colon. They may have a rosette configuration at one end.[43]

The main complications from this type of smuggling (other than the legal consequences involved) are bowel obstruction and acute drug toxicity. Bowel obstruction occurs in somewhat less than 10% of documented cases.[43] Acute drug overdose is a very serious risk to the smuggler if one or more of the condoms should rupture. There have been reports of sudden deaths from massive drug overdoses. Considering the large amount of smuggling that no doubt takes place by this means, the complication rate is probably infrequent.

Young children with an esophageal foreign body may present with mainly respiratory symptoms and not volunteer a history of foreign-body ingestion. Stridor, wheezing, and pneumonia can be unsuspected sequelae from an ingested, impacted foreign body in the hypopharynx, esophagus, or respiratory tree (Figs. 3-13 to 3-15).[39-40] Whenever there is a history of a foreign-body ingestion, whether in an adult or a child, the patient should be examined from the nasopharynx to the rectum. Often, there is ingestion of more than one object, and the search for foreign bodies should not be suspended just because one has been found. Children are especially prone to ingest objects in multiples.

Esophageal and bowel strictures may be produced by common prescription medications, such as potassium chloride or quinidine preparations. Most of the strictures develop in the middle or proximal area of the esophagus. Risk factors for esophageal caustic injury related to medications include older age, male sex, left atrial enlargement, and prior esophageal structural abnormality. Sustained-release formulations appear to increase the risk for injury.[44]

Children, mentally incapacitated adults, and suicidal persons may knowingly or inadvertently ingest one or more poisonous substances. Most medications and toxic agents are probably not radiopaque enough to be easily detected by routine imaging methods. However, many metals and their compounds are sufficiently opaque to be seen on plain abdominal radiographs.[45-49] These include barium, lead, arsenic, bismuth, thorium, and iodine compounds (Figs. 3-20 and 3-25 to 3-27).

Iron poisoning is a large problem in the pediatric age group because iron-containing medications are so widely used, and adults usually do not fully appreciate the potential toxicity of iron tablets.[49] Iron tablets that are intact, fragmented, or in a coarse powder form are usually visible in the stomach and small bowel (Fig. 3-20). However, if iron preparations are dissolved or form a fine suspension, they may not be sufficiently radiopaque to be recognizable. Thus, although potentially helpful, plain abdominal radiographs may not permit the diagnosis of iron ingestion or convincingly rule it out. Also, plain abdominal radiographs should not be relied upon to gauge the success of efforts to remove iron from the gastrointestinal tract.[49]

Interestingly, some industrial and research solvents, such as carbon tetrachloride, and some medications, such as chloral hydrate, phenothiazines, and enteric coated drugs, are often radiopaque.[46-48] *CHIPES* (chloral hydrate, heavy metals, iodides, phenothiazines, enteric coated drugs, solvents) is a good mnemonic for remembering classes of radiopaque compounds.[47]

FOREIGN-BODY INSERTIONS

The rectum, vagina, urethra, nose, and ear are favorite sites for insertion of foreign objects (Figs. 3-28 to 3-56). Patients may derive sexual pleasure from this, be mentally incompetent, or do it merely out of curiosity (Table 3-2).

Foreign bodies in the rectum, urethra, or bladder are most commonly introduced by the patient, though occasionally they are the result of a penetrating injury, past

Table 3-2   Foreign-Body Insertions

General Principles
1. Most insertions cause no significant injury
2. Minor mucosal injuries are common
3. Retained objects may be encrusted with mineral salts
4. Retained objects may perforate and travel to remote locations

Predisposed Patients
1. Children, especially those with emotional problems
2. Adults engaging in unusual sexual practices
3. Mentally retarded or incapacitated individuals
4. Patients undergoing instrumentation or surgery
5. Patients undergoing nontraditional medical therapy

Complications
1. Severe bleeding from mucosal injury
2. Edema preventing natural passage or easy removal of the object
3. Organ perforation with resultant hemorrhage, abscess formation, or sepsis.

surgery, or past instrumentation.[50-57] Their occurrence is more frequent in adults with mental illness or in children. Bladder foreign bodies are particularly prone to being a site for deposition of mineral salts with the formation of one or more bladder calculi (Fig. 3-39).[58]

Surprisingly, most foreign bodies inserted into the urethra or rectum do not cause significant injury even if they are large, sharp, or pointed. These tubular structures are capable of considerable expansion, and they are well lubricated by natural fluids. Patients also learn how to "dilate" these structures so that they will accommodate large objects. Common rectal foreign bodies that result from medical procedures going awry include thermometers (Fig. 3-37), rectal tubes, anal packs, light covers, enema tips and covers, suppository wrappers, and oral or topical medication used inappropriately in the rectum.[59]

The supine view of the abdomen is often the first film obtained to evaluate a patient with abdominal or pelvic pain with or without a history of a foreign-body insertion. If the object lies in the bladder, it will generally be oriented mediolaterally (Fig. 3-38). If it lies in the vagina or rectum, it will generally be oriented in a craniocaudal direction (Figs. 3-28, 3-29, and 3-31). This rule is probably more applicable in children than in adults because vaginal foreign objects may lie mediolaterally in adults. Oblique and lateral radiographs of the pelvis as well as endoscopy and contrast studies can help to determine the exact location of a foreign body.

Cleansing enemas are sometimes a source of complications for patients.[59] There can be mucosal injury from the enema fluid being too hot or too caustic. The enema tube or its protective sheath may be retained in the rectum or sigmoid, or the mucosa may be lacerated and perforated. Small retained colonic foreign bodies

Text continued on p. 94.

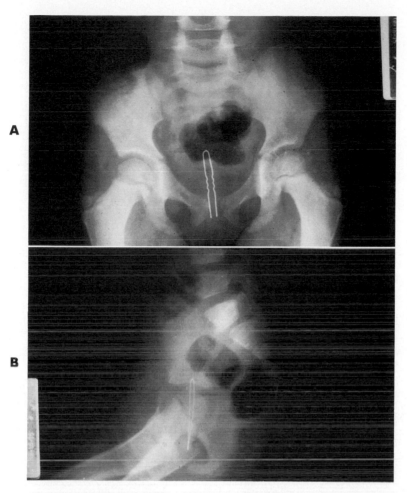

Fig. 3-28. Young child who inserted a bobby pin in her vagina. **A,** Frontal view. **B,** Lateral view. (Courtesy Dr. Laurie L. Fajardo, Tucson.)

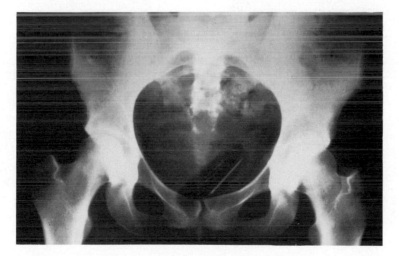

Fig. 3-29. Young woman who lost a comb in her vagina. (Courtesy Dr. Laurie L. Fajardo, Tucson.)

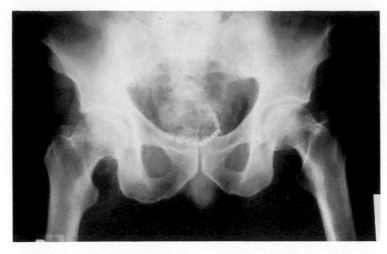

Fig. 3-30. Elderly woman who lost her false teeth in her vagina. (Courtesy Dr. Laurie L. Fajardo, Tucson.)

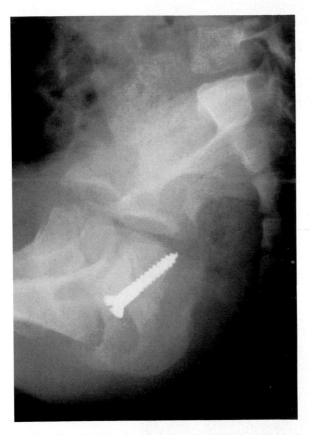

Fig. 3-31. Small child who developed chronic vaginitis because of a screw impacted in her vagina. (Courtesy Dr. George R. Barnes, Jr., Tucson.)

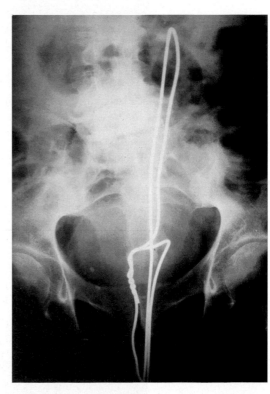

Fig. 3-32. Young woman who inserted a coat hanger into vagina and uterus in an attempted abortion. (Courtesy Dr. Laurie L. Fajardo, Tucson.)

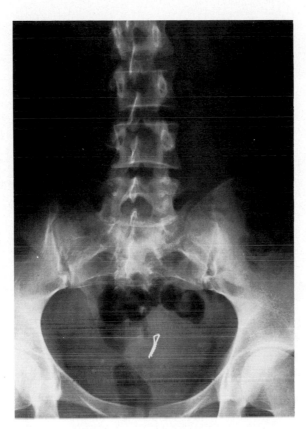

Fig. 3-33. A 19-year-old woman attempted an abortion with a bobby pin, which lodged in her uterus. A later abortion attempt by her was successful. (Courtesy Dr. George R. Barnes, Jr., Tucson.)

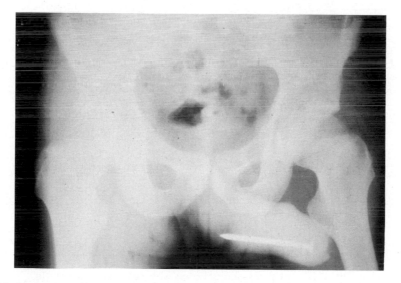

Fig. 3-34. Young man inserted a nail in his urethra. (Courtesy Dr. Laurie L. Fajardo, Tucson.)

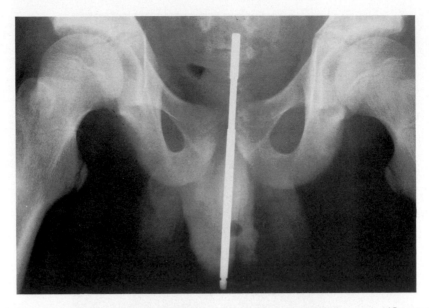

Fig. 3-35. Young man with a pen caught in the urethra and bladder neck. (Courtesy Dr. Laurie L. Fajardo, Tucson.)

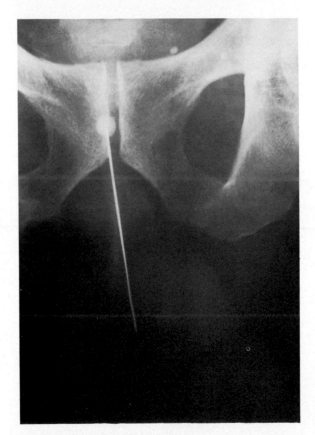

Fig. 3-36. Sixty-six-year-old man who inserted a hat pin in his penis and lost it deep in the bulbous urethra. (Courtesy Dr. Brahm B. Hyams, Montreal, Quebec.)

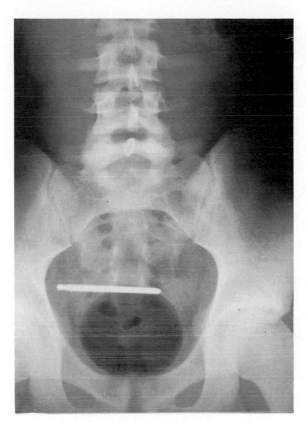

Fig. 3-37. Fifteen-year-old boy with rectal thermometer lying free in the peritoneum. Its origin was unknown. He denied inserting any foreign objects into his rectum or urethra. He had had no treatments or hospitalizations since 1 year of age. (Courtesy Dr. George R. Barnes, Jr., Tucson.)

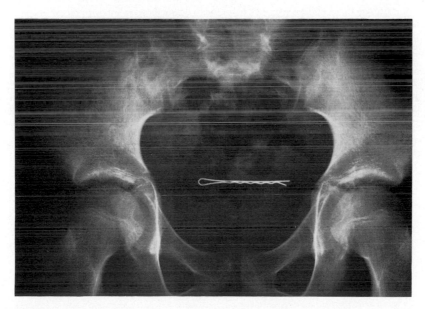

Fig. 3-38. Two-year-old child with a bobby pin in her bladder. (Courtesy Dr. George R. Barnes, Jr., Tucson.)

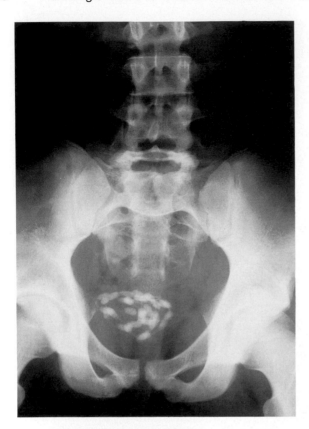

Fig. 3-39. Eighteen-year-old man with a bladder calculus that formed on fine telephone wire. Six months before this film he lost the wire in his bladder when he got an erection while inserting the wire into his urethra during masturbation. (Courtesy Dr. George R. Barnes, Jr., Tucson.)

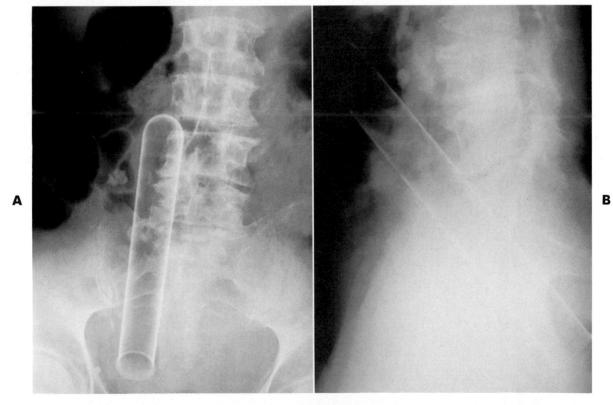

Fig. 3-40. Man, 71 years of age, with abdominal pain. He gave no other history. On rectal examination a consulting surgeon observed that the patient had very loose, redundant rectal mucosa. The surgeon was able to pull the test tube out. **A,** Frontal view. **B,** Lateral view. (Courtesy Dr. Donald Mar, St. Louis.)

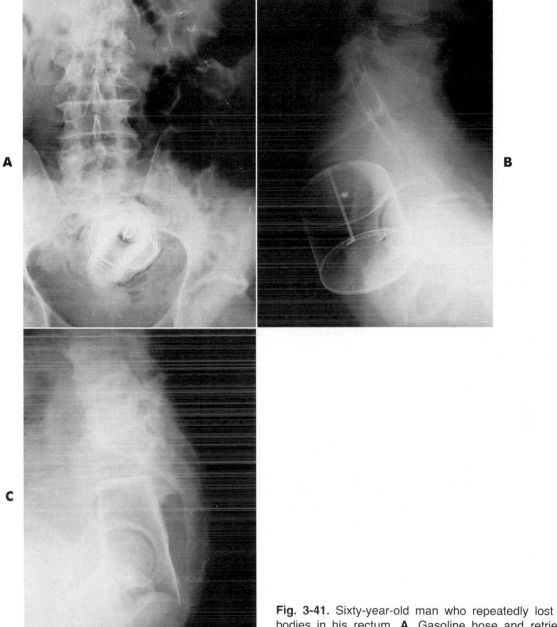

Fig. 3-41. Sixty-year-old man who repeatedly lost foreign bodies in his rectum. **A,** Gasoline hose and retriever. **B,** Condensed milk can. **C,** Drinking glass. (Courtesy Dr. George R. Barnes, Jr., Tucson.)

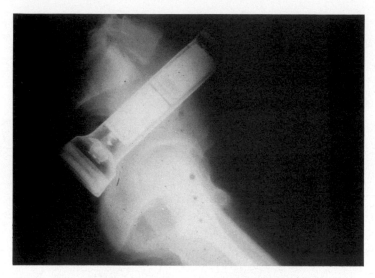

Fig. 3-42. Patient with a flashlight lodged in his rectum. (Courtesy Dr. Laurie L. Fajardo, Tucson.)

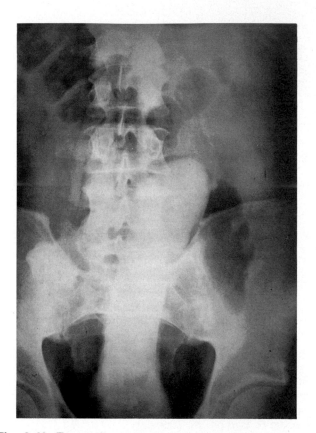

Fig. 3-43. Twenty-five-year-old man who sat on a dildoe. (Courtesy Dr. George R. Barnes, Jr., Tucson.)

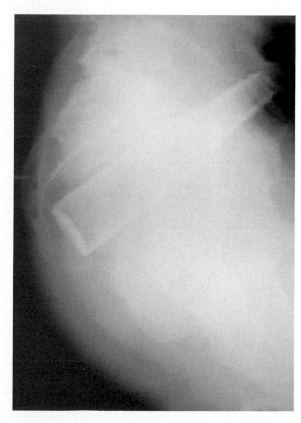

Fig. 3-44. Sixty-four year-old man with a soda bottle lodged in his rectum. (Courtesy Dr. George R. Barnes, Jr., Tucson.)

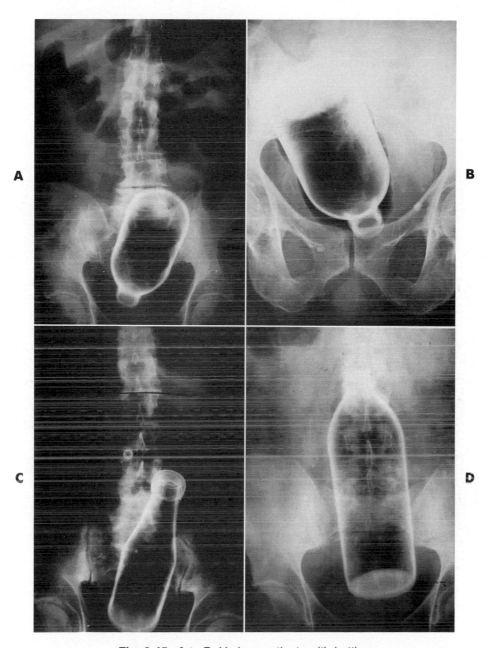

Fig. 3-45. A to **D,** Various patients with bottles.

Continued.

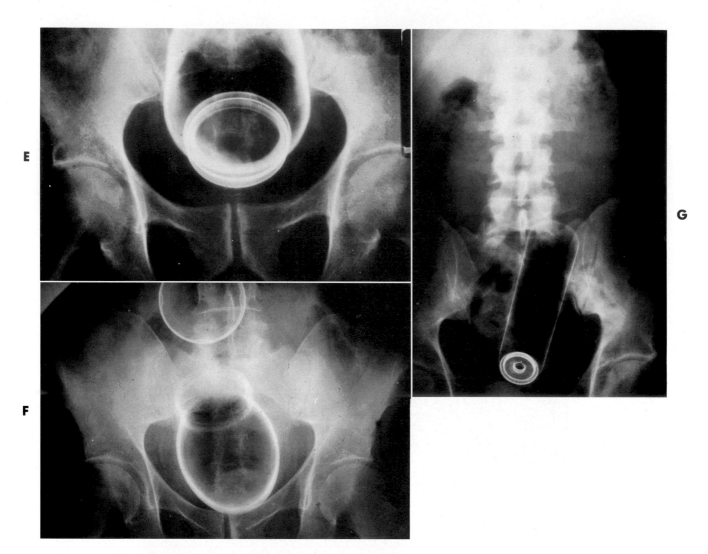

Fig. 3-45, cont'd. E, Mason jar; **F,** glass balls; and **G,** butane canister in the rectosigmoid portions of their colons.. (Courtesy Dr. Laurie L. Fajardo, Tucson.)

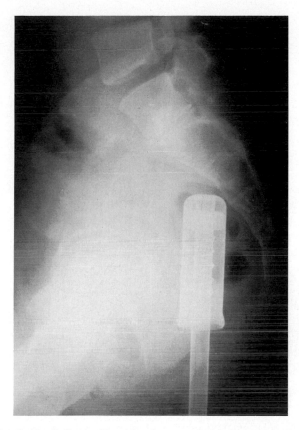

Fig. 3-46. Patient with a bicycle pump lodged in the rectum. (Courtesy Dr. Charles A. Rohrmann, Jr., Seattle.)

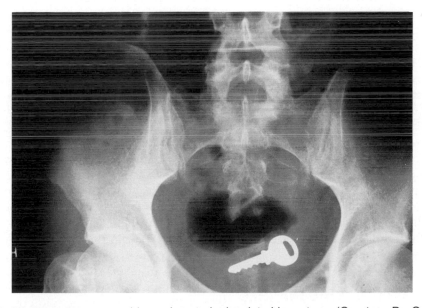

Fig. 3-47. Thirty-three-year-old man inserted a key into his rectum. (Courtesy Dr. George R. Barnes, Jr., Tucson.)

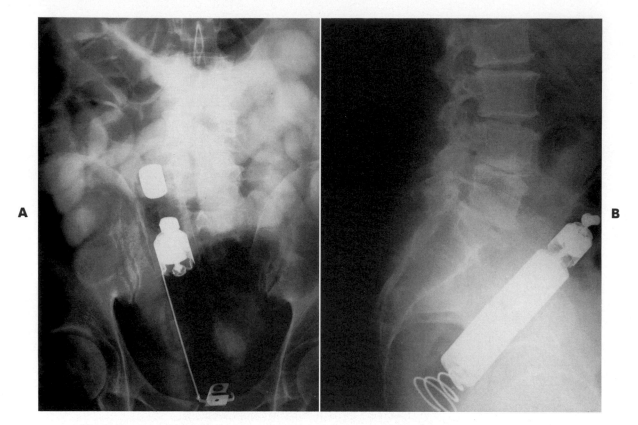

Fig. 3-48. Fifty-eight-year-old man inserted a battery-operated electric flare (normally used for directing traffic) into his rectum and was unable to retrieve it. **A,** Frontal view. **B,** Lateral view. (Courtesy Dr. George R. Barnes, Jr., Tucson.)

usually pass spontaneously. Large ones may induce enough wall edema or bowel atony that they cannot be passed naturally. In such instances, they must be removed by endoscopy, by perianal extraction during anesthesia, or by surgery with either direct removal of the object from the bowel or by laparotomy with anal delivery of the object.[59-62]

Retained rectal bodies may rarely form asymptomatic calcified fecaliths. More commonly, they cause acute and chronic discomfort and have the potential for producing severe bleeding, bowel obstruction, and perforation. Retained objects can also ascend higher into the colon, even going as far as the hepatic flexure. If they perforate the colon, they may lodge in the retroperitoneal tissues, induce localized contained abscesses, lie free within the peritoneum, or even travel to distant sites in the body.[59-65]

MISCELLANEOUS FOREIGN-BODY INJURIES

Even the most sheltered of persons has a life filled with a multitude of mostly minor injuries, including falls, cuts, abrasions, scratches, and burns. Everyone has been inadvertently injured by splinters, needles, thorns, and glass. The entire range of possible foreign body in-

juries cannot possibly be covered in this book. However, we can illustrate (Figs. 3-49 to 3-62) some common types of accidents and point out general principles concerning these injuries (Table 3-3). Ballistic injuries (Fig. 3-57) are, unfortunately, far too common in the United States and are covered in Chapter 19.

It is well recognized that most metallic materials (Figs. 3-49 to 3-51, 3-54, 3-55, and 3-57 to 3-59) are radiopaque on plain films. However, many radiologists and referring physicians do not realize that thorns, splinters, wooden fragments, and pieces of plastic are usually not sufficiently opaque to be visualized with plain radiography.[33-35, 66-67] On the other hand, glass of all types is radiopaque (Fig. 3-53).[33-34,65] Its opacity is not related to its lead content. Therefore, all substantially large pieces of glass should be visible on plain films.

The diagnosis of a nonopaque object may be difficult. Computed tomography and ultrasound offer hope in selected cases for visualization of a suspected foreign object in the superficial tissues of the body.[35,67-71] At ultrasound, foreign objects frequently give a localized, reproducible hyperechoic signal (Fig. 3-56). Needle localization techniques similar to those used for mammographic breast needle localization of nonpalpable lesions before surgical breast biopsy may on occasion aid in the surgical removal of a foreign object from the extremities or other superficial soft tissues of the body (Fig. 3-62).[72]

Most foreign-body injury to the extremities or other parts of the body involve common daily activities. Motor vehicle accidents and industrial accidents probably account for the majority of the cases. Infrequently, foreign objects may travel a great distance from their original site of entrance into the body (Fig. 3-57).

Some patients who practice sorcery or wizardry may insert wires, paper clips, and so forth in themselves to ward off evil spells (Fig. 3-60).[73] Patients undergoing instrumentation or surgery may experience an iatrogenic injury involving foreign material inserted into the body. Most acupuncture needles are temporarily inserted into the subcutaneous tissues of the body, but they may be deliberately or accidently left in place (Fig. 3-58).[74-78]

A very interesting form of injury results from the deliberate or accidental injection of metallic mercury into the body. Metallic mercury is very radiopaque and easily recognized on plain radiographs. It is most commonly seen with patients who ingest it deliberately as part of a suicide attempt or inadvertently ingest or aspirate it as a complication of long intestinal tube use (see Chapter 8). Metallic mercury in general is nontoxic. Mercury compounds and mercury vapor, on the other hand, are quite toxic.

Text continued on p. 105.

Table 3-3   Foreign-Body Injuries

General Principles

1. Opaque materials
   a. Glass
   b. Metal (except many aluminum objects)
   c. Some animal bone fragments
   d. Some soil and mineral fragments
2. Nonopaque materials
   a. Most wood and vegetable fragments
   b. Most plastic fragments
   c. Most thorns
3. Diagnosis may be difficult and require computed tomography, ultrasound, or special techniques to identify nonopaque materials in the body

Predisposed Patients

1. Children and mentally incompetent adults
2. Those with a history of recent injury, particularly motor vehicle accident victims, industrial workers, and trauma patients unable to give a history
3. Those with deviant sexual practices
4. Those who engage in wizardry or sorcery
5. Patients undergoing instrumentation or surgery
6. Patients undergoing nontraditional types of therapy
7. Patients subject to physical abuse

Complications

1. Pain, discomfort, swelling, tenderness
2. Cellulitis, abscess formation
3. Migration of foreign material to distant locations with potential vascular or nerve injury

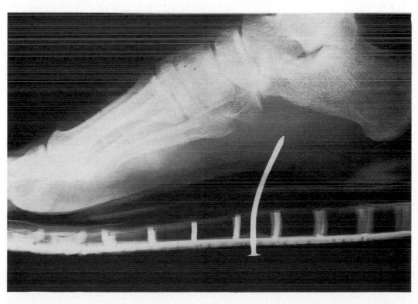

Fig. 3-49. Young man who stepped on a nail while wearing sandals. This radiograph was obtained to see if the nail had entered his calcaneus.

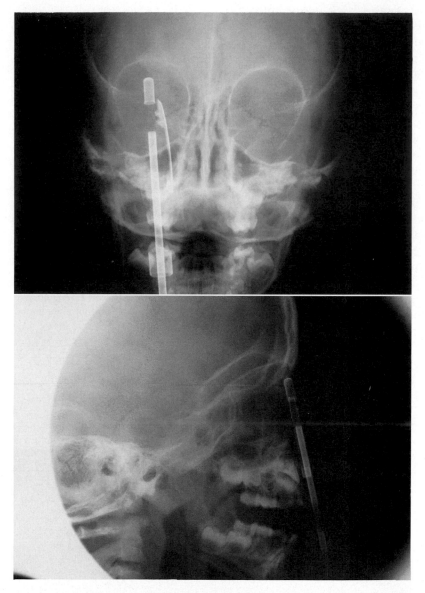

Fig. 3-50. Two-year-old boy was running with a ballpoint pen in his mouth when he fell down. The pen was jammed into the soft tissues of his face, entering his mouth under his upper lip. He recovered from his injuries without sequelae. **A,** Frontal view. **B,** Lateral view. (Courtesy Dr. George R. Barnes, Jr., Tucson.)

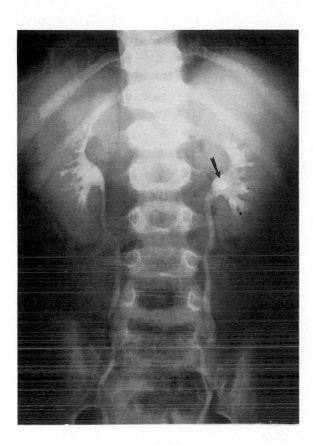

Fig. 3-51. This child presented with painless hematuria. There was a history of the child being shot in the back with a BB 2 years earlier. The BB, *arrow,* had lodged in the left kidney. (Courtesy Dr. George R. Barnes, Jr., Tucson.)

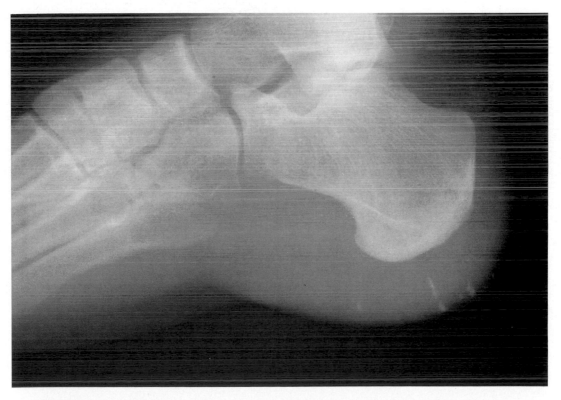

Fig. 3-52. Seventeen-year-old boy who was water skiing, came in on the dock, and unexpectedly encountered barnacles, pieces of which lodged in his left heel. Glass fragments would have a similar appearance. (Courtesy Dr. George R. Barnes, Jr., Tucson.)

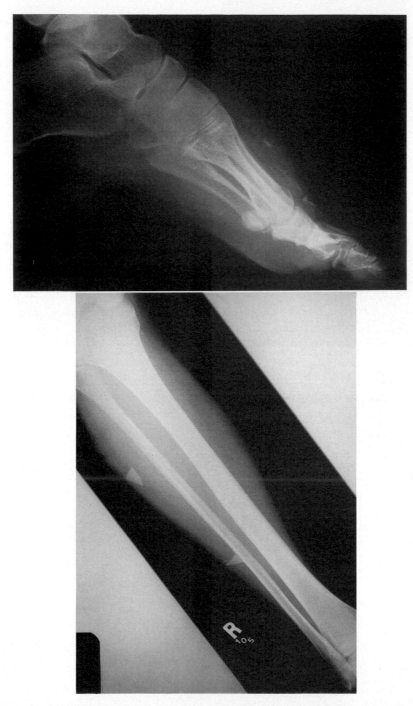

Fig. 3-53. A, Woman, 21 years of age, thrown out of a car during a motor vehicle accident suffering considerable soft-tissue damage to her left foot. The multiple opaque densities visible in the soft tissues of her foot represent gravel, dirt, and pieces of glass. **B,** Young woman with pieces of glass in her leg secondary to an automobile accident.

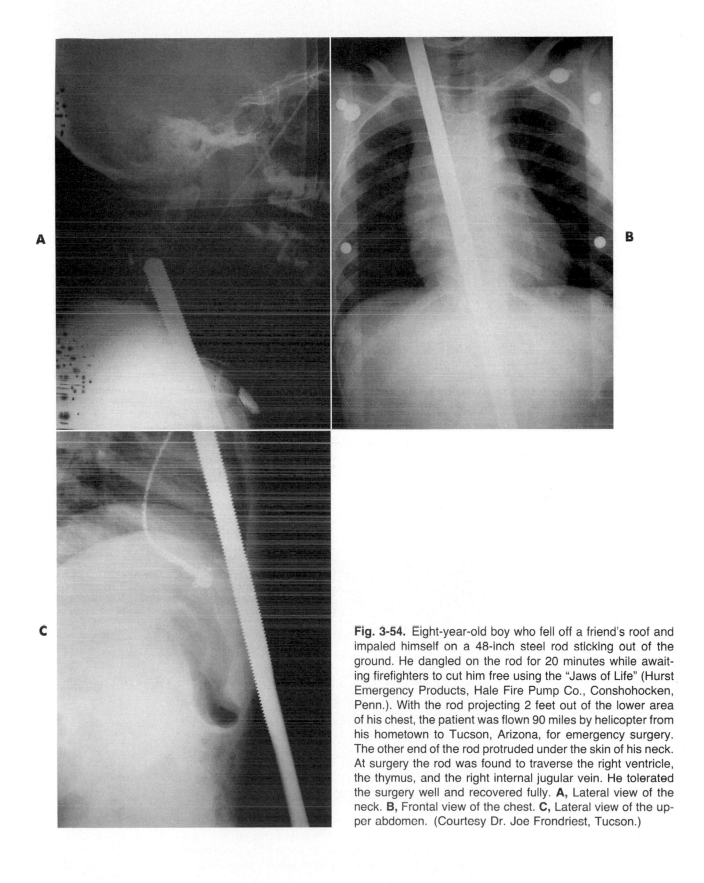

Fig. 3-54. Eight-year-old boy who fell off a friend's roof and impaled himself on a 48-inch steel rod sticking out of the ground. He dangled on the rod for 20 minutes while awaiting firefighters to cut him free using the "Jaws of Life" (Hurst Emergency Products, Hale Fire Pump Co., Conshohocken, Penn.). With the rod projecting 2 feet out of the lower area of his chest, the patient was flown 90 miles by helicopter from his hometown to Tucson, Arizona, for emergency surgery. The other end of the rod protruded under the skin of his neck. At surgery the rod was found to traverse the right ventricle, the thymus, and the right internal jugular vein. He tolerated the surgery well and recovered fully. **A,** Lateral view of the neck. **B,** Frontal view of the chest. **C,** Lateral view of the upper abdomen. (Courtesy Dr. Joe Frondriest, Tucson.)

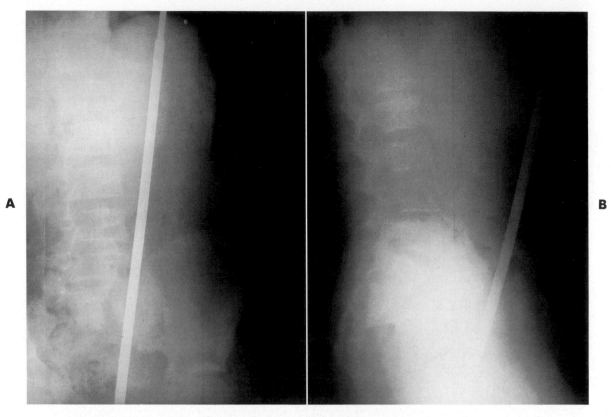

Fig. 3-55. Twelve-year-old boy who fell out of a tree onto a junk pile. A car antenna pierced his left buttock and came out next to his xiphoid. He walked home without trouble and had to calm his hysterical mother so that she could take him to the hospital. The antenna missed all the large vessels in the pelvis, abdomen, and chest but did rupture a portion of his colon. He required bowel repair and a temporary colostomy but recovered uneventfully. **A,** Frontal view. **B,** Lateral view.

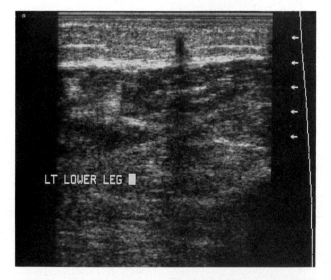

Fig. 3-56. Ten-year-old boy with tenderness and possible palpable foreign body in the soft tissues of his left leg. Ultrasound confirmed the presence of a foreign body (palm frond). (Courtesy Dr. Robert Gatenby, Huntingdon Valley, Pa.)

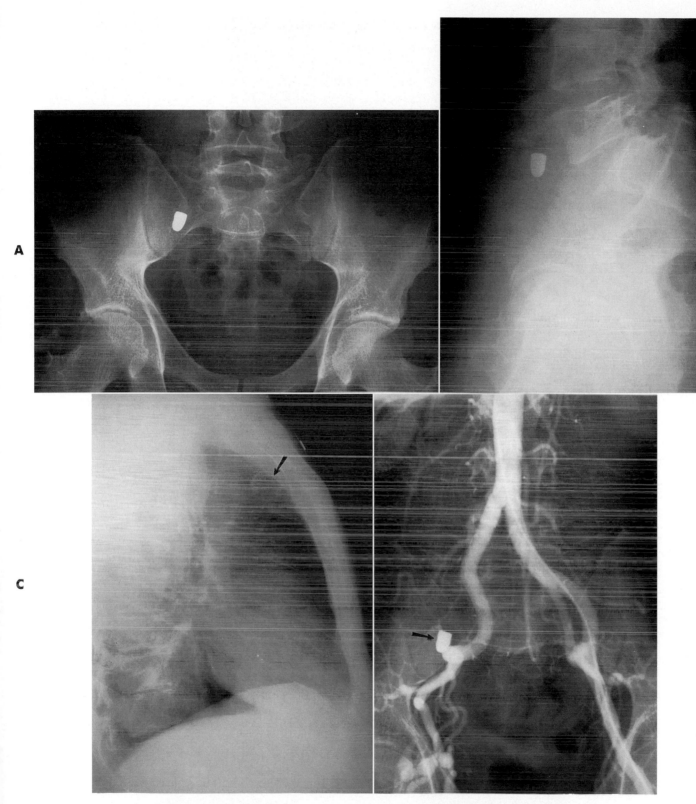

Fig. 3-57. Thirty-five-year-old man who at 13 years of age was shot in the chest on Mother's Day by his older brother. The bullet was not removed because "it was too close to the heart." Twenty-two years later the scout film for an upper gastrointestinal series showed a .32-caliber slug in his pelvis, **A** and **B.** A subsequent chest film, **C,** showed a calcification consistent with an aortic pseudoaneurysm, *arrow.* **D,** Elective angiography showed that the bullet, *arrow,* had migrated to the right iliac arterial system and had occluded the right external iliac artery. (Courtesy Dr. George R. Barnes, Jr., Tucson.)

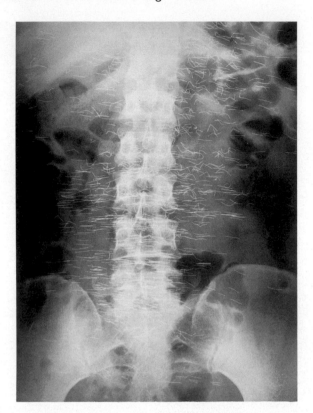

Fig. 3-58. Acupuncture needles in the paraspinal subcutaneous soft tissues of a 37-year-old Korean woman. The needle fragments were purposefully left in place. (Courtesy Dr. Joseph A. Alvarado, Tucson.)

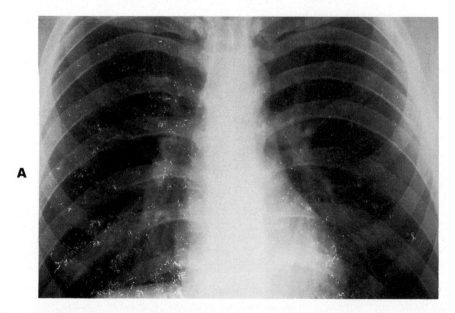

Fig. 3-59. Twenty-one-year-old man who had apparently injected himself with metallic mercury producing emboli to the lungs, **A** and **B,** and residual mercury deposits in his left antecubital fossa, **C** and **D.** (**A** and **B** from Peterson N et al: *AJR* 135:1079-1081, 1980; **C** and **D,** courtesy Dr. Charles A. Rohrmann, Jr., Seattle.)

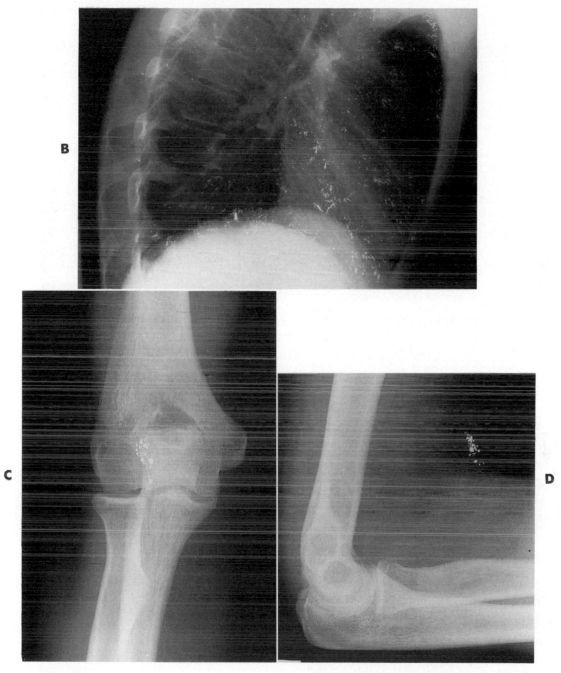

Fig. 3-59, cont'd.

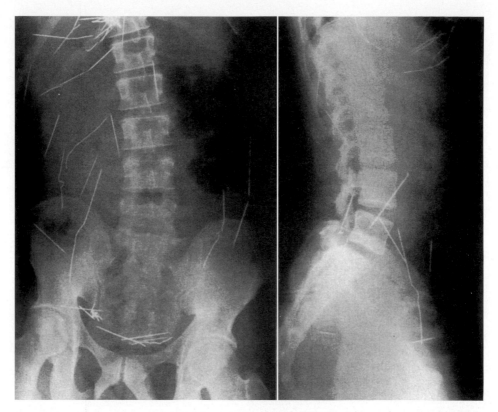

Fig. 3-60. **A,** Anteroposterior and, **B,** left lateral radiographs of the abdomen demonstrate scoliotic posture in a 33-year-old African man living in Gabon. One hundred sharp metal foreign bodies, such as needles and sharpened paper clips, were found scattered between his neck and pelvis, representing darts in an attempt to protect the patient from supposed evil spells and evil spirits. (From Desrentes M: *Radiology* 177(1):115-116, 1990.)

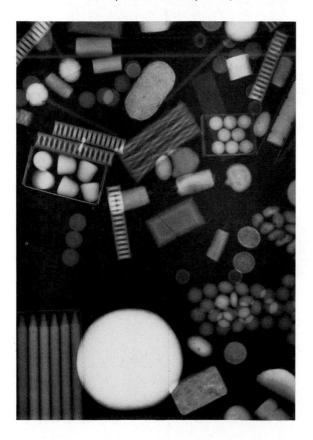

Fig. 3-61. Trick-or-treat candy. There are no hidden needles or razor blades. The candy and apple (not the crayons) were eaten without problems. Can you identify the various objects?

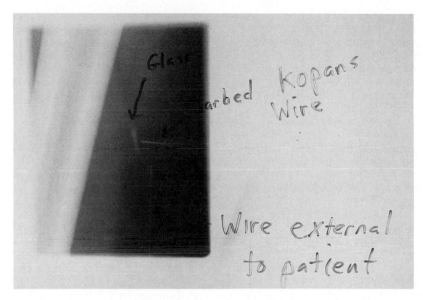

Fig. 3-62. Twenty-four-year-old woman with glass lodged in the left side of her thigh. It was visible on plain radiographs but not palpable. Needle-localization technique with a Kopans breast needle-localizing hookwire was used to locate the glass for easy surgical removal. The labeling on the illustration was not done by the author; it represents permanent ink writing placed on the radiograph by a radiology resident! It is always best to label such films with wax pencils rather than with permanent ink, which cannot be erased, because there may be a labeling error, or the film may be used in a future publication.

Deliberate injection of mercury subcutaneously or intravenously produces dramatic radiographic results (Fig. 3-59). Individuals may inject themselves in the mistaken belief that mercury increases their strength, or they may be drug abusers, or even attempting suicide.[79-82] At one time mercury was used as an anaerobic seal for arterial blood gas sampling during cardiac catheterization and as a seal for arterial blood gas sampling syringes and arterial pressure monitors. If the seal was broken, metallic mercury could be inadvertently injected into the arterial or venous system of the patient.[79,81] Infrequently, soft-tissue mercury deposits are also seen in patients who accidently break a mercury thermometer.

If mercury is injected into subcutaneous tissues (Fig. 3-59), it forms irregular globules and may remain in place for months to years. Sometimes it forms sterile abscesses with gradual extrusion of the mercury globules. If it is injected into the venous system, it will embolize to the lungs (Fig. 3-59). Here, it forms small globules in the peripheral branches of the pulmonary arterial tree. The mercury may also pool in the right ventricle. Differentiating aspirated metallic mercury from mercury embolism to the lungs is difficult from the chest radiograph alone. The diagnosis depends on the patient history, presence of mercury in the right ventricle or subcutaneous tissue of the arm or leg (favoring mercury embolism), or presence of mercury in the gastrointestinal tract (favoring mercury aspiration).[80-82]

Metallic mercury in the bronchial tree or in the pulmonary arterial tree is relatively "benign" and is usually not associated with symptoms.[79-82] The mercury may remain indefinitely but usually shows some slow clearing. If metallic mercury is injected into the arterial system, passes through the pulmonary capillary bed, or bypasses the lungs via a shunt, it can embolize in the systemic circulation, ending up in such locations as the cerebral vasculature, the coronary arteries, the spleen, kidneys, and distal phalanges.[79]

Halloween is a fun time of the year for children. Unfortunately, some individuals have taken delight in hiding needles, razor blades, and other harmful items in candy and food given out to trick or treaters. Plain film radiography of food and candy is surprisingly effective (Fig. 3-61) and can be used to identify harmful objects or to reassure parents that there is a low likelihood for a sharp object lurking in treats.

REFERENCES

1. Schwartz GF, Polsky HS: Ingested foreign bodies of the gastrointestinal tract, *Am Surg* 42:236-238, 1976.
2. Eldridge WW: Foreign bodies in the gastrointestinal tract, *JAMA* 178:665-667, 1961.
3. Maglinte DDT, Taylor SD, Ng AC: Gastrointestinal perforation by chickenbones, *Radiology* 130:597-599, 1979.
4. McPherson RC, Karlon M, Williams RD: Foreign body perforation of the intestinal tract, *Am J Surg* 94:564-566, 1957.
5. Maleki M, Evans WE: Foreign body perforation of the intestinal tract, *Arch Surg* 101:475-477, 1970.

6. Selivanov V, Sheldon GF, Cello JP, Crass RA: Management of foreign body ingestion, *Ann Surg* 199:187-191, 1984.

7. Segal I, Nouri MA, Hamilton DG, et al: Foreign body ileitis: a case report, *S Afr Med J* 588:421-422, 1980.

8. Himadi GM, Fischer GJ: Magnetic removal of foreign bodies from the upper gastrointestinal tract, *Radiology* 123:226-227, 1977.

9. Balch CM, Silver D: Foreign bodies in the appendix, *Arch Surg* 102:14-20, 1971.

10. Price J, Dewar GA, Metreweli C: Airgun pellet appendicitis, *Australas Radiol* 32:368-370, 1988.

11. Muhletaler CA, Gerlock AJ Jr, Shull HS, Adkins RB Jr: The pill bottle desiccant: a cause of partial gastrointestinal obstruction, *JAMA* 242:1921-1922, 1980.

12. Jackson CL: Foreign bodies in the esophagus, *Am J Surg* 93:308-312, 1957.

13. Nandi P, Ong GB: Foreign body in the esophagus: review of 2394 cases, *Br J Surg* 65:5-9, 1978.

14. Chaikhouni A, Kratz JM, Crawford FA: Foreign bodies of the esophagus, *Am Surg* 51:173-179, 1985.

15. Vizcarrondo FJ, Brady PG, Nord HJ: Foreign bodies of the upper gastrointestinal tract, *Gastrointest Endosc* 29:208-210, 1983.

16. Bunker PG: The role of dentistry in problems of foreign bodies in the air and food passages, *J Am Dent Assoc* 64:782-787, 1962.

17. Kuhns DW, Dire DJ: Button battery ingestions, *Ann Emerg Med* 18:293-300, 1989.

18. Studley JGN, Linehan IP, Ogilvie AL, Dowling BL: Swallowed button batteries: Is there a consensus on management? *Gut* 31:867-870, 1990.

19. Jaffe RB, Corneli HM: Fluoroscopic removal of ingested alkaline batteries, *Radiology* 150:585-586, 1984.

20. Shaffer HA, Alfred BA, deLange EE, et al: Basket extraction of esophageal foreign bodies, *AJR* 147:1010-1013, 1986.

21. Volle E, Hand D, Berger P, Kaufman HJ: Ingested foreign bodies: removal by magnet, *Radiology* 160:407-409, 1986.

22. Bundred NJ, Blackie RAS, Kingsnorth AN, Eremin O: Hidden dangers of sliced bread, *Br Med J* 288:1723-1724, 1984.

23. Sutten G: Hidden dangers of sliced bread, *Br Med J* 288:1995, 1984.

24. Rivron RP, Jones DRB: A hazard of modern life, *Lancet* 2:334, 1983.

25. Jamison MH, Davis RWW, Maclennan I: A plastic bread-bag clip: cause of intermittent intestinal obstruction, *Br J Clin Pract* 37:402-403, 1983.

26. Guindi MM, Troster MM, Walley VM: Three cases of an unusual foreign body in small bowel, *Gastrointest Radiol* 12:240-242, 1987.

27. Maleki M, Evans WE: Foreign-body perforation of the intestinal tract: report of 12 cases and review of the literature, *Arch Surg* 101:475-477, 1970.

28. Ziter FM Jr: Intestinal perforation in adults due to ingested opaque foreign bodies, *Am J Gastroenterol* 68:382-385, 1976.

29. Schwartz JT, Graham DY: Toothpick perforation of the intestines, *Ann Surg* 185:64-66, 1977.

30. Gunn A: Intestinal perforation due to swallowed fish or meat bone, *Lancet* 1:125-128, 1966.

31. Ashby BS, Hunter-Craig ID: Foreign-body perforations of the gut, *Brit J Surg* 54:382-384, 1967.

32. Ngan JHK, Fox PJ, Lai ECS, et al: A prospective study on fish bone ingestion: experience of 358 patients, *Ann Surg* 211:459-462, 1990.

33. Tandberg D: Glass in hand and foot: Will x-ray film show it? *JAMA* 248:1872-1874, 1982.

34. Gordon D: Nonmetallic foreign bodies, *Br J Radiol* 58:574, 1985.

35. Fornage BD, Schemberg FL: Sonographic diagnosis of foreign bodies of the distal extremities, *AJR* 147:567-569, 1986.

36. Heller RM, Reichelderfer TE, Dorst JP, Oh KS: The problems with the replacement of copper pennies by aluminum pennies, *Pediatrics* 54:684, 1974.

37. Dorst JP, Reichelderfer TE, Sanders RC: Radiology of the proposed new penny, *Pediatrics* 69:224, 1982.

38. Eggli KD, Potter BM, Garcia V, et al: Delayed diagnosis of esophageal perforation by aluminum foreign bodies, *Pediatr Radiol* 16:511-513, 1986.

39. Smith PC, Swischuk LE, Fagan CV: Elusive and often unsuspected cause of stridor or pneumonia (esophageal foreign body), *AJR* 122:80-89, 1974.

40. Humphry A, Holland WG: Unsuspected esophageal foreign bodies, *J Can Assoc Radiol* 32:17-20, 1981.

41. Danielson KS, Hunter TB: Barium capsules, *AJR* 144:414, 1985.

42. Berger PE, Kuhn JP, Kuhns LR: Computed tomography and the occult tracheobroncheal foreign body, *Radiology* 134:133-135, 1980.

43. Beerman R, Nuñez D Jr, Wetli CV: Radiographic evaluation of the cocaine smuggler, *Gastrointest Radiol* 11:351-354, 1986.

44. McCord GS, Clouse RE: Pill-induced esophageal strictures: clinical features and risk factors for development, *Am J Med* 88:512-518, 1990.

45. Hilfer RJ, Mandel A: Acute arsenic intoxication diagnosed by roentgenograms, *N Engl J Med* 266:663-664, 1962.

46. Goldfrank LR, Howland MA, Kirstein RH: Arsenic. In: Goldfrank LR, Flomebaum NE, Lewin NA, et al, editors: *Toxicologic emergencies*. East Norwalk, Conn, 1986, Appleton-Century-Crofts, pp 609-618.

47. Spiegel SM, Hyams BB: Radiographic demonstration of a toxic agent, *J Can Assoc Radiol* 35:204-205, 1984.

48. Gray JR, Khalil A, Prior JC: Acute arsenic toxicity—an opaque poison, *J Can Assoc Radiol* 40:226-227, 1989.

49. Staple TW, McAlister WH: Roentgenographic visualization of iron preparations in the gastrointestinal tract, *Radiology* 83:1051-1056, 1964.

50. Busch DB, Starling JR: Rectal foreign bodies: case reports and a comprehensive review of the world's literature, *Surgery* 100:512-519, 1986.

51. Classen JN, Marten RE, Sabagal J: Iatrogenic lesions of the colon and rectum, *South Med J* 68:1417-1428, 1975.

52. Rosser C: Foreign bodies of the rectum, *Texas State J Med* 27:23-24, 1931.

53. Rebell FG: The problem of foreign bodies in the colon and rectum, *Am J Surg* 76:678-686, 1948.

54. Crass RA, Tranbaugh RF, Kudsk KA, Trundey DD: Colorectal foreign bodies and perforations, *Am J Surg* 142:85-88, 1981.

55. Kraker DA: Foreign bodies in the rectum and sigmoid, *Am J Surg* 29:449-450, 1935.

56. Fuller RC: Foreign bodies in the rectum and colon, *Dis Colon Rectum* 8:123-127, 1965.

57. Barone JE, Sohn N, Nelson TF: Perforations and foreign bodies of the rectum: report of 28 cases, *Ann Surg* 184:601-604, 1976.

58. Lebowitz RL, Vargas B: Stones in the urinary bladder in children and young adults, *AJR* 148:491-495, 1987.

59. Zelegman BE, Feinberg LE, Johnson ED: A complication of cleansing enema: retained protective shield of the enema tip, *Gastrointest Radiol* 11:372-374, 1986.

60. Richter RM, Littman L: Endoscopic extraction of an unusual colonic foreign body, *Gastrointest Endosc* 22:40-45, 1975.

61. Wolf L, Geracy K: Colonoscopic removal of balloons from the bowel, *Gastrointest Endosc* 24:41-44, 1977.

62. Eftaiha M, Hambrick E, Abcarian H: Principles of management of colorectal foreign bodies, *Arch Surg* 112:691-695, 1977.

63. Lau JTK, Ong GB: Broken and retained rectal thermometers in infants and young children, *Aust Pediatr J* 17:93-94, 1981.

64. Morales L, Rovida J, Mongrad M, et al: Intraspinal migration of rectal foreign body, *J Pediatr Surg* 18:634-635, 1983.

65. Buzzard AJ, Waxman BP: A long standing much travelled foreign body, *Med J Aust* 1:600, 1979.

66. deLacey G, Evans R, Sandin B: Penetrating injuries: How easy is it

to see glass (and plastic) on radiographs? *Br J Radiol* 58:27-30, 1985.

67. Spouge AR, Weisbrod GL, Herman SJ, Chamberlain DW: Wooden foreign body in the lung parenchyma, *AJR* 154:999-1001, 1990.

68. Bodne D, Quinn SF, Cochran CF: Imaging foreign glass and wooden bodies of the extremities with CT and MRI, *J Comput Assist Tomogr* 12:608-611, 1988.

69. Gooding AW, Hardiman T, Sumers M, et al: Sonography of the hand and foot in foreign body detection, *J Ultrasound Med* 6:441-447, 1987.

70. Brewer TE, Leonard RB: Detection of retained wood following trauma, *NC Med J* 47:575-577, 1988.

71. Roberts CF, Leehey PJ III: Intraorbital wood foreign body mimicking air at CT, *Radiology* 185:507-508, 1992.

72. Meyer JE, Kopans DB, Mueller PR: Preoperative localization of radiopaque foreign bodies, *Radiology* 144:179, 1982.

73. Desrentes M: Wizardry and radiography: a clinical case, *Radiology* 177:115-116, 1990.

74. Imray TJ, Hiramatsu Y: Radiographic manifestations of Japanese acupuncture, *Radiology* 115:625-626, 1975.

75. Schatz CJ, Fordham S: Acupuncture needles a "new" foreign body in the ear, *AJR* 127:688-689, 1976.

76. Glauten A, Austin JHM: Permanent subcutaneous acupuncture needles: radiographic manifestations, *J Can Assoc Radiol* 398:54-56, 1988.

77. Saenz L, Lee H, Mottram M: Permanent acupuncture needles, *JAMA* 240:1482-1483, 1978.

78. Behrstock BB, Petrakis NL: A case report: permanent subcutaneous gold acupuncture needles, *West J Med* 121:140-142, 1974.

79. Nadich TP, Bartelt D, Wheeler PS, Stern WZ: Metallic mercury emboli, *AJR* 117:886-891, 1973.

80. Wenzel V, Tuttle RJ, Zylak CJ: Intravenous self-administration of metallic mercury, *Radiology* 137:313-315, 1980.

81. Peterson N, Harvey-Smith W, Rohrmann CA Jr: Radiographic aspects of metallic mercury embolism, *AJR* 135:1079-1081, 1980.

82. Spizarny DL, Renzi P: Metallic mercury pulmonary emboli, *J Can Assoc Radiol* 38:60-61, 1987.

4

Medical Devices of the Head and Neck

. . . .

Mark T. Yoshino

This chapter contains examples of medical and surgical devices seen when one is imaging the central nervous system as well as devices found in the head and neck. As is the case elsewhere in the body, there are many devices placed in the head, neck, and spine. This chapter focuses on the most common ones. The specific device placed depends on both the needs of the patient and the experience and preference of the neurologic, orthopedic, or head and neck surgeon. An excellent source of information on the specific devices placed in any given hospital is the central supply department, which has specimens of items commonly used in that hospital, as well as catalogs containing a huge number of possible alternatives.

Usually a referring surgeon knows what sort of device is placed, and his or her question is, What is the location of the device and has it moved? For this reason, a thorough description of the location of the device is really more important than its actual name. A frequently asked and important question is, Is a specific device magnetic resonance (MR) compatible? (See Chapter 17.) Certain objects, such as intracranial aneurysm clips, cochlear implants, and ocular metallic foreign bodies, are definitely contraindications to an MR examination.[1] Many aneurysm clips are not ferromagnetic and do not pose a hazard to the patient (though they do produce degradation of MR images), but unless the specific model and manufacturer of the clip is unequivocally known, it is risky to image patients with clips. Other metallic foreign bodies such as dental amalgam, ocular implants, cerebrospinal fluid shunts, as well as orthopedic rods and wires produce magnetic susceptibility artifacts on MR images but do not pose a hazard to the patient.[1]

BRAIN

Cerebrospinal Fluid (CSF) Shunts
(see also Chapter 8)

CSF diversions have been performed for nearly 100 years. Shunts to multiple anatomic spaces including the subaponeurotic space of the scalp, the venous sinuses, the mastoids, the thoracic duct, the pleural space, the right atrium, and the peritoneum and to various intraabdominal organs have been tried. Currently, the only commonly used drainage procedures are those to the peritoneum and atrium.[2] There may also be associated pressure valves and antisiphon devices.[3] Multiple complications of shunt placement, the commonest being obstruction, infection, and subdural hematoma, have been reported.[4-6] These are frequent indications for shunt imaging. Additionally, a CT scan may be obtained to determine the position of the shunt tip, as well change in location over time. Ideally the shunt tip should be near the foramen of Monroe, but in practice virtually any lateral intraventricular location is acceptable provided that the ventricles have not enlarged. Shunts are mostly nonmetallic, except some models that have metallic tips, connectors, and reservoirs (Figs. 4-1 to 4-3). Two tip configurations are commonly seen, a straight tip and an enlarged, bulbous tip, the Portnoy shunt, which is shaped like a honey dipper (Fig. 4-2).

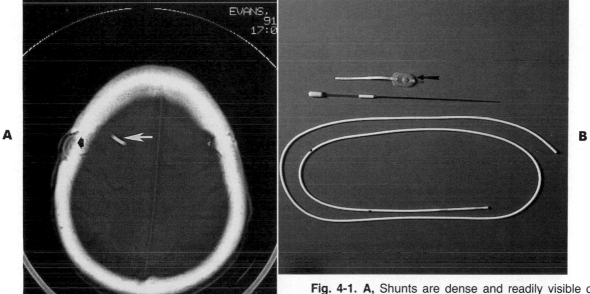

Fig. 4-1. A, Shunts are dense and readily visible on plain films or computerized tomographic (CT) scan. Notice the shunt, *white arrow,* in the right frontal lobe as well as subcutaneous reservoir, *black arrow.* **B,** This is a Pudenz type of ventriculoperitoneal shunt with introducer. Notice the reservoir, *arrow.*

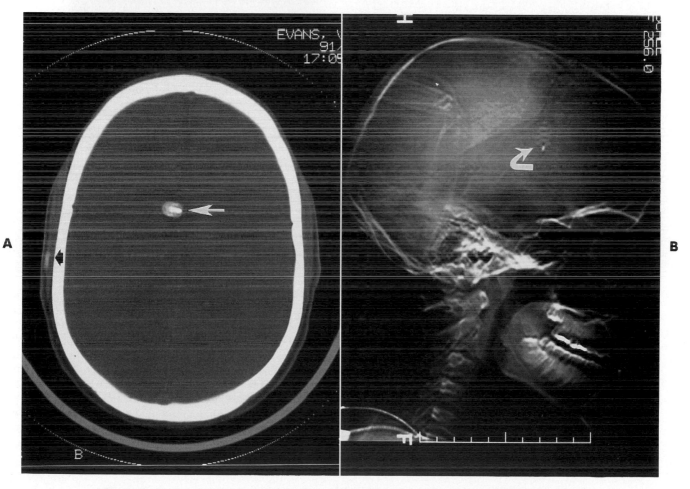

Fig. 4-2. A, The "honey-dipper" figuration of this shunt tip, *white arrow,* is characteristic of Portnoy shunts. Also notice the subcutaneous portions of this ventriculoperitoneal shunt, *black arrow.* **B,** This lateral scout film shows the tip of a Portnoy shunt, *arrow.*

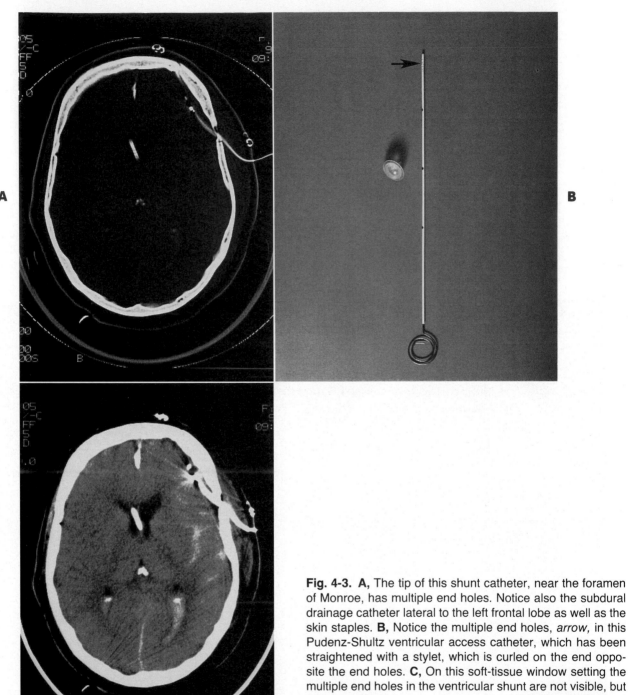

Fig. 4-3. A, The tip of this shunt catheter, near the foramen of Monroe, has multiple end holes. Notice also the subdural drainage catheter lateral to the left frontal lobe as well as the skin staples. **B,** Notice the multiple end holes, *arrow,* in this Pudenz-Shultz ventricular access catheter, which has been straightened with a stylet, which is curled on the end opposite the end holes. **C,** On this soft-tissue window setting the multiple end holes in the ventricular shunt are not visible, but the subdural drainage catheter and skin staples, though not seen as well as on bone windows, are adequately visualized. Intraventricular and left sylvian subarachnoid hemorrhage is apparent.

Subdural Drainage Catheters

Subdural hematomas are a common neurosurgical problem that may present with a wide variety of signs and symptoms.[7] Acute subdural hematomas are generally evacuated by craniotomy because the gelatinous clot is difficult to extract via burr holes.[8] Chronic, liquefied subdural hematomas are usually drained using burr holes and lavage. Subdural drainage catheters are commonly placed to diminish hematoma reaccumulation and allow the brain to re-expand (Figs. 4-3 and 4-4). Typically, straight-tipped ventricular catheters are utilized through burr holes.[9,10] If the hematoma appears loculated, or if there is insufficient response to one drainage catheter, multiple catheters may be placed. Catheters enter through a burr hole but, unlike ventricular shunts, drain to gravity externally. There is no long subcutaneous tunnel, or pressure or antisiphon valve. By definition subdural drainage catheters should be extra-axial. The tip should be in the location of the subdural hematoma documented preoperatively. Incomplete radiographic resolution of chronic subdural hematoma after burr hole evacuation at drainage is common, being seen in over one third of patients; however, most patients demonstrate complete or nearly complete resolution of their signs and symptoms, and thus these hematomas are followed and not reoperated.[9]

Radiotherapy Catheters

Primary malignant brain tumors remain a difficult therapeutic challenge. The mean survival time from di-

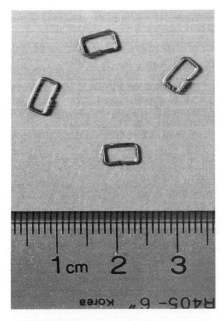

Fig. 4-4. Metallic skin staples such as these (Davis & Geck, Wayne, N.J.) are commonly used because they permit more rapid scalp closure and the resultant scar is esthetically acceptable because it is covered with hair.

agnosis still is between only 2 and 4 years, even with optimum therapy.[11] Additionally, metastatic disease to the brain is common, being seen in over 25% of patients with primary tumors elsewhere. Of these patients, over half die as a result of their intracranial metastases. Depending on the primary tumor histology, mean survival time from diagnosis of brain metastases is usually less than 1 year.[12] Chemotherapy has a limited effect in brain malignancy because most drugs do not cross the blood brain barrier in sufficient concentration to be effective.[13,14] Thus radiotherapy remains the primary nonsurgical treatment for brain malignancy.

External-beam whole-brain radiation is effective in controlling cerebral malignancy but is limited by the toxic effect of radiation on adjacent normal brain tissue. This means that total doses are limited to approximately 5500 rad.[15] For this reason, whole-brain radiation is often supplemented by lower "boost" doses either administered by finely collimated external beams or by implantation of radioactive seeds (brachytherapy). Typically the seeds are iodine 125, chosen because of its limited tissue penetration and low-energy gamma radiation, both of which serve to limit the radiated volume of brain and diminish exposure to others. The radioactive seed may be permanent or temporary. If temporary, the seeds are left in place between 5 and 8 days to achieve a desired dosage and then removed. The seeds are introduced and removed through catheters that are percutaneously placed in the lesion using CT guidance (Fig. 4-5). Serious complications occur in less than 5% of patients, but when the neurologic examination changes the status after catheter placement, hematoma and abscess need to be differentiated from radiation-induced edema. In this setting CT scans of the brain may be obtained with interstitial therapy seeds still in place. On CT examination the catheters are tubular structures extending from a burr hole into the tumor. The rims are radiodense and the centers radiolucent. Typically the catheters are made from Teflon or plastic and are of 14 or 16 gauge.[15,16] The tip of each catheter usually appears very dense but may not be if the iodine seed has not yet been placed (Fig. 4-5).

Endovascular Devices

Balloons

Percutaneously placed, detachable balloons are now an accepted method of occluding arteries as well as treating a variety of fistulas, the commonest being internal carotid to cavernous sinus.[17] Balloons are well suited to permanent vascular occlusion because the effect of occlusion may be determined in an awake patient while the balloon is still attached, meaning that if there are complications the balloon can be deflated and removed. Balloons are made of either silicone or latex. Silicone balloons can be filled with contrast or HEMA

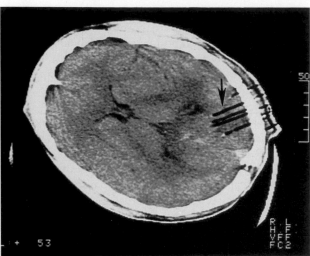

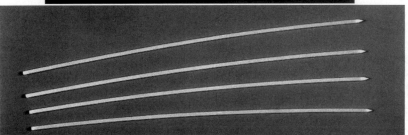

Fig. 4-5. A, These brachytherapy catheters, *arrow,* are low in density because they have not yet been loaded with radioactive seeds. **B,** Brachytherapy catheters.

(2-hydroxyethylmethacrylate). Latex balloons are filled with contrast medium. Thus the balloons are dense; however, they may not appear so on subtraction angiograms, where they may be subtracted out, or in plain films, where they do not appear dense compared to the adjacent skull base[18,19] (Fig. 4-6). In addition to noting the presence of the balloon, it is important to also carefully check for changes in size and position of the balloon.

Coils

Stainless and now platinum coils are also used to occlude fistulas, arteries, and the venous sinuses (Figs. 4-7 and 4-8). Platinum coils have the advantage of passing readily through microcatheters as well as being thrombogenic and biocompatible.[20] Often they do not assume a "coil" shape when they are actually deposited because they are in small vessels, which may not allow them to recoil completely.

Liquid Adhesives

Liquid adhesives (glue) are used to treat arteriovenous malformations (AVM), high-flow fistula, and occasionally tumors.[21] Butyl-cyanoacrylate is the embolic material. This is mixed with iophendylate and further opacified with tantalum powder. This mixture polymerizes quickly on contact with ionic substances such as blood, but it has a tendency to pass far distally into small

vessels, which it permanently occludes, forming a "cast" of the vascular abnormality and any other vessel that is filled (Fig. 4-9). The entire volume of glue deposited may not be visible on plain radiographs because the mixture has a tendency to settle, with more of the tantalum being present in one part of the mixture than elsewhere.[18]

Particles

The commonest particulate embolic agents are gelatin powder (Gelfoam, Upjohn, Kalamazoo, Michigan) and polyvinyl alcohol (PVA). The latter is the most commonly used agent, coming prepacked in containers with a selected range of particle sizes. The particles are not very radiopaque and therefore difficult to see on plain films or on CT. This means that they are infrequently noted on radiographs, especially because patients who receive particulate emboli are usually operated on shortly after embolization. However, if patients are imaged within a day or two of embolization, the thrombus caused by the particles may be seen on CT where it has the appearance of any other intravascular thrombus, that being a linear area of increased density in a vascular distribution.

Recording Electrodes

There are two types of intracranial recording electrodes. The first, called "depth electrodes," are placed

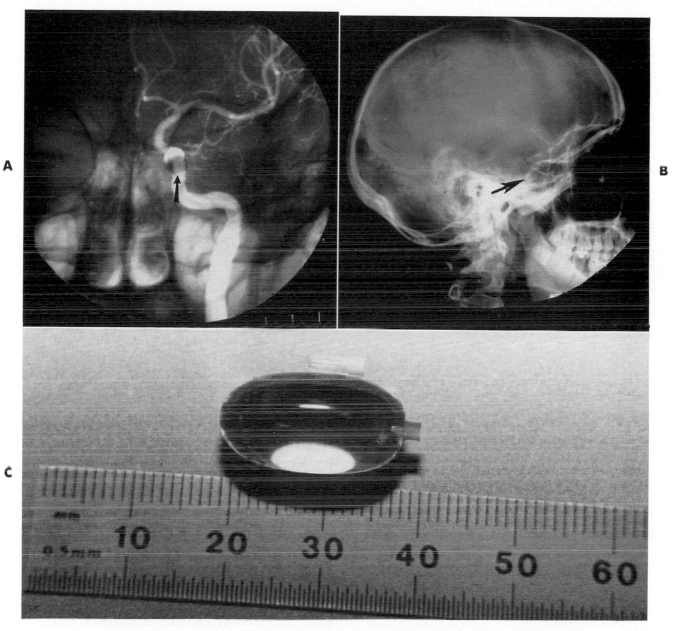

Fig. 4-6. A, The oval lucency projected over the cavernous carotid is a balloon, *arrow,* in the cavernous sinus. Even though it is filled with contrast medium, it is less dense than the adjacent artery, which is more densely opacified during angiography. **B,** The balloon, *arrow,* is difficult to see on this plane of the skull film, but as expected, it is in the area of the cavernous sinus. **C,** Silicone balloon (investigational device pending FDA review; manufactured by Interventional Therapeutics Corporation, San Francisco). These range in size from 6 to 21 mm in length.

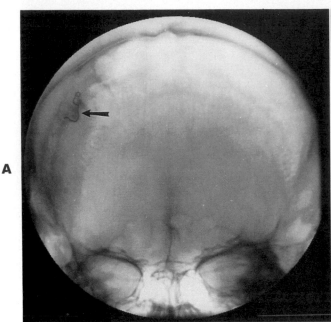

A

B

Fig. 4-7. A, This platinum coil, *arrow,* does not look circular because it has conformed to the shape of a small, distal middle cerebral artery branch. **B,** Platinum coils, such as these from Target Therapeutics (San Jose, Calif.), come in a variety of lengths, coil shapes, and diameters. The coils on the bottom have Dacron threads incorporated into them to increase thrombogenicity.

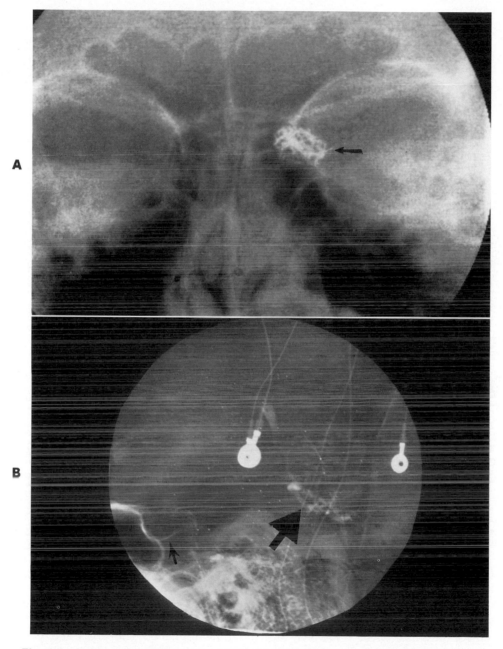

Fig. 4-8. A, This frontal view of the orbits shows multiple pieces of platinum wire, *arrow,* coiled in the left cavernous sinus to occlude a carotid cavernous fistula. **B,** The cyanoac- rylate glue, *arrow,* occluding this arterial venous malformation has conformed to the shape of the underlying vessels and is somewhat stellate. (Courtesy Gary Duckwiler, UCLA School of Medicine, Los Angeles.)

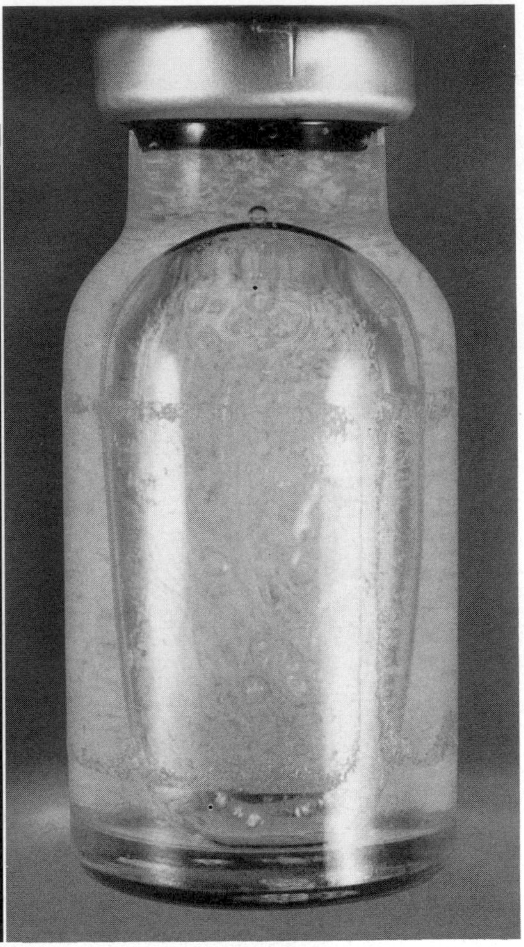

Fig. 4-9. A, Polyvinyl alcohol (PVA) is not dense and is difficult to see on CT scan. However, if the patient is imaged immediately after embolization, the clot produced by PVA can be seen as a linear area of increased density, *arrow.* **B,** The polyvinyl alcohol in this bottle (placed on its side and seen from above it) has been recently shaken, making the entire solution appear opaque.

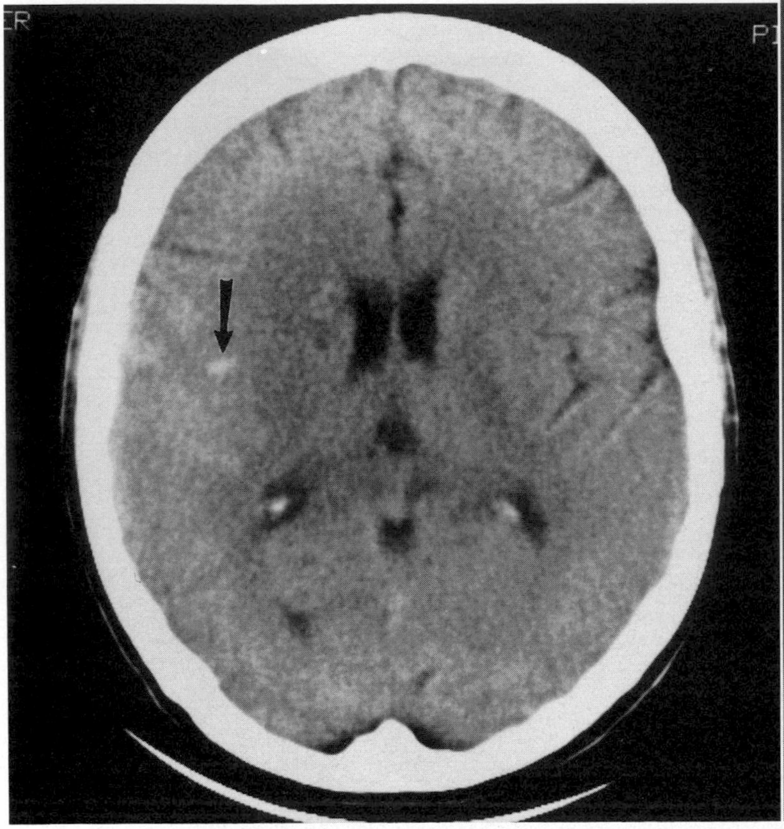

in the brain substance. These range from 0.5 to 3.0 mm in diameter and may be made of either wire or polyethylene. The commonest metals used for the electrodes are stainless steel, platinum, and platinum-iridium alloys.[22] Typically, these electrodes are placed bilaterally for sampling six or eight sites on each side.

Extra axial electrodes are also used. These may be placed either subdurally or epidurally; most commonly they are subdural (Fig. 4-10, *A*). These electrodes are either strips of four to six electrodes, or grids containing an 8 × 8 matrix of electrodes embedded in a Silastic sheet. The grid type of electrode must be placed through a craniotomy and is therefore usually placed unilaterally. The strip electrodes, which can be placed through burr holes, are often placed bilaterally. Radiographically, electrodes are readily seen as they are by necessity at least partially metallic.[23]

Cerebellar Electrodes

The cerebellum may be stimulated to diminish spasticity associated with cerebral palsy. This procedure is somewhat controversial and is infrequently performed. Cerebellar stimulation is achieved by placement of an electrode array, commonly a strip of eight electrodes (Avery Laboratories, Glen Cove, NY) over the cerebellar hemispheres. The leads and electrodes are quite dense and readily seen on plain film or CT examinations (Fig. 4-10, *B* and *C*). The leads connecting the electrodes with the necessary implantable generator not infrequently break (17% in one series)[24] and should be checked in addition to noting the electrode position and appearance of the underlying cerebellum.

Aneurysm Clips

Cerebral aneurysm clips come in a variety of sizes and shapes (Fig. 4-11). Initially, they were hand bent from

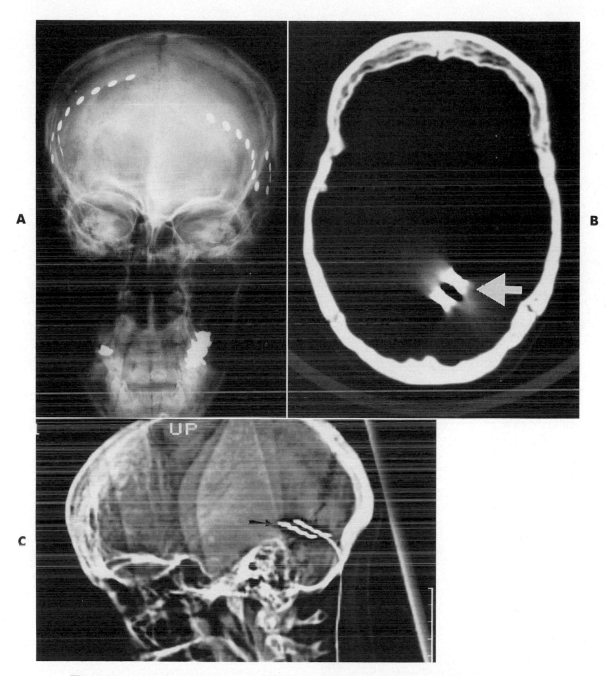

Fig. 4-10. Recording electrodes. **A,** Bilateral subdural recording electrodes. These are the strip type of electrode. The plastic and tiny wires connecting the electrodes are too thin to be seen, and hence the individual electrodes appear discontinuous on plain film examination. **B,** The cerebellar stimulators are easily seen in the posterior fossa, *arrow.* **C,** Cerebellar stimulators. These are dense and readily seen, *arrow.*

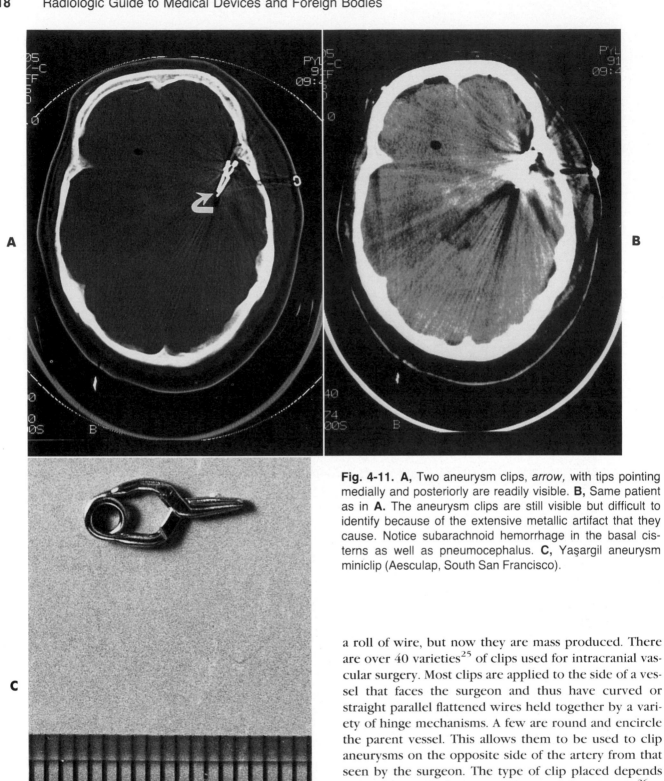

Fig. 4-11. A, Two aneurysm clips, *arrow,* with tips pointing medially and posteriorly are readily visible. **B,** Same patient as in **A.** The aneurysm clips are still visible but difficult to identify because of the extensive metallic artifact that they cause. Notice subarachnoid hemorrhage in the basal cisterns as well as pneumocephalus. **C,** Yaşargil aneurysm miniclip (Aesculap, South San Francisco).

a roll of wire, but now they are mass produced. There are over 40 varieties[25] of clips used for intracranial vascular surgery. Most clips are applied to the side of a vessel that faces the surgeon and thus have curved or straight parallel flattened wires held together by a variety of hinge mechanisms. A few are round and encircle the parent vessel. This allows them to be used to clip aneurysms on the opposite side of the artery from that seen by the surgeon. The type of clip placed depends on preference and past experience of the surgeon.[26]

Clips are made from stainless steel and other alloys as well as tungsten. They are all radiodense, but especially the older clips may change position in strong magnetic fields and thus are a contraindication to MRI. The most commonly used clips are the Yaşargil-Aesculap clips.[26] These have either straight or curved blades and a rounded spring in the hinge posteriorly.

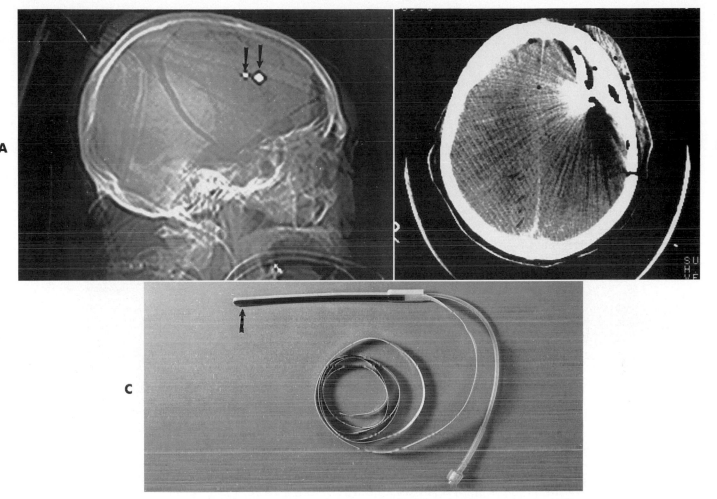

Fig. 4-12. A, Cerebral blood flow probe. Blood flow probes contain two gold thermistors, readily visible at the tips of the arrows. **B,** Blood flow probe. The beam-hardening artifact produced by the gold tips makes the probe apparent but obscures detail. **C,** Thermodynamic blood probe (Flowtronics, Phoenix, Ariz.). The distal surface containing the two thermistors, *arrow,* is placed directly on a gyrus.

Cerebral Blood Flow Probes

Regional cerebral blood flow can be continuously monitored in vivo using thermal diffusion probes. The clinical utility of this technology is not entirely established, but, in general, diminished cerebral blood flow is associated with increased intracranial pressure, except in patients with malignant cerebral edema who have elevated pressures and flows. Currently, there is clinical research designed to determine whether changes in cerebral blood flow can be used to help differentiate between disorders of autoregulation and cerebral edema and thus help determine which therapy or combinations of therapies (hemodilution, induced hypertension, hyperventilation, mannitol, barbiturates, and calcium antagonists) will be most effective in the acutely brain-injured patient.[27] The probes consist of a Silastic sheath with two gold plates, each containing a

thermistor (Fig. 4-12). Cerebral blood flow is measured by thermal diffusion, with the distal plate being heated while the proximal plate is held at a neutral temperature (the gradient between the plates is inversely proportional to cerebral blood flow).[28] Because the thermistors contain gold, they are very dense and easy to recognize in the subdural space, where they produce significantly more artifact than the usual subdural drainage catheter does. However, because the probe is in direct contact with gyri, the presence of extra-axial fluid collection can be inferred from the distance between the probe and the inner table of the skull.

SPINE

This section covers common devices found in the spine. Usually, these are internal stabilization devices, such as anterior and posterior cervical plates, wires, and

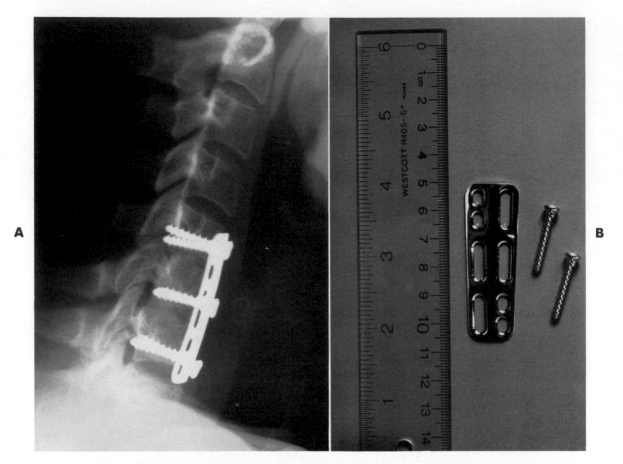

Fig. 4-13. A, Anterior cervical fusion plate. Notice the superior and inferior screws, which in this case extend slightly beyond the cortex of the posterior margins of the fifth and seventh vertebral bodies. **B,** Cervical bone plate and screws (Aesculap, South San Francisco).

assorted lumbar rods and rectangles; however, dorsal column stimulators and halo vests are also seen when the spine is being imaged and are discussed here.

Cervical Spine

Most devices found in the cervical area of the spine are placed there to treat instability, usually from trauma, but occasionally from tumor, infection, or prior laminectomy. In the past, prolonged immobilization with cervical traction was the method of choice to stabilize the spine and allow for healing. This approach is rarely used today because it is poorly tolerated by most patients and has an unacceptable incidence of systemic complications, such as pulmonary emboli[29] from prolonged bedrest. For this reason, a variety of approaches to cervical spine stabilization have been devised. These include anterior and posterior cervical plating, interbody fusion, and sublaminar wiring.

Anterior interbody fusion using bone dowels or plugs was popularized by Cloward and Smith and Robinson.[29-31] These techniques are still widely used to treat cervical diskogenic degenerative disease; however, when there is ligamentous injury, as is frequently seen with trauma, these methods alone do not provide adequate stabilization.[32]

Anterior cervical plates

Because anterior interbody fusion is unstable in patients with ligamentous injuries, a variety of anterior cervical fusion plates to supplement the bone plugs and dowels have been developed.[33-36] All anterior cervical plates are similar in design and use (Fig. 4-13). The most common and best known is the Caspar plate. They vary between 28 and 72 mm in length and may thus span two or three vertebral bodies. These plates are anchored to the underlying vertebral bodies with screws, which should enter the anterior cortex of each vertebral body and be seated in the posterior cortex without impinging on the cord. To prevent loosening, the screws should be at least 2 mm from the adjacent end plates. In severely osteopenic bone they are occasionally supplemented by acrylate.[36] All anterior cervical

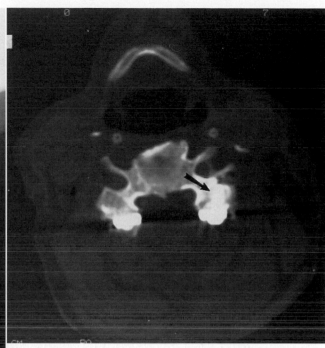

Fig. 4-14. **A,** Posterior cervical plates and screws. **B,** Posterior cervical plates and screws. Notice the placement of the screw, *arrow,* into the articular mass, lateral to the spinal canal and dorsal to the vertebral artery.

plates are opaque and thus visible on routine radiographs. The position and stability of the plates, as well as evidence of loosening and infection, must be evaluated radiographically. Additionally, signs of progressive diskogenic degenerative changes in the adjacent disk spaces need to be searched for because these are commonly seen after surgery.[37]

Type 2 odontoid fractures are unstable and frequently do not heal adequately with external fixation (a halo vest). For this reason, internal fixation is often performed, especially when there is need for reduction, evidenced by displacement of the odontoid fracture fragment more than 4 mm anteriorly upon the body of C2. Posterior wires are commonly used for this purpose. They achieve satisfactory fusion rates, but neck rotation is frequently limited. Because of this, an anterior approach utilizing a compression pin placed caudally and then cephalad through the body of C2, the fracture line, and into the dens has been employed.[38] These screws are characteristic in their appearance and readily identified from their location.

Posterior cervical plates

When anterior decompression of the thecal sac is not required, posterior stabilization with a plate and screw provides an excellent means of achieving stability. These plates limit extension as well as flexion. Posterior cervical plates are fixed to the underlying vertebral bodies by screws in the articular masses (Fig. 4-14). These are typically angled 20 to 30 degrees laterally and cephalad to avoid the adjacent thecal sac, exiting nerve roots, and vertebral arteries. The plates themselves are always bilateral and are slightly curved to help maintain the normal cervical lordosis. Current plates are made of vitallium, an alloy of cobalt, chromium, and molybdenum. This alloy is less corrosive than stainless steel and has the additional advantage of being MRI compatible, though significant magnetic susceptibility artifact is still produced.[29,39]

Posterior wiring

Spinal fixation with posterior cervical wires is most effective in limiting flexion and poor in preventing rotation and in treating patients who have compression of the anterior surface of the thecal sac; however, this technique is less complicated than anterior cervical fusion and plating and is reported to have fewer complications. Variations of posterior wiring have been used for over 50 years and are commonly seen today. Generally, 20-gauge stainless steel wire is used, but those at 18, 22, and 24 gauge are also employed. All wires are dense and easily visualized on radiographs (Fig. 4-15). Most are stainless steel, though some are made of vitallium, but this is not frequently used because it tends to break more easily. There are many specific techniques of wiring. Variations include wires under the lamina, over the lamina, and through holes drilled in the facets or spinous processes. Intralaminar or spinous bone grafts may be placed in addition to the wires.[40] Complications are unusual, but wire fracture, erosion through predrilled holes in facets, lamina, or spinous processes, as well as overall loss of cervical spine reduction are occasionally seen on plain films. Additionally, CT, which is most helpful with intrathecal contrast, may demonstrate posterior cervical cord compression from sublaminar wires that are too ventral in location.[41]

Lumbar Spine

Rods

Lumbar fusion procedures have been performed since the turn of this century. Initially only bone grafts were used, and many fusions are still done in this manner; however, now a variety of devices are used to supplement the bony grafts by providing immediate stability, improved fusion rates, and rapid patient mobilization.[42] Harrington and Knodt rods are both commonly used today.[41] Both have hooks, which allow these devices to either distract or compress the spine, depending on the direction in which the hooks are placed. The Harrington rods have flanged ends, which allow the rods to be contoured to the lumbar area of the spine (Fig. 4-16). The Knodt rods are threaded and can be bent less, meaning that they are used for more limited fusions.[43] All rods are very dense and easily visualized. Stability and location of rods and hooks as well as maintenance of spinal alignment should be evaluated. Additionally, evidence of pseudoarthrosis or rod fracture should be sought, though these complications are rare, occurring in 0.5% and 1% of patients respectively.[44]

Screws and plates

Thoracolumbar stabilization rods were initially developed in the 1950s and have a long record of success; however, all rods have the disadvantage of sublaminar hooks, which may potentially compress the thecal sac. Additionally, because they span multiple vertebral segments, all tend to cause a loss of normal lumbar lordosis. These problems led to the development of segmen-

tal pedicle fixation. In these devices, screws that are placed through the pedicles into the vertebral bodies are connected with rods or plates.[41] Several systems are now available. Steffee, Edwards, Roy Camille, and Cotrell-Dubousett devices are systems commonly used today.[41,45,46] The Cotrell devices use rods to connect to the pedicular screws, whereas in the Steffee apparatus flat plates connect the screws (Fig. 4-17). Screw size is determined by the pedicle, but typically screws are 5 to 6 mm thick and 45 mm long. Steffee plates range in size from 44 to 196 mm.[47] Screw placement is critical, and imaging studies can help to determine whether or not the screws have broken through the pedicles or pulled out of the vertebral bodies.

An advantage to the posterior screw and plate fixation devices is that both the vertebral body and posterior elements are fixed by one system. Complication rates are low in experienced hands, with less than a 0.6% infection rate and a 0.2% incidence of nerve root damage. However, the procedures are lengthy, averaging more than 4 hours, and special surgical training is required.[47]

Other screws are occasionally seen in the lumbar spine. The Zielke rod and screw fixation device consists of a unilateral plate affixed to the lateral portion of adjacent vertebral bodies by screws. Additionally, screws without plates may be found in the lumbar spine. In Buck's fusion, bilateral pars interarticularis fractures are fixed with bilateral translaminar to pedicle screws, whereas in the Boucher type of fusion, screws are directed inferiorly through the cephalad facets of a vertebra into the pedicles of the more distal vertebra.[48,49]

Rectangles

Rectangular spinal fixation devices are also found. Luque and Hartshill rectangles are held to the adjacent vertebrae with sublaminar wires (Fig. 4-18). These are mechanically very strong and have the additional advantage in that they may be contoured.[41]

Spinal Column Stimulators

Percutaneously introduced epidural wires or surgically placed electrodes may be found adjacent to the thecal sac. Generally, these are adjacent to the dura, but occasionally they are placed in the subarachnoid space.[50-52] Most commonly, these stimulators are used to treat intractable pain, but occasionally they are used to diminish spasticity.[53,54] The mechanisms of action of these stimulators are not completely known, but one hypothesis is that they act by increasing the activity of pain-inhibitory fibers.[55] Approximately one half of patients receiving spinal-column stimulation obtain good or excellent relief, though success rates vary depending on the location of the electrodes, the cause of the pain, and specific stimulation parameters (that is, am-

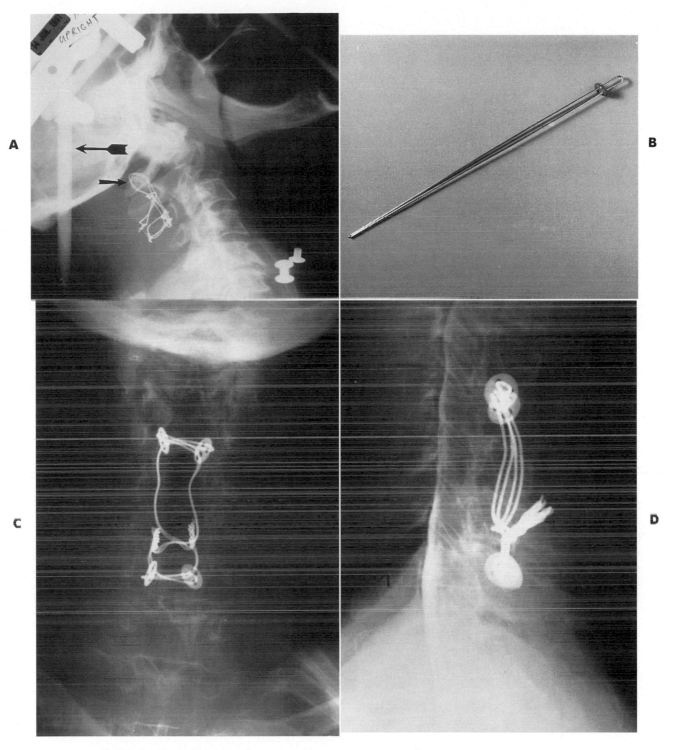

Fig. 4-15. A, Sublaminar wires, *small arrow,* from C1 to C3. Notice the metastasis destroying the C2 vertebral body as well as the halo vest, *large arrow.* **B,** Posterior cervical wire and button (Wisconsin wire, Zimmer, Warsaw, Indiana). The wire has not yet been bent to shape. **C,** Status of posterior cervical wires from C4 to C7 after laminectomy. **D,** Posterior cervical wires. Lateral view of same patient shown in **C** but shortly after cervical myelogram.

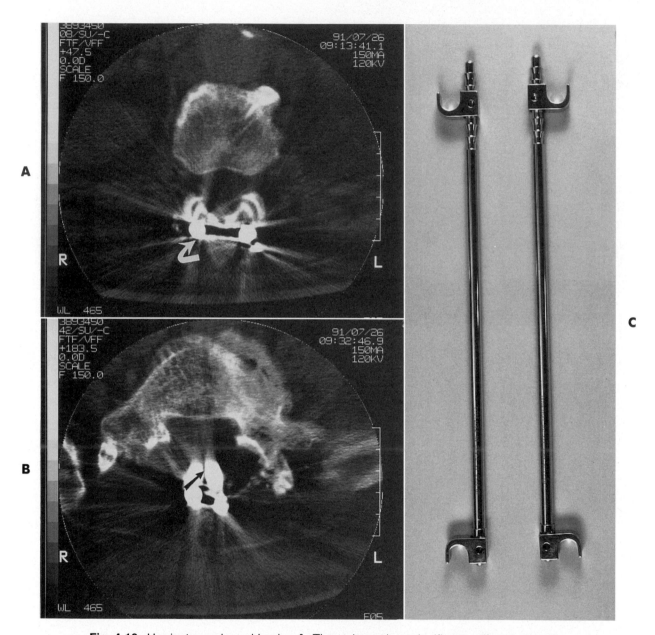

Fig. 4-16. Harrington rods and hooks. **A,** The rods produce significant artifact, but generally the thecal sac adjacent to the rods, *arrow,* can be evaluated. **B,** The sublaminar hooks produce more artifact than the rod, *arrow,* and often obscure the underlying thecal sac. **C,** With the hooks facing out, as in this case, the rods can be used for distraction.

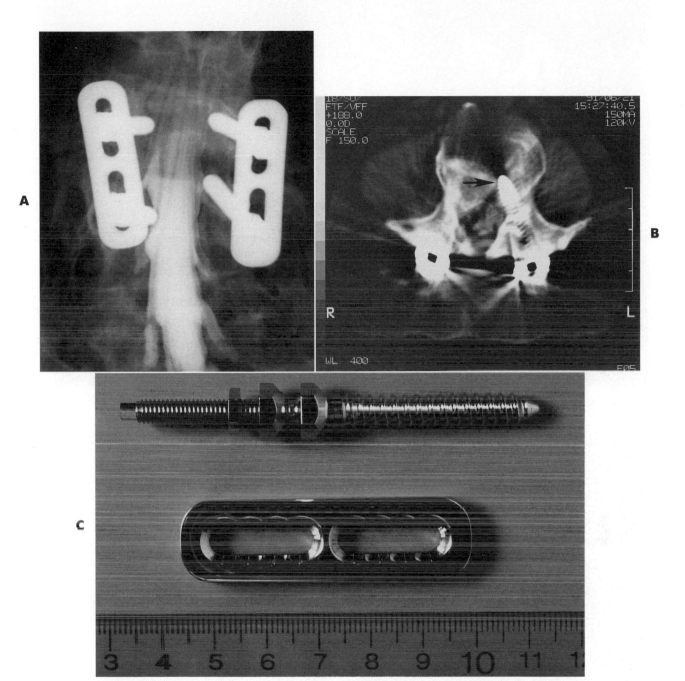

Fig. 4-17. Steffee plates and screws. **A,** The peduncular screws and plates produce extensive artifact on CT scan, meaning that myelography is often necessary for proper evaluation of these patients postoperatively. **B,** Steffee plates and screws, *arrow.* The thecal sac is seen unusually well in this patient immediately after myelogram. The screw should extend through the pedicle into the vertebral body, without exiting the vertebral body, fracturing the pedicle, or compressing the medially located exiting nerve roots. **C,** Steffee plate and screw (Acromed, Cleveland). **D,** Oblique and, **E,** lateral views of 27-year-old woman who had a tumor resected from the upper thoracic spine. Steffee plates and screws were placed for spine stabilization, Gold foil, *arrows,* was also inserted into the surgical bed to protect the spinal cord before the patient underwent radiation therapy.

Continued.

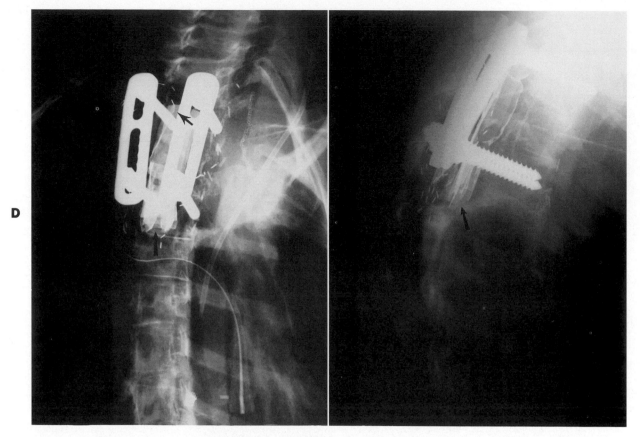

D　　　　　　　　　　　　　　　　　　　　　　　　　　E

Fig. 4-17, cont'd. For legend see p. 125.

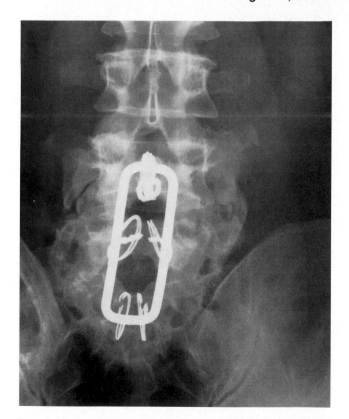

Fig. 4-18. Hartshill rectangle held in place by sublaminar wires. The inferior wires are fractured. However, the bony fusion was solid, and spinal alignment was maintained.

plitude, frequency, and duration of impulse).[54]

Stimulator epidural wires and electrodes are metallic and easily seen on radiographs (Fig. 4-19). Electrodes are enmeshed in a Teflon or plastic matrix that is not visible, meaning that the electrodes may look like a set of unconnected metallic dots.[51] Pain relief generally decreases with time after electrode placement, possibly secondary to envelopment of the electrodes by reactive fibrous tissues,[52] but other causes of diminished effectiveness, such as broken or knotted wires, should be sought.

Cervical Collars and Halo Vests

External cervical immobilization devices can be divided into three types: collars, braces, and halo vests. There are two types of collars. The first, the soft foam collar covered by cotton, is least effective in controlling neck motion and is primarily useful as a reminder to the patient that neck motion is to be avoided. A second type of collar, the Philadelphia collar, is molded from plastic and has chin and occipital supports. This provides more support and is only a little less comfortable than the soft collar, but it still does not provide adequate stabilization for most fractures.

Cervical braces all share certain characteristics. They have chin and occipital supports that are connected to a thoracic vest by metal rods. These provide good resistance to flexion but are less effective in preventing

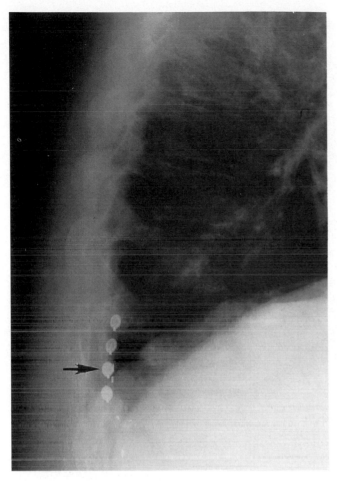

Fig. 4-19. Dorsal column stimulator, *arrow*. The individual electrodes do not appear connected because the wire to them has been removed. These stimulators are in the usual position, dorsal to the cord. Occasionally, they may be found anterolaterally as well.

extension. The four most common braces are the four-poster, the cervicothoracic, the Somi, and the Yale braces.[56]

The last type of cervical immobilization device is the halo vest (Fig. 4-20). In this orthosis, a metallic ring (the halo) is fixed to the outer table of the skull by screws. This halo is connected to a padded fiberglass or plastic thoracic cast by metal rods (the struts). This provides the best cervical fixation in all three planes but still does allow minimal motion, typically less than 5% of normal.[57] Usually halo vests are used for unstable fractures and dislocations. Old fractures, incompletely reduced injuries, and pathologic fractures as well as injuries with subluxed facets are relative contraindications to external fixation. These patients usually proceed directly to open reduction and operative fixation.[58,59] Overall, there are few complications from halo fixation; however, radiographs should be examined for evidence of

pin loosening or infection, loss of cervical alignment, and slippage of the halo vest reflected in change in position of the uprights or ring.

HEAD, EYE, EAR, NOSE, AND THROAT (HEENT) DEVICES

Gastric and Tracheal Tubes

Endotracheal, tracheostomy, orogastric, nasogastric, and oral airways may all be seen on cervical radiographs (Figs. 4-21 and 4-22). Both tracheal and gastric tubes may be placed through the nose. Nasotracheal and nasogastric tubes overlap in size, but tubes less than 5 mm in diameter are nasogastric. The walls of these tubes have a low density, but there is usually a high-density stripe, easily seen on plain films or CT. Foley or other balloon catheters can also be seen in the nose. These are placed for treatment of epistaxis.[60] The balloon is usually filled with water and can mimic other low-density masses.

Orotracheal and orogastric tubes as well as oral airways enter the mouth. Oral airways are H- or oval-shaped in cross section. These are made of plastic or rubber and can have variable density but are usually radiopaque (see Fig. 4-20). Orotracheal tubes are placed for a short term or emergency intubation, but nasotracheal tubes are preferred in other situations.[61] Tracheal tubes are anterior to gastric tubes and can be unequivocally identified if they are seen to pass between the vocal cords (see Fig. 4-22). If the tip of the endotracheal tube has a cuff, the balloon should not be inflated over one and a half times the diameter of the trachea because doing so leads to ischemic necrosis and tracheomalacia.[62]

Tracheostomy tubes are inserted for patients in need of long-term mechanical ventilation (see Fig. 4-22, *D*). Usually, they are placed between the second and third tracheal rings. Occasionally, a cricothyroid incision is performed in an emergency situation, though this does carry a higher risk of vocal chord damage. The tubes inserted in this manner look similar to the routinely placed tracheostomy tubes. Both types are made of dense plastic or metal and are thus readily visible.

Orbital Prostheses

Orbital defects after enucleation are repaired with custom-made prostheses. First, a mold of the defect is fabricated and then a silicone implant is cast and tinted to match the patient's skin.[63,64] Ocular prostheses are placed in the orbital prosthesis or directly into the globe remnant in the case of evisceration. These are made either of glass or acrylic resin, but resin is preferred because there is decreased breakage and better tissue compatibility, durability, and color match.[65] Generally, ocular prostheses are custom made for the individual

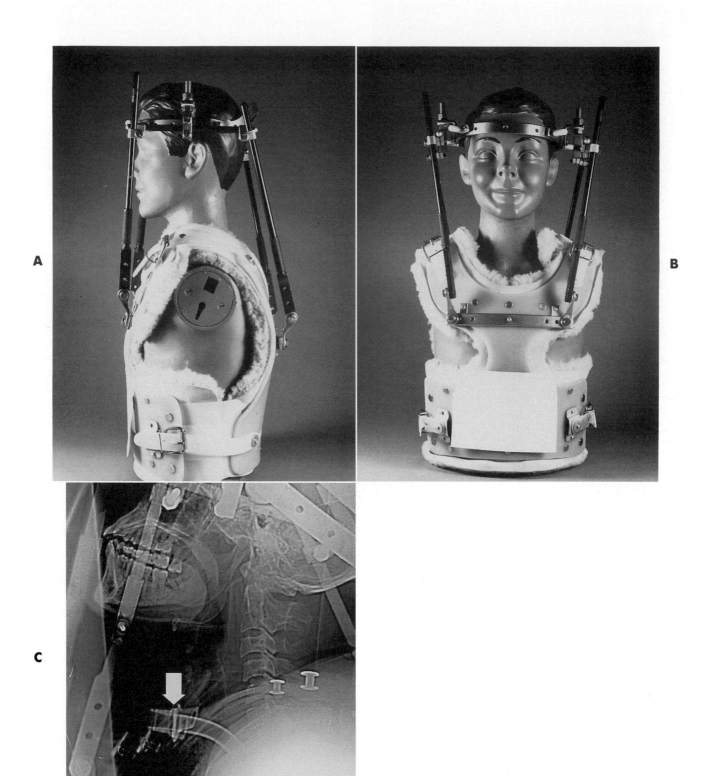

Fig. 4-20. Frontal, **A,** and lateral, **B,** views of a halo vest and brace. Notice the four metallic uprights connecting the halo ring around the skull to the vest. **C,** Halo vest in place in patient with tracheostomy tube, *arrow.*

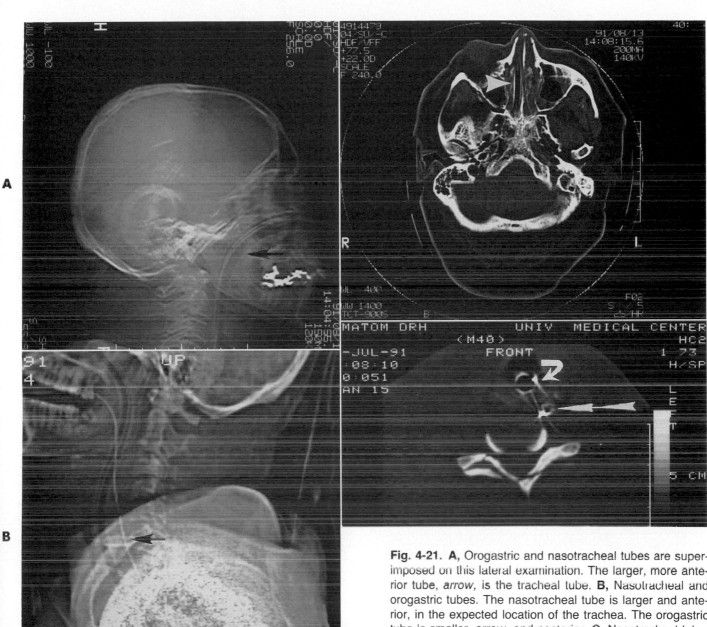

Fig. 4-21. A, Orogastric and nasotracheal tubes are superimposed on this lateral examination. The larger, more anterior tube, *arrow,* is the tracheal tube. **B,** Nasotracheal and orogastric tubes. The nasotracheal tube is larger and anterior, in the expected location of the trachea. The orogastric tube is smaller, *arrow,* and posterior. **C,** Nasotracheal tube. The edge of this right-sided tube, *arrowhead,* is dense and therefore seen between the air in the tube and the fluid-filled nasal cavity. **D,** Endotracheal *(curved arrow)* and nasogastric *(straight arrow)* tubes. Notice the size difference of these tubes. The tracheal tube is anterior. Facet and lamina fractures are present as well.

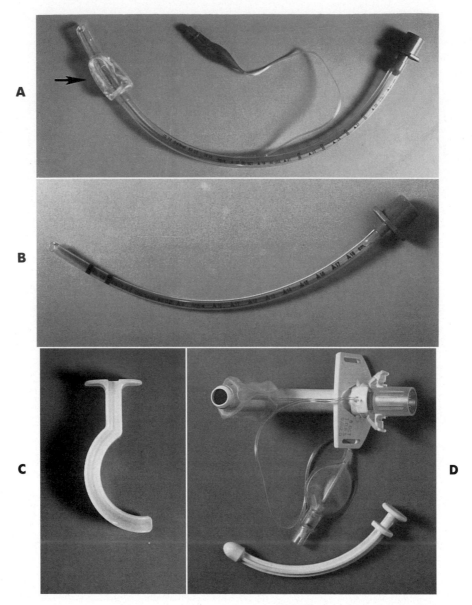

Fig. 4-22. A, Endotracheal tube (Sherwood, St. Louis). When placed in a patient the cuff, *arrow,* is filled with air and appears lucent. **B,** Uncuffed endotracheal tube (Argyle; now Sherwood, St. Louis). **C,** Oral airway. **D,** Cuffed tracheostomy tube (Shiley, Irvine, Calif.).

patient. Stock protheses are available but infrequently used because a large and expensive inventory is required to match iris color, and the result is seldom as good as with custom-made devices. Occasionally, plastic scleral shells can be seen. These are cosmetic devices most commonly used to treat patients with phthisis bulbi or microphthalmia.[66] Because the protheses are custom made, they are all different, but upon imaging they are readily visualized, the surgical defects being obvious and the protheses apparent. Generally, globes have low density, but the appearance is variable (Fig. 4-23).

Hearing Aids

Between 5% and 10% of the population is hearing impaired. Usually, this hearing loss is idiopathic in nature and the treatment is symptomatic, involving hearing aids, which amplify sound. These devices are nonselective and increase the volume but not the clarity of sound.[67,68] Most hearing aids consist of a behind-the-ear unit and an ear mold. The behind-the-ear unit contains a microphone, battery, and speaker, as well as volume and on/off controls. The ear molds, which are made of acrylic polymer, are fitted to occlude the external auditory canal, though there may be vent hole drilled in the

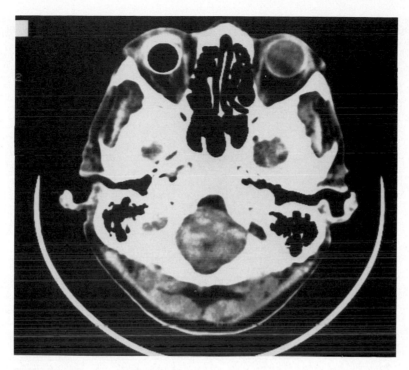

Fig. 4-23. Right ocular prosthesis. These are generally left in place for weeks and not removed before imaging.

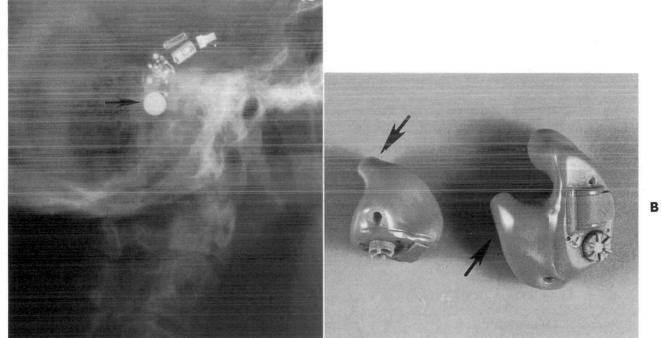

Fig. 4-24. A, Typical hearing aid with a behind-the-ear compartment containing a battery *(arrow),* microphone, and amplifier. The ear mold has been removed. **B,** These hearing aids incorporate the microphone, battery, and amplifier into the ear mold, *arrows.*

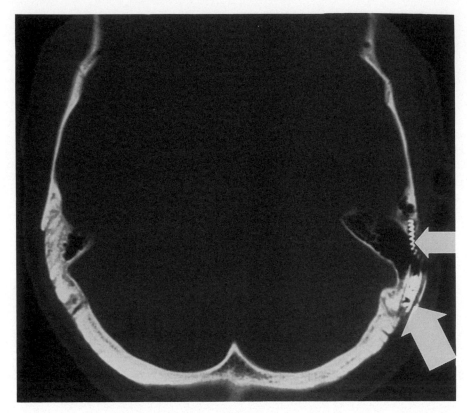

Fig. 4-25. Cochlear implant. This axial computed tomographic scan shows the receiver/ stimulator *(large arrow)* lying in a groove cut into the mastoid portion of the temporal bone. The wire leaving the receiver/stimulator *(small arrow)* passes into the cochlea and forms the electrodes. (Courtesy Dr. Steve Bessen, Tucson.)

ear mold to diminish the sensation of blockage and improve patient comfort.[69,70] Although over 1% of the population owns hearing aids,[67] they are uncommonly seen on imaging, because they are routinely removed before the studies are obtained (Fig. 4-24).

At times, one may see cochlear implants (Fig. 4-25), which are used to treat sensorineural hearing loss. They consist of a microphone stimulator located on the skin next to the pinna. This is connected to an externally located induction coil. Underneath the microphone stimulator is an internally located coil implanted in bone. The coil is connected to the scala tympani by a thin wire through the round window.[71] The stimulator may have either a single electrode or, more typically, multiple electrodes mounted on the same wire in the cochlea.

Even with high-resolution CT, it is difficult to determine the exact location of the stimulator wire in the cochlea. However, the subcutaneous coil and the wire through the round window that connects to the cochlear electrode are readily visible.

REFERENCES

1. Shellock FG, Curtis JS: MRI imaging and biomedical implants, materials, and devices: an updated review, *Radiology* 180(2):541-550, 1991.
2. Pudenz RH: The surgical treatment of hydrocephalus: an historical review, *Surg Neurol* 15(1):15-26, 1981.
3. Portnoy HD, Schulte RR, Fox JL, et al: Anti-siphon and reversible occlusion valve for shunting in hydrocephalus and preventing post-shunt subdural hematomas, *J Neurosurg* 38:729-738, 1973.
4. Hoffman HJ, Duffner PK: Extraneural metastases of central nervous system tumors, *Cancer* 56:1778-1782, 1985.
5. Lovell MA, Ross GW, Cooper PH: Gliomatosis peritonei associated with a ventriculoperitoneal shunt, *Am J Clin Pathol* 91:485-487, 1989.
6. Raimondi AJ: Shunts, indications, problems, and characteristics, *Child's Nerv Syst* 4:321-324, 1988.
7. Black DW: Subdural hematoma, *Postgrad Med* 78(1):107-114, 1985.
8. Markwalder TM, Seiler RW: Chronic subdural hematomas: to drain or not to drain? *Neurosurgery* 16(2):185-188, 1985.
9. Camel M, Grubb RL: Treatment of chronic subdural hematoma by twist-drill craniotomy with continuous catheter drainage, *J Neurosurg* 65:183-187, 1986.
10. Wakai S, Hashimoto K, Watanabe N, et al: Efficacy of closed system drainage in treating chronic subdural hematoma: a prospective comparative study, *Neurosurgery* 26(5):171-173, 1990.

11. Larson DA, Gutin PH, Leibel SA, et al: Stereotaxic irradiation of brain tumors, *Cancer* 65:792-799, 1990.

12. Praudos M, Leibel S, Barnett CM, Gutin P: Interstitial brachytherapy for metastatic brain tumors, *Cancer* 63:657-660, 1989.

13. Heros DO, Kasdon DL, Chun M: Brachytherapy in the treatment of recurrent solitary brain metastases, *Neurosurgery* 23(6):733-737, 1988.

14. Willis BK, Heilbrun MP, Sapozink MD, McDonald RR: Stereotaxic interstitial brachytherapy of malignant astrocytomas with remarks on post plantation computed tomographic appearance, *Neurosurgery* 23(3):348-354, 1988.

15. Ostertag CB: Stereotaxic interstitial radiotherapy for brain tumors, *J Neurosurg Sci* 33(3):83-89, 1989.

16. Gutin PH, Phillips T, Hosobuchi Y, et al: Permanent and removable implants for the brachytherapy of brain tumors, *Int J Radiat Oncol Biol Phys* 7:1371-1381, 1981.

17. Serbinenko FA: Balloon catheterization and occlusion of major cerebral vessels, *J Neurosurg* 41:125 145, 1974.

18. Eskridge JM: Interventional neuroradiology, *Radiology* 172:991-1006, 1989.

19. Hieshima GB, Grinnell VS, Mehringer CM: A detachable balloon for therapeutic transcatheter occlusions, *Radiology* 138:227-228, 1981.

20. Yang PJ, Halbach VV, Higashida RT, Hieshima GB: Platinum wire, a new transvascular embolic agent, *AJNR* 9.547-550, 1988.

21. Berenstein A, Choy IS: Therapeutic angiography of the head and neck. In Tavares J, Ferrucci JJ, editors: *Radiology* 3(100):1-6, Philadelphia, 1990, Lippincott.

22. Morris HH, Luders XX: Electrodes. In Gotman J, Ives JR, Gloor P, editors: *Long term monitoring in epilepsy*, Amsterdam, 1985, Elsevier.

23. Spencer SS: Intracranial recording. In Spencer SS, Spencer DD, editors: *Surgery for epilepsy*, London, 1991, Blackwell Scientific.

24. Davis R, Engle H, Kudzma J, et al: Update of chronic cerebellar stimulation for spasticity and epilepsy, *Appl Neurophysiol* 45:44-50, 1982.

25. Fox JL: Vascular clips for the microsurgical treatment of stroke, *Stroke* 7(5):489-500, 1976.

26. Yaşargil MG, Vise WM, Bader DCH: Technical adjuncts in neurosurgery, *Surg Neurol* 8:331-336, 1977.

27. Dickman CA, Carter LT, Baldwin HZ, et al: Continuous regional cerebral blood flow monitoring in acute cranial cerebral trauma, *Neurosurgery* 28(3):467-472, 1991.

28. Wei D, Saidel GM, Jones SC: Optimal design of a thermistor probe for surface measurement of cerebral blood flow, *IEEE Trans Biomed Engineering* 37(12):1159-1172, 1990.

29. Cooper PR, Cohen A, Rosiello A, Coslow M: Posterior stabilization of cervical spine fractures and subluxations using plates and screws, *Neurosurgery* 23(3):300-305, 1988.

30. Cloward RB: Anterior approach for removal of ruptured cervical discs, *J Neurosurg* 15:602-614, 1958.

31. Smith GW, Robinson RA: The treatment of cervical spine disorders by anterior removal of the intervertebral disk and interbody fusion, *J Bone Joint Surg* (Am) 40A:607-624, 1958.

32. Harris T: Cervical spine fixation, *Neurosurg Rev* 12:521-524, 1989.

33. Bohler J, Gaudernak T: Anterior plate stabilization for fracture-dislocation of lower cervical spine, *J Trauma* 20:203-205, 1980.

34. Lesoin F, Viaud C, Jomin M: Universal plate for anterior cervical spine osteosynthesis, *Acta Neurochir* (Wien) 70:60-61, 1985.

35. Oliveria JC: Anterior plate fixation of traumatic lesions of the lower cervical spine, *Spine* 12(4):324-329, 1986.

36. Tippets RH, Apfelbaum RI: Anterior cervical fusion with the Caspar instrumentation system, *Neurosurgery* 22(6):1008-1013, 1988.

37. Gore DR, Gardner GM, Sepic SB, Murray MP: Roentgenographic findings following anterior cervical fusion, *Skeletal Radiol* 15:556-559, 1986.

38. Esses SI, Bednar DA. Screw fixation of odontoid fractures and nonunions, *Spine* 16(10 suppl):S483-485, 1991.

39. Churney WB, Sonntag VKH, Douglas RA: Lateral mass posterior plating and facet fusion for cervical spine instability, *BNI Q* 7(2)2-11, 1991 (Barrow Neurological Institute, Phoenix, Arizona).

40. Stauffer ES: Wiring techniques of the posterior cervical spine for the treatment of trauma, *Orthopedics* 11(11):1543-1548, 1989.

41. Clockard HA, Ransford AO: Stabilization of the spine, *Adv Tech Stand Neurosurg* 17:159-188, 1990.

42. Egnatchik JG: Lumbar spine stabilization: techniques, *Clin Neurosurg* 36:159-167, 1990.

43. Selby D: The Knodt rod. In White AH, Rothman RH, Ray CD, editors: *Lumbar spine surgery*, St. Louis, 1982, Mosby.

44. Dickson JH, Erwin WD, Rossi D: Harrington instrumentation and arthrodesis for idiopathic scoliosis, *J Bone Joint Surg* 72(5)A:678-683, 1990.

45. Luque ER: Interpeduncular segmental fixation, *Clin Orthoped Rel Res* 203:54-57, 1986.

46. Steffee AD, Biscup RS, Sitkowski DJ: Segmental spine plates with pedicle screw fixation, *Clin Orthoped Rel Res* 203:45-53, 1986.

47. Allison RE, Amundson G: Spinal fixation using the Steffee pedicle screw, *AORN* 49:1016-1030, 1989.

48. Boucher HH: A method of spinal fusion, *J Bone Joint Surg* 41(2)B:248-259, 1959.

49. Buck JE: Direct repair of the defect in spondylolisthesis, *J Bone Joint Surg* 52(3)B:432-437, 1970.

50. Burton C: Dorsal column stimulation, optimization of application, *Surg Neurol* 4:171-175, 1975.

51. Larson SJ, Sances A, Cusic JF, et al: A comparison between anterior and posterior spinal implant systems, *Surg Neurol* 4:180-186, 1975.

52. Richardson RR, Siqueira EB, Cerullo LJ: Spinal epidural neurostimulation for treatment of acute and chronic intractable pain: initial and long term results, *Neurosurgery* 5(3):344-348, 1979.

53. Campos RJ, Dimitrijevic MR, Sharkey PC, Sherwood AM: Epidural spinal cord stimulation in spastic spinal cord injury patients, *Appl Neurophysiol* 50:453-454, 1987.

54. Mundinger F, Neumuller H: Program stimulation for control of chronic pain and motor diseases, *Appl Neurophysiol* 45:102-111, 1982.

55. Ray CD: Electrical and chemical stimulation of the CNS by direct means for pain control: present and future, *Clin Neurosurg* 28:564-588, 1981.

56. Johnson RM, Owen JR, Hart DL, Callahan RA: Cervical orthoses, *Clin Orthoped* 154:34-45, 1981.

57. Whitehill R, Richman JA, Glaser JA: Failure of immobilization of the cervical spine by halo vest, *J Bone Joint Surg* 68A:326-332, 1986.

58. Bucholz RD, Cheung C: Halo vest versus spinal fusion for cervical injury: evidence from an outcome study, *J Neurosurg* 70:84-892, 1989.

59. Kostuik JP: Indications for use of the halo immobilization, *Clin Orthoped* 154:46-50, 1981.

60. Price DB: Tubes in the alimentary and respiratory tracks: appearances on CT scans of the head and neck, *AJR* 156:1047-1051, 1991.

61. Stoelting RK: Endotracheal intubation. In Miller RD, editor. *Anesthesia*, ed 2, New York, 1986, Churchill-Livingstone.

62. Ravin CE, Handel DB, Kariman K: Persistent endotracheal tube cuff over extension: a sign of tracheomalacia, *AJR* 137:408-409, 1981.

63. Shifman A, Levin AC, Levy M, Depley JB: Prosthetic restoration of orbital defects, *J Prosthet Dent* 42:543-546, 1979.

64. Wolfaardt JF, Hacqueboard A, Els JM: A mold technique for construction of orbital protheses, *J Prosthet Dent* 50(2):224-226, 1983.

65. Cain JR: Custom ocular protheses, *J Prosthet Dent* 48(6):690-694, 1982.

66. Dortzbach RK, Woog JJ: Choice of procedure: enucleation, evisceration for prothesis fitting over globes, *Ophthalmology* 92(9):1249-1255, 1985.
67. Pichora-Fuller MK, Corbin H, Raiko K, Alberti PW: A review of current approaches to aural rehabilitation, *Int Rehabil Med* 5:58-66, 1983.
68. Wasson JH, Gall V, McDonald R, Liang MH: The prescription of assisted devices for the elderly: practical considerations, *J Gen Intern Med* 5:46-54, 1990.
69. Cocoran AL: A very basic introduction to hearing aids, *Int Rehabil Med* 5(2):79-81, 1983.
70. Mackenzie K, Browning GG, McClymont LG: Relationship between earmold venting, comfort and feedback, *Br J Audiol* 23(4):335-337, 1989.
71. Berliner KI, House WF. The cochlear implant program: an overview, *Ann Otol Rhinol Laryngol* 91(suppl 91):11-14, 1982.

5

Dental Devices

· ·

Stephen Harkins
Luis Cueva

Hundreds of materials and devices are utilized routinely by dentists and dental technicians. Although there are many variations in composition of specific dental materials, the majority fall into five general categories: acrylic resins, porcelain, alloplastic materials, alloy metals, and other miscellaneous materials.[1]

The acrylic dental materials fall into two subcategories: resin-based acrylics and composite-based acrylics. Resin-based acrylics are used in dentures, removable orthodontic appliances, bite guards, temporomandibular joint orthotic appliances, temporary crowns/bridges, and denture teeth. Resin-based acrylics are usually radiolucent. Composite-based acrylics are used in tooth-colored restorations and tooth veneers. Composite-based acrylics are usually radiolucent but may appear slightly radiopaque depending on filler materials added to the composite for strength and color.

Porcelain dental materials are usually found in fixed crowns, bridges, veneers, and denture teeth. Porcelain is more radiopaque than acrylic polymer is and has a radiopacity similar to that of the enamel on natural teeth.

Alloplastic dental materials consist of silicones, tetrahydrofluorocarbons (Teflon), and hydroxyapatites. Silicone and Teflon prosthetic implant materials were used extensively on TMJ and facial reconstruction surgery in the past decade. Silicone and Teflon alloplastic materials are radiolucent but were often fixed in position with steel wire ligatures. Hydroxyapatite implants are used to supplement bone defects in the jaw as well as in facial bones and in tooth implants. Hydroxyapatite has a radiopacity similar to that of dense bone.

Dental metal alloy materials may contain varying combinations of gold, platinum, palladium, silver, copper, chromium, zinc, mercury, and other metals. Dental alloys are most commonly used in dental restorations, crowns, bridges, denture frameworks, orthodontic appliances/retainers, wire ligatures, bone plates/screws, and TMJ/mandibular implant devices. All dental metal alloys are radiopaque.

Miscellaneous dental materials and devices include dental cements and sealers, root canal fillings, dental instruments, and disposable items that can be accidentally swallowed or aspirated during dental treatment. Disposable items such as cotton rolls, 2 × 2 inch gauze sponges, and rubber and plastic mouth props are radiolucent. Dental cements, sealers, and root canal fillings are usually slightly radiopaque. Dental probes, mirrors, filling and carving instruments, scalpel blades, tooth clamps, handpiece burs, and root canal instruments are usually radiopaque.

Figs. 5-1 to 5-3 are radiographic examples of primary, mixed, and permanent dentitions. Figs. 5-4 to 5-15 are radiographic examples of common dental devices.[2]

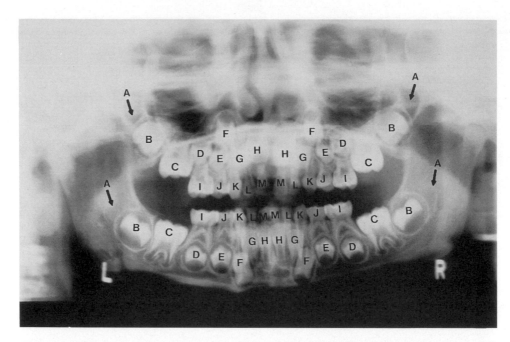

Fig. 5-1. Primary (deciduous/baby) dentition in 4-year-old child. The secondary/permanent/adult dentition is impacted. *A,* Developmental tooth follicle of third molar (wisdom tooth); *B,* impacted second permanent molar (12-year molar); *C,* impacted first permanent molar (6-year molar); *D,* impacted second permanent premolar (second bicuspid); *E,* impacted first permanent premolar (first bicuspid); *F,* impacted permanent canine (cuspid); *G,* impacted permanent lateral incisor; *H,* impacted permanent central incisor; *I,* primary second molar (baby/deciduous second molar); *J,* primary first molar (baby/deciduous first molar); *K,* primary canine (baby/deciduous canine); *L,* primary lateral incisor (baby/deciduous lateral incisor); *M,* primary central incisor (baby/deciduous central incisor).

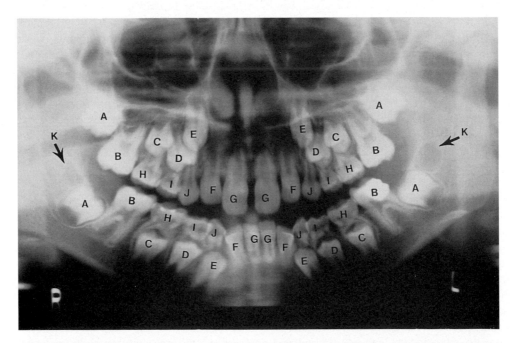

Fig. 5-2. Mixed dentition of an 8-year-old child (28 permanent teeth + 12 retained primary teeth). *A,* Impacted second molar (12-year molar); *B,* first molar (6-year molar); *C,* impacted second premolar (second bicuspid); *D,* impacted first premolar (first bicuspid); *E,* impacted canine (cuspid); *F,* lateral incisor; *G,* central incisor; *H,* second primary molar (second deciduous molar); *I,* first primary molar (first deciduous molar); *J,* primary canine (deciduous cuspid); *K,* developmental follicle for third molar.

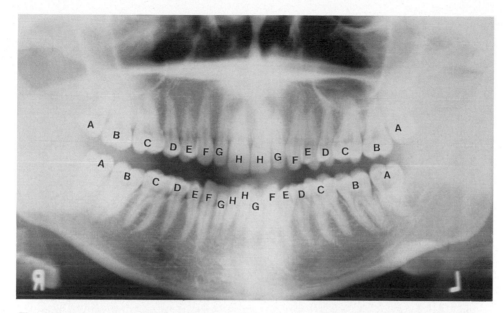

Fig. 5-3. Full adult dentition in a 20-year-old adult (32 secondary or permanent teeth). *A,* Third molar (wisdom tooth); *B,* second molar (12-year molar); *C,* first molar (6-year molar); *D,* second premolar (second bicuspid); *E,* first premolar (first bicuspid); *F,* canine (cuspid); *G,* lateral incisor; *H,* central incisor.

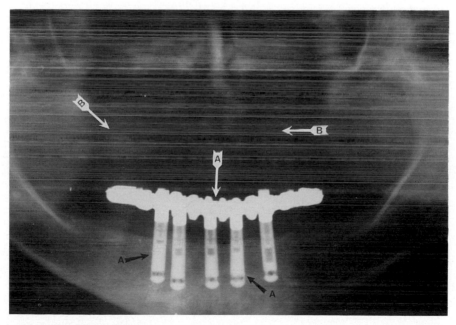

Fig. 5-4. *A,* Osseointegrated dental implants with fixed dental bridgework; *B,* maxillary denture with acrylic teeth.

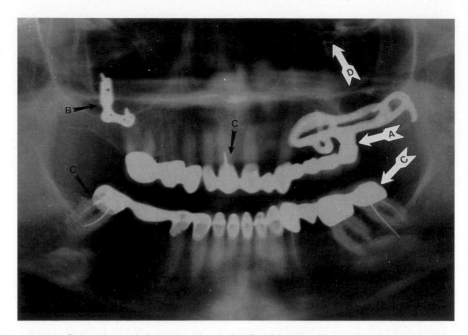

Fig. 5-5. *A,* Subperiosteal dental implant with fixed bridge; *B,* bone plate with screws; *C,* fixed dental bridgework with root canal fillings; *D,* fixation wire.

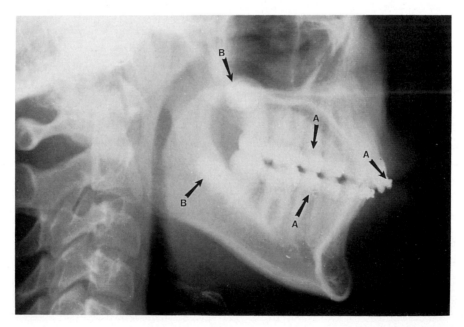

Fig. 5-6. Lateral view. *A,* Fixed orthodontic appliances (braces); *B,* impacted third molars (wisdom teeth).

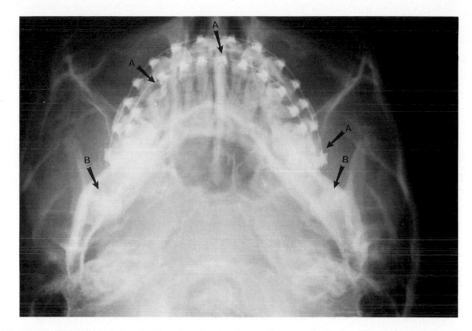

Fig. 5-7. Occipital view. *A,* Fixed orthodontic appliances (braces); *B,* impacted third molars (wisdom teeth).

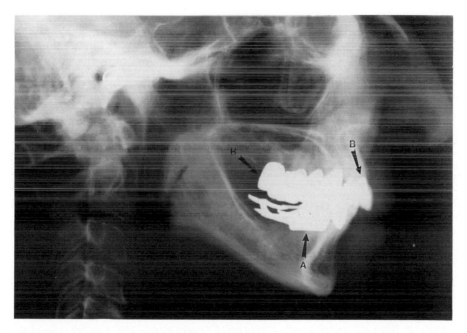

Fig. 5-8. *A,* Removable partial denture framework (partial); *B,* dental crowns (caps).

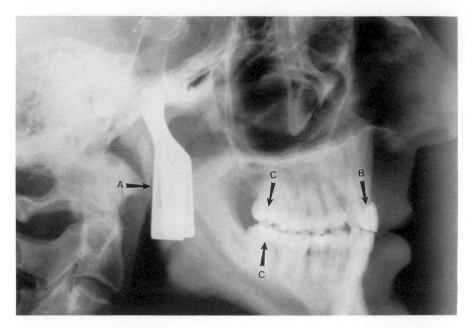

Fig. 5-9. *A,* Temporomandibular joint (TMJ) prothesis (condyle implant); *B,* dental crowns; *C,* dental alloy restoration (amalgam).

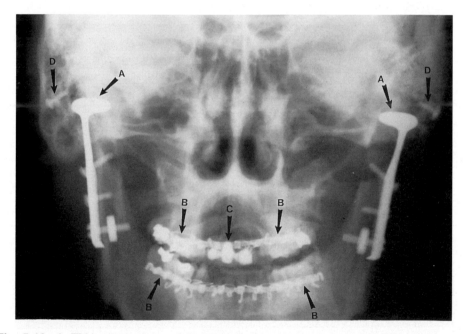

Fig. 5-10. *A,* TMJ prosthetic condyle implant; *B,* orthodontic arch bars; *C,* porcelain veneer dental crowns (caps); *D,* fixation screws (bone screws).

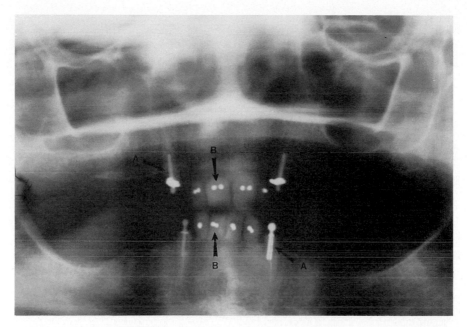

Fig. 5-11. *A*, Root canal fillings with denture retention posts; *B*, porcelain denture teeth with pins.

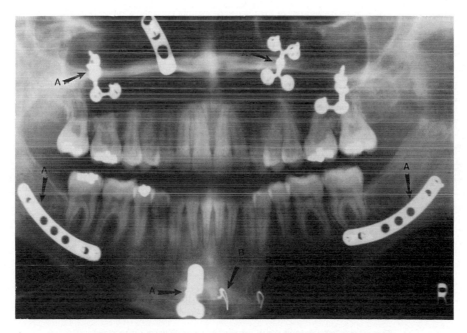

Fig. 5-12. *A*, Bone plates with screws; *B*, bone ligature wire.

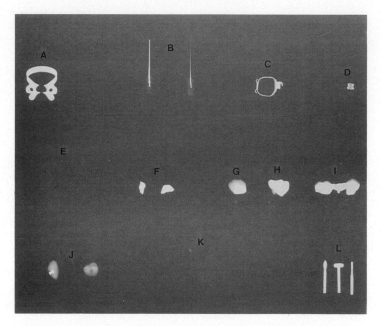

Fig. 5-13. *A,* Rubber dam tooth clamp; *B,* root canal instruments (reamers); *C,* orthodontic band; *D,* orthodontic bracket; *E,* cotton roll; *F,* dental restorations (fillings); *G,* porcelain veneer crown (porcelain cap); *H,* cast gold crown (gold cap); *I,* cast metal bridge; *J,* denture teeth; *K,* gauze sponge; *L,* dental handpiece burs (drill bits).

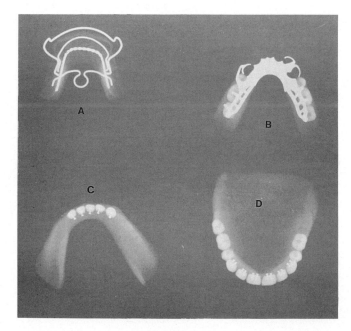

Fig. 5-14. *A,* Removable orthodontic retainer (retainer); *B,* removable partial denture (partial); *C,* mandibular denture with porcelain anterior teeth/acrylic posterior teeth (lower plate); *D,* maxillary denture with porcelain teeth (upper plate).

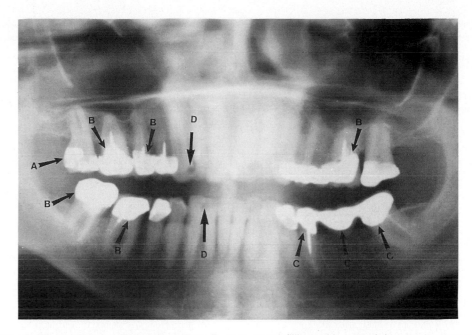

Fig. 5-15. *A,* Alloy dental restoration; *B,* root canal filling with porcelain veneer crowns and posts; *C,* fixed bridge pontic with abutment crowns; *D,* dental composite (acrylic) restoration (tooth-colored fillings).

REFERENCES

1. Phillips R: *Skinner's science of dental materials,* ed 9, Philadelphia, 1991, Saunders.

2. Stafne E: *Stafne's oral radiographic diagnosis,* ed 5, Philadelphia, 1985, Saunders.

6

Medical Devices of the Thorax

James R. Standen

Radiography of the chest accounts for approximately 40% of the work load of a diagnostic radiology department in a modern general hospital. The proliferation of intensive care units (ICUs) and the advances in the management of the very ill have greatly increased the numbers of examinations performed at the patient's bedside. A daily chest radiograph is standard practice in most ICUs, and any change in the patient's condition, or an intervention, can lead to several more studies. As a result, chest radiography in these very sick patients provides images of medical devices in great numbers.[1,2]

EXTRATHORACIC DEVICES

Most life-assisting devices are, of course, within the patient's heart, blood vessels, lungs, or pleura. Tubing, clamps, syringes, and other apparatus often lie on or under the patient and are imaged with the chest during the radiographic examination. These are usually easy to recognize and of no great importance. Patients may also lie on trauma boards, foam mattresses, or other similar supports (Fig. 6-1). Other devices such as a shoulder prosthesis (Fig. 6-2) or a halo apparatus (Fig. 6-3) are often well enough visualized on chest films to detect significant abnormalities.

Ventilator support tubing is almost always visible somewhere on a chest film, as are attachments, such as temperature and humidity sensors (Fig. 6-4). ECG electrodes (Fig. 6-5) are now so ubiquitous that even healthy newborns rarely escape having them applied. The usual positions are shown in Fig. 6-5. A versatile device commonly used in cardiac patients being transported by helicopter or ambulance is the external pacemaker/defibrillator. An electrode plate of one such unit is seen overlying the heart in Fig. 6-6.

Breast prostheses are usually composed of a polyurethane envelope filled with either silicone gel (Fig. 6-7) or saline (Fig. 6-8) (see also Chapter 7). Leakage of silicone into the adjacent soft tissues is sometimes visible radiographically (Fig. 6-9). Breast reconstruction after mastectomy may require the gradual preparation of a pocket suitable for the prosthesis, using a tissue expander (Fig. 6-10).

PLEURAL DEVICES

Thoracostomy (chest) tubes are commonly used for evacuating fluid or air from the pleural space. They vary from 10 to 40 French in size, depending on the viscosity of the material to be evacuated and the preferences of the individual physician involved in the management of the case.[3-5] The tube is usually placed anterosuperiorly for pneumothoraces and posteroinferiorly for fluid collections. The normally positioned tube lies on the surface of the expanded lung, between the visceral and parietal pleurae (Figs. 6-11 and 6-12). Notice that the tube in Fig. 6-12 is not optimally positioned for drainage of pleural fluid. A 12 French pigtail catheter for urokinase treatment of empyema is shown in Fig. 6-13.

If the thoracostomy tube is not accomplishing its task of adequate fluid drainage or reexpansion of a collapsed lung secondary to a pneumothorax, the tube is probably malpositioned. To assess the position of a tube accurately, one may have to obtain both frontal and lateral views of the chest or even use a chest computed tomogram.[6-8]

A chest tube may enter an interlobar fissure. With apposition of the visceral pleura of the two lobes, the end and side holes of the tube may become obstructed and

Text continued on p. 155.

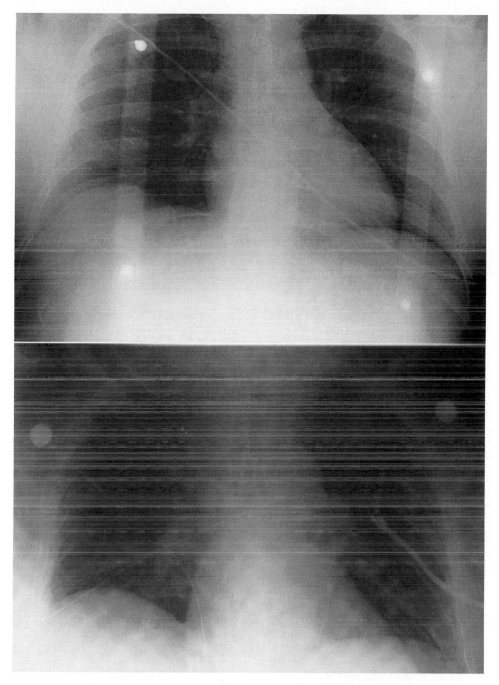

Fig. 6-1. A, Patient lying on a trauma board. The parallel densities on either side of the chest and the metallic screws are part of the board and should not be confused with material lying on or within the patient. **B,** Patient lying on a foam mattress. Do not confuse with a photographic Moiré pattern.

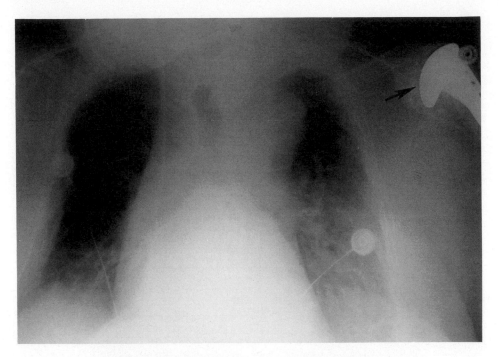

Fig. 6-2. Metallic left shoulder prosthesis, *arrow.*

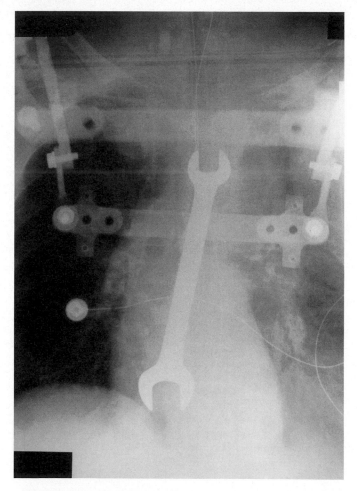

Fig. 6-3. Halo apparatus (with emergency wrench close at hand) for cervical spine stabilization.

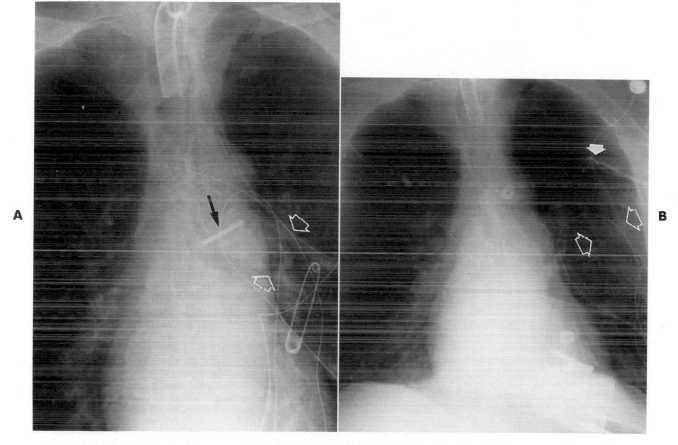

Fig. 6-4. A, Respirator tubing, *open arrows,* with mercury thermometer for monitoring temperature of inspired gas, *closed arrow.* **B,** Respirator tubing, *open arrows,* with electronic temperature probe, *closed arrow.*

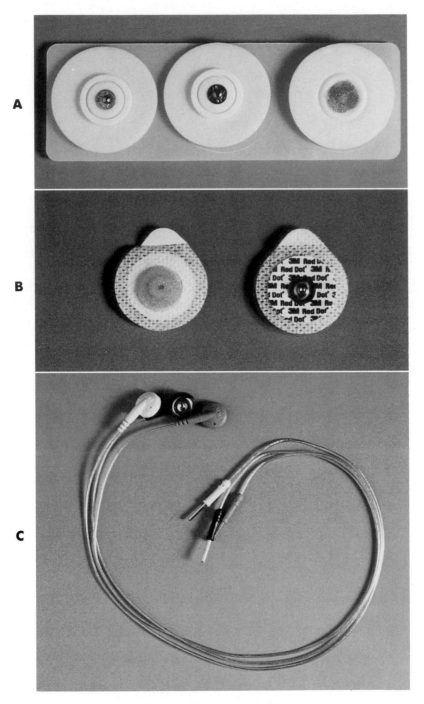

Fig. 6-5. A and **B,** Electrocardiogram (ECG) monitoring electrodes. **C,** ECG lead wires.

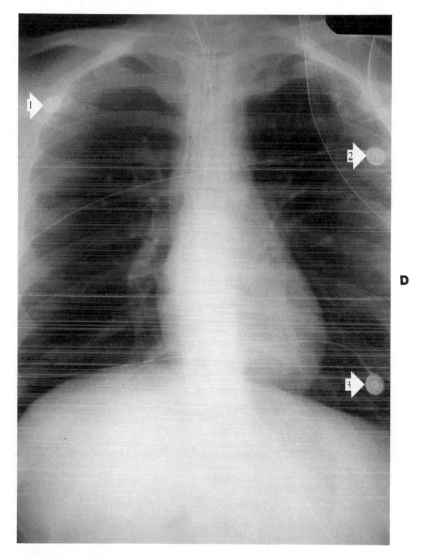

Fig. 6-5, cont'd.   **D,** ECG monitoring electrodes *(1* to *3)* in usual position on chest wall.

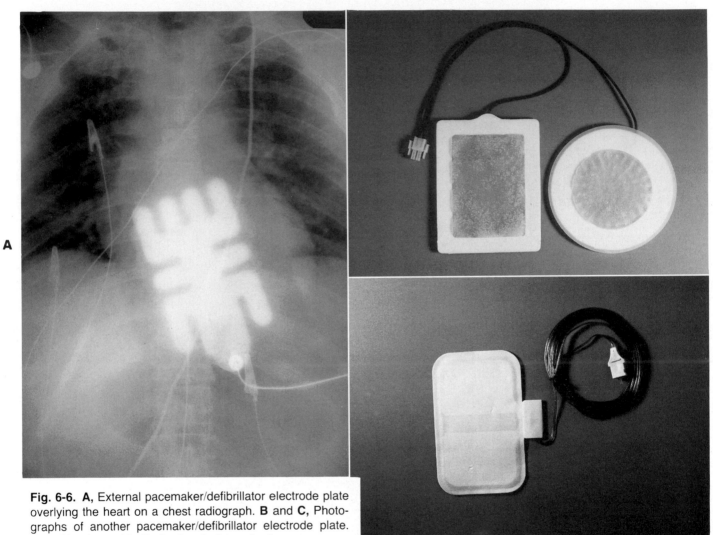

Fig. 6-6. A, External pacemaker/defibrillator electrode plate overlying the heart on a chest radiograph. **B** and **C,** Photographs of another pacemaker/defibrillator electrode plate. The side pictured in **C** attaches to the patient.

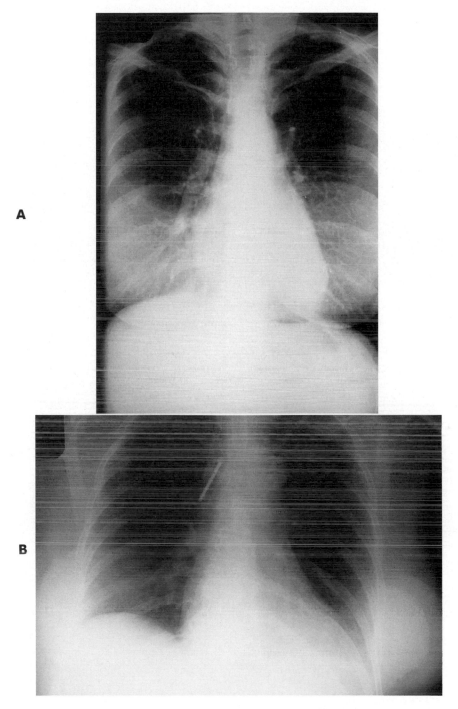

Fig. 6-7. Silicone gel breast implants in two different patients

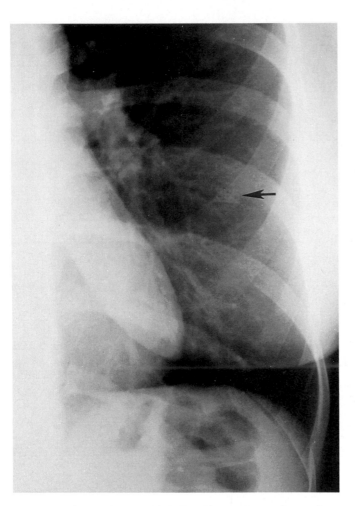

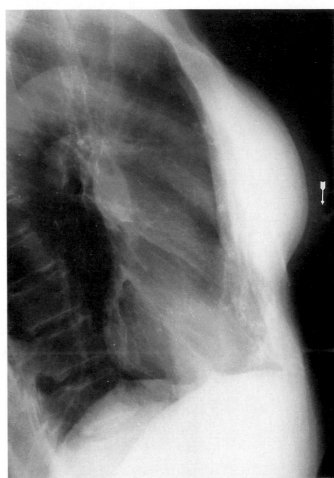

Fig. 6-8. Saline breast implant with opaque unit number "365" visible over anterior fifth rib, *arrow*.

Fig. 6-9. Lateral view showing leakage, *arrow,* into subcutaneous tissues from silicone gel breast implant.

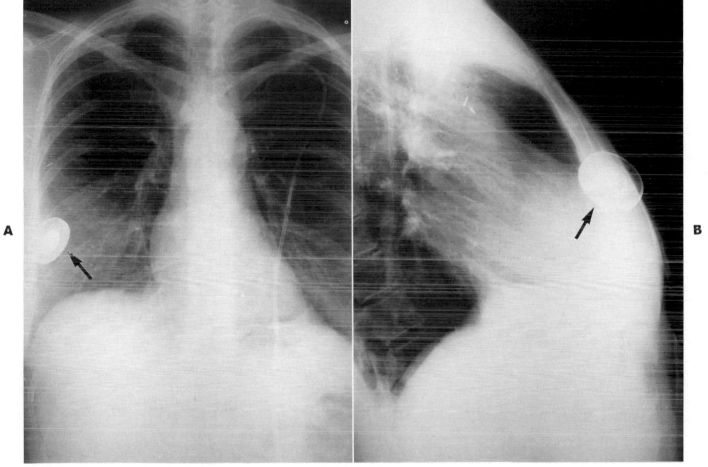

Fig. 6-10. Frontal, **A,** and lateral, **B,** views showing tissue expander, *arrow,* for subsequent breast reconstruction.

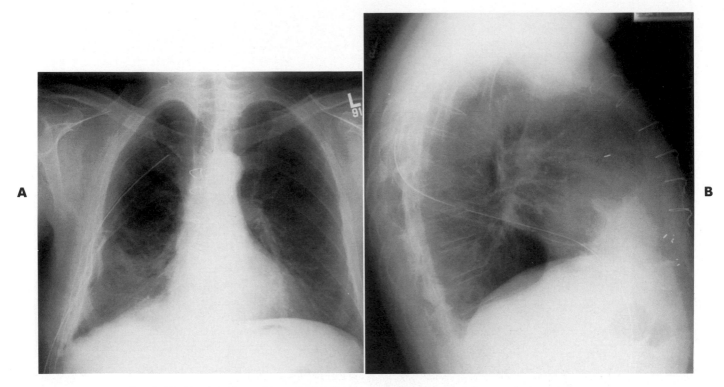

Fig. 6-11. Frontal, **A,** and lateral, **B,** views with thoracostomy tube passing posterosuperiorly on the surface of the lung from axillary entry site.

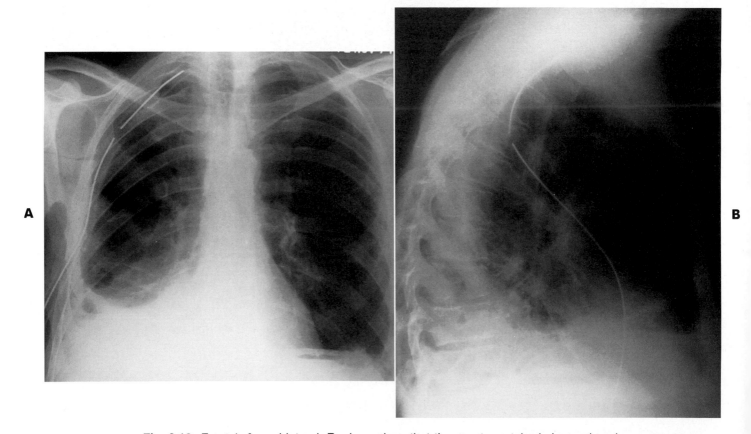

Fig. 6-12. Frontal, **A,** and lateral, **B,** views show that thoracostomy tube is in good position for treatment of pneumothorax but not for effusion.

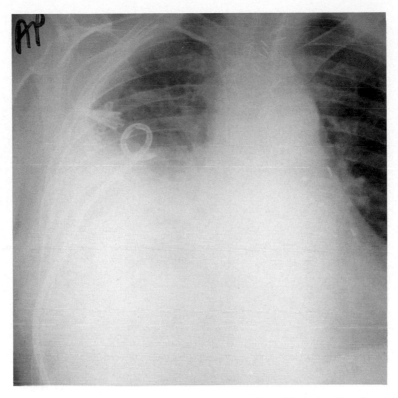

Fig. 6-13. Frontal view of the chest after fluoroscopically guided pigtail catheter insertion into a loculated right empyema for instillation of urokinase and fluid drainage.

the tube rendered ineffective (Figs. 6-14 and 6-15). Malposition of chest tubes in lung parenchyma or subcutaneous soft tissues is not uncommon, particularly if a trocar technique of insertion is employed and there are underlying pleural adhesions (Fig. 6-16). The proximal port of the chest tube may be in a superficial location outside the pleural cavity, or the tube may become kinked. The tube can also become occluded if its tip lies against the mediastinum.

In the preantibiotic era, a variety of pleural devices were used in the treatment of tuberculosis. These include "Ping-Pong ball plombage" (Fig. 6-17) and wax plombage (Fig. 6-18). Their appearance is quite surprising, and they may occasionally be encountered in an older patient.

TRACHEAL AND ESOPHAGEAL DEVICES

(See also chapters 4 and 8.)

Endotracheal intubation is a lifesaving procedure, but it can also be life threatening if the tube is incorrectly positioned. In an adult, the tip of the tube should be situated approximately 5 cm above the tracheal carina, so that excursions of 2 cm upwards or downwards (with neck extension or flexion) can be safely accommodated.[9]

The carina may not be visible on every film, but the aortic "knob" usually is. The carina is just caudal to the aortic arch, so that if the tip of the endotracheal tube (ETT) is just above the aortic "knob," it is in good position, midway between the vocal cords and the carina (Fig. 6-19). When advanced too far, the ETT usually enters the right main bronchus, causing various combinations of hyperinflation and atelectasis of the two lungs, depending on the positions of the end and side holes (Figs. 6-20 to 6-22).

Sometimes, a double-lumen endotracheal tube is deliberately used for differential ventilation of the two lungs to accommodate differences in compliance between them (Fig. 6-23). Besides being placed into the right bronchus, endotracheal tubes can also be inadvertently placed in the esophagus (Fig. 6-24) or in the soft tissues of the neck (Fig. 6-25).

Nasogastric tubes and feeding tubes are frequently visualized passing through the mediastinum on their way to the stomach and intestines (Fig. 6-26) (see also Chapters 2, 4, and 8). Examples of other, more specialized gastrointestinal tubes sometimes seen on chest radiographs are shown in Figs. 6-27 and 6-28. Not infrequently, chest radiographs reveal unexpected foreign bodies and medical devices in abnormal locations (Figs. 6-29 to 6-35) (see also Chapter 3).

Text continued on p. 169.

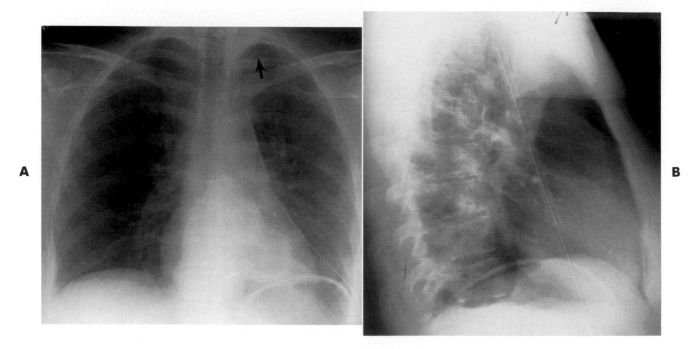

Fig. 6-14. Frontal, **A,** and lateral, **B,** views of the chest show a chest tube in the left major fissure with residual pneumothorax, *arrow,* at the apex.

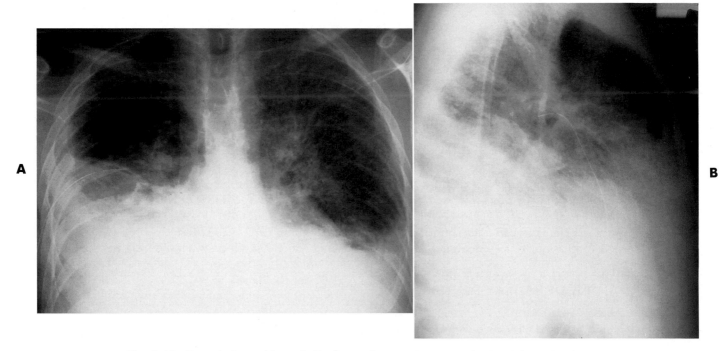

Fig. 6-15. Frontal, **A,** and lateral, **B,** views show a chest tube in the right major fissure with considerable remaining pleural effusion.

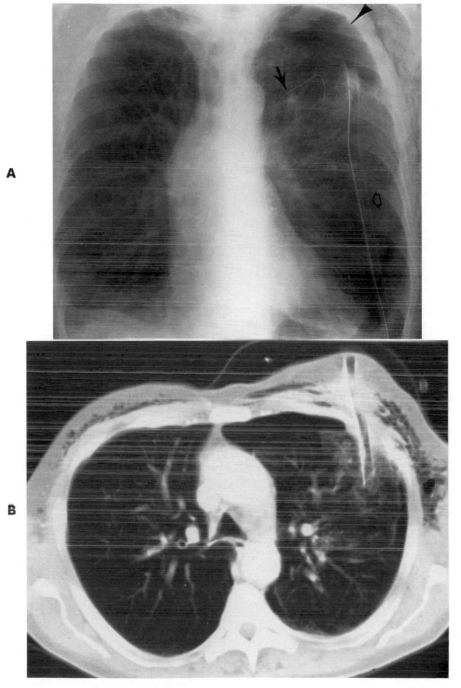

Fig. 6-16. Frontal, **A,** view shows residual pneumothorax, *arrowhead,* with large-bore *(open arrow)* and small-bore *(closed arrow)* tubes present. CT sections, **B** and **C,** show that the large tube is impaled in the left lung and the small tube is in the chest wall.

Continued.

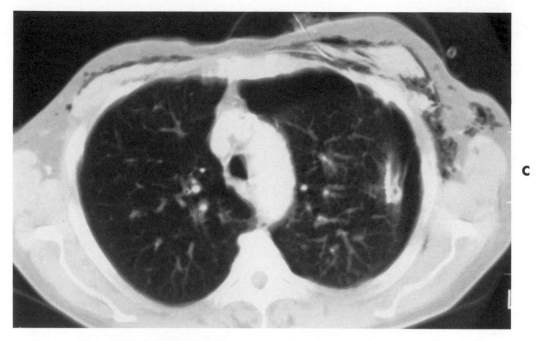

Fig. 6-16, cont'd.

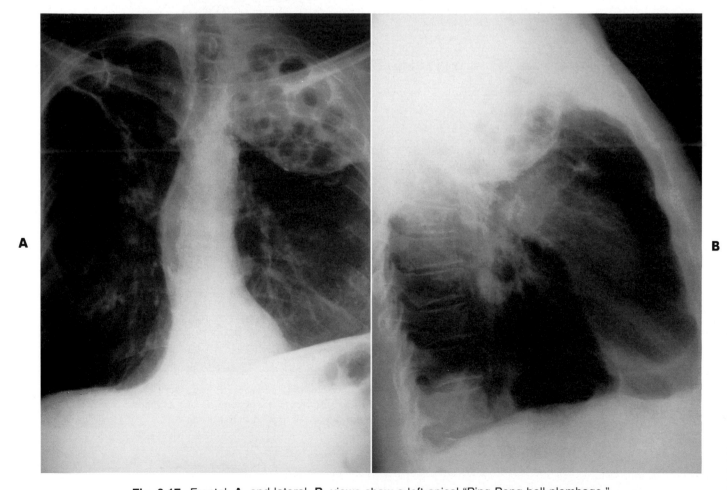

Fig. 6-17. Frontal, **A,** and lateral, **B,** views show a left apical "Ping-Pong ball plombage."

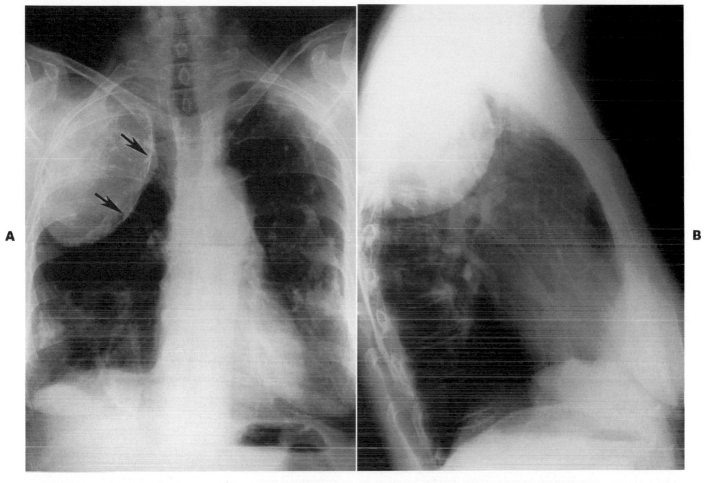

Fig. 6-18. Frontal, **A,** and lateral views, **B,** show a right apical oleothorax (wax plombage). Extensive pleural calcification includes the surface of the wax ball, *arrows.*

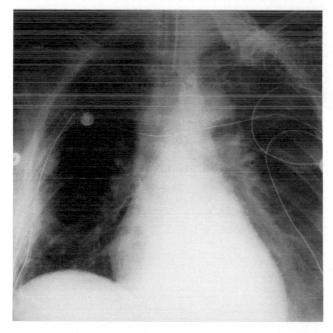

Fig. 6-19. The tip of the endotracheal tube is slightly above the aortic arch and well above the carina, in a good position.

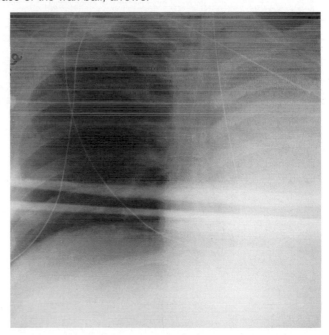

Fig. 6-20. The endotracheal tube tip is in the right bronchus intermedius with hyperinflation of the right lung and atelectasis of the left lung.

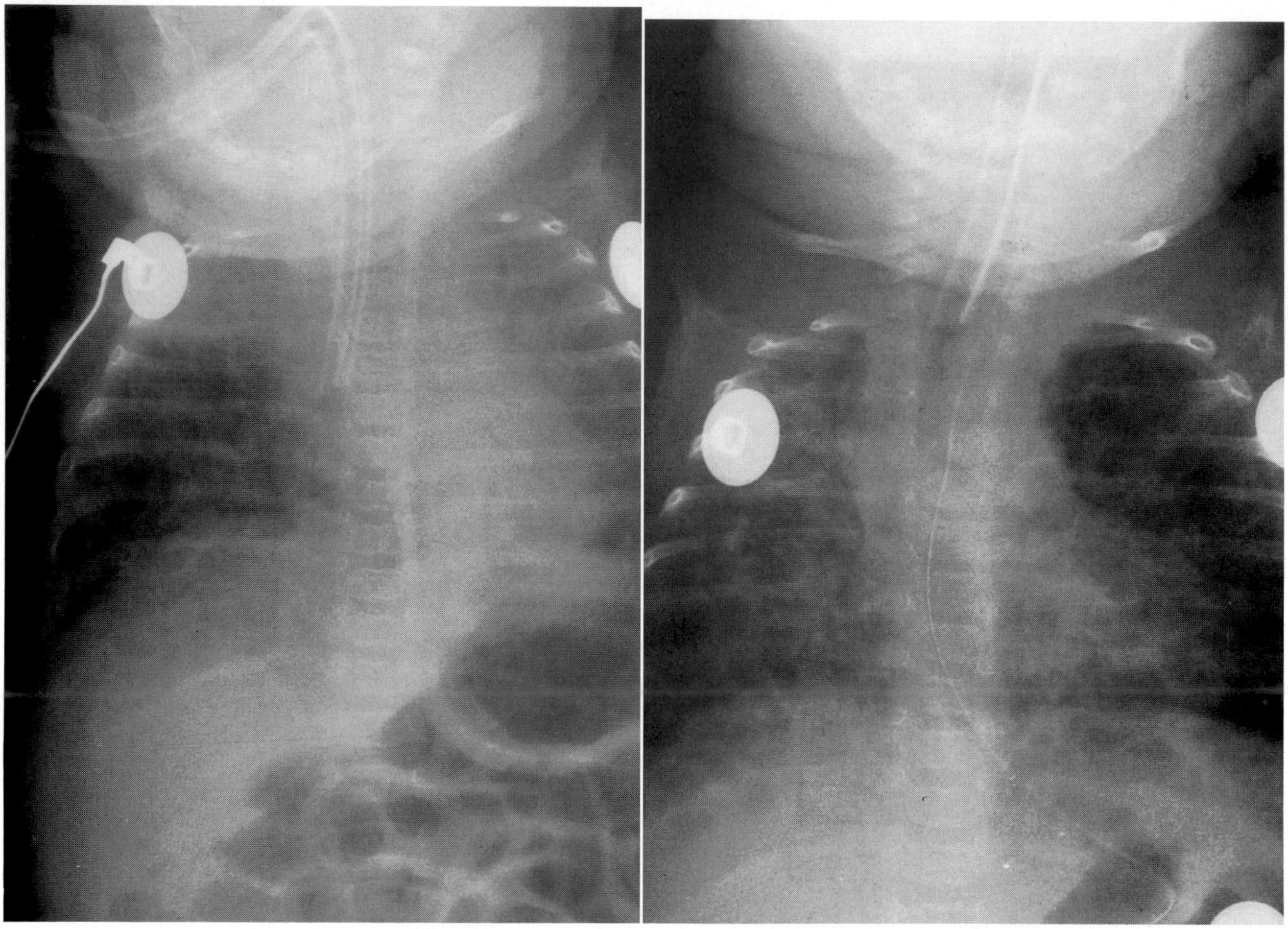

Fig. 6-21. A, Endotracheal tube tip in the right main bronchus of an infant producing right upper lobe atelectasis. **B,** The tube has been repositioned with reexpansion of the right upper lobe.

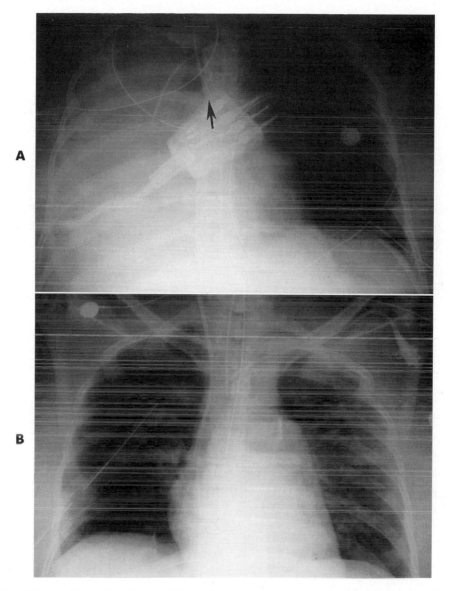

Fig. 6-22. A, There is collapse of the right lung because of selective intubation of the left main bronchus (behind ECG connector block, *arrow*). **B,** Thoracostomy tube is inserted on the right for supposed massive hemothorax. Repositioning of the endotracheal tube allowed the right lung to reinflate.

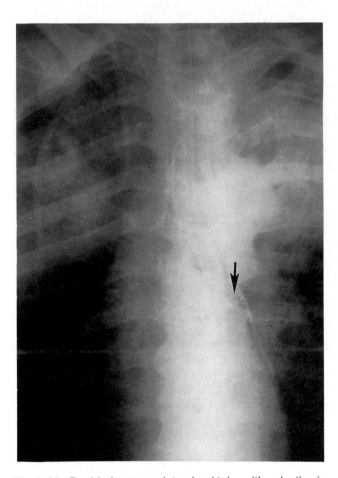

Fig. 6-23. Double-lumen endotracheal tube with selective intubation of the left main bronchus, *arrow*.

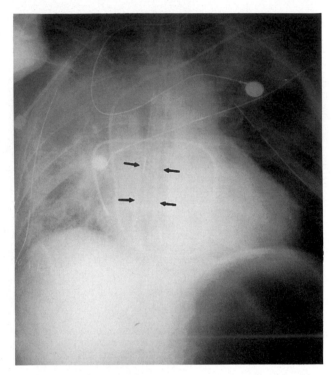

Fig. 6-24. Double-lumen endotracheal tube in distal esophagus with cuff inflated, *arrows.* Pronounced gastric dilatation has resulted.

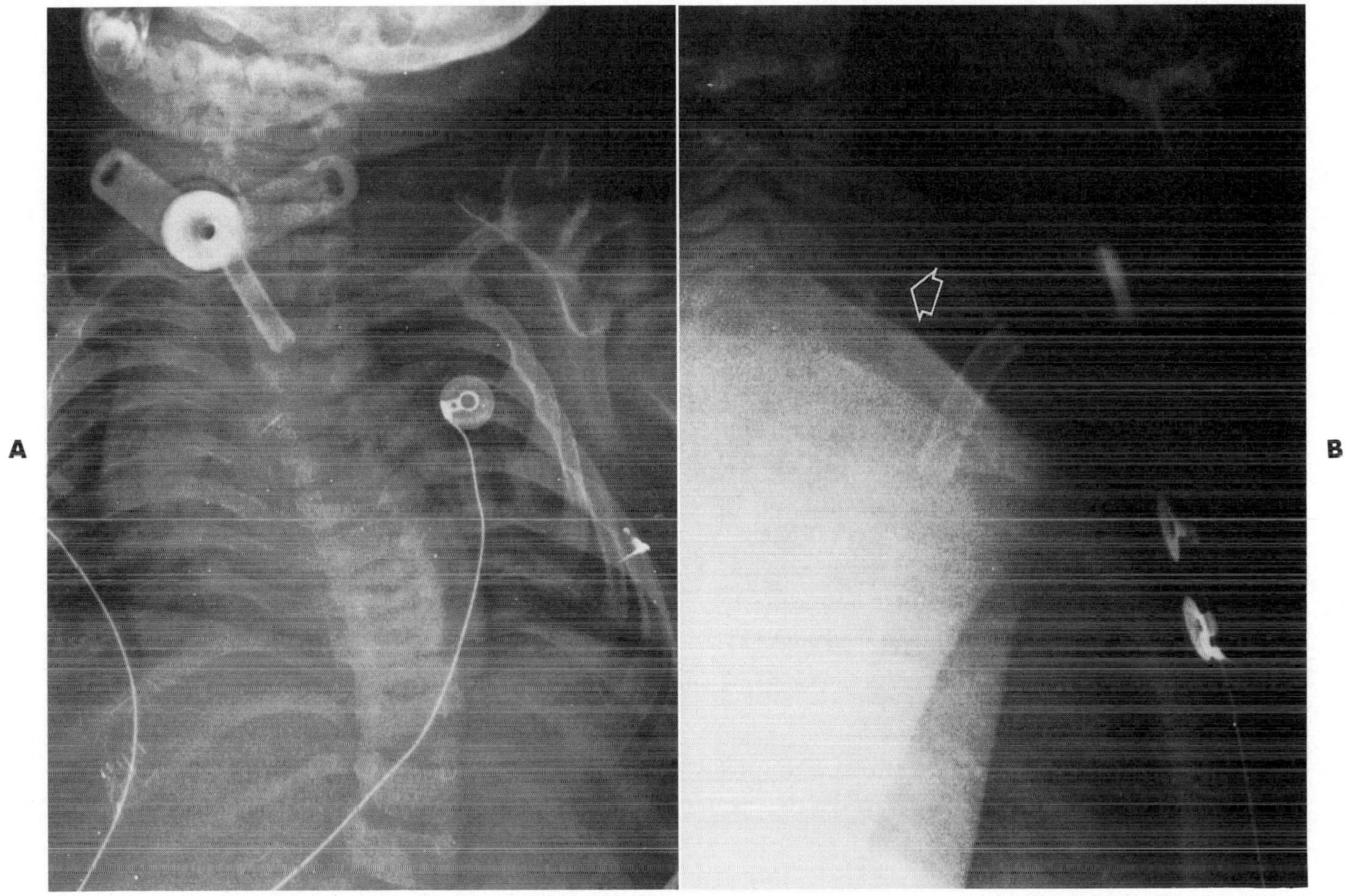

Fig. 6-25. Incorrect placement of a tracheostomy tube. **A,** The tip of the tracheostomy tube is to the left of the trachea on the frontal view. **B,** The tip of the tube is anterior to the trachea, *arrow,* on the lateral view.

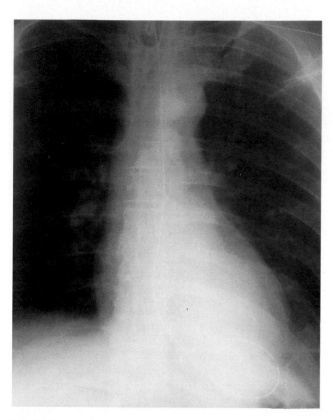

Fig. 6-26. Nasogastric tube with opaque linear marker. The tube passes through the esophagus to loop in the fundus of the stomach.

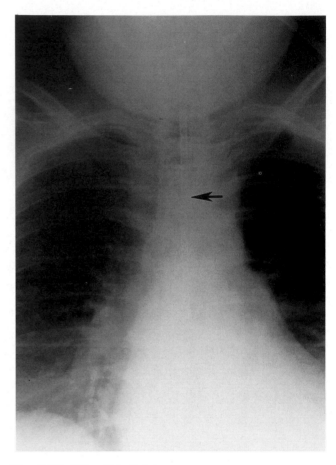

Fig. 6-27. Miller-Abbott tube, *arrow,* passing through the esophagus.

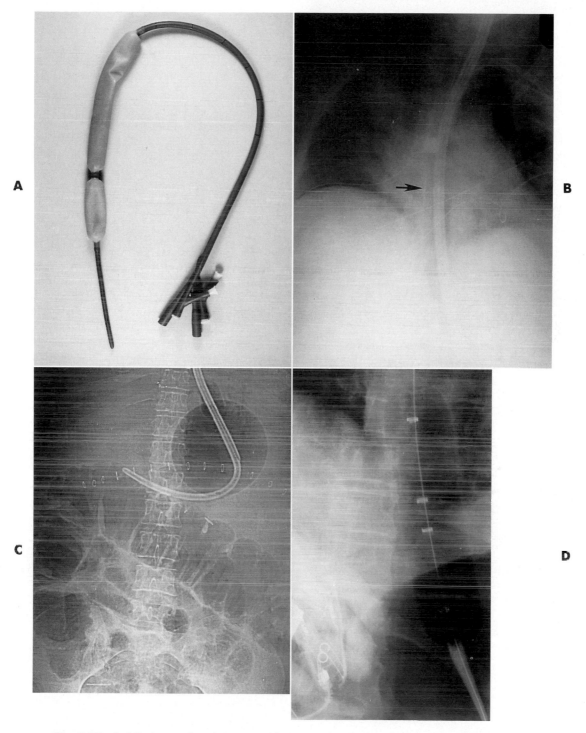

Fig. 6-28. A, Minnesota four-lumen esophagogastric tamponade tube (Davol). This tube is similar to a Sengstaken-Blakemore tube. **B,** Sengstaken-Blakemore tube in the esophagus. The inflated balloon, *arrow,* compresses varices. **C,** The balloon in the stomach when retracted against the gastric cardia stabilizes the position of the Sengstaken-Blakemore tube. **D,** Balloon dilatation of distal esophageal stricture.

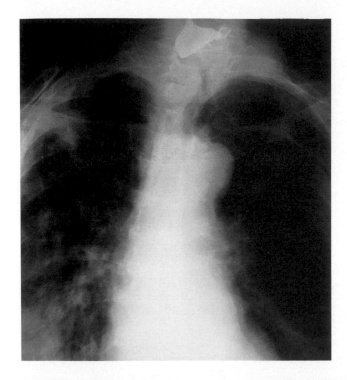

Fig. 6-29. Dental appliance lying in the hypopharynx.

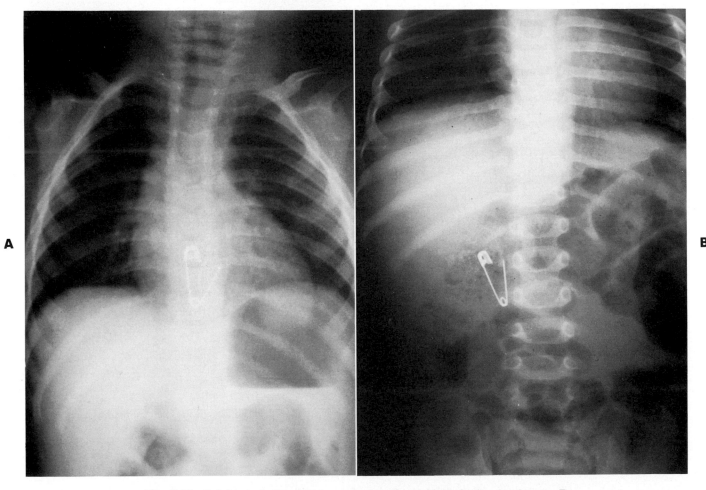

A

B

Fig. 6-30. Safety pin in the distal esophagus, **A,** and later in the duodenum, **B.**

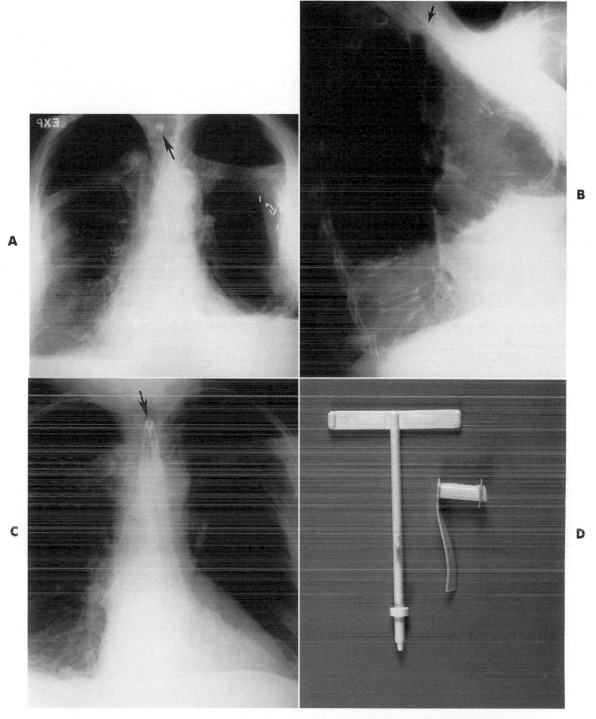

Fig. 6-31. Tracheoesophageal voice prosthesis, *arrow,* on frontal, **A,** and lateral, **B,** chest views. **C,** Dislodged prosthesis in the right bronchus intermedius. It was recovered with a bronchoscope and reinserted in the fistula kept open with a soft catheter. **D,** Photograph of the prosthesis, *top,* and inserting apparatus, *bottom.*

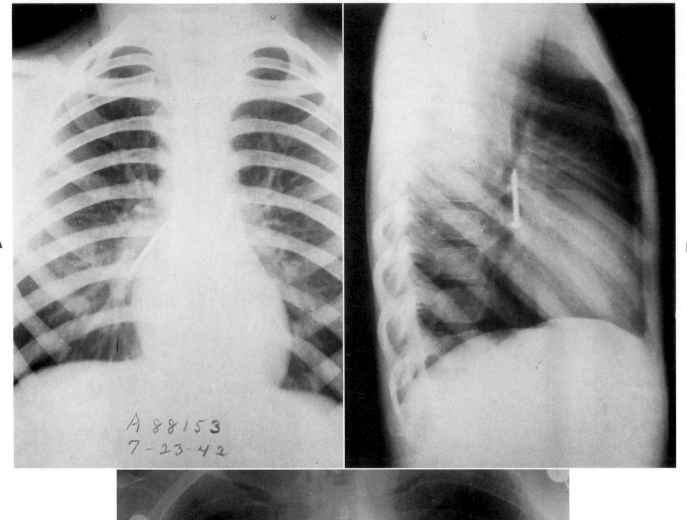

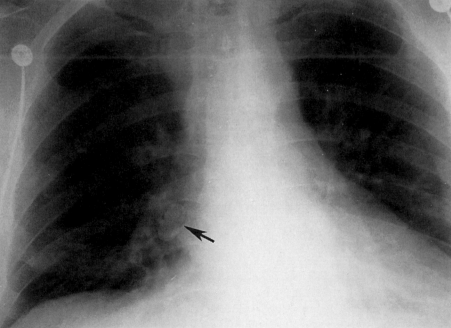

Fig. 6-32. Foreign bodies in right lower lobe bronchus. Roofing nail: frontal, **A,** and lateral, **B,** views. **C,** Potassium chloride pill, *arrows.* (**C,** Courtesy Dr. Jennifer Harvey, Tucson, Arizona.)

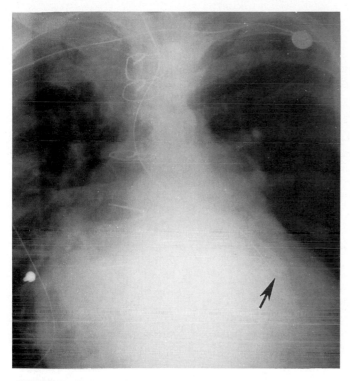

Fig. 6-33. Nasogastric tube, *arrow,* in left lower lobe bronchus.

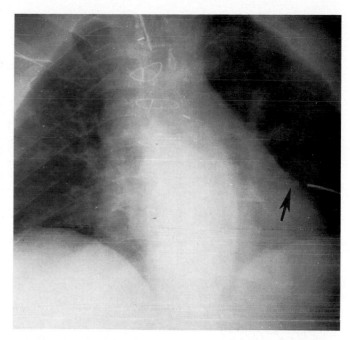

Fig. 6-34. Feeding tube, *arrow,* in left lower lobe bronchus.

VASCULAR DEVICES

Vascular catheters of various types are now routinely used for monitoring of hemodynamic function, for performance of hemodialysis, and for administration of fluids, medications, and nutrition (Fig. 6-36). Some catheters are designed for short-term use in the postoperative or intensive care unit setting, whereas others are implanted for long-term use, as in cancer patients.[10-12] Venous devices are usually inserted, either percutaneously or surgically, via the subclavian, internal jugular, or femoral veins. Arterial devices usually enter via the femoral artery, but sometimes the brachial or axillary route is employed.[13-15]

Central venous pressure (CVP) catheters typically have one to three lumens and are constructed out of medical-grade silicone or polyurethane. The nomenclature for CVP catheters is confusing and inconsistent in daily use. For example, the terms Hickman, Broviac, Leonard, and Hohn are trademarks of C.R. Bard, Inc. Cordis sheath is a trademark of the Cordis Corporation. However, in many medical centers, these terms have come to represent generically any CVP catheter, no matter its actual construction, manufacturer, or particular use.

Swan-Ganz is a registered trademark of Baxter International. This term has come to represent any type of multilumen catheter used for measuring hemodynamic

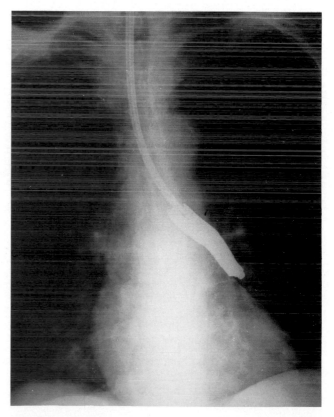

Fig. 6-35. Mercury bag of Miller-Abbott tube in left lower lobe bronchus.

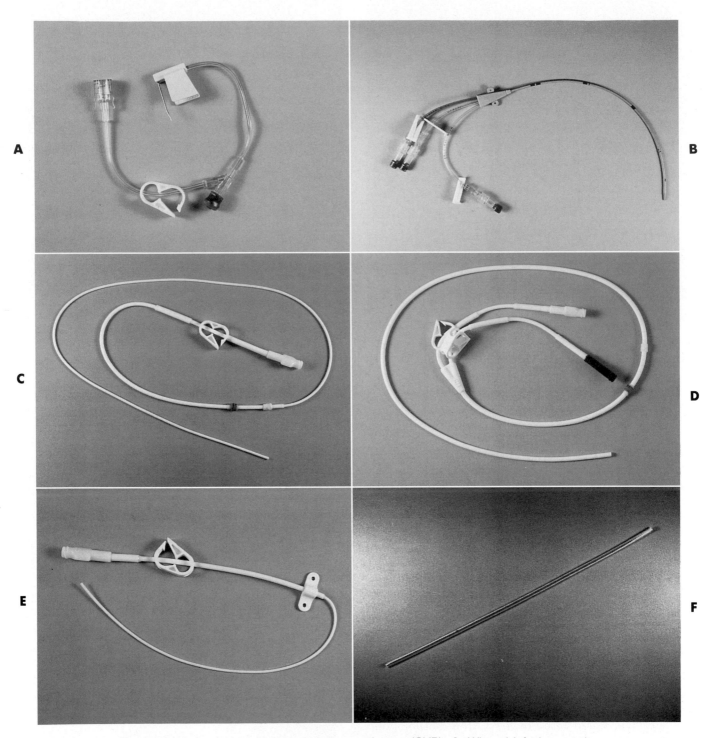

Fig. 6-36. Various types of central venous catheters (CVP). **A,** Winged infusion set designed to hook into any CVP line (Churchill Medical Systems). **B,** Triple-lumen CVP catheter (Cook). **C,** Single-lumen Broviac catheter (Davol). **D,** Double-lumen Hickman catheter (Davol). **E,** Hohn CV catheter (Davol). **F,** Cordis sheath (Cordis Corp.).

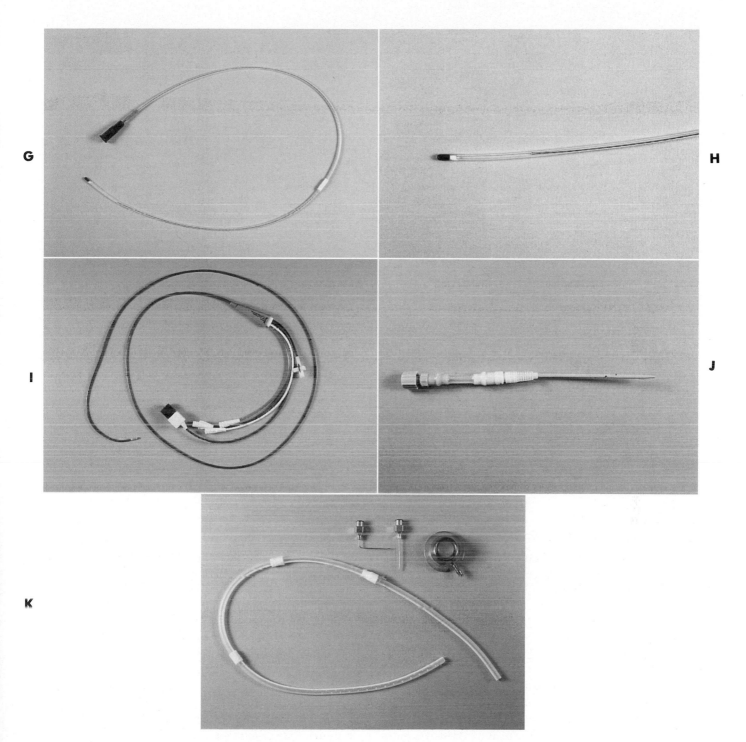

Fig. 6-36, cont'd. G, Groshong catheter (Davol). **H,** Close-up view of Groshong catheter tip. **I,** Swan-Ganz catheter (Baxter). **J,** Hemodialysis catheter (Argon). **K,** Subcutaneous port (Davol).

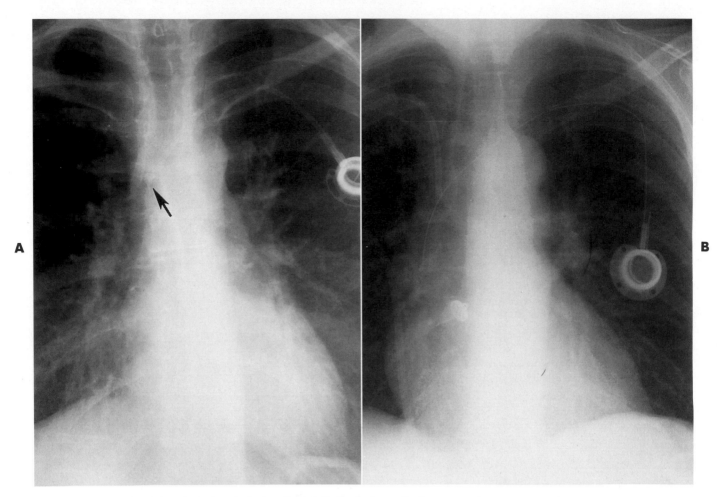

Fig. 6-37. A, Left subclavian Port-A-Cath device with tip, *arrow,* in upper superior vena cava. **B,** Left subclavian Groshong catheter connected to Port-A-Cath infusion port.

pressures and cardiac output. The Groshong (trademark of Bard Access Systems) catheter is noted for its unusual closed, rounded tip. Near the tip in the side of the catheter is a three-position valve. The valve is designed to allow fluid to flow in and out through the valve, but it remains closed when it is not in use. This catheter does not require routine clamping or heparin solution to keep it open. It does require periodic flushing with 0.9% normal saline solution.

There is also a variety of implantable access devices (subcutaneous ports), most commonly represented by the Port-A-Cath, a trademark of Pharmacia Deltec, Inc. Such devices are designed for easy, long-term access to the vascular system or peritoneal cavity. Port access is accomplished by percutaneous needle insertion. The port itself typically sits in the infraclavicular fossa, over the upper abdomen, or over the lower ribs. The port is usually connected to a central venous catheter or to an arterial catheter and can be used for the instillation of fluids, medications, chemotherapeutic agents, paren-

teral nutritional solutions, and blood products. It can also be used for the withdrawal of blood samples.

A central venous catheter is ideally positioned in the superior vena cava for the monitoring of pressure or infusion of medication and food (Figs. 6-36 to 6-40). A catheter tip positioned in the right atrium increases the risk of perforation and cardiac arrhythmia[16] (Fig. 6-41). The same holds true for dialysis catheters (Fig. 6-42).

Flow-directed balloon-tipped catheters (Swan-Ganz) are now widely used for monitoring circulatory hemodynamics (Figs. 6-43 to 6-46). Accurate measurement of pulmonary arterial wedge pressure in a supine patient requires the catheter tip to be in the lower lobe (zone 3 of West) so that left atrial pressure, not alveolar pressure, is measured.[17,18] Other types of catheters, of course, may also be positioned in pulmonary vessels (Fig. 6-47).

Over a period of time, Swan-Ganz catheters may migrate toward the periphery of the pulmonary bed and become lodged in a small pulmonary artery. This can

Text continued on p. 178.

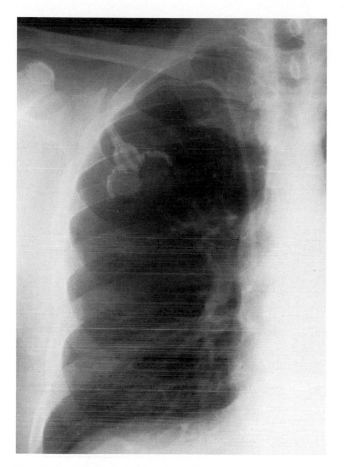

Fig. 6-38. Right subclavian Dual-Chamber Port-A-Cath device.

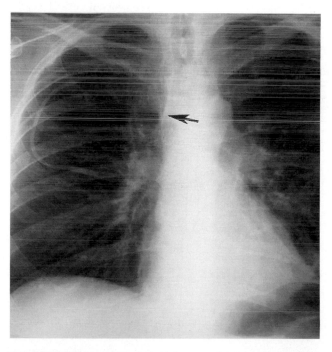

Fig. 6-39. Right subclavian Hohn coaxial venous catheter, *arrow*.

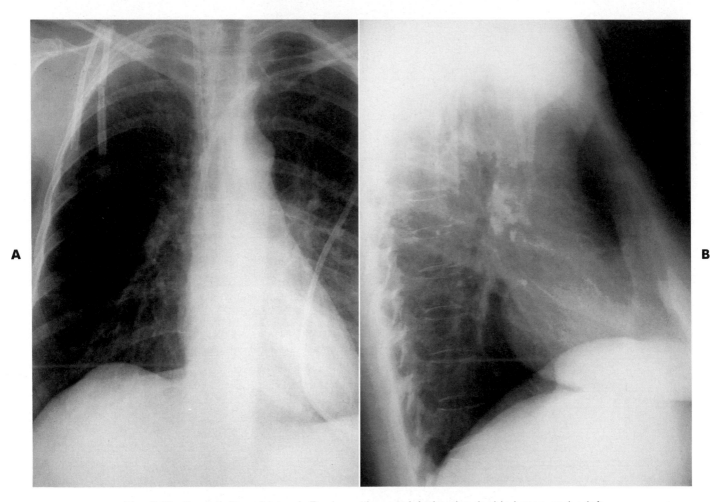

Fig. 6-40. Frontal, **A,** and lateral, **B,** views show a right jugular double-lumen and a left subclavian triple-lumen catheter in a bone marrow transplant patient.

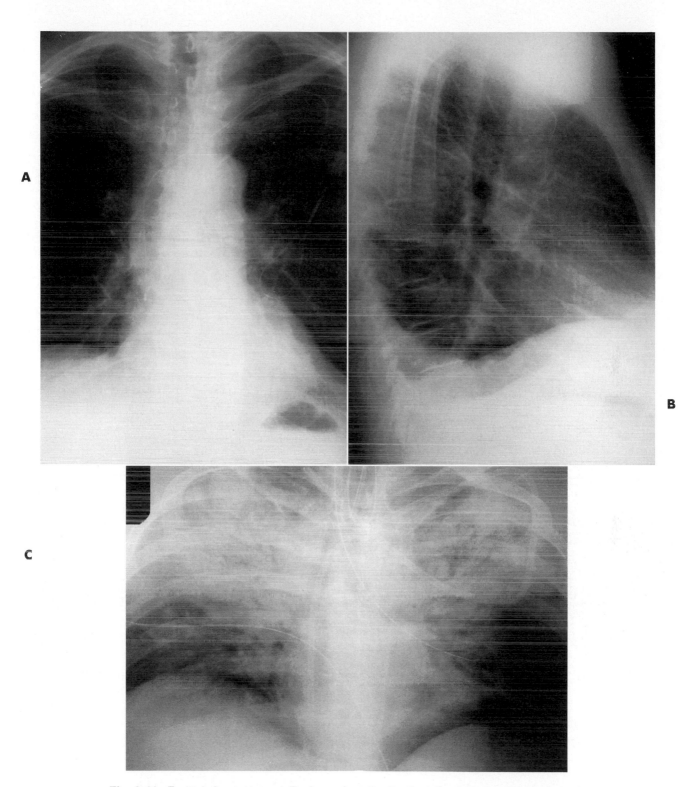

Fig. 6-41. Frontal, **A,** and lateral, **B,** views show the tip of a left subclavian Groshong catheter in the upper part of the right atrium. **C,** Another patient with central venous catheter tip in the lower right atrium.

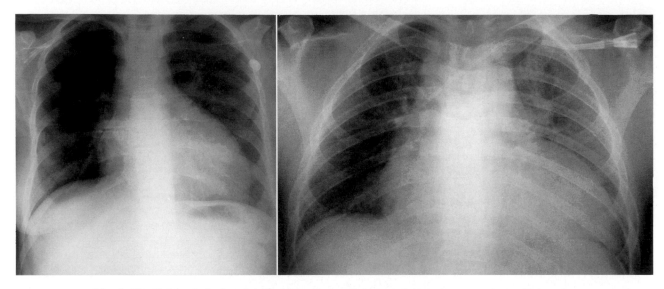

Fig. 6-42. Right subclavian double-lumen hemodialysis catheters in two patients. The catheter tips are in the superior vena cava.

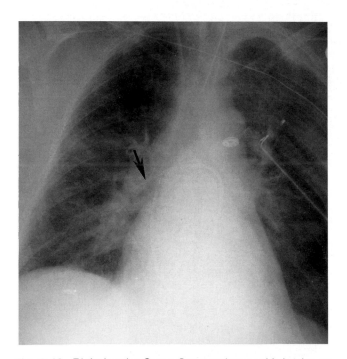

Fig. 6-43. Right jugular Swan-Ganz catheter with its tip, *arrow,* in the right lower pulmonary artery.

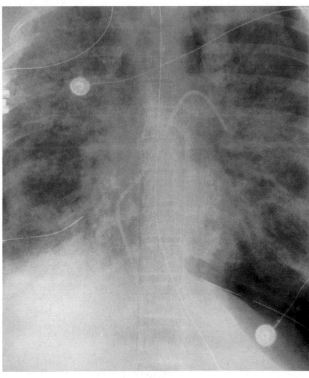

Fig. 6-44. Swan-Ganz catheter in the left pulmonary artery via the inferior vena cava.

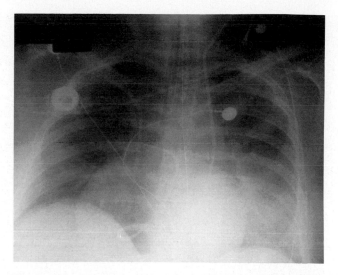

Fig. 6-45. Left jugular Swan-Ganz catheter passes through a persistent left superior vena cava into the coronary sinus, through the right atrium and right ventricle, and into the right pulmonary artery.

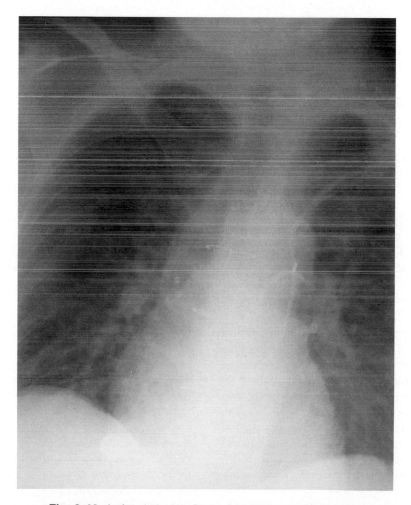

Fig. 6-46. Left subclavian Swan-Ganz catheter also passes through a left superior vena cava.

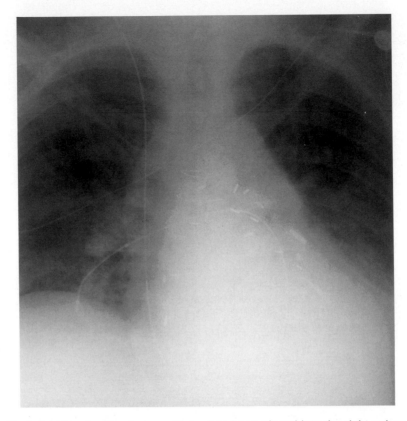

Fig. 6-47. A right jugular Mewissen catheter has been placed into the right pulmonary artery for urokinase infusion.

cause vessel injury by prolonged occlusion or by over-distension of the vessel when the catheter balloon is inflated. Also, pulmonary infarction can result from this situation. The period of time during which the balloon remains inflated and wedged should be limited, particularly in patients with pulmonary hypertension. A central location of the catheter tip near the lung hilum helps prevent pulmonary artery perforation and is a good parking position for the catheter when it is not being used to measure pulmonary arterial wedge pressure.

Complications of catheter insertion vary with the catheters used and the sites employed.[2,11-14,19-22] Catheter malposition usually involves the catheter passing into a tributary vessel rather than the one sought. The internal jugular vein (Fig. 6-48), the azygous arch, and the internal mammary vein (Fig. 6-49) are common examples of this type of malpositioning. A congenital anomaly can produce an unusual catheter course and position (Fig. 6-50). Arterial puncture may lead to an abnormal catheter position with pulsatile flow in the catheter (Fig. 6-51).

Pneumothorax is a common complication of unsuccessful attempts at subclavian or low jugular catheter insertion. Nerve injury is usually a complication of improper puncture technique. Vessel lacerations and perforations can produce hematomas, hemothoraces, and infusion of fluid into the mediastinum or other inappropriate space (Figs. 6-52 to 6-56). Looping of catheters (Fig. 6-57) may lead to knotting (Fig. 6-58). Pinching off of catheters and catheter shearing usually occur at the site of entry and suture fixation[21] (Fig. 6-59).

CARDIAC DEVICES

The heart has probably fostered more development of sophisticated medical interventions than all other organs combined. Coronary artery angioplasty, coronary bypass grafts, the surgical correction of congenital cardiac defects, and even cardiac transplantation are no longer considered novel, experimental procedures. Heart pacemakers, valve prostheses, and artificial hearts are sophisticated biomedical engineering products that have drastically altered the course of many cardiac disorders. Since chest radiography is commonly employed in the assessment of patients with heart disease, the radiologic recognition of cardiac devices and of the problems associated with them are important for all involved in the care of these patients.

Text continued on p. 185.

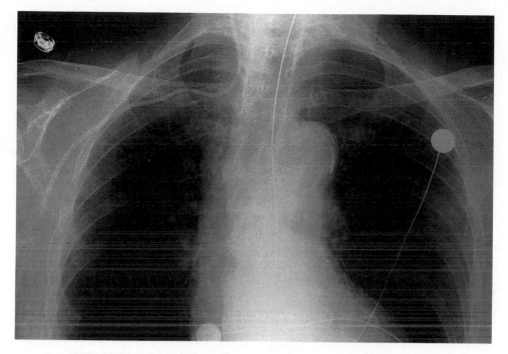

Fig. 6-48. Subclavian venous catheter going into the right internal jugular vein.

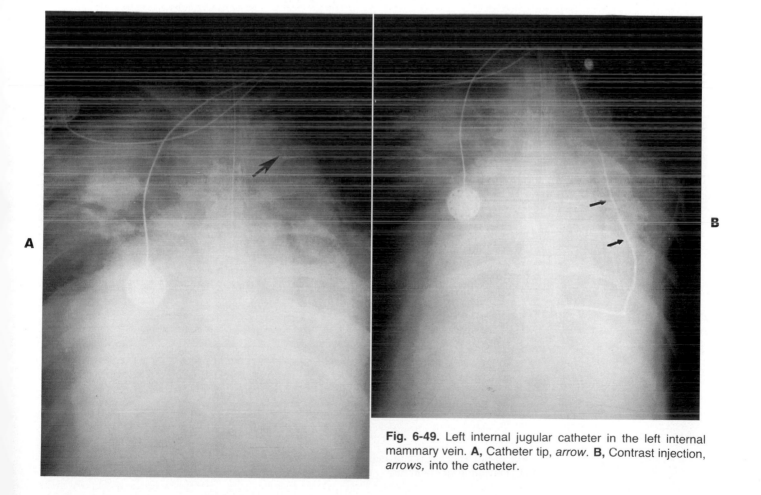

Fig. 6-49. Left internal jugular catheter in the left internal mammary vein. **A,** Catheter tip, *arrow.* **B,** Contrast injection, *arrows,* into the catheter.

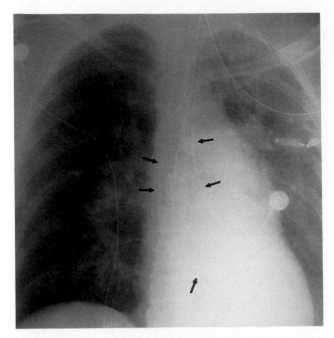

Fig. 6-50. Left subclavian Swan-Ganz catheter, *arrows,* passes through an ostium primum atrial septal defect and the left ventricle to the ascending aorta. It occulted the left sub-clavian artery when the balloon was inflated.

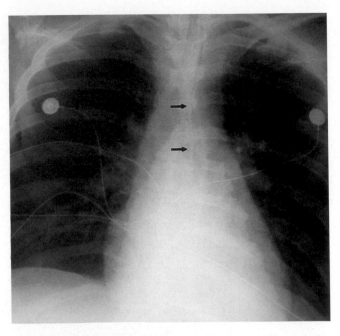

Fig. 6-51. Right subclavian catheter, *arrows,* in the subclavian artery and ascending aorta.

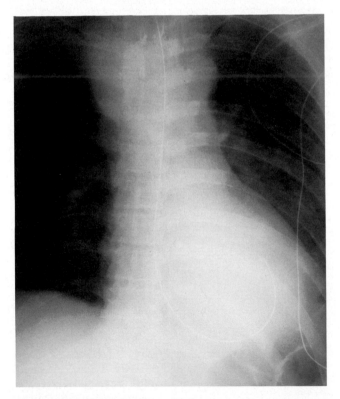

Fig. 6-52. Right superior mediastinal hematoma after right subclavian artery puncture.

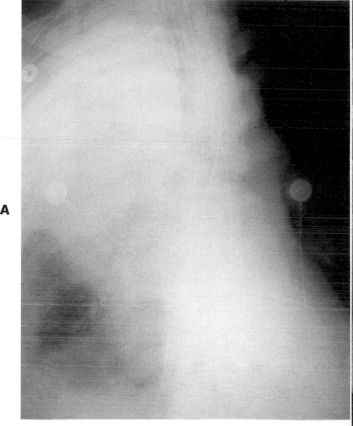

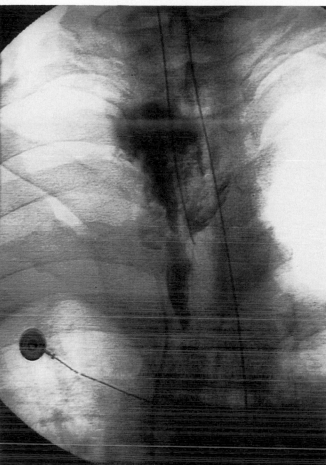

Fig. 6-53. A, Large right hemothorax after laceration of the right internal jugular vein at an attempted Swan-Ganz catheter insertion. **B,** Contrast extravasation from the jugular vein at venography.

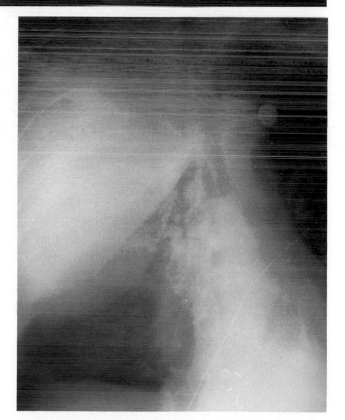

Fig. 6-54. Large right extrapleural hematoma from avulsion of the right internal mammary artery near its origin during subclavian dialysis catheter insertion.

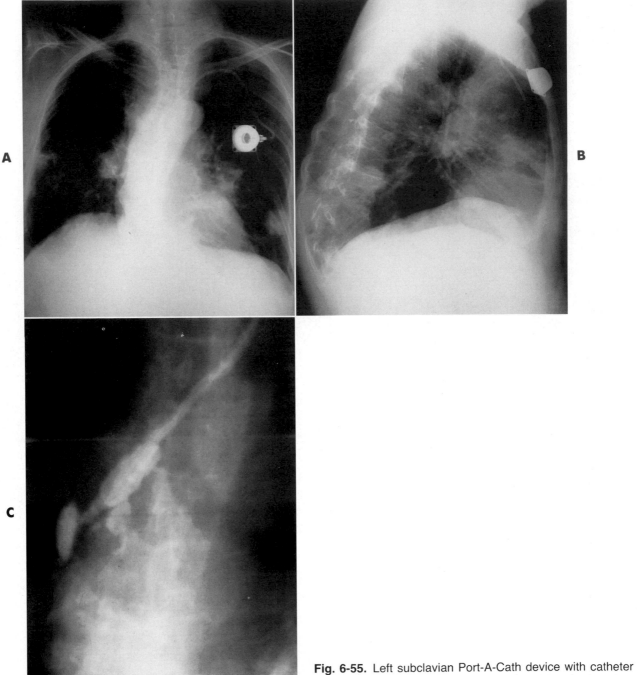

Fig. 6-55. Left subclavian Port-A-Cath device with catheter tip in the anterior mediastinum in an extravascular location. Frontal, **A,** and lateral, **B,** views. **C,** Contrast injection.

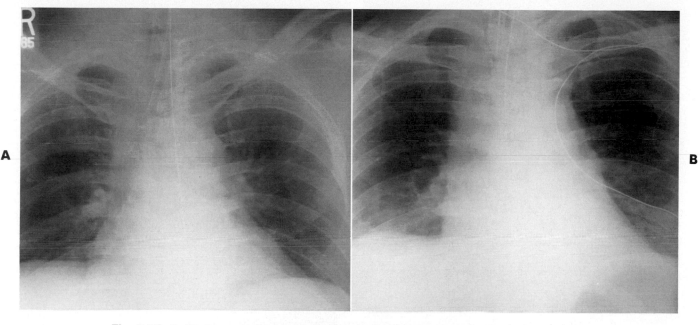

Fig. 6-56. A, Radiograph obtained immediately after left subclavian catheter insertion. **B,** Radiograph after overnight infusion of 1200 ml of fluid into the mediastinum. Notice the mediastinal widening.

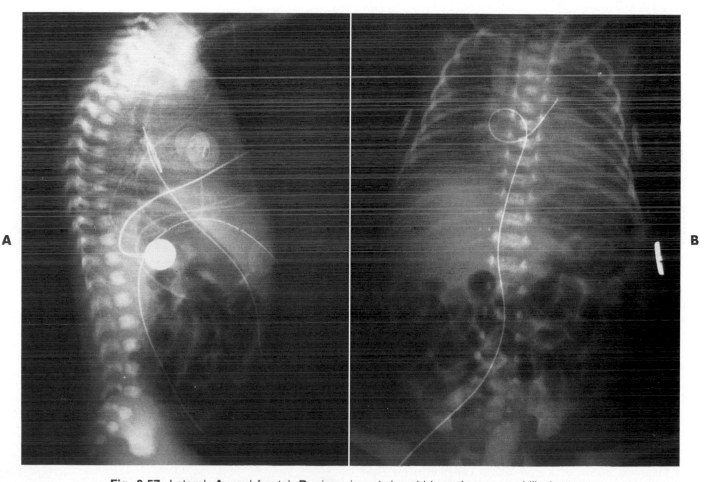

Fig. 6-57. Lateral, **A,** and frontal, **B,** views in a 1-day-old boy show an umbilical artery catheter looped in the right atrium and then passing to the left atrium.

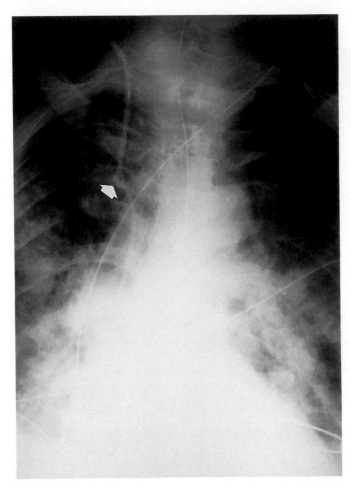

Fig. 6-58. Knot, *arrow,* in right jugular Swan-Ganz catheter.

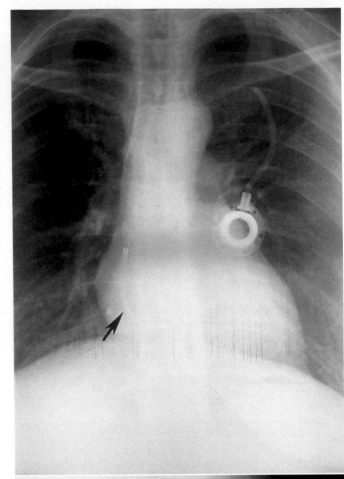

A

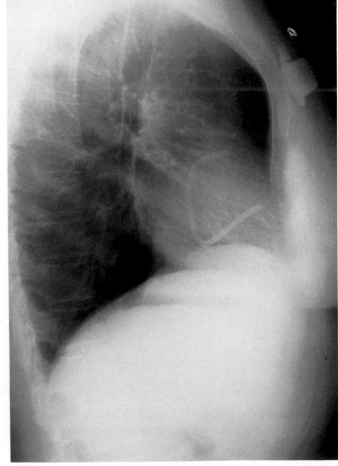

B

Fig. 6-59. Frontal, **A,** and lateral, **B,** chest radiographs show a fragment, *arrow,* of a Port-A-Cath catheter in the right atrium and right ventricle. The fragment was successfully removed via the inferior vena cava with a guidewire snare.

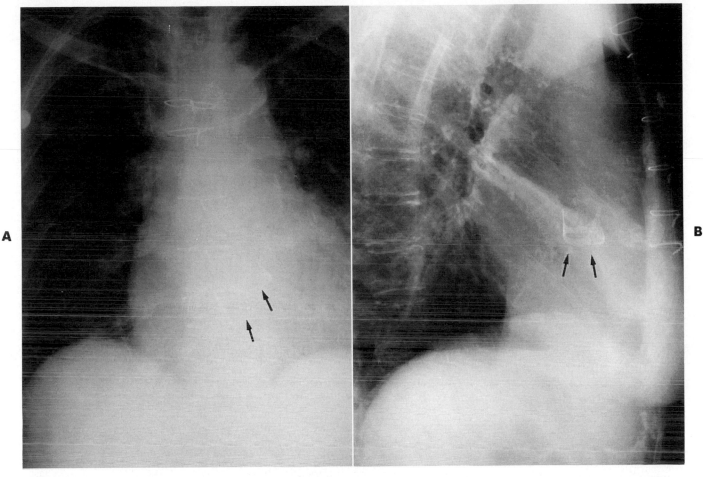

Fig. 6-60. Frontal, **A,** and lateral, **B,** views show Ionescu-Shiley pericardial valve prosthesis (xenograft) in the aortic position, *arrows.*

Heart Valves

Heart valve prostheses have been used successfully since the 1960s, with more than 50 different models having been introduced in the interval. There are two basic types of valve prosthesis, mechanical and biological. Mechanical valves are composed of metals, polymers, and ceramics. They are basically an occluder moving passively with changes in pressure and flow within the heart. Most require lifelong anticoagulation. Biologic valves contain tissue from human cadavers (homografts), porcine aortic cusps, or bovine pericardium (xenografts). They are less durable than mechanical valves, with some deterioration frequent at 5 years, but they do not usually require anticoagulation.

Because of the number and the complexity of the heart valves that have been introduced over the years, this chapter cannot explore them in depth. Some of the more common and important findings associated with heart valves are illustrated in Figs. 6-60 to 6-66. For a more thorough coverage of the subject, refer to the excellent review of Steiner[23] and articles listed in the Bibliography, p. 215.

Cardiac Pacemakers

A cardiac pacemaker is composed of two main elements: (1) a pulse generator and (2) lead wires with electrodes for contact with the endocardium or myocardium. Cardiac pacemakers were first used clinically in the 1960s, with stainless steel electrodes sewn directly onto the myocardium and attached to a fixed-rate pulse generator implanted in the subcutaneous tissues of the upper abdomen. Since then, there have been many advances, including small-caliber fracture-resistant transvenous leads and programmable dual-chamber atrioventricular pulse generators.

Mercury-zinc and nickel-cadmium batteries have been replaced by lithium iodide ones with much greater longevity. The radiology of cardiac pacemakers has been thoroughly reviewed by Steiner and his colleagues to which you are referred for more complete coverage.[24] (See also articles and books listed in the Bibliography, p. 215.) A modern pulse generator with a short length of lead is shown in Fig. 6-67. A single-lead intramyocardial pacer electrode may be appropriate in one patient (Fig. 6-68), whereas a right atrial–left ventricular syn-

Text continued on p. 195.

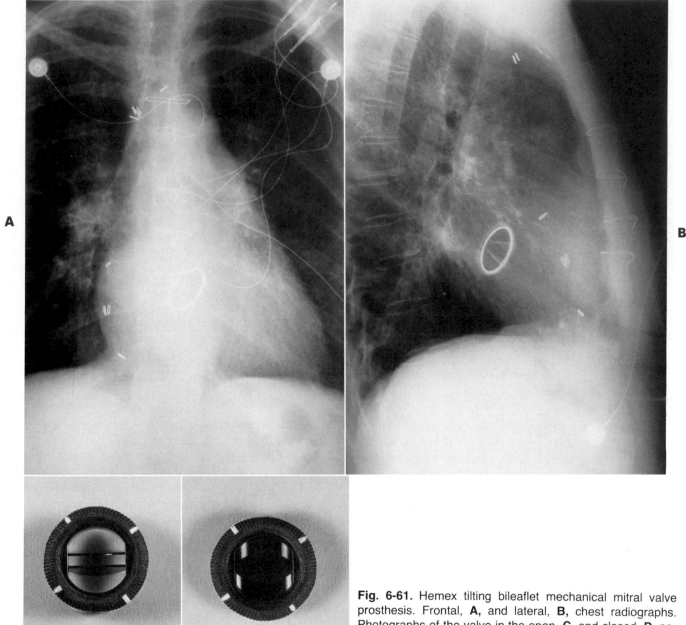

Fig. 6-61. Hemex tilting bileaflet mechanical mitral valve prosthesis. Frontal, **A,** and lateral, **B,** chest radiographs. Photographs of the valve in the open, **C,** and closed, **D,** positions.

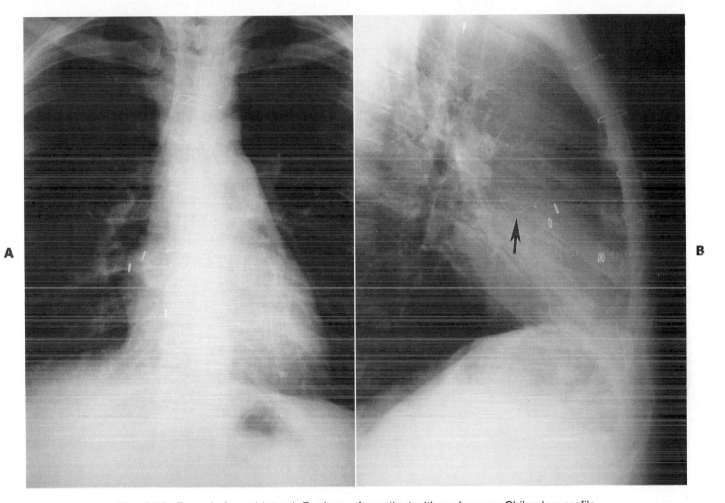

Fig. 6-62. Frontal, **A,** and lateral, **B,** views of a patient with an Ionescu-Shiley low-profile bovine pericardial aortic valve prosthesis. Wire arcs of the base ring are well seen in the lateral view, **B,** *arrow,* but obscured by the spine on the frontal view.

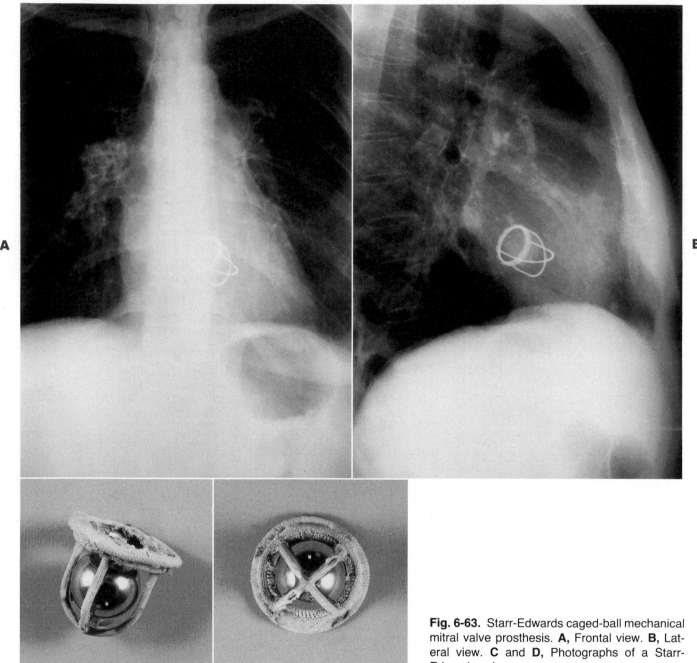

Fig. 6-63. Starr-Edwards caged-ball mechanical mitral valve prosthesis. **A,** Frontal view. **B,** Lateral view. **C** and **D,** Photographs of a Starr-Edwards valve.

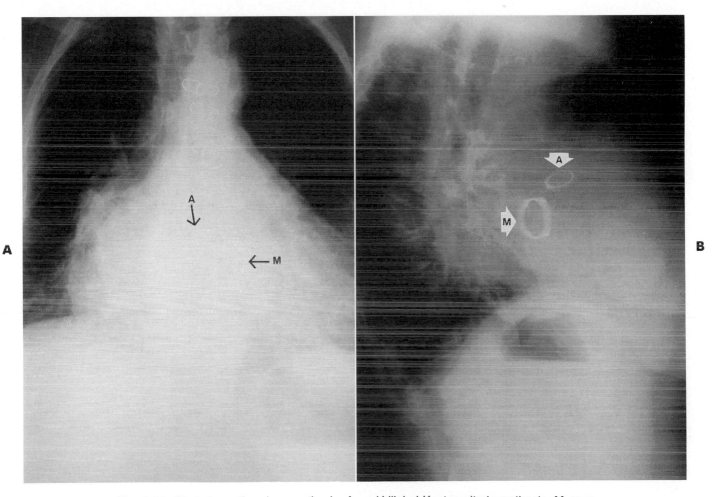

Fig. 6-64. St. Jude aortic valve prosthesis, *A,* and Lillehei-Kaster mitral prosthesis, *M,* seen better on the lateral view than on the frontal view. **A,** Frontal view. **B,** Lateral view.

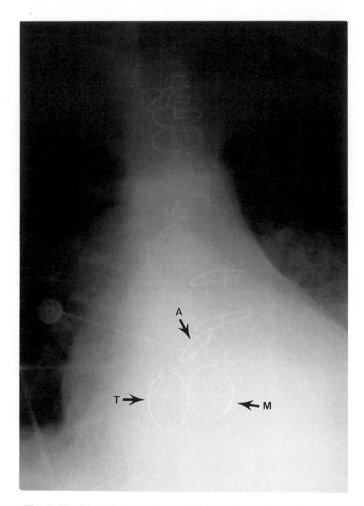

Fig. 6-65. Metallic base rings of Hancock porcine valve prostheses in the tricuspid, *T;* mitral, *M;* and aortic, *A,* positions.

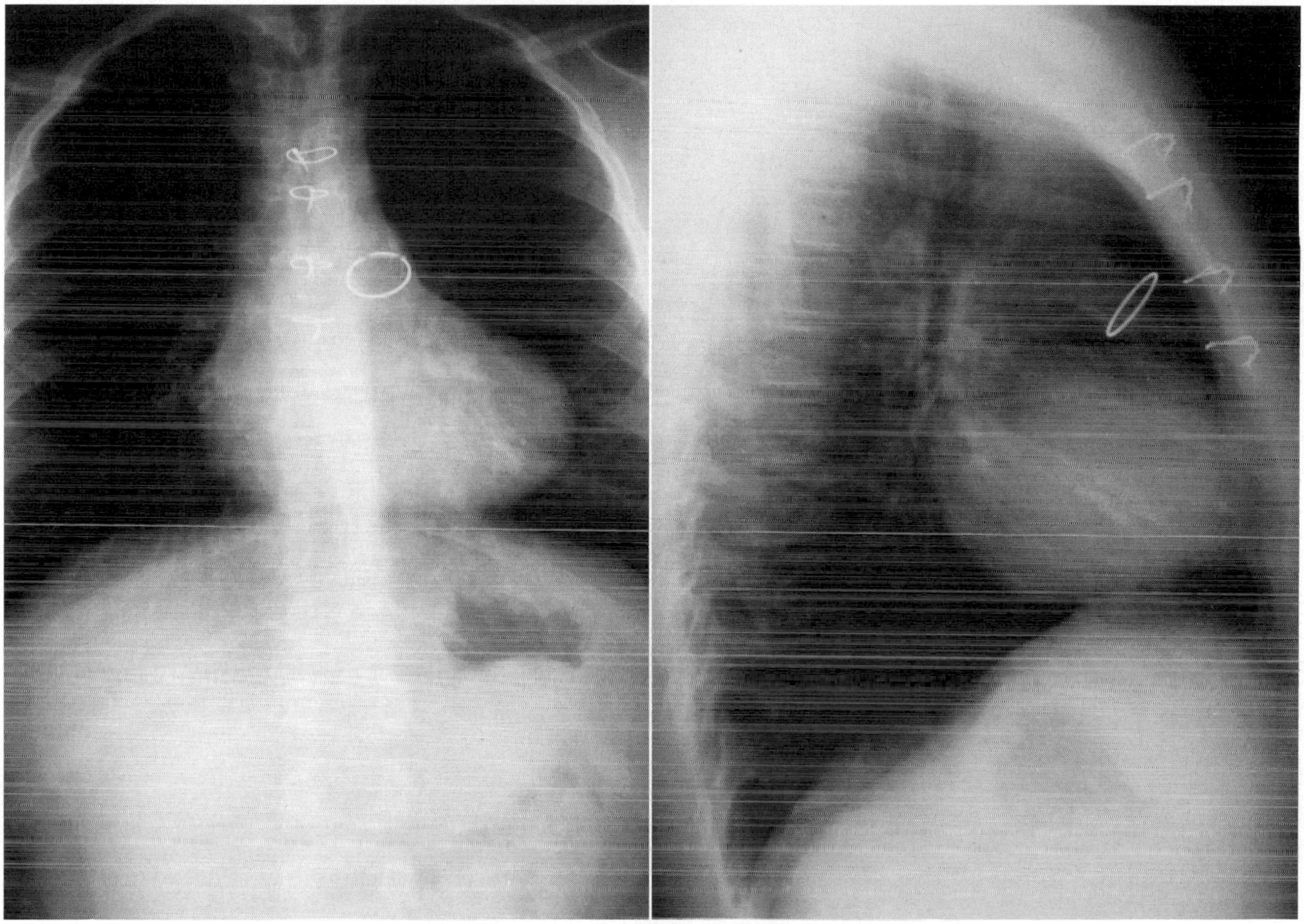

Fig. 6-66. Frontal, **A,** and lateral, **B,** views showing a Hancock porcine valve prosthesis in Rastelli conduit from the right ventricle to the pulmonary artery.

Continued.

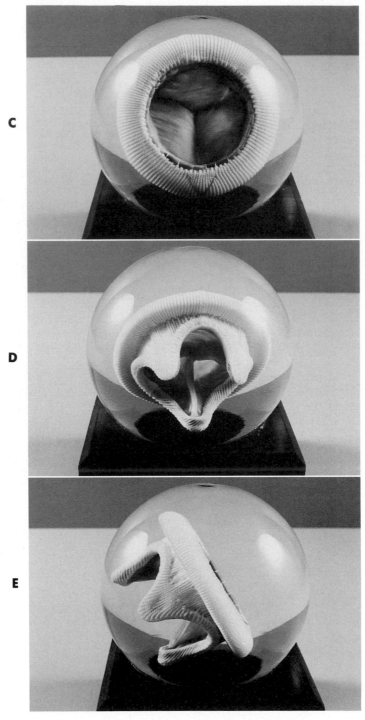

Fig. 6-66, cont'd. C to E, Three photographic views of a Hancock porcine valve prosthesis.

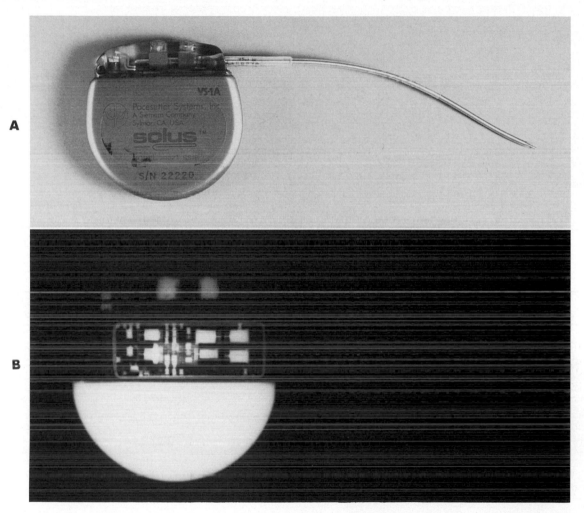

Fig. 6-67. Photograph, **A,** and radiograph, **B,** of Solus pulse generator by Pacesetter (Siemens).

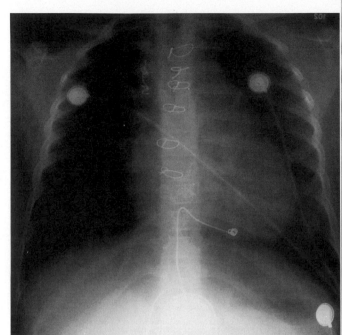

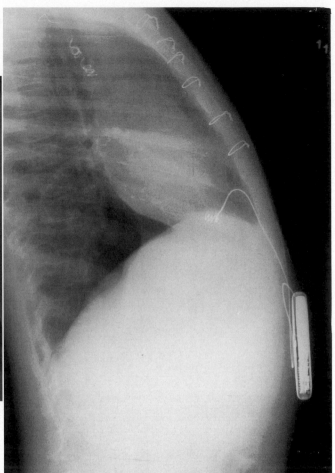

Fig. 6-68. Frontal, **A,** and lateral, **B,** views of a single-electrode epicardial "corkscrew" subxiphoid pacemaker implantation.

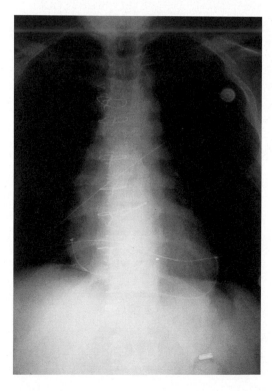

Fig. 6-69. Intrapericardial atrioventricular synchronous epicardial subxiphoid pacing apparatus.

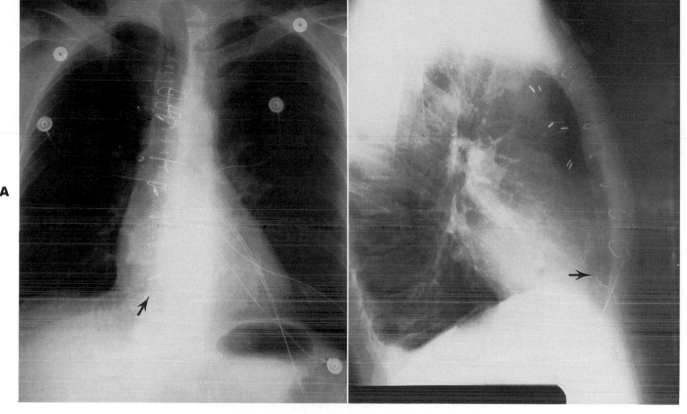

Fig. 6-70. Frontal, **A,** and lateral, **B,** views of temporary epicardial pacemaker leads, *arrow,* in a patient with recent cardiac surgery.

chronous intrapericardial transthoracic device is indicated in another (Fig. 6-69).

Temporary, easily removable epicardial electrodes are now commonly placed at the time of cardiac surgery for immediate pacemaker access, should the need arise. The leads are simply pulled out through the incision when the patient is discharged from the hospital (Fig. 6-70). Transvenous (perivenous) pacemaker leads are the most common today, inserted via the subclavian or jugular vein under local anesthesia (Figs. 6-71 and 6-72).

Mechanical fixation devices (such as plastic tines) have greatly reduced the incidence of dislodged pacemaker leads, often a significant problem in their early development.[25] With fluoroscopic control of implantation, malposition of leads is uncommon. Placement in the coronary sinus is now rarely deliberate (Fig. 6-73). A position too far to the left may indicate perforation of the interventricular septum (Fig. 6-74).

Once the electrode is properly positioned, with satisfactory thresholds of power for pacing and sensing, the pulse generator is connected and placed in a subcutaneous pocket in the chest wall (see Figs. 6-71 to 6-73). If the pocket is too large, the generator may retract the lead from the endocardium, particularly if the patient twists it around in the pocket ("twiddler's syndrome"). A unipolar pacemaker, in which one surface of the pulse generator is the anode, can also change position in a large pouch. If the pacemaker is flipped, the subcutaneous anode comes to lie against the pectoralis muscle. Pectoralis myopotentials can mimic those of the heart and inhibit demand pacemaker function. Pacing of the muscle rather than of the heart can also occur in this situation ("counterclockwise syndrome")[26] (Fig. 6-75).

Lead fracture is now rarely seen because of improvements in the flexibility of the metal alloys used in electrode construction. Even when they are broken, the ends frequently do not separate, and so the radiograph does not show the fracture. Electronic testing has largely replaced radiography in cases of suspected lead malfunction.

The automatic implantable cardioverter defibrillator (AICD) consists of two shocking electrodes, two sensing electrodes, and a generator implanted in the abdominal wall. It is being increasingly used for the long-term treatment of ventricular arrhythmias and is easily recognized on chest films[27-29] (Figs. 6-76 and 6-77).

Text continued on p. 203.

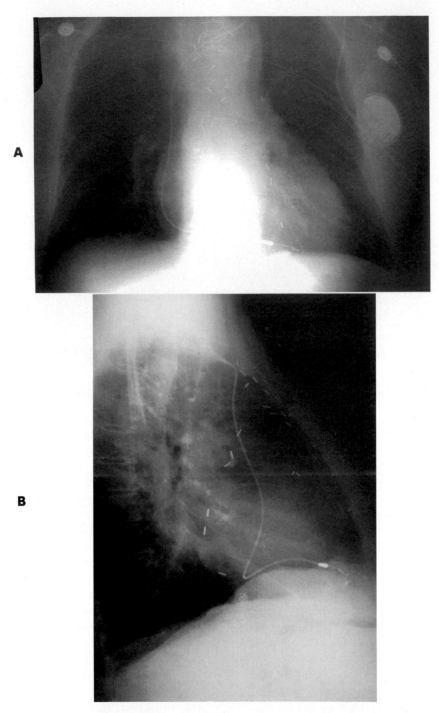

Fig. 6-71. Frontal, **A,** and lateral, **B,** views showing a transvenous pacemaker lead with electrode at or near the apex of the right ventricle.

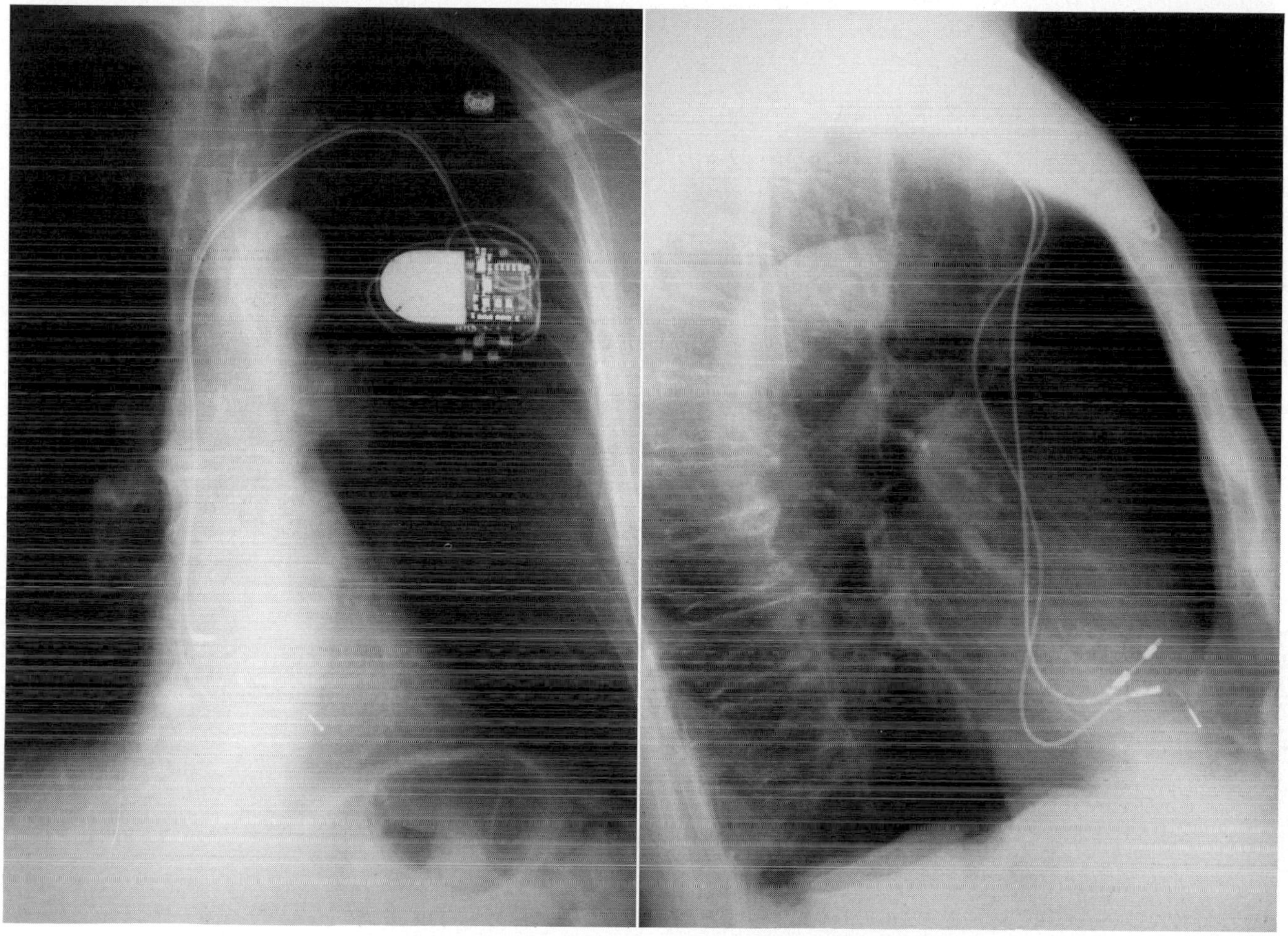

Fig. 6-72. Frontal, **A,** and lateral, **B,** views showing a transvenous atrioventricular sequential pacer with one electrode in the right atrial appendage and the other at the right ventricular apex.

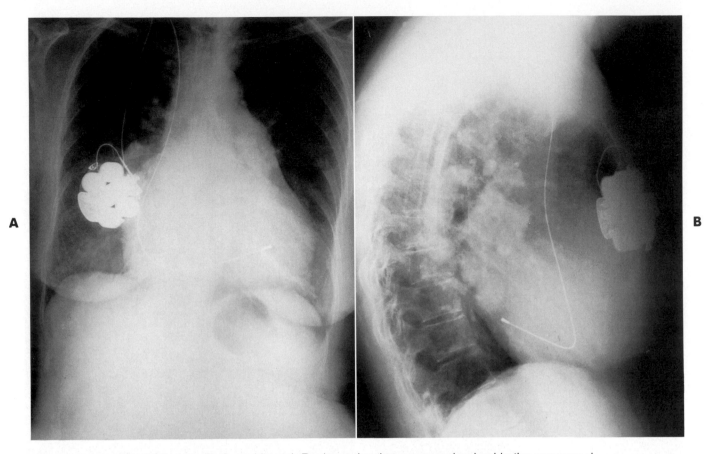

Fig. 6-73. Frontal, **A,** and lateral, **B,** views showing a pacemaker lead in the coronary sinus. The electrode is above the right ventricular apex on the frontal view and much posterior to it on the lateral view.

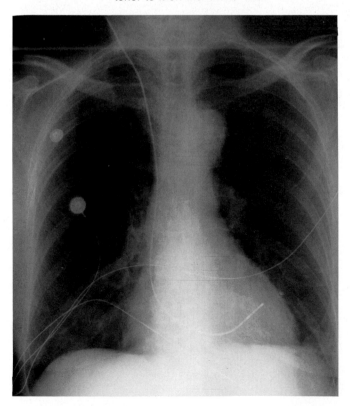

Fig. 6-74. Frontal view of temporary pacemaker lead pacing the left ventricle in a patient with a fresh anterior myocardial infarction.

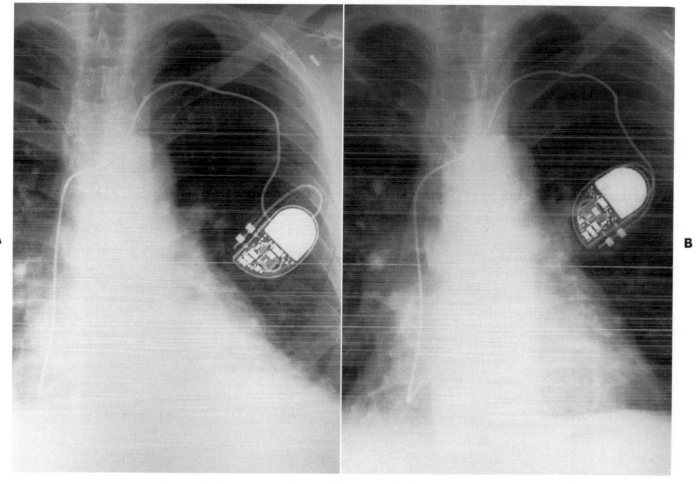

Fig. 6-75. Initial position, **A,** and position when the pacemaker stimulates the pectoralis muscle, **B.** The pulse generator has undergone a 180-degree flip.

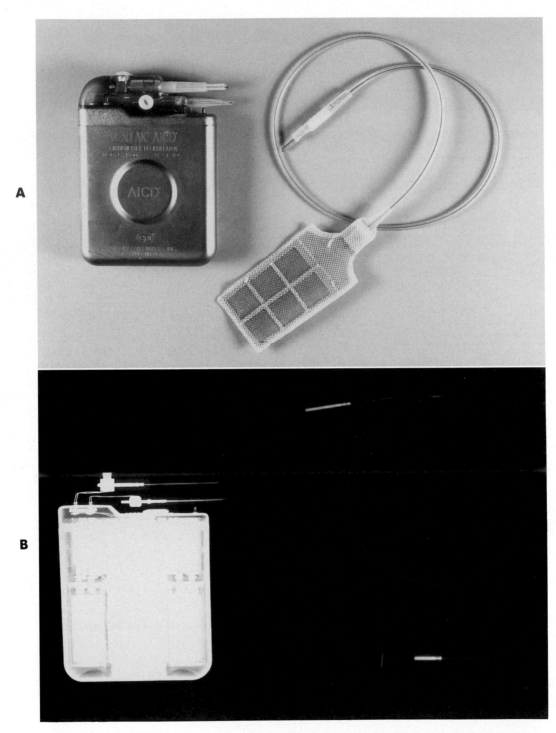

Fig. 6-76. Photograph, **A,** and radiograph, **B,** of automatic implantable cardioverter defibrillator (AICD) device. Generator, *left,* and titanium mesh patch electrode, *right.*

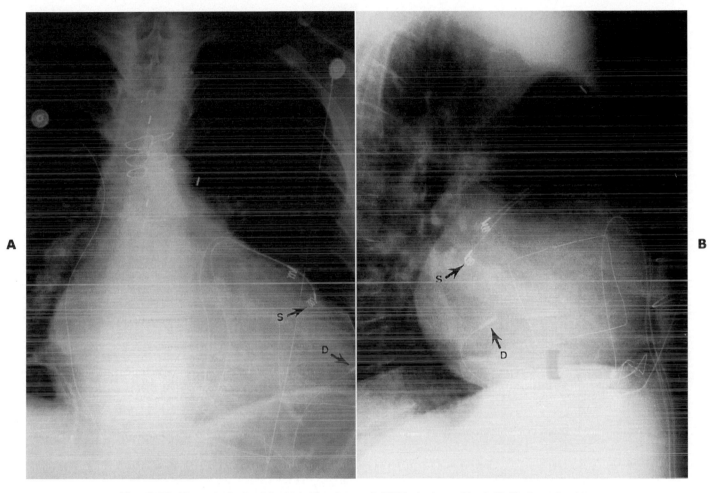

Fig. 6-77. Frontal, **A,** and lateral, **B,** views of AICD device with defibrillating shocking electrodes, *D,* on right atrium and left ventricle and epicardial sensing electrodes, *S,* in the left ventricle.

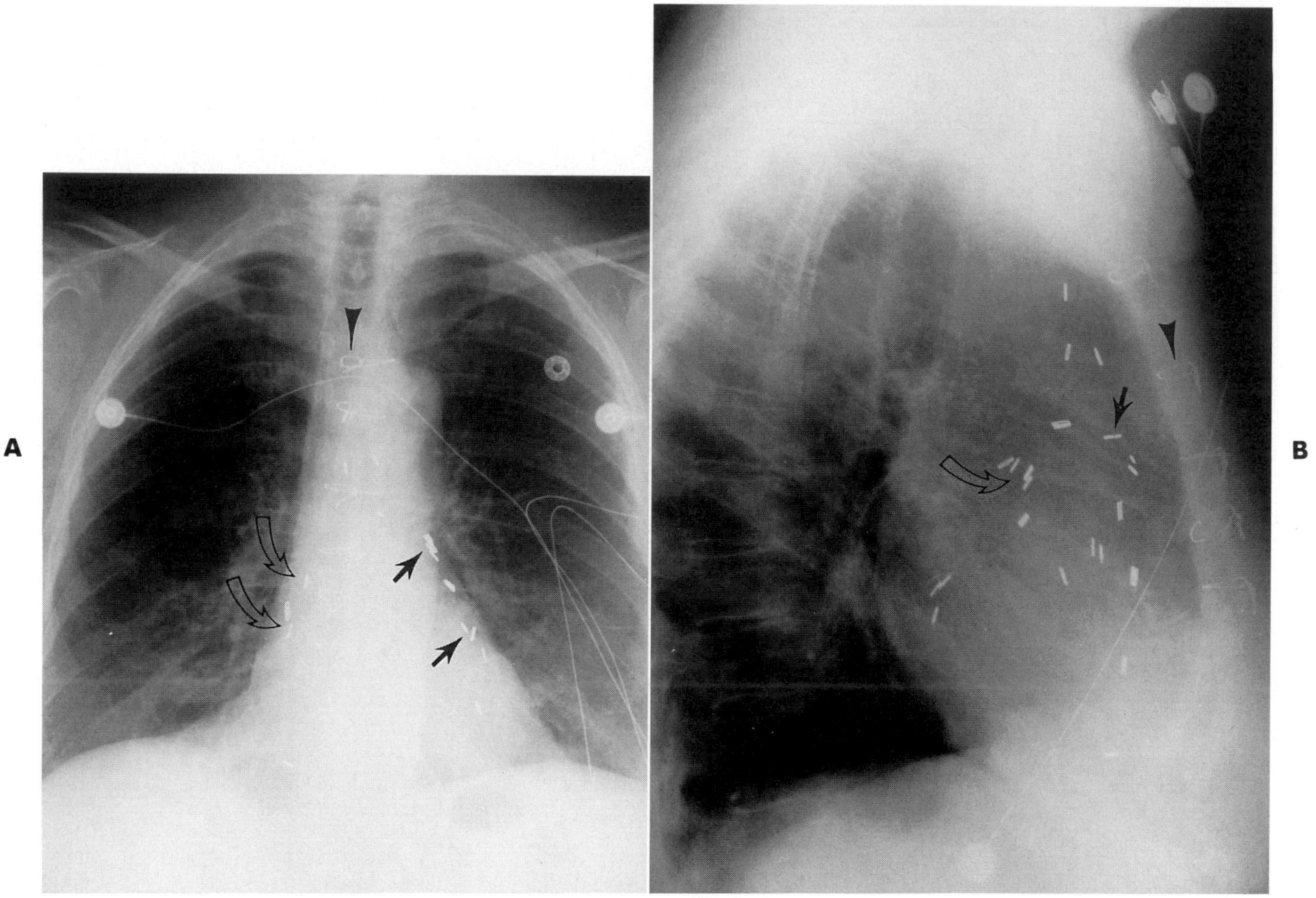

Fig. 6-78. Frontal, **A,** and lateral, **B,** views showing sternal wires *(arrowhead),* vascular clips of saphenous vein bypass graft to the right coronary artery *(curved open arrows),* and those of the left internal mammary graft to left anterior descending artery *(solid arrows).*

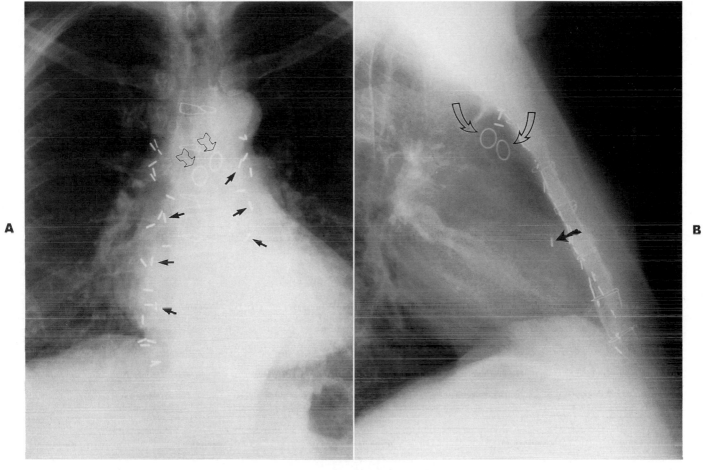

Fig. 6-79. Frontal, **A,** and lateral, **B,** views showing vascular clips of bilateral (left and right) internal mammary artery bypass grafts, *solid arrows,* and marker rings on the ascending aorta around the ostia of two saphenous vein bypass grafts, *open arrows.*

CORONARY ARTERY SURGERY

(See also Chapter 10.)

Since 1967, when the first aortocoronary saphenous vein bypass graft was performed, direct myocardial revascularization has gained wide acceptance. Surgical techniques have evolved and been refined over the years, and they can vary considerably from center to center, which is reflected in the variety of devices seen in the postoperative chest films of these patients.

Median sternotomy is the usual surgical approach, and the use of sternal wires is the common method of fixation of the two sternal segments (Figs. 6-78 to 6-81). Vascular clips are used to occlude tributary branches of saphenous vein grafts and anterior intercostal branches of the internal mammary arteries. There may be a few clips or a great many, depending on the number and types of grafts used (Figs. 6-78 to 6-80).

Some surgeons place markers on the adventitia of the ascending aorta to indicate the proximal anastomoses of the bypass grafts. These markers, which facilitate subsequent graft angiography, vary considerably from center to center and even from surgeon to surgeon (Figs. 6-79 to 6-81).

CIRCULATORY ASSIST DEVICES

The high mortality of cardiogenic shock continues to spur efforts to develop mechanical support for the circulatory system. Most devices currently available provide temporary assistance until the damaged heart can recover, or a donor heart becomes available for transplantation.[30-33] Permanent implantable artificial hearts may soon be a reality.[34-35]

The intra-aortic counterpulsation balloon device is used to support the circulation after cardiac surgery or acute myocardial infarction until the heart recovers adequate function of its own. The device consists of an inflatable balloon approximately 25 cm long mounted on a catheter which is introduced via a femoral artery.

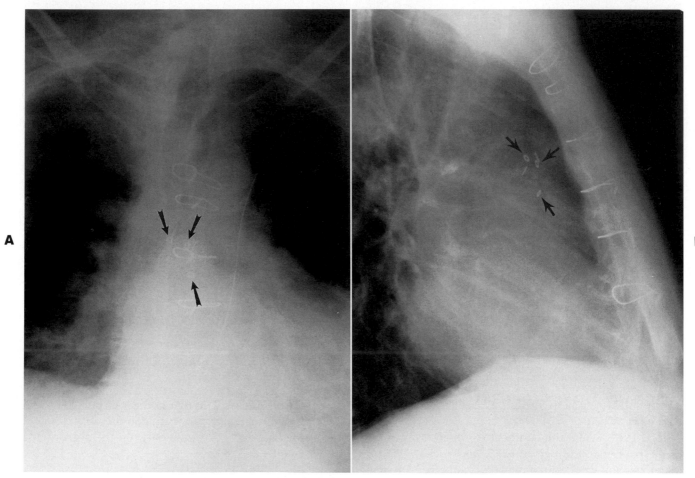

Fig. 6-80. Frontal, **A,** and lateral, **B,** views with small washers positioned immediately above the ostia of three saphenous vein bypass grafts, *arrows.*

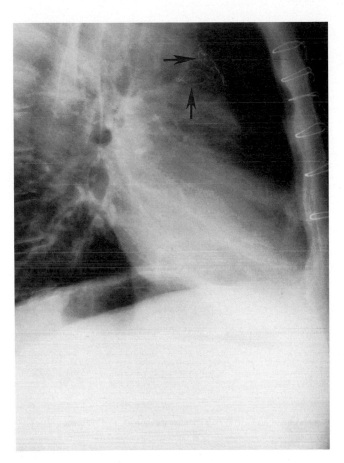

Fig. 6-81. Lateral radiograph with wire loop markers around the ostia of saphenous vein bypass grafts, *arrows.*

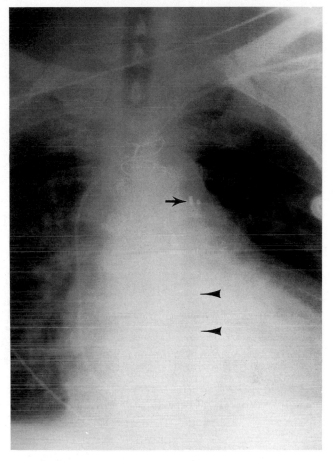

Fig. 6-82. Frontal view showing metal tip, *arrow,* of intra-aortic balloon pump (IABP) in the upper descending thoracic aorta. Gas in the balloon is faintly seen through the heart, *arrowheads.*

The tip of the catheter is placed just distal to the left subclavian artery in the descending thoracic aorta (Fig. 6-82). The balloon is inflated with gas (carbon dioxide) during ventricular diastole to augment diastolic coronary artery perfusion and reduce left ventricular afterload. This improves cardiac function by both increasing the oxygenation and decreasing the work requirements of the myocardium.

Ventricular assist devices (VAD) may be univentricular or biventricular. For example, the Novacor left ventricular assist device (Fig. 6-83) is an implantable electrically driven pump that takes blood through a Dacron conduit from the apex of the left ventricle and pumps it through another Dacron conduit to the aorta. The device is implanted subcutaneously in the left upper abdomen, with power lines and sensors exiting through the right lower quadrant to connect with a control console. Its main use has been as a bridge to cardiac transplantation.[36]

The extracorporeal nonimplantable devices may also be univentricular or biventricular. One example is the Symbion Biventricular assist device, which has a diaphragm in each ventricular unit propelled by compressed air (Fig. 6-84). Implantation usually requires cardiopulmonary bypass. Blood from the right or left atrium is withdrawn to the pump with unidirectional mechanical valves at the inflow and outflow ports. The outflow conduit is a Dacron graft anastomosed to the ascending aorta or pulmonary artery. These devices can provide long periods of support for one or both ventricles, they are relatively easy to implant, and they are commercially available.

The total artificial heart requires removal of the native heart. It serves as a bridge to cardiac transplantation but occasionally becomes the permanent circulatory support for the rest of the patient's life. The best known is probably the Jarvik heart, a pneumatically driven biventricular device completely replacing the native heart within the pericardial sac (Figs. 6-85 and 6-86). The polyurethane ventricles contain a diaphragm

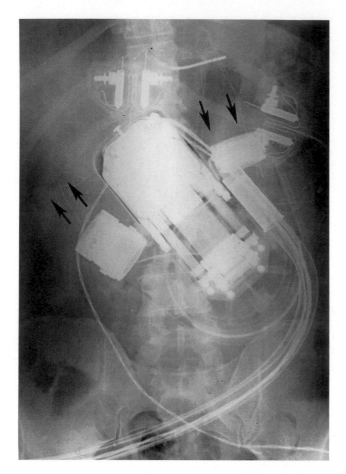

Fig. 6-83. Frontal film of the abdomen with Novacor left ventricular assist device implanted in the abdominal wall. The Dacron conduits to and from the heart are nonopaque, *arrows*. There is no hint of the device on chest films.

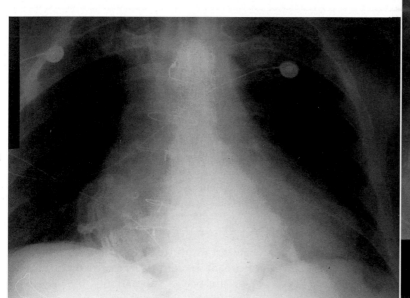

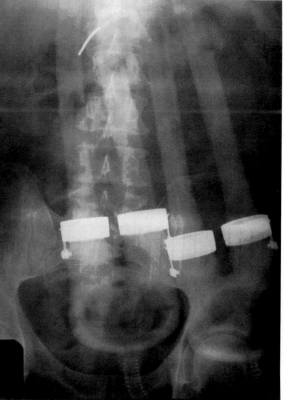

Fig. 6-84. Frontal chest, **A,** and abdominal, **B,** radiographs of biventricular assist device lying on the patient's abdomen. Conduits connect it to the two atria, aorta, and pulmonary artery. The conduits are not radiopaque.

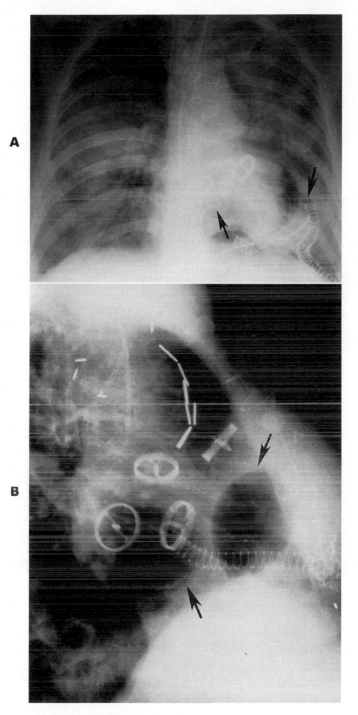

Fig. 6-85. Frontal, **A,** and lateral, **B,** views showing a Jarvik-7/70 heart with its four prosthetic valves and coil-reinforced polyurethane tubing carrying pulses of compressed air to the two artificial ventricles, *arrows.*

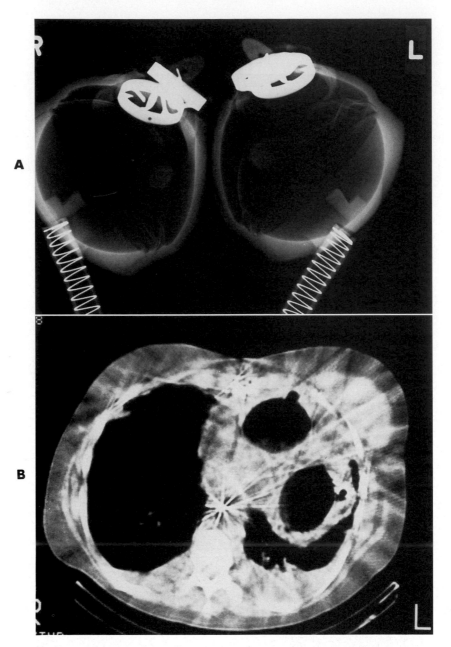

Fig. 6-86. A, Radiograph of Jarvik-7/70 device. **B,** CT scan of implanted Jarvik-7/70 device.

that retracts during diastole, drawing blood from the atria, and then is displaced forward by compressed air during systole, forcing blood into the aorta and pulmonary artery. This device is used when there is global cardiac dysfunction not likely to be reversible, with good prospects of cardiac transplantation within a few weeks.

Circulatory assistance devices will continue to improve with newer materials, miniaturization, and new power sources. Fully portable left ventricular assist devices are now a reality, and a totally implantable artificial heart will undoubtedly be developed in the foreseeable future.

MISCELLANEOUS DEVICES

From time to time, other medical devices not commonly found in this location or not well known are seen on chest radiographs. A few examples are shown (Figs. 6-87 to 6-92), including Gianturco coils, remote telemetry ECG monitoring devices, and a Sideris atrial septal defect patch device.

Left atrial catheters (LACs) are sometimes seen after cardiac surgery.[37] They are used to monitor left atrial pressure, provide a ready access for blood samples, or provide a route for the instillation of medicine. A left

Text continued on p. 214.

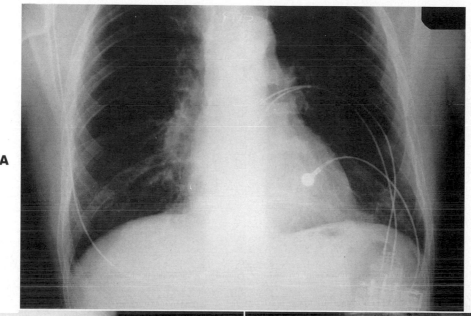

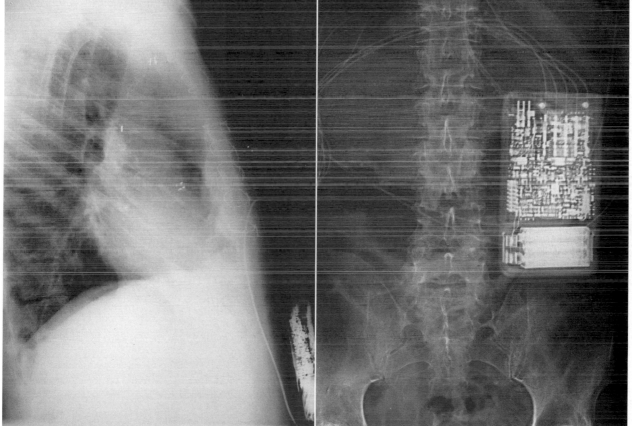

Fig. 6-87. Frontal, **A,** and lateral, **B,** chest radiographs show ECG electrodes on the chest connected to a telemetry transmitter strapped to the patient's abdomen. **C,** Remote ECG telemetry device strapped to abdomen.

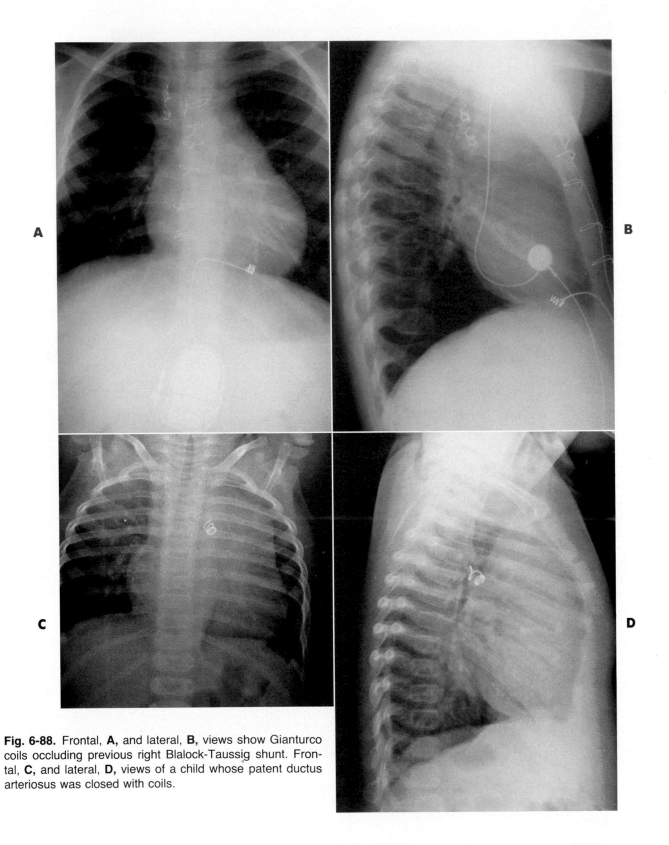

Fig. 6-88. Frontal, **A,** and lateral, **B,** views show Gianturco coils occluding previous right Blalock-Taussig shunt. Frontal, **C,** and lateral, **D,** views of a child whose patent ductus arteriosus was closed with coils.

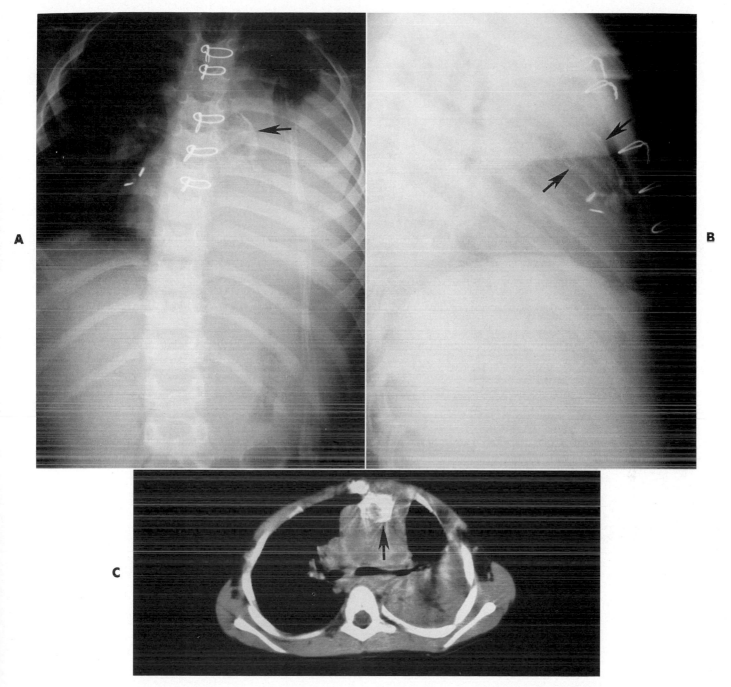

Fig. 6-89. Frontal, **A,** and lateral, **B,** views show calcification in a Rastelli right ventricle to pulmonary artery conduit, *arrows*. Axial CT scan, **C,** shows dense calcification of the conduit between the heart and sternum, *arrow*.

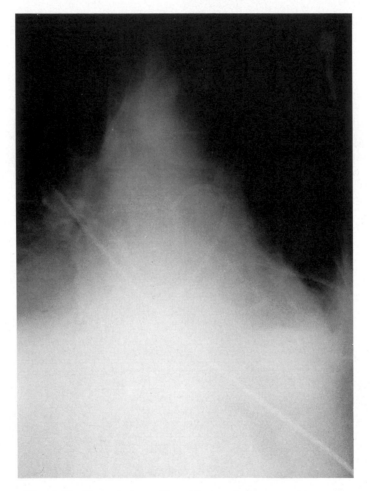

Fig. 6-90. Frontal chest film with two drainage catheters in the pericardial sac.

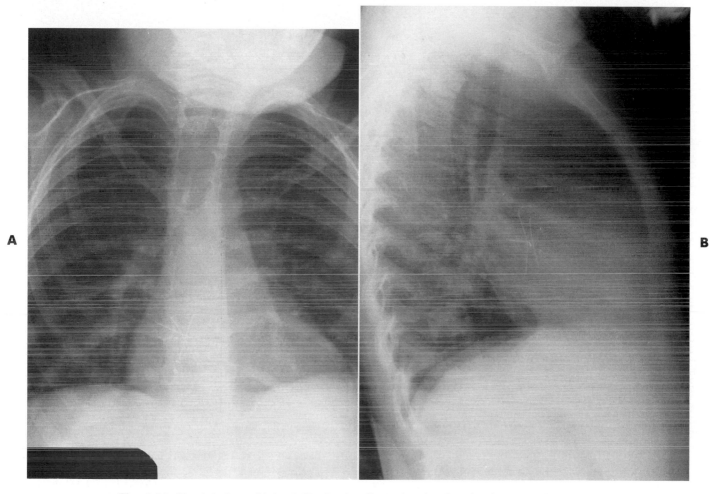

Fig. 6-91. Frontal, **A,** and lateral, **B,** chest radiographs showing the three metal struts of Sideris atrial septal defect patch device.

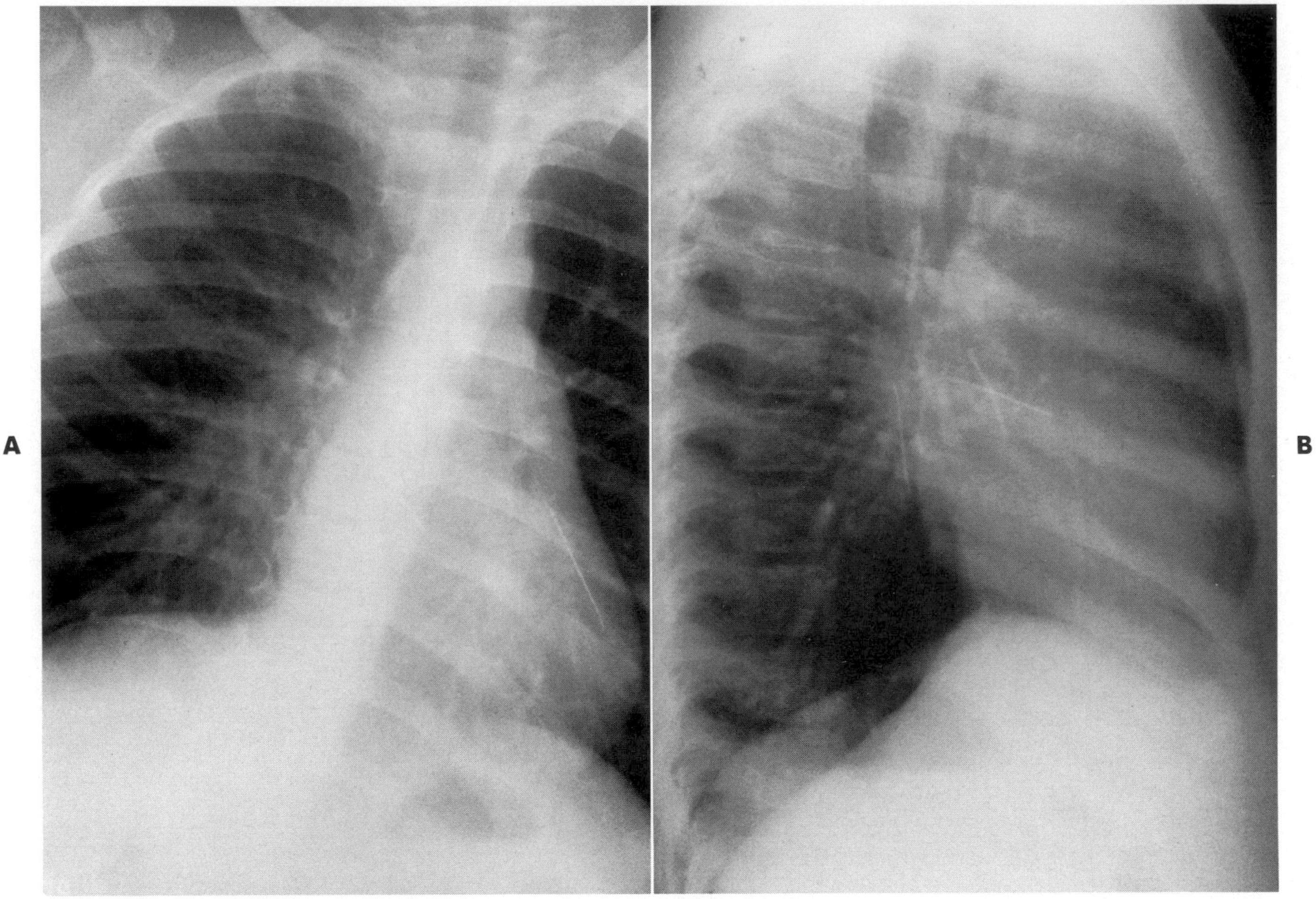

Fig. 6-92. Frontal, **A,** and lateral, **B,** chest radiographs showing detached right atrial component of the Sideris device in left lower lobe pulmonary artery branch.

atrial catheter is typically inserted at the end of cardiac surgery with the aid of a needle placed into the right superior pulmonary vein near its junction with the left atrium.[37] The needle is removed, and the catheter is held in place by loose sutures in the left atrium. The catheter's proximal end is brought out through the chest wall. Left atrial catheters are usually retained only for short periods. On radiographic studies, they typically appear as thin metallic lines in the left atrium. As with all other catheters, there are a number of possible complications with the use of LACs, including catheter malposition, breakage, infection, distant embolization, cardiac tamponade, and interference with the proper functioning of a prosthetic heart valve.[37]

REFERENCES

1. Ravin CE, Putman CE, McLoud TC: Hazards of the intensive care unit, *AJR* 126:423-431, 1976.
2. Wechsler RJ, Steiner RM, Kinori I: Monitoring the monitors: the radiology of thoracic catheters, wires and tubes, *Semin Roentgenol* 23:61-84, 1988.
3. Miller KS, Sahn SA: Chest tubes: indications, technique, management and complications, *Chest* 91:258-264, 1987.
4. Millikan JS, Moore EE, Steiner E, et al: Complications of tube thoracostomy for acute trauma, *Am J Surg* 140:738-741, 1980.
5. Daly RC, Mucha P, Pairolero PC, Farnell MB: The risk of percutaneous chest tube thoracostomy for blunt thoracic trauma, *Ann Emerg Med* 14:865-870, 1985.
6. Fraser RS: Lung perforation complicating tube thoracostomy: pathologic description of three cases, *Hum Pathol* 19:518-523, 1988.
7. Stark DD, Federle MP, Goodman PC: CT and radiographic assessment of tube thoracostomy, *AJR* 141:253-258, 1983.
8. Webb WR, LaBerge JM: Radiographic recognition of chest tube malposition in the major fissure, *Chest* 85:81-83, 1984.

9. Goodman LR, Conrardy PA, Laing F, Singer MM: Radiographic evaluation of endotracheal tube position, *AJR* 127:433-434, 1976.

10. Kaufman JL, Nissenblatt MJ: New options for central venous access in cancer chemotherapy: multiple lumen catheters, *Am Surg* 52:105-107, 1986.

11. Abraham E, Shapiro M, Podolsky S: Central venous catheterization in the emergency setting, *Crit Care Med* 11:515-517, 1983.

12. Baigrie RS, Morgan CD: Hemodynamic monitoring: catheter insertion techniques, complications and trouble-shooting, *Can Med Assoc J* 121:885-892, 1979.

13. Katz JD, Cronau LH, Barash PG, Mandel SD: Pulmonary artery flow-guided catheters in the perioperative period: indications and complications, *JAMA* 237:2832-2834, 1977.

14. McLoud TC, Putman CE: Radiology of the Swan-Ganz catheter and associated pulmonary complications, *Radiology* 116:19-22, 1975.

15. Hayson EA, Ravin CE, Kelly MJ, Curtis A McB: Intra-aortic counterpulsation balloon: radiographic considerations, *AJR* 128:915-918, 1977.

16. Dunbar RD, Mitchell R, Lavine M: Aberrant location of central venous catheters, *Lancet* 1:711-715, 1981.

17. Kubicka RA, Smith C: A primer on the pulmonary vasculature, *Med Radiogr Photogr* 61:14-28, 1985.

18. Henry DA, LeBolt S: Invasive hemodynamic monitoring: radiologists' perspective, *RadioGraphics* 6:535-572, 1986.

19. Scott WL: Complications associated with central venous catheters: a survey, *Chest* 94:1221-1224, 1988.

20. Weiner P, Sznajder I, Plavnick L, et al: Unusual complications of subclavian vein catheterization, *Crit Care Med* 12:538-539, 1984.

21. Hinke DH, Zandt-Stastny DA, Goodman LR, et al: Pinch off syndrome: a complication of implantable subclavian venous access devices, *Radiology* 177:353-356, 1990.

22. Hunt R, Hunter TB: Cardiac tamponade and death from perforation of the right atrium by a central venous catheter (Letter to the editor), *AJR* 151:1250, 1988.

23. Steiner RM, Olintz G, Morse D, et al: Radiology of cardiac valve prostheses, *RadioGraphics* 8:277, 1988.

24. Steiner RM, Tegtmeyer CJ, Morse D: The radiology of cardiac pacemakers, *RadioGraphics* 6:373-375, 1986.

25. Felice R, Hutton L, Klein G: Cardiac pacemaker leads: a radiographic perspective, *J Can Assoc Radiol* 35:20-23, 1984.

26. Karis JP, Ravin CE: Counterclockwise exit of cardiac pacemaker leads: sign of pulse-generator flip, *Radiology* 174:711-712, 1990.

27. Goodman LR, Troup PJ, Thorsen MK, Youker JE: Automatic implantable cardioverter-defibrillator: radiographic appearance, *Radiology* 155:571-573, 1985.

28. Lurie AL, Udoff EJ, Reid PJ: Automatic implantable cardioverter-defibrillator: appearance and complications, *AJR* 145:723-725, 1985.

29. Goodman LR, Almassi GH, Troup PJ, et al: Complications of automatic implantable cardioverter-defibrillators, *Radiology* 170:447-452, 1989.

30. Pierce WS: Artificial hearts and blood pumps in the treatment of profound heart failure, *Circulation* 68:883-888, 1983.

31. Hill JD: Bridging to cardiac transplantation, *Ann Thorac Surg* 47:167-171, 1989.

32. Ott RA, Mills TC, Eugene J, Gazzaniga AB: Clinical choices for circulatory assist devices, *ASAIO Trans* 36:792-798, 1990.

33. Magovern JA, Pierce WS: Mechanical circulatory assistance before heart transplantation. In Baumgartner WA, Reitz BA, Achuff SC, editors: *Heart and heart-lung transplantation,* Philadelphia, 1990, Saunders, pp 73-85.

34. Davis PK, Rosenberg G, Snyder AJ, Pierce WS: Current status of permanent total artifical hearts, *Ann Thorac Surg* 47:172-178, 1989.

35. Poirier VL: Can our society afford mechanical hearts? *ASAIO Trans* 37:540-544, 1991.

36. Portner PM, Oyer PE, Pennington DG, et al: Implantable electrical left ventricular assist system: bridge to transplantation and the future, *Ann Thorac Surg* 47:142-150, 1989.

37. Leitman BS, Naidich DP, McGuinness GM, McCauley DI: The left atrial catheter: its uses and complications, *Radiology* 185:611-612, 1992.

BIBLIOGRAPHY

Bodnar E, Frater R, editors: *Replacement cardiac valves,* New York, 1992, McGraw-Hill.

Landay MJ, Estrera AS, Bordlee RP: Cardiac valve reconstruction and replacement: a brief review, *RadioGraphics* 12:659-671, 1992.

Spirn PW, Gross GW, Wechsler RJ, Steiner RM: Radiology of the chest after thoracic surgery, *Semin Roentgenol* 23:9-31, 1988.

McGovern EM, Trastek VF, Pairolero PC, Payne S: Completion pneumonectomy: indications, complications, and results, *Ann Thorac Surg* 46:141-146, 1988.

Landay MJ, Mootz AR, Estrera AS: Apparatus seen on chest radiographs after cardiac surgery in adults, *Radiology* 174:477-482, 1990.

Carter AR, Sostman HD, Curtis AM, Swett HA: Thoracic alterations after cardiac surgery, *AJR* 140:475-481, 1983.

Katzberg RW, Whitehouse GH, deWeese JA: The early radiologic findings in the adult chest after cardiopulmonary bypass surgery, *Cardiovasc Radiol* 1:205-215, 1978.

Goodman LR: Postoperative chest radiograph. II. Alterations after major intrathoracic surgery, *AJR* 134:803-810, 1980.

Mandell VS, Nimkin K, Hoffer FA, Bridges ND: Devices for transcatheter closure of intracardiac defects, *AJR* 160:179-184, 1993.

7

Medical Devices and Foreign Bodies of the Breast

Laurie L. Fajardo

Various types of implants and medical devices as well as common and uncommon foreign bodies may be found within the breast. This chapter summarizes the range of medical devices as well as foreign bodies and uncommon materials that may manifest themselves in the breast radiographically.

BREAST IMPLANTS

Mammary prostheses are the most common implanted medical devices found in the breast. In the United States, only intraocular lenses, sutures, and dental materials are more frequently used than augmentation breast prostheses. Approximately 150,000 women undergo augmentation mammoplasty annually in the United States. The properties and characteristics of breast implants vary from manufacturer to manufacturer. They are produced with silicone or polyurethane envelopes that can be with a single or double lumen. The outer envelope may be either smooth or textured, and they are filled with saline or silicone fluid or gel. Several representative types of implants are illustrated in Figs. 7-1 to 7-5.

Requests for screening and diagnostic mammography

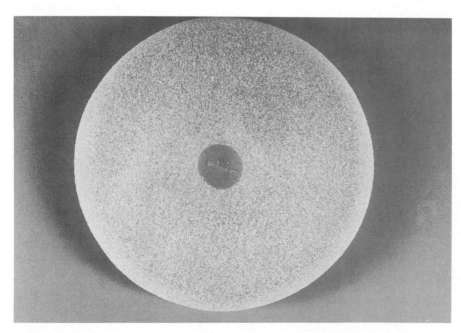

Fig. 7-1. Textured envelope, saline solution–filled breast implant.

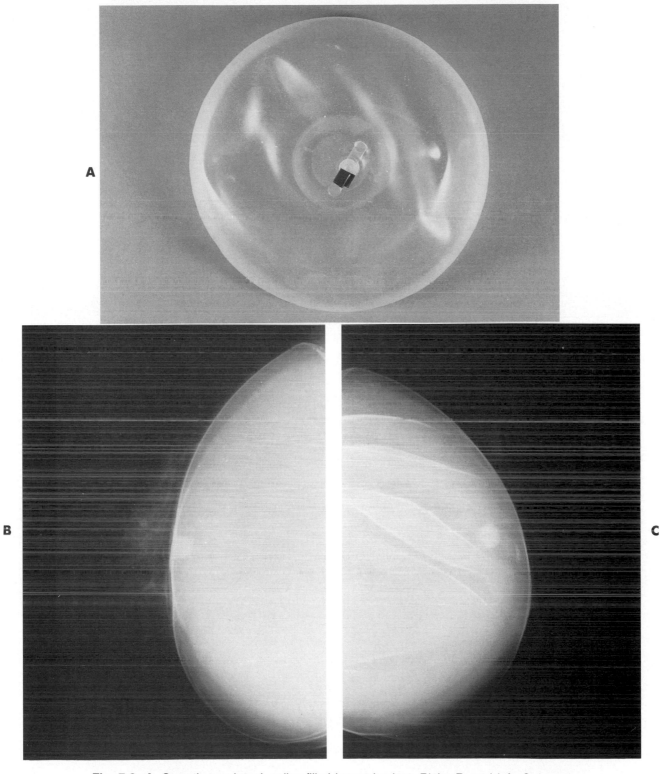

Fig. 7-2. A, Smooth-enveloped, saline-filled breast implant. Right, **B,** and left, **C,** lateral views of a 55-year-old woman with a saline-filled breast implant. Notice the nozzle for adding or withdrawing fluid.

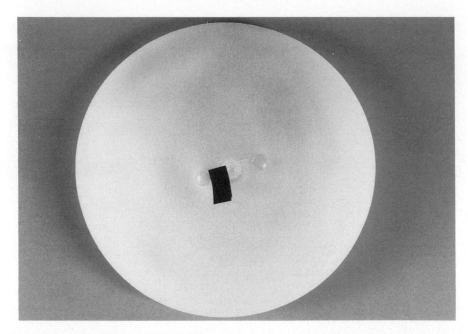

Fig. 7-3. Smooth, polyurethane-enveloped, silicone-filled breast implant.

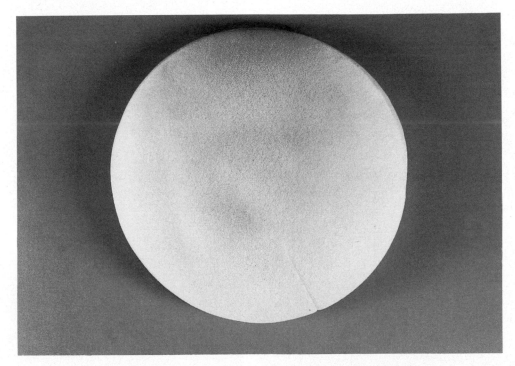

Fig. 7-4. Textured-envelope, silicone-filled breast implant.

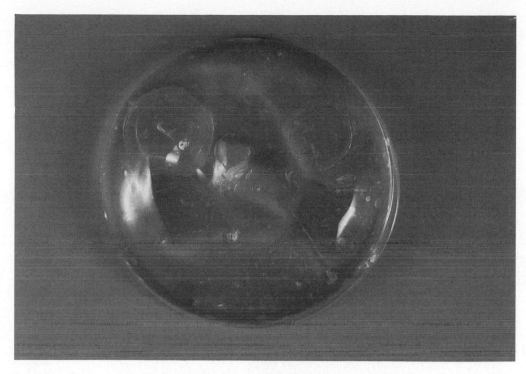

Fig. 7-5. Double-lumen, silicone-filled breast implant.

in women who have undergone augmentation mammo-plasty are frequent and increasing. Problems related to imaging of the breast with augmentation implants in-clude difficulty in viewing the entire breast parenchyma and the need for detecting any leakage of the breast-prosthesis contents or collapse of the implant.[1]

Imaging of the Augmented Breast

Augmentation breast prostheses may be placed either anterior (Fig. 7-6) or posterior (Fig. 7-7) to the pecto-ralis muscle.[2] The sensitivity of standard mammo-graphic techniques is likely to be lower in these pa-tients, and therefore special compression views have been described for improving the mammographic eval-uation of at least part of the augmented breast[1] (Fig. 7-8).

Leakage and Collapse of Implants

The diagnosis of leaking or ruptured breast implants may be associated with physical findings, such as breast nodules, decreased breast size, asymmetry, tenderness, and a softer texture.[3] Additionally, when Porex smooth-walled silicone gel-filled implants are used, the outer layer of silicone sheeting may separate from the under-lying silicone layer. This "delamination" is similar to the peeling of the layers of an onion. When this occurs, a freely movable or floating breast mass may be present, representing the shed lamina of the silicone implant.[4]

Mammographic characteristics of ruptured or leaking breast implants include:

1. Lobular or spherical densities adjacent to or sepa-rate from the implant, representing extravasated silicone gel globules[5,7] (Fig. 7-9).
2. Ill-defined border or irregular density of the im-plant
3. Decreased size of the implant (Fig. 7-10)

It is well known that fibrous capsules may form within the breast around an augmentation implant. It is proba-ble that many broken implants are undiagnosed because they are asymptomatic and the implant contents remain within the fibrous capsule. Additionally, when closed capsulotomy is performed to disrupt a fibrous capsule, a tear within the fibrous capsule may allow herniation of an intact breast implant. This does not necessarily im-ply impending rupture of the implant envelope.[8]

RECONSTRUCTION MAMMOPLASTY

After mastectomy, breast reconstruction can be ac-complished in several ways, including a reconstruction breast prosthesis (Fig. 7-11), or a transverse rectus ab-dominis muscle flap (TRAM flap, Fig. 7-12). Patients who have had silicone injections for augmentation of the breast are found to have very dense breasts with multi-ple small nodules representing silicone granulomas.[9] These patients may develop extensive round or cyst-like calcifications. The deposits may be related to fat necro-

Text continued on p. 226.

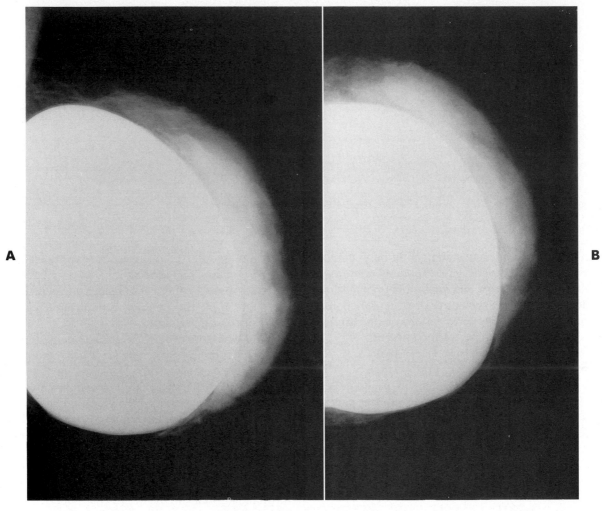

Fig. 7-6. Pre–pectoral augmentation breast prosthesis. **A,** Left lateral view. **B,** Left cra-niocaudal view.

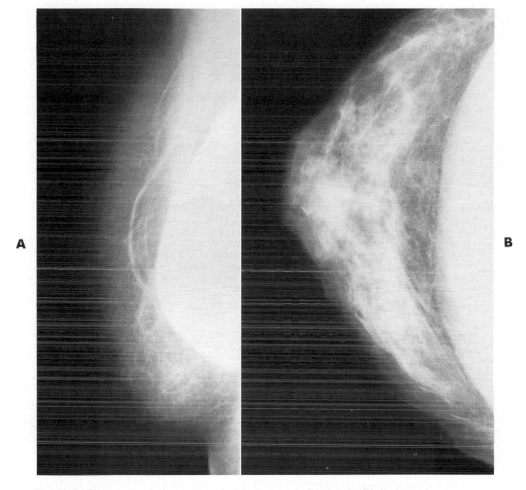

Fig. 7-7. Retropectoral augmentation breast prosthesis. **A,** Right lateral view. **B,** Right craniocaudal view.

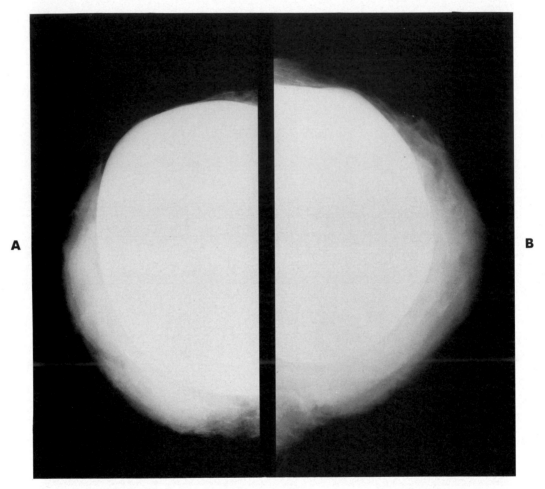

Fig. 7-8. A patient with augmentation breast prostheses imaged with modified positioning to improve the amount of breast tissue seen. **A,** Right craniocaudal view. **B,** Left craniocaudal view.

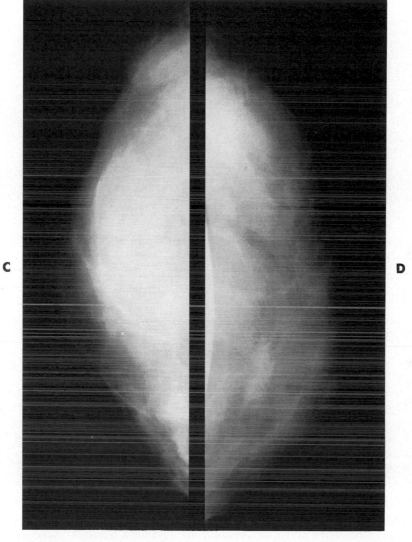

Fig. 7-8, cont'd. Right, **C,** and left, **D,** pinch views. By displacing the implant posteriorly against the chest wall and pulling the breast tissue over and in front of the implant, better breast compression and visualization of more parenchyma is achieved.

A   B   C

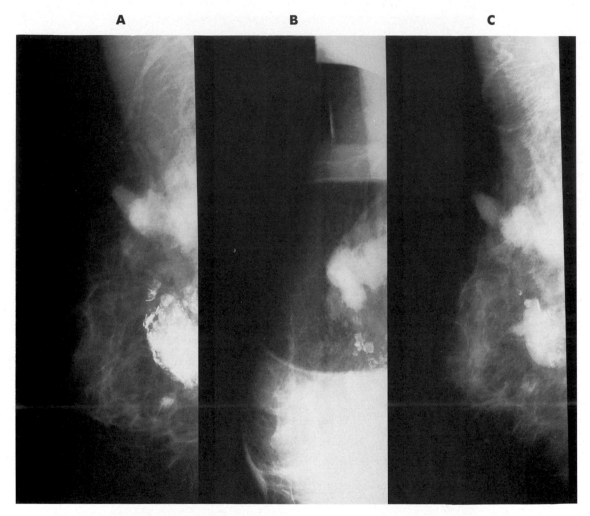

Fig. 7-9. Right lateral view. This patient experienced collapse of her saline-filled breast implant approximately 18 months before this mammogram. Although she initially reported fullness and tenderness within her breast, these symptoms gradually improved. The extravasated saline appears to have been completely resorbed and only the collapsed implant envelope is visualized mammographically.

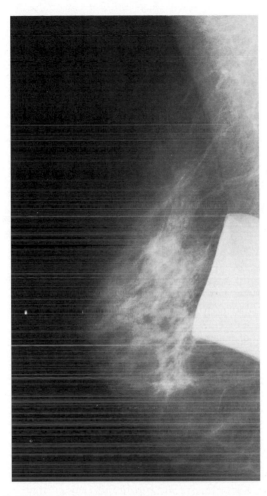

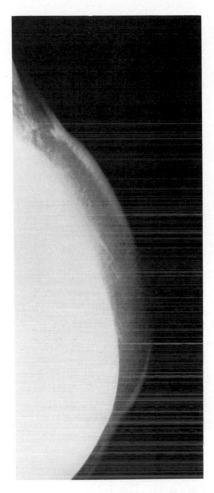

Fig. 7-10. Silicone implant rupture. After rupture and removal of a single-envelope, silicone gel–filled implant inserted some years ago this patient demonstrates a chronic granulomatous reaction caused by the dissemination of silicone within the breast parenchyma. Hard, palpable nodules were present on physical examination of this patient. **A,** Right lateral view. Notice the calcified mass posteriorly in the central part of the breast and the granulomatous mass in the right axilla. **B,** Coned compression view of the right axilla. **C,** Oblique right craniocaudal view.

Fig. 7-11. Left lateral view. Reconstruction breast implant after left modified radical mastectomy.

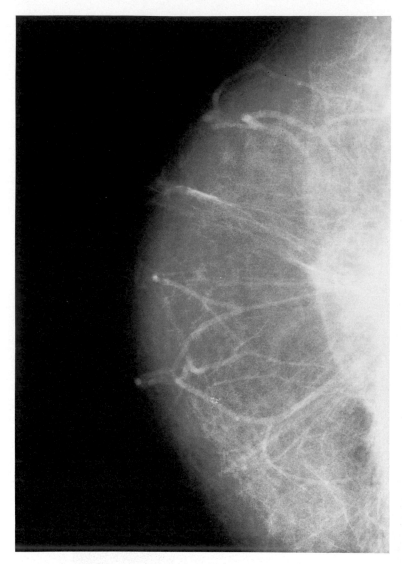

Fig. 7-12. Right craniocaudal view. Transverse rectus abdominis muscle flap (TRAM flap) after right modified radical mastectomy. This procedure involves dissecting free a portion of the rectus abdominis muscle, fascia, vascular supply, and overlying skin. The flap is anastomosed to the mastectomy defect, creating an artificial breast. A recognized complication of this procedure is compromise of the vascular supply, with resultant fat and skin-edge necrosis. Mammographic findings in patients with TRAM flaps include skin thickening along the anastomotic line and irregular microcalcifications (not seen in this patient). These microcalcifications coarsen over time and are the result of ischemic fat necrosis, not tumor recurrence.

sis and foreign-body reaction as well as to the presence of the silicone itself (Fig. 7-13).

RADIOGRAPHIC MANIFESTATIONS OF FOREIGN BODIES IN THE BREAST

Metallic and nonmetallic foreign bodies in the breast are well depicted on mammography (Figs. 7-14 to 7-18). These include foreign bodies that are external to the breast such as talcum powder, deodorant, skin tattoos, metallic cosmetic preparations and dermal pharmaceutical preparations. Foreign bodies within the breast include medically related devices such as surgical clips, surgical drains, and Dacron cuffs of Hickman catheters.[10] After heavy metal injections, such as gold for rheumatoid arthritis, radiodense metallic particles may be visualized within reticuloendothelial cells found in the intramammary and axillary lymph nodes.[11] Various nonmedical metallic foreign bodies such as bullet fragments may also be visualized on the mammogram.

External (Dermal) Foreign Bodies

Talcum powder, deodorant, cosmetic preparations and various creams and ointments may contain zinc oxide, silica, or alumina. These substances may simulate microcalcifications within the breast because they appear as very fine granular densities on the mammogram. In the case of deodorant, the densities appear in areas of the axillary folds (Fig. 7-14). When there is suspicion that a calcification-like density may represent a mammographic artifact, imaging should be repeated after careful cleansing of the skin surface. When metal-based inks are impregnated into the skin, as with tattooing, similar artifacts may appear on the mammogram (see Fig. I-6, *B* and *C*). In addition, pharmaceutical vehicles for transcutaneous delivery of medications may also be depicted on the mammogram (Fig. 7-15).

Medically Related Foreign Bodies in the Breast

Surgical clips may be found in the bed of a previous biopsy site, particularly if the mass is suspicious for car-

Text continued on p. 232.

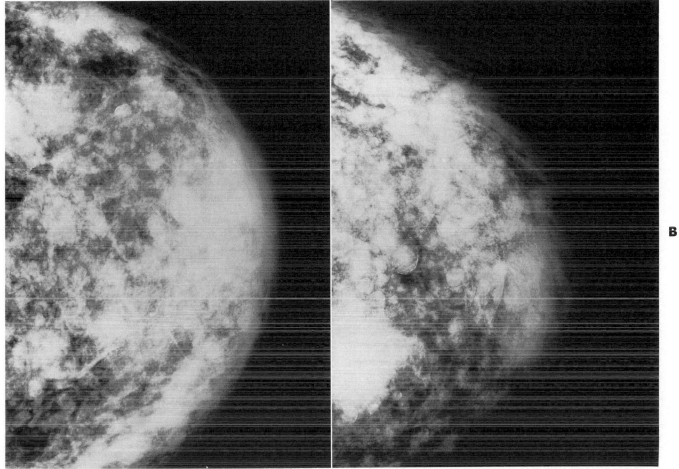

Fig. 7-13. Left craniocaudal, **A,** and lateral, **B,** views demonstrating the sequelae of silicone injections. Multiple ringlike calcific densities are present, representing fat necrosis, oil cysts, or injected silicone. The generalized increased breast density is presumably attributable to retained silicone, a noticeable foreign-body reaction, fibrosis, and fat necrosis. Because the parenchyma becomes very dense, mammographic imaging is difficult, and the detection of early carcinoma is limited.

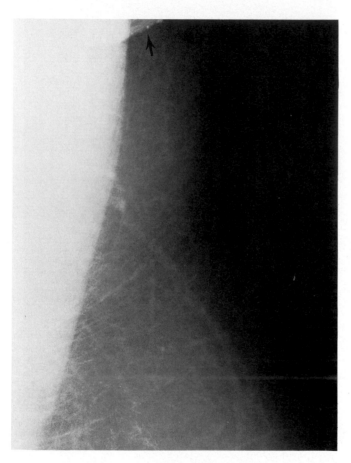

Fig. 7-14. Metallic, clustered densities, *arrow,* in the axillary folds on this coned oblique medial lateral projection of the left breast represent deodorant artifact.

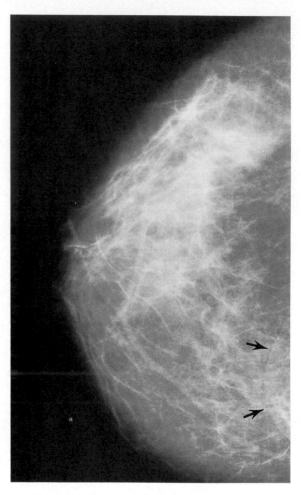

Fig. 7-15. The smooth, radiolucent density, *arrows,* seen in the medial portion of the right breast on this craniocaudal projection represents a Catapres medication patch.

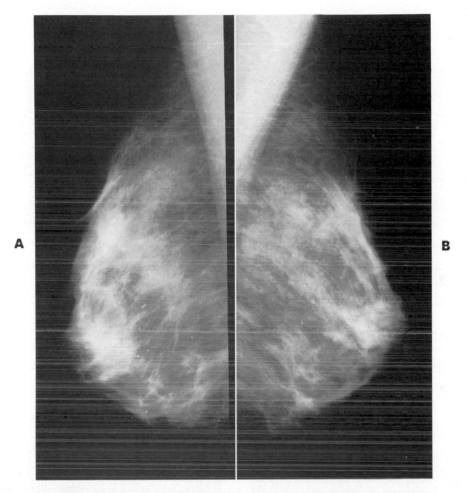

Fig. 7-16. Right, **A,** and left, **B,** views performed on Oct. 25, 1991, reveal diffuse small radiodensities simulating benign microcalcifications. When comparison was made to the patient's prior study of Sept. 28, 1990 (not shown), no such densities were present. On breast physical examination, it was noted that the patient had a "glistening" appearance to the skin. However, she denied having applied any cosmetic or other preparation to her skin. On further questioning, it was found that she had just returned from vacationing in Maui, Hawaii. The mammographic artifacts were found to represent small granules of sand that had become imbedded in her skin and, after cleansing, were no longer present on a repeat mammogram.

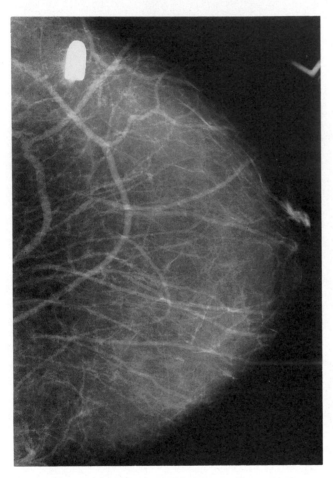

Fig. 7-17. A metallic foreign body in the upper outer quadrant of the right breast represents a bullet, after a gun wound 1 year previously.

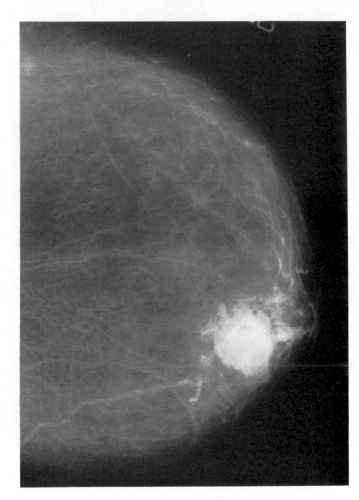

Fig. 7-18. For legend see opposite page.

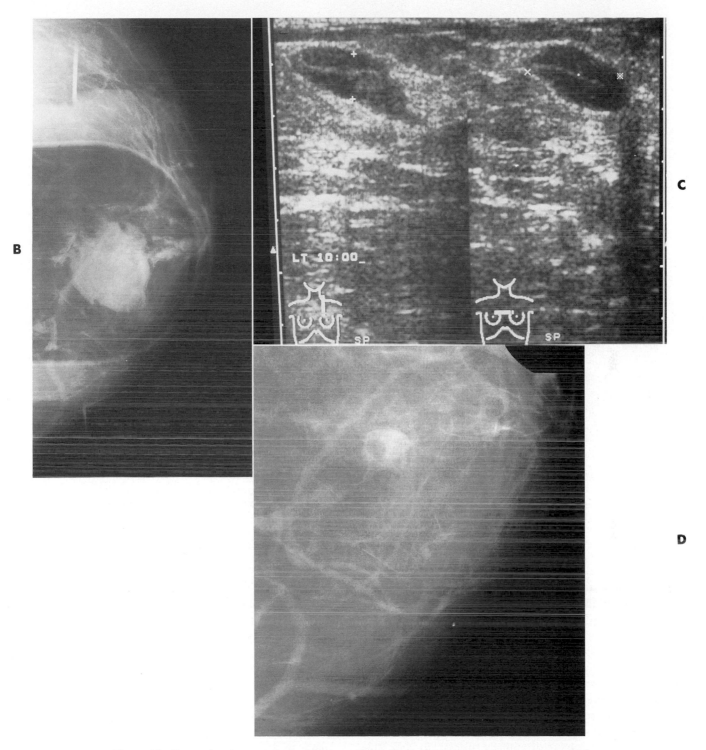

Fig. 7-18. Breast hematoma. Left oblique medial lateral, **A,** and coned left craniocaudal, **B,** views show a 2.5 cm, high-density irregular mass. This patient reported recent trauma to the breast. On ultrasound examination, **C,** the mass demonstrates low-level echos within it as well as a septation. On a follow-up mammographic examination 1 month later, **D,** the mass has considerably decreased in size and shows a small lucency within it consistent with a resolving breast hematoma.

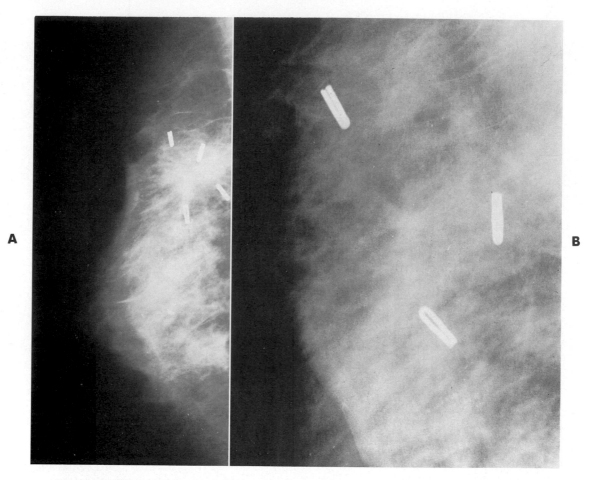

Fig. 7-19. A, Right oblique medial lateral mammographic view demonstrates skin thickening and a postoperative distortion from a recent breast biopsy. **B,** A cone magnification view of the surgical site reveals no retained microcalcifications and again shows surgical clips. The clips are placed in the deep portions of the surgical site to aid in delivery of therapeutic radiation to the tumor bed.

cinoma. These are placed by the surgeon to aid the radiation oncologist in delivering "booster" doses of radiation therapy to the tumor bed (Fig. 7-19).

Other foreign bodies that may be found in the breast include a retained surgical drain (Fig. 7-20) after breast surgery or a retained Dacron cuff that remains in the breast after removal of a Hickman catheter[10] (Fig. 7-21). Hickman catheters are constructed of silicone and have a proximal Dacron felt cuff that anchors the catheter to the subcutaneous tissue. Most commonly, they are inserted into the cephalic or axillary subclavian vein. The catheter is threaded through a subcutaneous tunnel to its entry point into the vein. The Dacron cuff, located in the subcutaneous tunnel, serves to anchor the catheter in the subcutaneous tissue and provide a physical barrier to infection.[12] The Dacron cuff elicits a fibrous reaction in the surrounding tissue and therefore is often left behind after removal of the catheter.

Intranodal Gold Deposits

Rarely, intramammary and axillary lymph nodes may demonstrate microcalcifications because of metastatic breast carcinoma.[13] However, a similar finding may be seen in patients with rheumatoid arthritis who have undergone chrysotherapy.[11] In these cases, the multiple punctate opacities within the lymph nodes represent gold deposits that have accumulated within reticuloendothelial cells of the lymph nodes (Figs. 7-22 to 7-24). Because some 50% of the gold injected for therapy remains in the body, the possibility of intranodal gold deposits should not be ignored in the diagnosis of suspicious radiographic densities in patients who have a history of gold injections. Often, gold deposition involves multiple nodes and is seen bilaterally.

Text continued on p. 238.

Fig. 7-20. A, Left lateral view. **B,** Left craniocaudal view. A retained Dacron cuff, *arrow,* is seen in the lower inner quadrant of the left breast. These devices are generally of radiographic density between that of water and that of calcium. They are often palpable on physical examination as firm, thick subcutaneous nodules.

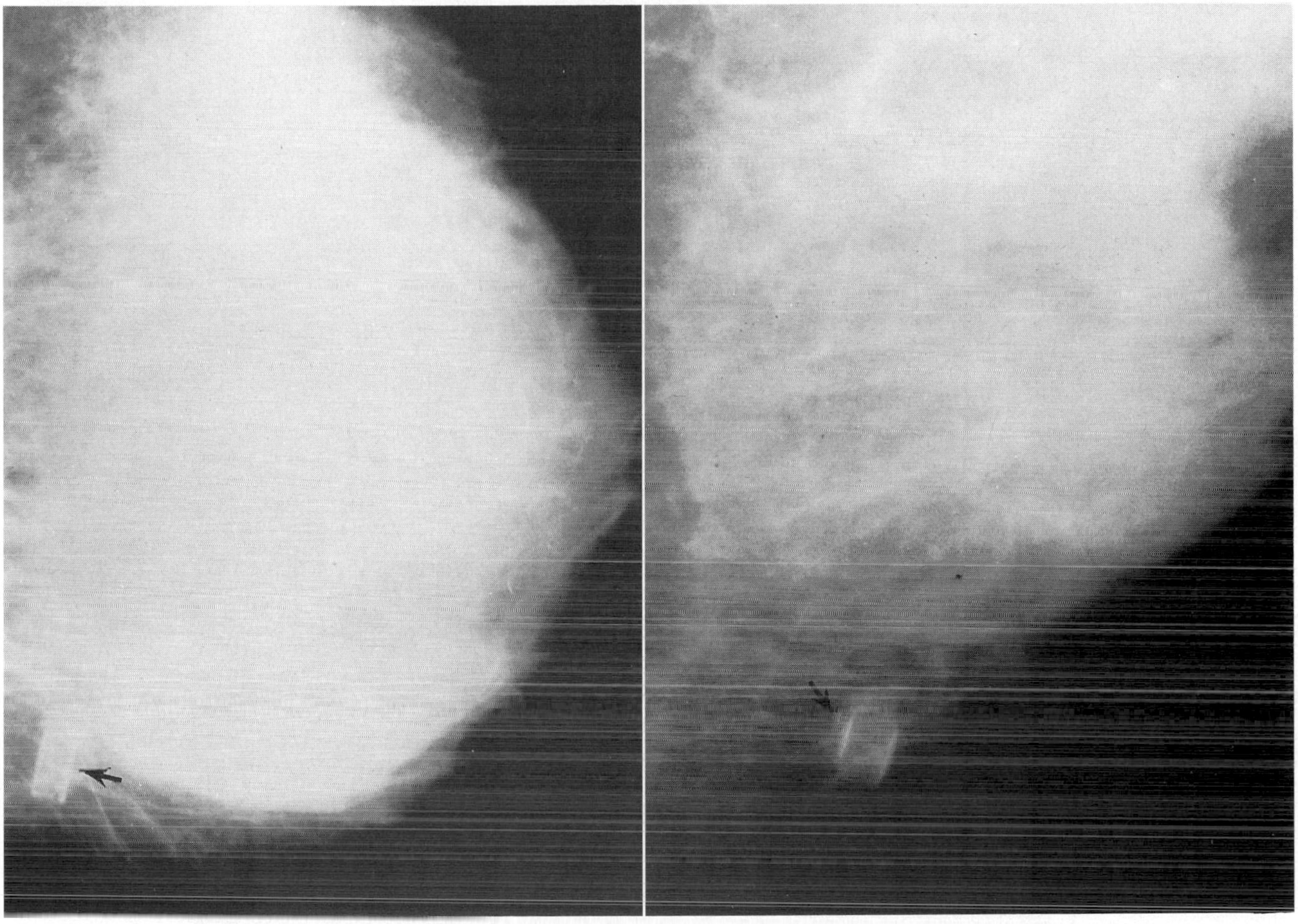

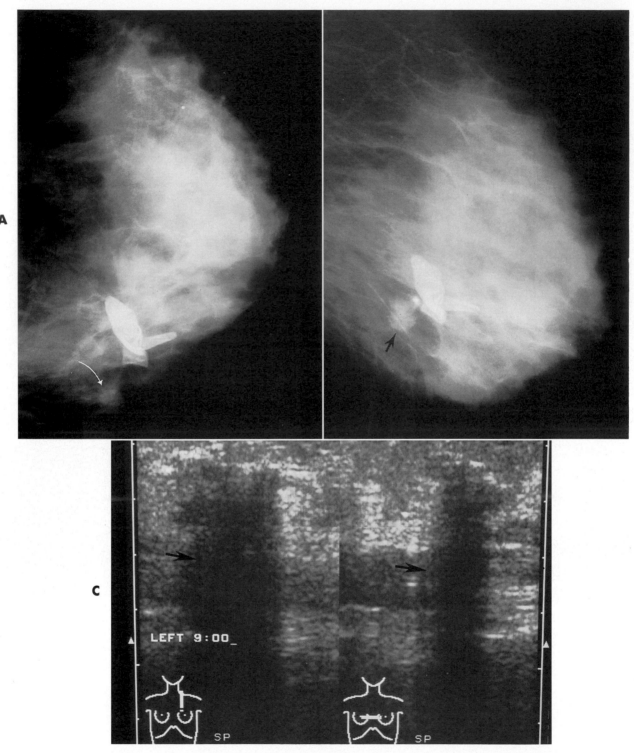

Fig. 7-21. Left oblique medial lateral, **A,** and craniocaudal, **B,** mammographic views demonstrate a retained surgical Penrose drain in the lower inner quadrant of the left breast. Also seen is a 1 cm spiculated mass adjacent to the retained drain *(arrow),* which represents a small carcinoma that was missed on surgical biopsy. **C,** Ultrasound examination of this area of the breast was difficult because of the presence of the surgical drain, which caused acoustic shadowing, *arrows.*

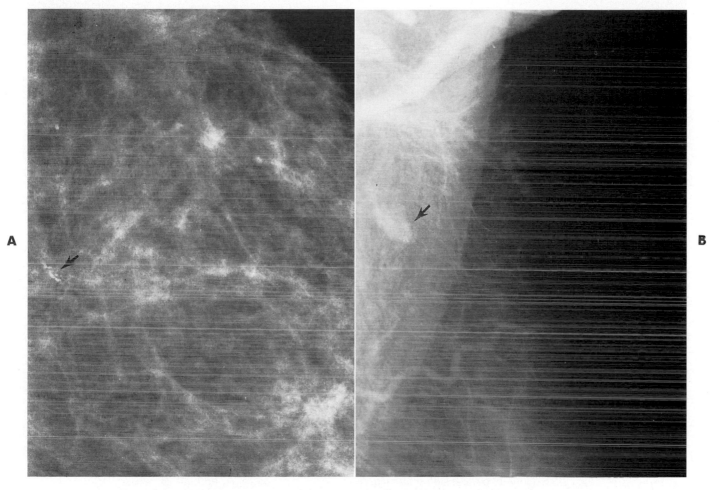

Fig. 7-22. Intramammary, **A,** and axillary, **B,** nodal accumulations of gold, *arrow,* in a patient with rheumatoid arthritis who had received prior chrysotherapy.

Fig. 7-23. Coned compression mammographic views of the right, **A,** and left, **B,** axillary regions demonstrating punctate intranodal gold deposits, *arrows,* bilaterally that simulate microcalcifications. This patient also had a history of rheumatoid arthritis and prior gold therapy.

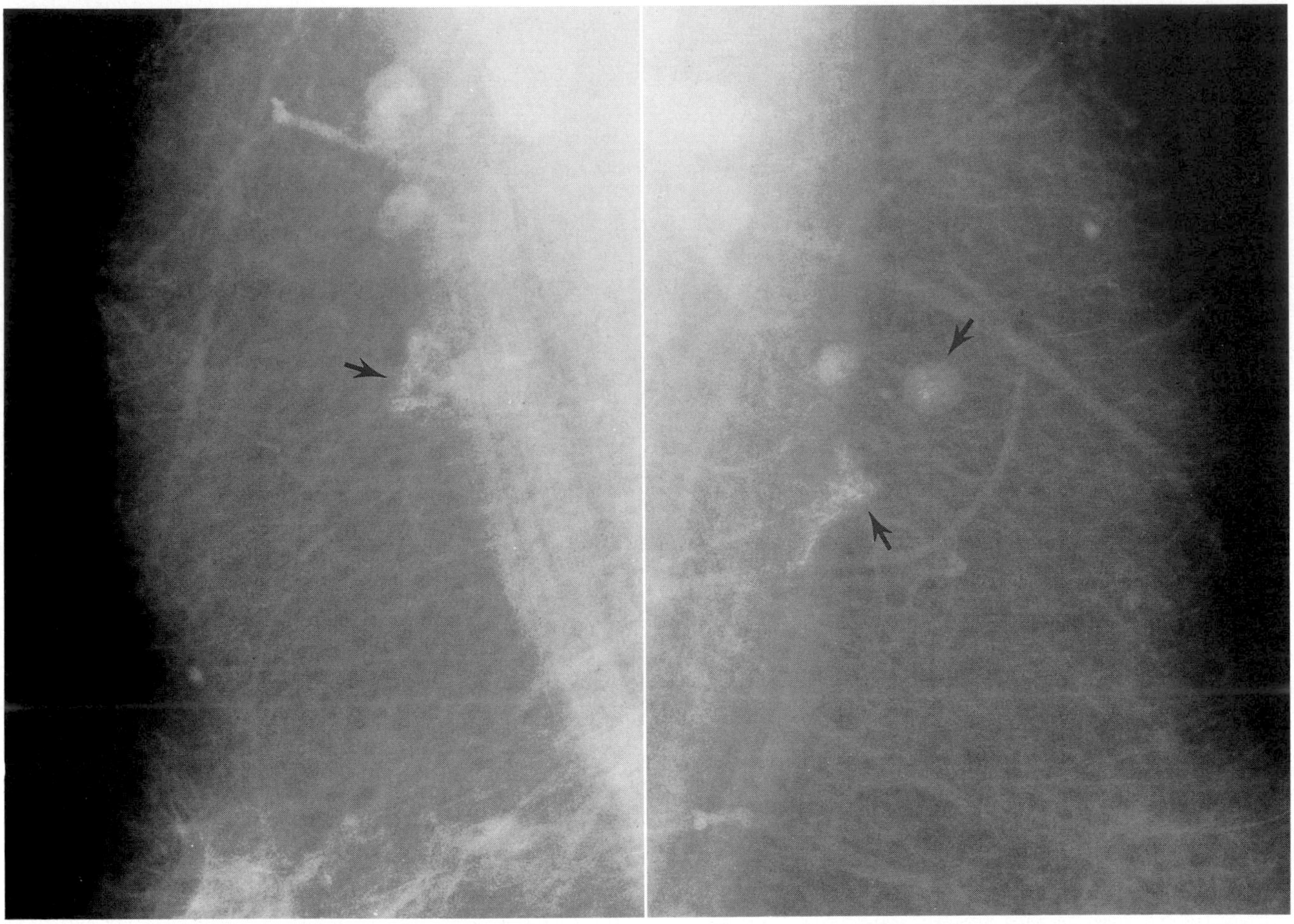

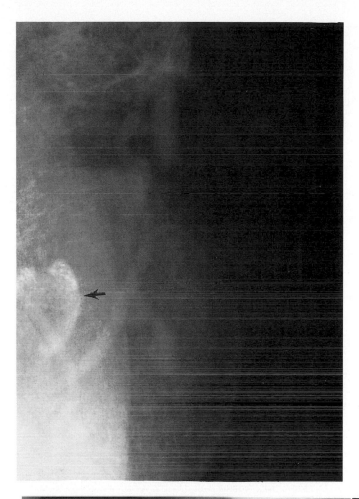

Fig. 7-24. Coned compression view of the left upper breast in a patient with rheumatoid arthritis shows punctate metallic densities within the low-lying left axillary lymph nodes, consistent with intranodal gold deposition.

Fig. 7-25. Right oblique medial lateral, **A,** and right craniocaudal, **B,** views of the breast show a pseudomass, *arrows,* at the base of the breast on the craniocaudal view. This finding represents a small portion of the normal pectoralis muscle, which may be seen on the well-positioned and compressed craniocaudal view.

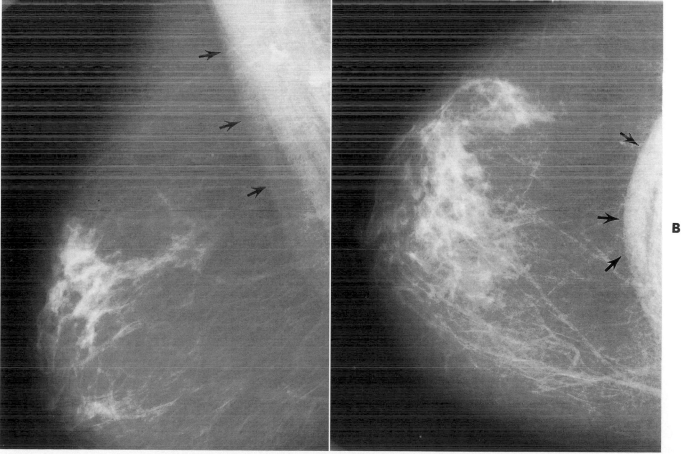

A   B

PSEUDOMASSES IN THE BREAST; BREAST IMPLANT REMOVAL

Occasionally, the pectoralis muscle (composed of the pectoralis major and minor) is partially visualized on the mammogram as a distinct, posteriorly located density (Fig. 7-25). Because it is not seen in its entirety, it may simulate a malignant breast mass.[14] Experience with mammography and familiarity with this normal variation of anatomy, which may mimic a mass, will avoid misdiagnosis

Silicone gel breast implants have recently undergone considerable scrutiny from various lay and medical groups concerning their safety.[15] This is for several reasons, including the complications associated with implant use (malposition, bleeding, rupture of the envelope, contracture formation, leakage, infection, and allergic reaction) as well as their obscuration of breast tissue during mammography.[15] There is also the question of the body's long-term reaction from continuous exposure to the silicone polymers used in breast implants and many other medical devices.

Some women have elected to have their implants removed because of complications with their implants or because of their concerns with implant safety. The mammographic appearance of the breasts may be difficult to interpret after implant removal if one does not know that implants were previously in place. After removal of submammary implants, there may be bilateral symmetric soft-tissue masses posterior to the breast glandular tissue. These masses and accompanying calcifications can sometimes simulate significant lesions and cause unnecessary concern.[16]

REFERENCES

1. Eklund GW, Busby RC, Miller SH, Job JS: Improved imaging of the augmented breast, *AJR* 151:469-473, 1988.
2. Biggs TM, Yarish RS: Augmentation mammaplasty: retropectoral versus retromammary implantation, *Clin Plast Surg* 15:549-555, 1988.
3. Andersen B, Hawtof D, Alani H, Kapetansky D: The diagnosis of ruptured breast implants, *Plast Reconstr Surg* 84:903-907, 1989.
4. Jones FR: Porex smooth-walled silicone gel–filled breast implants, *Plast Reconstr Surg* 87(3):588, 1991 (letter).
5. Hausner RJ, Schoen FJ, Pierson KK: Foreign-body reaction to silicone gel in axillary lymph nodes after an augmentation mammaplasty, *Plast Reconstr Surg* 62:381-384, 1978.
6. Leibman AJ, Kruse B: Breast cancer: mammographic and sonographic findings after augmentation mammoplasty, *Radiology* 174:195-198, 1990.
7. Hawes DR: Collapse of a breast implant after mammography, *AJR* 154:1345, 1990 (letter).
8. Smith DS: False-positive radiographic diagnosis of breast implant rupture: report of two cases, *Ann Plast Surg* 14:166-167, 1985.
9. Minagi H, Youker JE, Knudson HW: The roentgen appearance of injected silicone in the breast, *Radiology* 90:57-61, 1968.
10. Beyer GA, Thorsen MK, Shaffer KA, Walker AP: Mammographic appearance of the retained Dacron cuff of a Hickman catheter, *AJR* 155:1203-1204, 1990.
11. Bruwer A, Nelson GW, Spark RP: Punctate intranodal gold deposits simulating microcalcifications on mammograms, *Radiology* 163:87-88, 1987.
12. Bjeletich J, Hickman RO: The Hickman indwelling catheter, *Am J Nurs* 80:62-65, 1980.
13. Helvie MA, Rebner M, Sickles EA, Oberman HA: Calcifications in metastatic breast carcinoma in axillary lymph nodes, *AJR* 151:921-922, 1988.
14. Meyer JE, Stomper PC, Lee RR: Pectoralis muscle simulating a breast mass, *AJR* 152:481-482, 1989.
15. Steinbach BG, Hardt NS, Abbitt PL, et al: Breast implants, common complications, and concurrent breast disease, *RadioGraphics* 13:95-118, 1993.
16. Stewart NR, Monsees BS, Destouet JM, Rudloff MA: Mammographic appearance following implant removal, *Radiology* 185:83-85, 1992.

8

Medical Devices of the Abdomen and Pelvis

Tim B. Hunter
Welland O. Short

There are many devices found in the abdomen and pelvis. These range from nasogastric tubes to ureteral stents and pessaries. They can generally be divided into three broad categories: gastrointestinal (GI) devices, genitourinary (GU) devices, and miscellaneous devices that pass through the abdomen and pelvis en route to somewhere else or are intended for applications that do not concern GI or GU processes. Examples of the latter types of devices include ventriculoperitoneal shunts, umbilical catheters, and nerve stimulation catheters. This chapter illustrates a variety of abdominal and pelvic devices, grouping them into the above three categories.

GASTROINTESTINAL DEVICES

Esophageal Stents

Patients with carcinoma of the esophagus suffer from difficulty with swallowing, pooling of secretions, aspiration of fluid and food, and severe nutritional deficiency. Various surgical and endoscopic procedures have been devised for bypassing the tumor, obturating a tracheoesophageal fistula, placing a stent through an obstructing tumor, or significantly reducing a tumor's bulk.[1-5] A well-known surgical stent for palliation of an esophageal malignancy is the Celestin tube. The standard Celestin tube is a nylon-reinforced latex tube 28.5 cm in length and has a diameter of 1.5 cm. The upper portion is larger, being a somewhat tulip-shaped funnel with a length of 3.5 cm and a diameter of 2.8 cm.[1] The tube can be placed surgically or endoscopically and is often sutured into place.

The insertion of a Celestin tube is a procedure with little patient risk. Nevertheless, it is associated with a very significant incidence of subsequent morbidity, ranging to nearly 100%, and its use is not advocated for most patients.[1] Some of the complications associated with Celestin tube use include severe gastroesophageal reflux, aspiration pneumonitis, tube obstruction, tube migration, respiratory distress from tube compression of the trachea, esophageal perforation, and tube erosion into the aorta.[1]

More recent transendoscopic palliative therapy of esophageal malignancies include laser therapy, bipolar electrocoagulation therapy (BICAP), insertion of stents, and coaxial passage of bougies and balloons over endoscopically placed guide wires.[2] Bougienage can control symptoms temporarily, but most patients ultimately require ablative therapy with laser techniques or BICAP.

Stents are infrequently used; their prime indications are to bypass an esophagorespiratory fistula or to palliate a patient who has failed other therapy[2] (Figs. 8-1 to 8-3). Esophageal stent placement is critical and requires careful patient evaluation and close cooperation between the gastroenterologist and the radiologist.[2]

If the stent crosses the gastroesophageal junction, reflux may become a problem. The stent can become obstructed by herniating normal mucosa or by tumor growth around its lumen. Food and foreign bodies may obstruct a stent, and it may become kinked. Stents can also migrate proximally or distally and perforate the

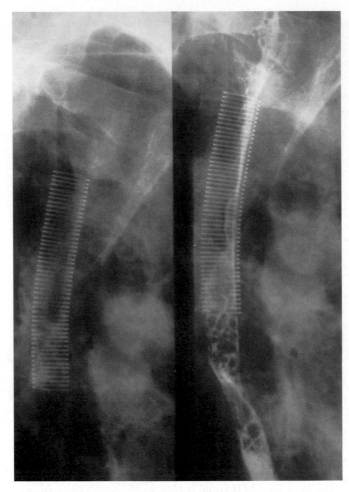

Fig. 8-1. Sixty-five-year-old man with advanced carcinoma of the esophagus. A Silastic (silicone elastomer) esophageal stent was passed through the tumor in the midportion of the esophagus.

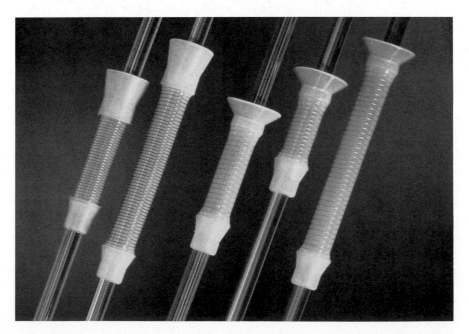

Fig. 8-2. Various esophageal prostheses. (Courtesy Wilson-Cook Medical Inc., Winston-Salem, N.C.)

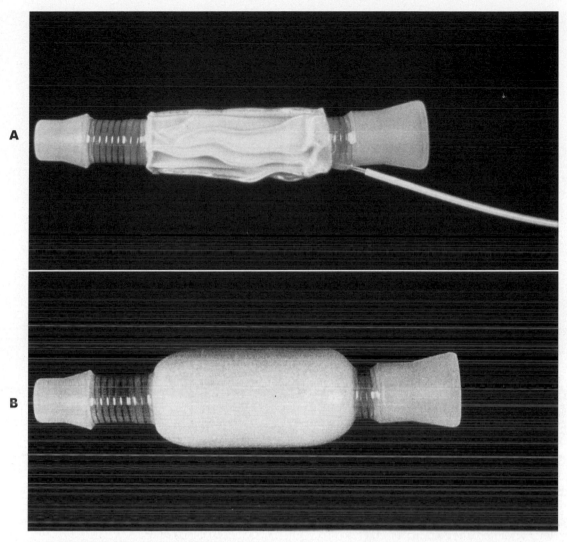

Fig. 8-3. Esophageal balloon prosthesis. **A,** Balloon deflated. **B,** Balloon inflated. (Courtesy Wilson-Cook Medical Inc., Winston-Salem, N.C.)

esophagus.[1-5] If the cricopharyngeus muscle is carefully avoided and short stents are used that do not cross the gastroesophageal junction, stent complications may be reduced.[2]

Plain chest and abdominal radiography are useful for evaluating possible stent complications, such as migration, or perforation with the development of pneumomediastinum. However, contrast studies and computed tomography may be indicated in more complex cases. CT may be the procedure of choice for the detection of perforation and for the distinction between intratumoral perforation and free esophageal perforation.[2]

Long Intestinal Tubes; Gastrostomy Tubes

Intestinal tubes have long been used to decompress the stomach and large and small bowel, to obtain fluid samples, and to provide an access route for patient nutrition. They come in various lengths and configura-

tions. The large-bore, somewhat stiff tubes, such as the traditional nasogastric tube, are used for temporary bowel decompression and fluid sampling. The small, flexible, soft feeding tubes are used for long-term (days to weeks) patient feedings.

A common long intestinal tube is the Miller-Abbott tube, which is a double-lumen radiopaque rubber tube. One lumen is used for bowel decompression, and the other lumen provides a route to inject mercury into the weighted balloon at the end of the tube. The weighted mercury balloon helps peristalsis "pull" the tube farther distally in the intestinal tract. The Cantor tube is similar to the Miller-Abbott tube except that it has only one lumen.

Complications of long intestinal tubes are infrequent but should be recognized by the physician. There are three major types of problems associated with intestinal tube use: (1) obstruction, (2) tube breakage, knot-

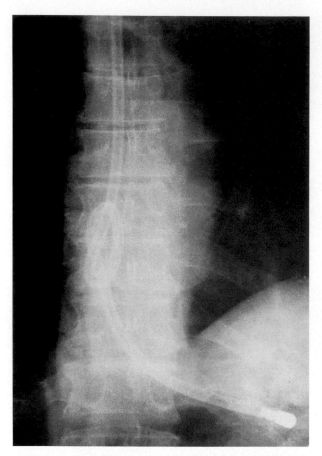

Fig. 8-4. Sixty-one-year-old male with knotted Miller-Abbott tube. It was withdrawn with gentle traction. When the tube reached the back of his throat, the knotted portion was pulled through his mouth and cut off. The rest of the tube was then pulled out through his nose. (From Hunter TB, Fon GT, Silverstein ME: *Am J Gastroenterol* 76:256-261, 1981.)

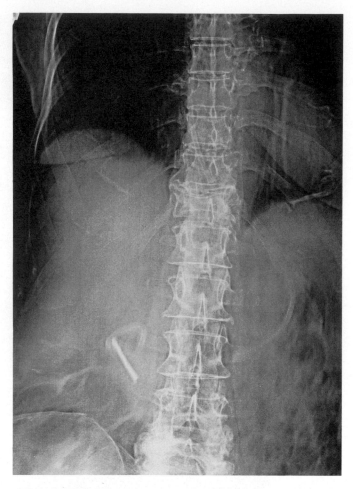

Fig. 8-5. Seventy-year-old woman with overlapping loops of her feeding tube, a potentially dangerous situation. The tube did not become knotted in this instance.

ting, or mercury spillage, and (3) gut perforation. There is also a variety of usually minor, somewhat frequent problems associated with intestinal tubes, such as nasal irritation, nasal ulceration, sinusitis, serous otitis media, pharyngitis, and gastroesophageal reflux.[6]

Tube knotting is always a potential problem (Figs. 8-4 and 8-5). It is probably more likely to occur with long indwelling tubes where there can be multiple, overlapping coils of the tube. Kinking of the tube and coiling back upon itself are predisposing conditions for knotting. It is always wise to avoid multiple coiled loops with a tube. If there is a potential for circular continuity of the gastrointestinal tract, as in a patient with a gastrojejunostomy, it is possible for the tube to coil back on itself in a circular fashion and thereby tie itself with loops of bowel and the stomach in a knot requiring surgical correction.[7-9]

If fluoroscopy or plain radiographs show there is excessive tube coiling or indicate that there is a knotted tube, the tube should be managed carefully. Forceful,

rapid retraction of the tube may tighten a knot further or lead to knotting where it did not originally exist. In rare instances, there could even be reverse intussusception produced.[10]

An interesting potential complication of intestinal tubes is gaseous distension of the tube bag (Fig. 8-6). Gases can gradually diffuse into the mercury balloon and inflate it after several days. The inflation can become large enough to impact the balloon in the bowel lumen and produce intestinal obstruction. This is not very common and tends to occur if the tube has been present in the gut for more than 10 days.[11,12] This is best prevented by perforating the balloon or mercury bag with a small 24- or 25-gauge needle before insertion of the intestinal tube into the patient. The small needle hole will allow for equilibration of intestinal and balloon atmospheres but will not allow significant leakage of the mercury.[9]

There are several ways to treat a gas-distended tube balloon or mercury bag. If the distension is not great,

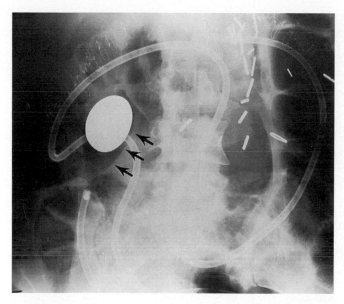

Fig. 8-6. Thirty-six-year-old female being fed an elemental jejunal diet through a Cantor tube. Gaseous distension of her tube bag, *arrows,* was noticed after several days. The tube was removed by gentle traction. (From Hunter TB, Fon GT, Silverstein ME: *Am J Gastroenterol* 76:256-261, 1981.)

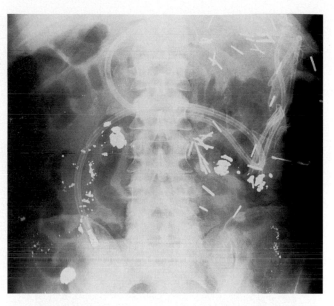

Fig. 8-7. Spillage of mercury into the gut after rupture of a mercury bag on a long intestinal tube. This caused the patient no problems.

the tube may be gently retracted and removed from the patient. If not, the balloon can be percutaneously punctured with a small Chiba type of needle.[12] In extreme cases, surgery or the use of a hyperbaric chamber may be necessary.

It is theoretically possible for an intestinal tube to produce intussusception. The tube tip or mercury bag can serve as a lead point for either forward intussusception or reverse intussusception at the time of tube removal.[13,14] Narrowing of the bowel from adhesions, inflammatory bowel disease, or tumors may predispose some patients to developing intussusception associated with an intestinal tube.

Spillage of metallic mercury from the rupture of a tube bag is an interesting complication of tube use (Fig 8-7). The bag may rupture because of problems with tube placement, it may rupture for unknown reasons, or medication may inadvertently be placed in the wrong portion of a double-lumen tube. Metallic mercury is generally considered a relatively nontoxic substance. It passes through the gastrointestinal tract without trouble. Even if it lodges in the bowel or appendix for long periods, it usually causes no symptoms (Fig. 8-8). If the metallic mercury is converted to absorbable divalent mercury, systemic mercury poisoning can result.[15]

Aspiration of metallic mercury is rare but may take place during tube passage with rupture of the mercury bag (Fig. 8-9). Some patients even attempt suicide by ingesting mercury and aspirate part of it. The mercury is readily visualized in the lungs as metallic clumps that

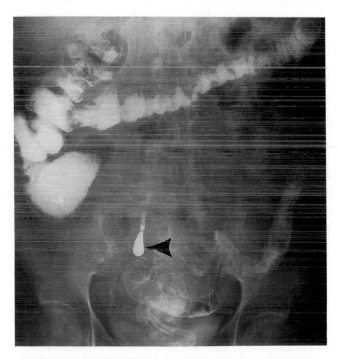

Fig. 8-8. Fifty-seven-year-old woman with metallic mercury visualized in her appendix, *arrowhead,* during a barium enema. This caused her no symptoms. It had resulted from rupture of a Miller-Abbott tube mercury bag 6 months previously. (From Hunter TB, Fon GT, Silverstein ME: *Am J Gastroenterol* 76:256-261, 1981.)

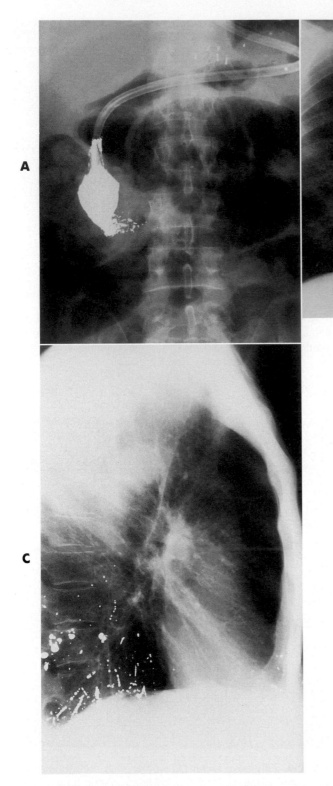

lie in dependent portions of the tracheobronchial tree.[7,16-19] It can be hard to differentiate from embolic metallic mercury pulmonary embolism in the pulmonary arterial bed (see Chapter 3). The mercury remains in the lungs for long periods as it is slowly cleared. It usually does not harm the patient, but metallic mercury anywhere in the body does have the potential for severe systemic toxicity if the mercury is converted into its poisonous salts or inhaled as a warmed vapor.

A very rare complication of Miller-Abbott tubes is the inadvertent injection of contrast material or feedings into the mercury balloon with noticeable overdistension to the balloon rather than balloon rupture and mercury spillage.[20] This can potentially lead to bowel obstruction, acute bowel rupture, or bowel necrosis if it is not recognized promptly.

Gut perforation from tube passage or use is fortunately rare. It appears to be most common in infants during the passage of feeding tubes[21] (Fig. 8-10). Duodenal perforations in infants sometimes take place because of loss of plasticity of the tube over time and the fixed position of the duodenal loop. Tube materials can harden and chemically change after prolonged contact with gastric and intestinal juices. Plastic nasogastric tubes should therefore be changed frequently.

If intubation is to be used for prolonged periods, a specially designed feeding tube (see below) or a gastrostomy or jejunostomy tube should be used. These tubes obviate or minimize irritation to the mucosa of the nasopharynx, hypopharynx, esophagus, and stomach because of their smaller size and softer materials. They are less likely to cause perforation because of these considerations or because of their well-controlled positioning.

Fig. 8-9. Fifty-four-year-old man who needed a long intestinal tube for bowel decompression before surgery. The mercury bag on his Miller-Abbott tube ruptured sometime during tube insertion spilling mercury into his gut, **A,** and also leading to his aspirating elemental mercury. **B** and **C,** The mercury was visible in his lungs 6 months after his hospital discharge. (From Hunter TB, Fon GT, Silverstein ME: *Am J Gastroenterol* 76:256-261, 1981.)

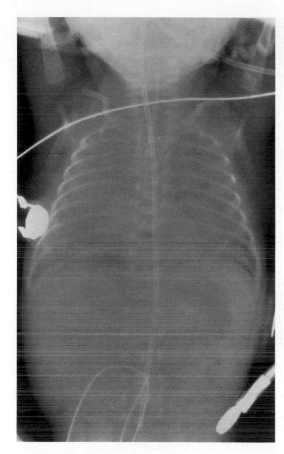

Fig. 8-10. Neonate with respiratory distress syndrome. An oral gastric tube was placed for feeding, but a routine radiograph showed it lying outside the normal course of the intestinal tract. The tube had probably perforated the gut at the gastroesophageal junction and entered the retroperitoneum. It was removed, and the patient was treated conservatively, recovering fully from his respiratory disease and tube injury. (From Hunter TB, Fon GT, Silverstein ME: *Am J Gastroenterol* 76:256-261, 1981.)

Tubes can find their way into all sorts of places (Fig 8-11). It is not unusual for them to coil in the mouth, hypopharynx, or nasopharynx, or for them to enter the trachcobronchial tree. It is dangerous to administer food, fluid, or contrast material to a patient through an intestinal tube unless the tube's location has been confirmed by radiographs or fluoroscopy to be in the stomach or bowel. All indwelling tubes cause local inflammation and gastroesophageal reflux. They can lead to local hemorrhage and inflammation as well.[22]

Endotracheal tubes and alimentary tract tubes are usually visualized on plain chest and abdomen films or at fluoroscopy. However, they may sometimes be present in patients undergoing CT, magnetic resonance imaging, and ultrasound studies. Physicians should be familiar with the appearance of various airway and alimentary tubes on these imaging modalities to better recognize tube misplacement and tube-related injuries.[23]

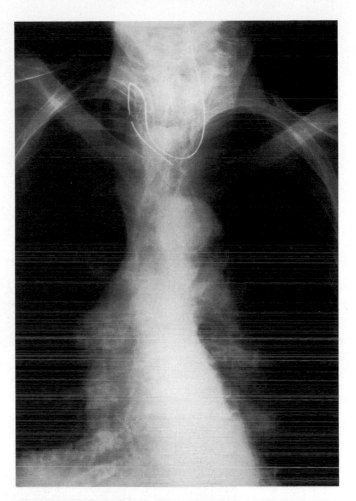

Fig. 8-11. Elderly male with a nasogastric tube coiled in a large Zenker's diverticulum.

Gastrostomy and jejunostomy tubes (Figs. 8-12 to 8-14) are placed in patients who need long-term assisted feedings.[24-34] Often, these patients have an obstruction or neuromuscular problems that render them unable to swallow effectively. The complications that can result from percutaneously endoscopically or surgically placed gastrostomy and jejunostomy tubes include perforation, stomal leakage, tube prolapse with intestinal or gastric obstruction, pneumatosis, stomach and bowel ulceration, fistula formation, and gastric torsion.[24-26] The most frequent complication appears to be gastrostomy tube prolapse into the duodenum, which generally can be corrected by retraction of the deflated tube into the stomach under fluoroscopy.[26] Extrusion of a percutaneous endoscopic gastrostomy (PEG) tube or a surgically placed gastrostomy tube into a fistulous tract is also possible.[27] There can be external migration of the PEG tube with impaction along the wall of the stomach or the anterior abdominal wall.[27-32] This may result from too much traction on the tube, and it can lead to ischemia and pressure necrosis.

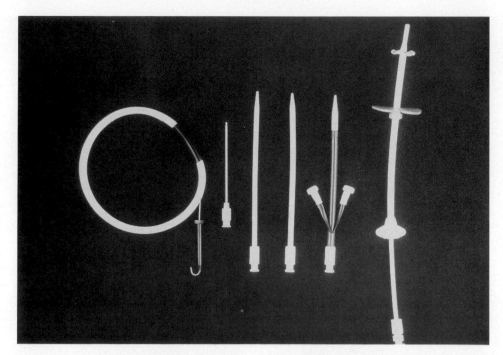

Fig. 8-12. Malecot Russell Gastrostomy set. (Courtesy Wilson-Cook Medical Inc., Winton-Salem, N.C.)

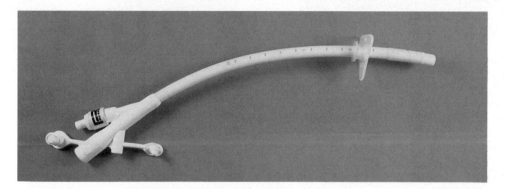

Fig. 8-13. Versa-Peg Gastrostomy Kit (Ross).

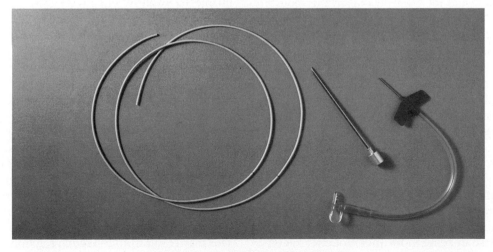

Fig. 8-14. Jejunostomy kit (Surgitek).

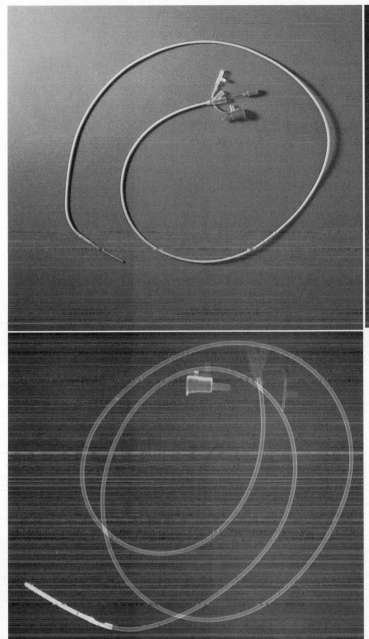

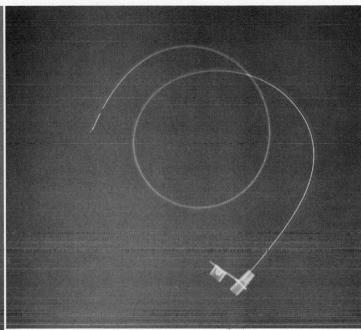

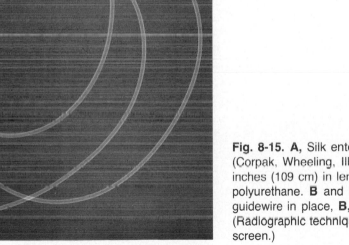

Fig. 8-15. A, Silk enteral feeding tube weighted with stylet (Corpak, Wheeling, Ill.). The tube pictured is 8 French 43 inches (109 cm) in length. It is composed of medical-grade polyurethane. **B** and **C,** Radiographs of the tube with the guidewire in place, **B,** and with the guidewire removed, **C.** (Radiographic technique: 47 kVp, 4 mAs, Quanta 3 film and screen.)

Feeding Tubes

New small-bore enteric tubes, such as the Entriflex and Dobbhoff tubes (Biosearch Medical Products, Somerville, N.J.), the Flexiflow tubes (Ross Laboratories, Columbus, Ohio), the Silk (Corpak, Wheeling, Illinois), and products by Argyle-Sherwood and the Frederick-Miller tube by Cook are now used to feed chronically ill patients[35-56] (Figs. 8-15 and 8-16). Older large-bore tubes constructed from polyethylene or polyvinyl chloride harden if left in the bowel for a long period and predispose the patient to mucosal injury and perforation.[48,50] The newer feeding tubes are constructed of biocompatible plastic, silicone, or other suitable materials and have greatly improved patient tolerance and permit extended use. They often have flexible metallic tips that are radiopaque, and they are usually introduced with the aid of a thin, slightly stiff metallic stylet, or sometimes they are passed over a guide wire.[48,53,55,56]

The preferred location for feeding tubes is beyond the stomach and proximal duodenum, preferably in the distal duodenum or proximal jejunum (Figs. 8-17 and 8-18). This is to prevent buildup of feedings within the

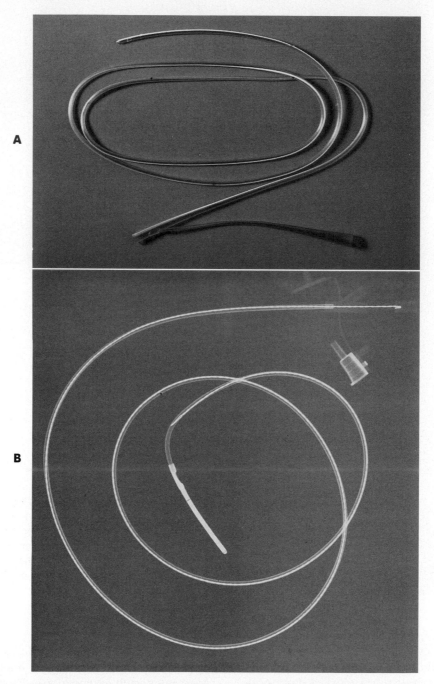

Fig. 8-16. A, Argyle Indwell feeding tube (Sherwood Medical, St. Louis). The tube pictured is radiopaque, 8 French (2.7 mm), 20 inches (51 cm) long, and composed of nonstiffening polyurethane compound. **B,** Radiograph of a small pediatric feeding tube. (Radiographic technique same as in Fig. 8-15.)

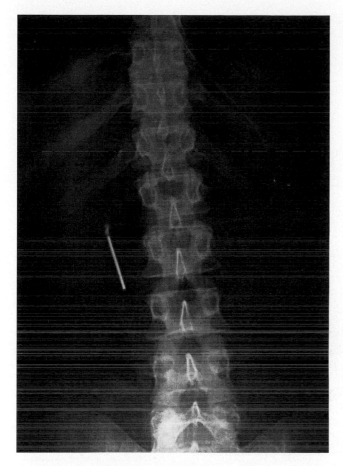

Fig. 8-17. Twenty-two-year-old woman with feeding tube tip in the descending portion of her duodenum. A more distal location is preferred and may result from bowel peristalsis moving the tube along. Proximal locations predispose to reflux of feeding solutions into the stomach.

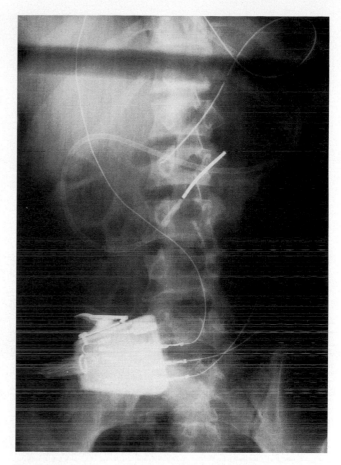

Fig. 8-18. Good positioning of a feeding tube near the duodenojejunal junction. An even more distal positioning is desirable.

stomach leading to aspiration and poor propulsion of feedings to the small bowel where they are absorbed.[51,54] Because of their thin, flexible nature, feeding tubes tend to coil easily and may be difficult to pass beyond the stomach (Fig. 8-19).

The Entriflex tube has a flexible tip 2.7 mm in diameter. The Dobbhoff tip is 5.9 mm in diameter. The tips of both of these tubes are composed of tungsten segments coated in a self-lubricating polyurethane.[42] The Flexiflow tube has a tip diameter of 4.3 mm and is composed of a soft tungsten-impregnated material.[42] The long section of all feeding tubes proximal to their tips is flexible and self-lubricating and has an external diameter of approximately 2.5 mm. The tubes are supposed to be opaque, but they can be difficult to visualize (see Chapter 2). Generally, only their tips are sufficiently opaque to be readily visualized. The wire stylets used to stiffen the tubes during insertion are radiopaque.

Feeding tubes are not without their problems, and many complications have been associated with their

use, including aspiration pneumonitis (Fig. 8-20), intestinal perforation, pneumothorax, transpleural tube passage, tracheobronchial intubation, and other injuries resulting from tube malposition.[35-46] These complications are best recognized by visualization of the tube along its entire course, which can be very difficult to do because of the relatively poor opacity of the tubes. Neurologically impaired patients may be at greater risk of complications. In these individuals it is probably wise for the feeding tube to be inserted under fluoroscopic control.[42] For patients who are neurologically intact this is probably not needed on a routine basis.[47]

Endoscopic Retrograde Cholangiopancreatography (ERCP)

ERCP (Figs. 8-21 to 8-28) requires both skilled endoscopy and good radiologic technique.[57-59] If a radiologist is not available for the procedure to either perform it or coordinate the imaging, a radiologic technologist specially trained for the procedure is essential. In

Text continued on p. 257.

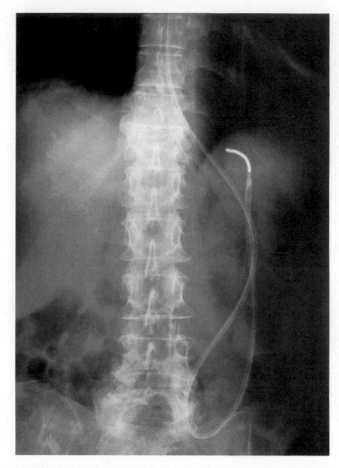

Fig. 8-19. Seventy-year-old woman with a feeding tube coiled in her stomach.

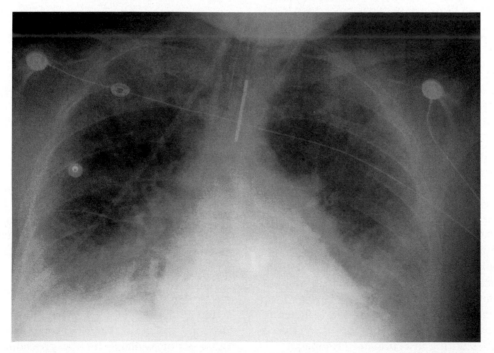

Fig. 8-20. Forty-eight-year-old woman with adult respiratory disease syndrome. Her feeding tube tip is located in the proximal part of her esophagus, a dangerous position predisposing the patient to aspiration of feedings.

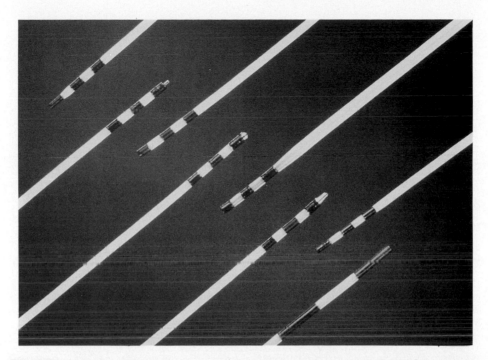

Fig. 8-21. Various endoscopic retrograde cholangiopancreatographic (ERCP) catheters used for cannulation of the biliary and pancreatic ductal systems. (Courtesy Wilson-Cook Medical Inc., Winston-Salem, N.C.)

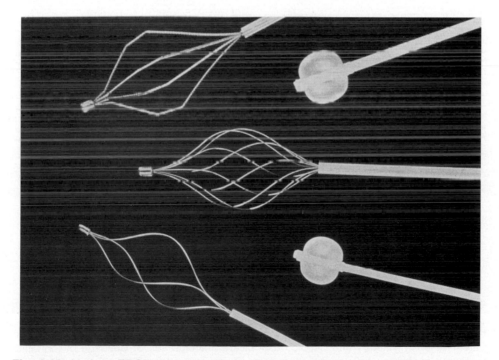

Fig. 8-22. Various ERCP stone extraction devices including a soft multifilament basket, balloon extraction device, eight-wire basket stone extractor, and a three-wire basket. (Courtesy Wilson-Cook Medical Inc., Winston-Salem, N.C.)

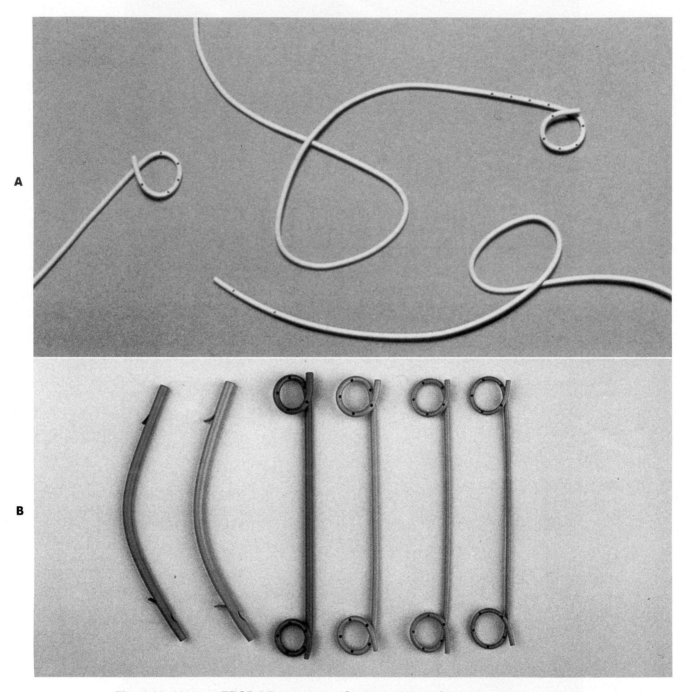

Fig. 8-23. Various ERCP biliary stents. (Courtesy Wilson-Cook Medical Inc., Winston-Salem, N.C.) **A,** Liguory endoscopic nasal biliary drainage set for drainage of the biliary system through use of an indwelling catheter. **B,** Zimmon endoscopic biliary stents (pigtail ends). Cotton-Leung biliary stent (curved with single fins).

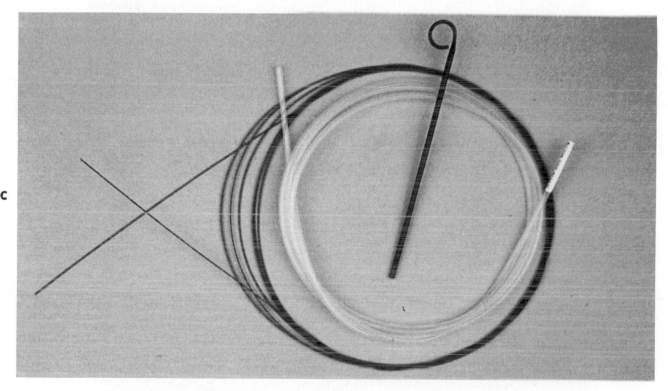

Fig. 8-23, cont'd.   C, Soehendra endoscopic biliary stent set.

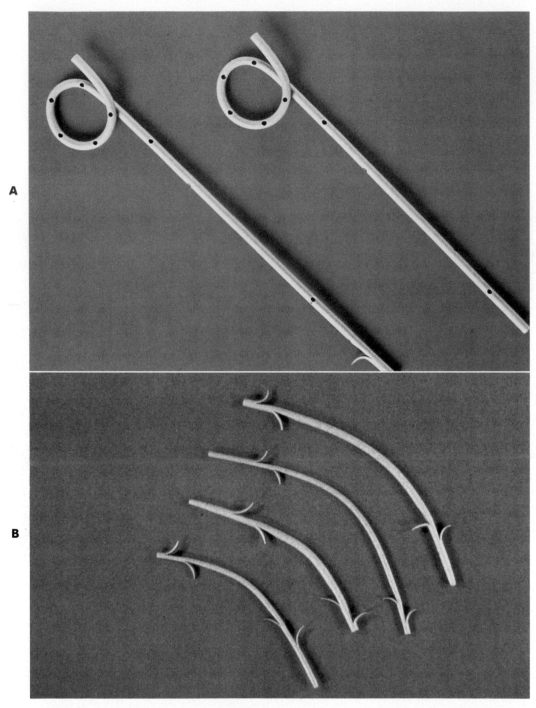

Fig. 8-24. Pancreatic stents. **A,** Zimmon Endoscopic Pancreatic Stent. (Courtesy Wilson-Cook Medical Inc., Winston-Salem, N.C.) **B,** Geenen pancreatic stents.

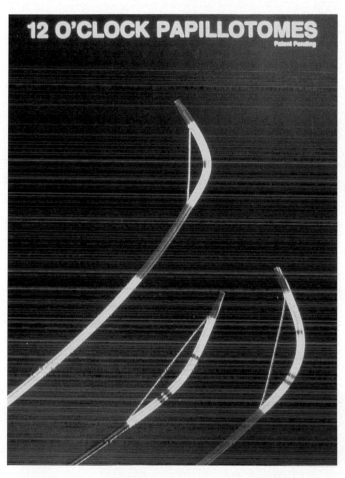

Fig. 8-25. Various papillotomes. (Courtesy Wilson-Cook Medical Inc., Winston-Salem, N.C.)

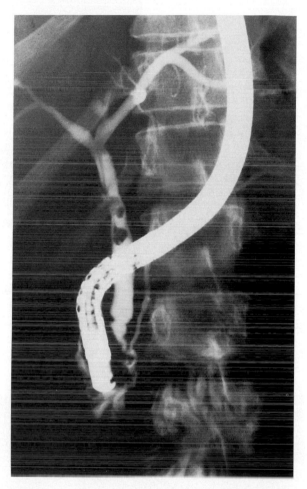

Fig. 8-26. ERCP in a 26-year-old woman after cholecystectomy shows streaming of contrast material with a flow defect in the common hepatic duct as well as three lucencies that represent retained gallstones in the common bile duct. Sometimes air bubbles can have a similar appearance.

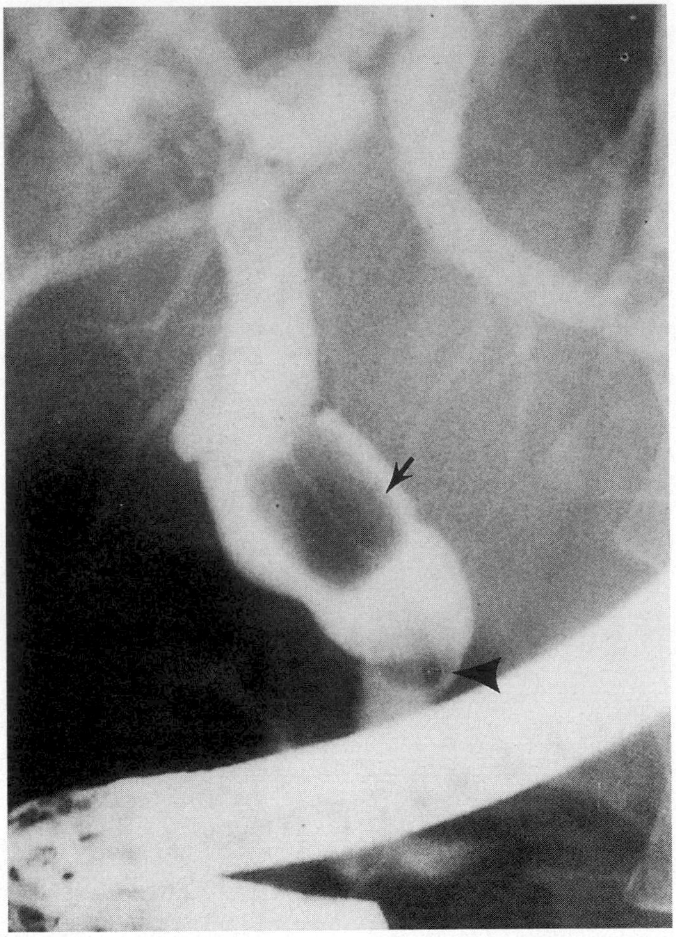

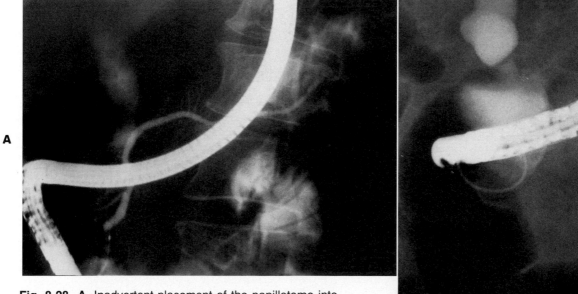

Fig. 8-27. A balloon-tipped catheter, *arrow,* is used to help extract a retained calculus, *arrowhead,* in the common bile duct.

Fig. 8-28. A, Inadvertent placement of the papillotome into the main pancreatic duct. This could cause grievous injury to the patient. **B,** Proper placement of the papillotome across the sphincter of Oddi.

most instances standard ionic water-soluble contrast agents are used at 30% to 50% strength. If too concentrated a contrast mixture is used, small stones may be hidden, and it becomes more difficult to visualize catheters and guide wires.

Radiographs show more detail than the fluoroscopic image on the screen. The appearance of contrast excretion by the kidney means that there has been either some extravasation of contrast or excessive injection of contrast into the pancreas with acinarization (opacification of the pancreatic parenchyma). Acinarization is to be avoided because it increases the risk for the subsequent development of pancreatitis.

Sometimes balloon occlusion techniques are used to better opacify the biliary system. Balloon-tipped catheters are useful for stone retrieval and for occlusion of the biliary system (Fig. 8-27). A balloon-tipped catheter may be passed proximally into the hepatic duct (ideally proximal to the cystic duct) and then inflated to occlude the duct. This allows better contrast opacification of the duct because higher filling pressures can be achieved with less drainage from the ductal system.

Common artifacts include air bubbles and streaming (Fig. 8-26). Air bubbles may be difficult to differentiate from bile duct stones. Air bubbles usually have a typical round configuration, are very lucent, line up in a single column, and "float" in the contrast and bile, whereas stones will have a more polygonal shape and "sink" in the bile and contrast mixture (Fig. 8-26). However, thick bile and dense contrast material may inhibit stone and air bubble movements, and they may be difficult to differentiate. It is always best in any type of biliary procedure (ERCP, transhepatic cholangiography, operative cholangiography, or T-tube cholangiography) to exercise extreme care to avoid the introduction of air bubbles.

There is usually about 30% magnification on the radiographs. Therefore the actual size of the dilated ducts, tumors, and stones has to be corrected accordingly. One can best estimate this by correlating the known size of an object, such as the endoscope, which is often 12 mm in diameter, with its size on the radiographs.

The radiologist, endoscopist, and other involved physicians should be aware of the radiographic appearance, proper placement, and use of specialized ERCP equipment, including papillotomes, drainage catheters, balloon catheters, and wire baskets (see Figs. 8-21 to 8-25 and 8-28).

GENITOURINARY DEVICES

Urinary Stents

(See also Chapter 12.)

Stents are used in various portions of the urinary tract to traverse benign and malignant strictures, bypass areas of dehiscence, bypass obstructing calculi, and help with fistula healing.[60-66] The most commonly used are ureteral stents (Fig. 8-29). They may be inserted percutaneously in an antegrade fashion, or they may be inserted at cystoscopy in a retrograde fashion. Sometimes they are placed at surgery, and occasionally a combination of cystoscopy and fluoroscopy is used to help in the placement of stents in complicated cases.

Polyurethane stents are widely used, especially with cystoscopic insertion techniques, because urologists and other physicians involved in these procedures are most familiar with them. Polyurethane and polyethylene stents have potentially serious problems with brittleness, bladder inflammation, encrustation, and bleeding.[63-68]

Silicone, C-Flex copolymer (Cook), and Percuflex biocompatible copolymer (Medi-tech) stents are softer and have fewer problems with patient discomfort and encrustation. They can be left in place for periods of 6 to 12 months.[63-66,69,70] Six months is the maximum recommended period for polyurethane stents to be left in place before they alter their physical characteristics from constant exposure to urine.[71] The softer stents may, however, be considerably harder to place.[65]

A double pigtail design (Fig. 8-29) is a popular stent configuration because it holds the stent in place well. One pigtail resides in the renal pelvis and the other in the bladder. A properly functioning ureteral stent permits antegrade flow of urine from the renal pelvis through the stent into the bladder.[72] Stent failure in the

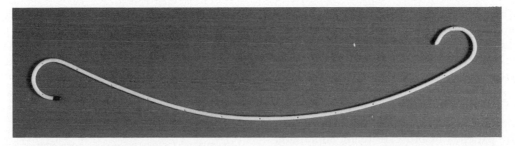

Fig. 8-29. Surgitek All Silicone Double-J ureteral stent. The stent pictured is 7 French in diameter and 24 cm in length.

first day after insertion usually is secondary to obstructing blood clots and debris. Late stent failure results from encrustation and side-hole occlusion.[67,72]

Recently, stenting has been introduced for urethral strictures.[73] Urethral strictures are a very common problem and generally are the sequelae of infection or trauma. They are treated by a variety of methods including mechanical dilatation and endoscopic and open reconstructive urologic procedures. In selected cases, a metallic stent (Urolume or Wallstent by American Medical Systems, Minnetonka, Minn.) has been successfully used for the treatment of urethral strictures.[73] The stent is woven in the form of a tubular mesh composed of a superalloy. It comes in various sizes and was developed originally for arterial and venous endovascular use but has also found application in the management of biliary obstruction.[73-77]

For urethral strictures stents with a length of 2 to 3 cm and a diameter of about 14 mm have been used.[73] The stents are designed to be flexible and self-expanding. The stent holds the stricture open while the mucosa of the urethra grows over and through the stent mesh. These types of stents are also used for treatment of prostatic outflow obstruction and detrusor sphincter dyssynergia.[73,78-80]

Stent success depends on accurate placement of the stent across the area of narrowing. Sometimes there is a hyperplastic mucosal response that may simulate a recurrent obstruction. This tends to resolve with no therapy in 4 to 6 months.[73]

Suprapubic Cystostomy

Suprapubic cystostomy, whether surgically or percutaneously placed, is used for the treatment of acute urinary retention, if standard urethral bladder catheterization is difficult or dangerous, and for long-term urinary tract drainage. Small-diameter trocar suprapubic percutaneous catheter placement is generally safe and effective for the short term.[81-84] Long-term bladder drainage is not so amenable to percutaneous techniques because the smaller catheters used in percutaneous procedures tend to plug more easily and are difficult to keep in place for any length of time.[85]

Surgical placement of large (20 to 30 French) suprapubic catheters is common for those situations in which a patient will need permanent or long-term urinary drainage.[86] There are various methods for long-term bladder drainage, including indwelling catheter, intermittent catheterization, transurethral sphincterotomy with continuous condom drainage, and suprapubic cystostomy.[86-88] The method chosen depends on a patient's particular problem and health status and the experience of the patient's health care team. Suprapubic cystostomy is best tolerated by those patients who cannot tolerate intermittent catheterization.[86]

The trocar method of percutaneous placement of suprapubic cystostomy catheters generally uses 8- to 12-French Silastic catheters (Figs. 8-30 and 8-31) for temporary urinary diversion.[86] More permanent placement of larger percutaneous suprapubic catheters has been described and will no doubt become more common.[86,89] Infection, hemorrhage, and bladder calculus formation are well-known possible complications of any type of bladder catheterization.

Foley Catheters

The Foley catheter is one of the most common devices inserted into patients (Fig. 8-32). Its use is probably exceeded in numbers only by intravenous lines and needles and external devices, such as oxygen lines and ECG leads. Foley catheters come in a large variety of sizes and are usually readily visible on plain radiographs. The balloon used to anchor the catheter can be filled with either sterile saline solution or water or with air and be distended up to a volume of 30 cc, depending on a particular catheter's design. The balloons are usually visible on plain films and are readily evident at CT and ultrasound. Some newer catheter designs suffer from poor visibility, with only the tip being readily radiopaque.

Foley catheters are used to decompress a distended bladder, collect urine, or monitor patient urine output, or are inserted as part of a radiographic or urologic study. There are Foley catheters that have a temperature probe built into them, allowing for simultaneous monitoring of the patient's body temperature. The soft design of most Foley catheters causes fairly little tissue trauma, and they are associated with a low rate of complications. Overdistension of the catheter balloon may cause its rupture and produce tissue injury. Distension of the balloon in the urethra (Fig. 8-33) can also potentially produce significant injury and is to be avoided. Occasionally, the balloons on self-retaining urinary catheters fail to deflate, necessitating some extraordinary method for their decompression.[90,91]

Penile Prostheses*

There are more than a dozen different types of penile prostheses in use[92-113] (Table 8-1).

The history of penile prostheses has recently involved a series of advancements in two main areas: (1) the development of more durable and inert synthetic materials and (2) the mechanisms by which they are designed to function.[92-113]

---

*The material for this section was adapted from Hovsepian DM, Amis ES: Penile prosthetic implants: a radiographic atlas, *RadioGraphics* 9(4):707-716, 1989.

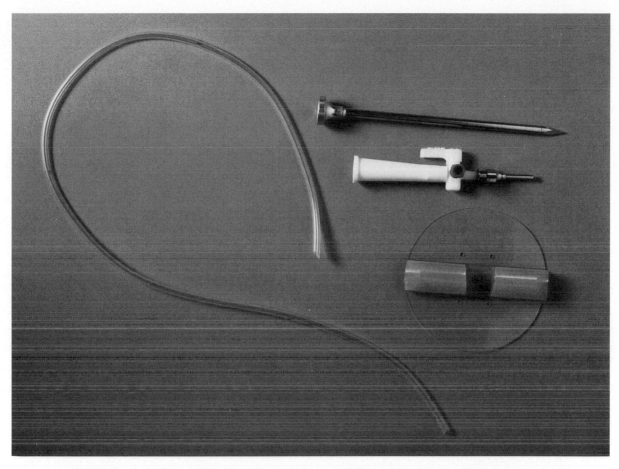

Fig. 8-30. Dow Corning Cystocath Suprapubic Drainage System. This is a standard trocar suprapubic system that temporarily places a small silicone elastomer catheter.

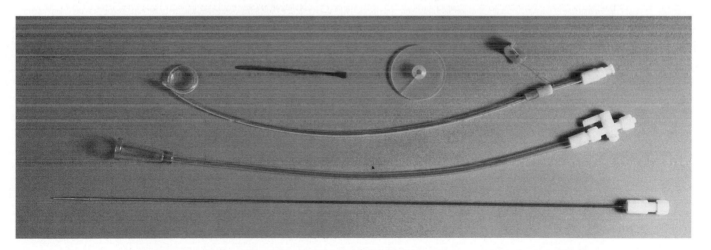

Fig. 8-31. Loop Suprapubic Catheter Set (Cook, Spencer, Ind.). The system pictured uses a 12 French, 23 cm loop catheter with a radiopaque stripe. There is a 14 French, 30 cm connecting tube.

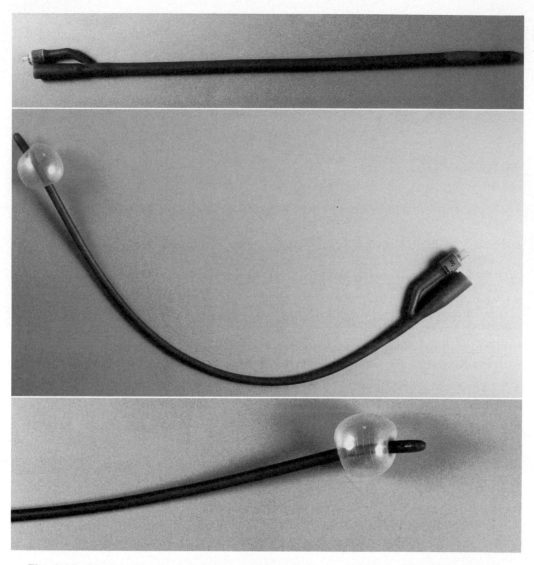

Fig. 8-32. Typical Foley catheter (Bard Urological, Covington, Ga.). **A,** Balloon deflated. **B** and **C,** Balloon inflated. The soft rubber catheter has end holes for urine drainage and a balloon near the end for retention of the catheter in the bladder. The small side channel is for instilling air or fluid to distend the balloon. The main channel is for bladder drainage.

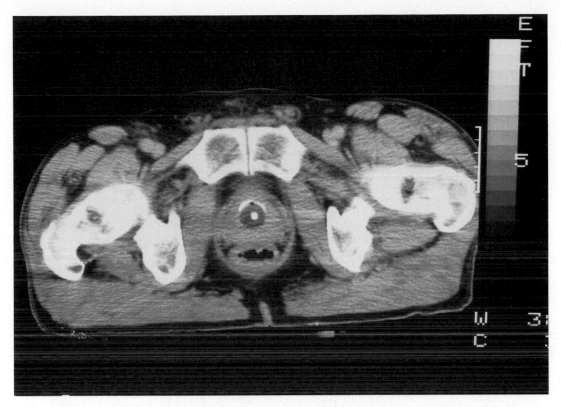

Fig. 8-33. Foley catheter balloon distended in the urethra of a patient undergoing an abdominal CT scan. The patient suffered no significant injury.

Table 8-1   Penile Prosthetic Implants

Semirigid	Inflatable
Solid Silicone	*Distant Reservoir*
Small-Carrion	AMS 700 (Scott)
Finney Flexi-Rod	AMS 700CX (Scott)
Finney Flexi-Rod II	Mentor "3-piece"
	Mentor GFS
	Uni-Flate 1000
Malleable	
Jonas	*Self-contained*
AMS 600	Flexi-Flate
Mentor	Flexi-Flate II
Positionable	AMS Hydroflex
DuraPhase	
OmniPhase	

Semirigid penile prostheses

Solid silicone. The first synthetic prostheses employed acrylic materials and, later, silicone. The earliest attempts were troubled by migration, patient discomfort, and failure of the materials.[94] Since then, many improvements in design and materials have produced a variety of semirigid implants (Fig. 8-34). They enjoy widespread use because they are relatively inexpensive, re-

liable, and easy to implant.[100] Often requiring only local or regional anesthesia, they are inserted after dilatation of the corpora cavernosa by saline solution or a mechanical dilator.

Malleable prostheses. The ESKA Jonas Silicone-Silver malleable penile prosthesis (Bard Urological, Covington, Ga.) (Fig. 8-35) was devised to further improve concealability and satisfactory function by the addition of a core of silver wire. Being malleable, it was also claimed that it simplified treatment in the case of Peyronie's disease; that is, a corporoplasty was no longer needed to correct erectile deformities.[106] This also holds true for other prostheses, including some inflatable models.

The Mentor prosthesis (Mentor Corporation, Goleta, Calif.) is a malleable prosthesis that contains a stainless steel wire core (Fig. 8-36). The wire is coiled in a spiral, which is intended to reduce metal fatigue.

Positionable prostheses. The DuraPhase and OmniPhase (Dacomed, Minneapolis, Minn.) prostheses have an outer coating of silicone elastomer but differ from the previously described prostheses in the design of the core. The braided wire used in the malleable models has been replaced by a series of articulating plastic (polysulfone) segments. In the DuraPhase prosthesis, a central tensioning cable is connected at both ends

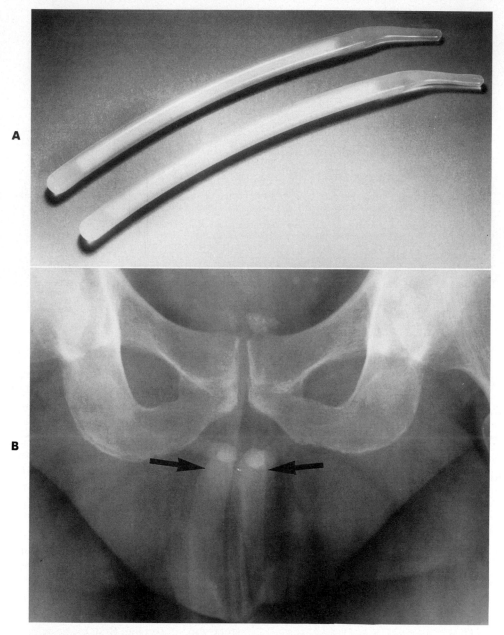

Fig. 8-34. Photograph, **A,** and radiograph, **B,** of the Small-Carrion prosthesis. The cylindrical implants are faintly visible in the corpora cavernosa, *arrows*. (Courtesy of Mentor Corp., Goleta, Calif.)

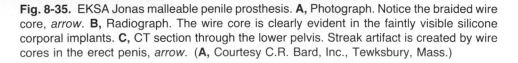

Fig. 8-35. EKSA Jonas malleable penile prosthesis. **A,** Photograph. Notice the braided wire core, *arrow.* **B,** Radiograph. The wire core is clearly evident in the faintly visible silicone corporal implants. **C,** CT section through the lower pelvis. Streak artifact is created by wire cores in the erect penis, *arrow.* (**A,** Courtesy C.R. Bard, Inc., Tewksbury, Mass.)

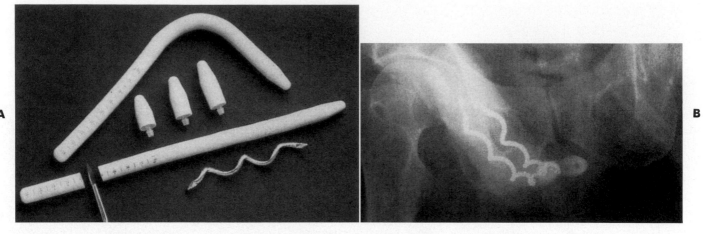

Fig. 8-36. Mentor malleable prosthesis. **A,** Photograph. Notice the spiral wire core. **B,** Radiograph. The prosthesis has a "corkscrew" appearance and dense proximal end caps. (**A,** Courtesy Mentor Corp., Goleta, Calif.; **B,** courtesy Dr. Richard L. Fein, N. Miami, Fla.)

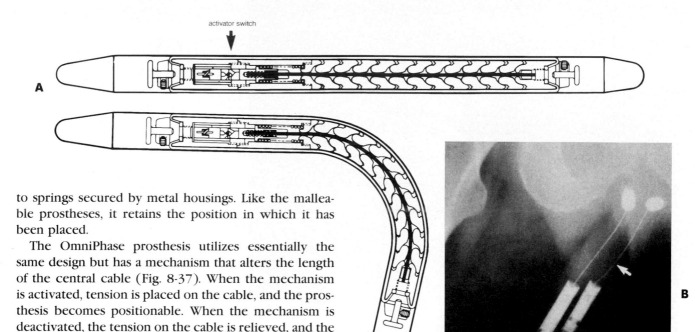

to springs secured by metal housings. Like the malleable prostheses, it retains the position in which it has been placed.

The OmniPhase prosthesis utilizes essentially the same design but has a mechanism that alters the length of the central cable (Fig. 8-37). When the mechanism is activated, tension is placed on the cable, and the prosthesis becomes positionable. When the mechanism is deactivated, the tension on the cable is relieved, and the prosthesis returns to flaccidity.

Inflatable penile prostheses

The inflatable prostheses can be divided into two types: (1) distant reservoir and (2) self-contained systems. The essential mechanism of operation is the same; fluid is pumped into distensible cylinders implanted in the corpora cavernosa. A series of valves regulates the flow in and out of the corporal implants. These devices are more complex than the semirigid prostheses and therefore have an additional set of problems that may arise. They are also considerably more expensive and difficult to implant. Nevertheless, they are quite popular because of near-natural performance.

Fig. 8-37. OmniPhase prosthesis. **A,** Diagram of prosthesis activator switch, *arrow.* **B,** Radiograph of prosthesis. Distal activator switch, *large arrow,* shortens tensioning cable, *small arrow,* to render previously flaccid prosthesis positionable. The articulating plastic segments that surround the wire are not visible. (**A** and **B,** Courtesy Dacomed Corp., Minneapolis.)

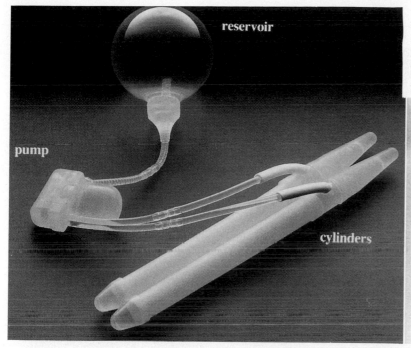
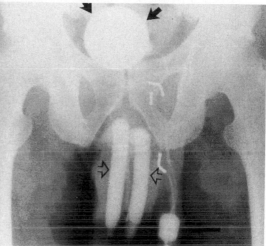

Fig. 8-38. AMS 700 (Scott) inflatable prosthesis. **A,** Photograph. **B,** Radiograph The abdominal reservoir *(short arrows),* scrotal pump *(long arrow),* and corporal implants *(open arrows)* are clearly demonstrated. The tubing and connectors are also easily seen. (**A,** Courtesy of American Medical Systems, Minnetonka, Minn.)

Distant reservoir prostheses. The first inflatable prosthesis was introduced in 1973 by Scott and co-workers.[111] It consisted of a reservoir placed in the abdomen, two pumps implanted in the scrotum, and two inflatable corporal inserts. The original design has continued to evolve, with the consolidation of the two pumps into a single unit (Fig. 8-38). A more recent model, the AMS 700CX, has additional reinforcement of the corporal cylinders in order to reduce the incidence of leakage and aneurysmal dilatation.[97]

In 1982, the Mentor corporation introduced a similar "3-piece" inflatable prosthesis (Fig. 8-39). It consists of an abdominal reservoir, a scrotal pump, and inflatable corporal cylinders. Modifications have been made since its introduction, primarily in the tubing and connections. The Mentor GFS prosthesis eliminates the need for an abdominal operation by consolidation of the reservoir and pump into a single unit, the "Resi-pump," which is implanted in the scrotum (Fig. 8-40). This "2-piece" system, like the "3-piece" Mentor and AMS 700 prostheses, requires assembly in the operating room. The hydraulic fluid is usually sterile saline, which cannot be seen radiographically.[96]

The Uni-Flate 1000 (Surgitek) prosthesis has its pump and reservoir made into a single unit, which is implanted in the scrotum (Fig. 8-41). Unlike the other inflatable prostheses, it is supplied as a prefilled and preassembled system. The hydraulic fluid is nonradiopaque sterile saline.

Self-contained inflatable prostheses. The self-contained inflatable prostheses are similar to the semirigid prostheses because they contain only corporal implants. Erection is achieved when fluid is transferred from a reservoir chamber to an inflatable segment. They are also similar to the semirigid devices because concealment can sometimes be difficult.

The Hydroflex (American Medical Systems) self-contained penile prosthesis has a reservoir located in the proximal end of the prosthesis. Valves located distally control the flow in and out of the centrally located inflation chamber (Fig. 8-42). As with other fluid-containing systems, leakage has been reported.[108]

The Flexi-Flate penile implant (Surgitek) is a coaxial system. A pump at the distal tip transfers the fluid from an outer reservoir chamber to an inflatable inner cylinder. A modified model, the Flexi-Flate II (Fig. 8-43) is also available.

Radiographic evaluation of penile prostheses

Care should be taken to ensure that the entire system is included, especially in those models with abdominal reservoirs. Evaluation should generally include radiographs of the lower abdomen, pelvis, and the scrotum. Soft-tissue technique and oblique views are often

Text continued on p. 271.

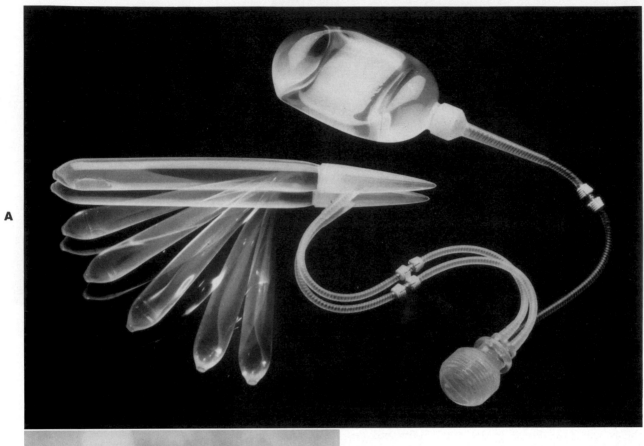

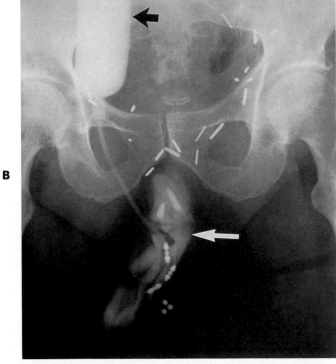

Fig. 8-39. Mentor inflatable prosthesis. **A,** Photograph. **B,** Radiograph. The abdominal reservoir, *black arrow,* is filled, whereas the corporal inserts, *white arrow,* are in the deflated state. The conical proximal ends of the corporal implant are clearly seen, as are the tubing and connectors, but the scrotal pump is visible only as three rounded opacities in the lower portion of the radiograph. (**A,** Courtesy Mentor Corp., Goleta, Calif.; **B,** courtesy Dr. Richard L. Fein, N. Miami, Fla.)

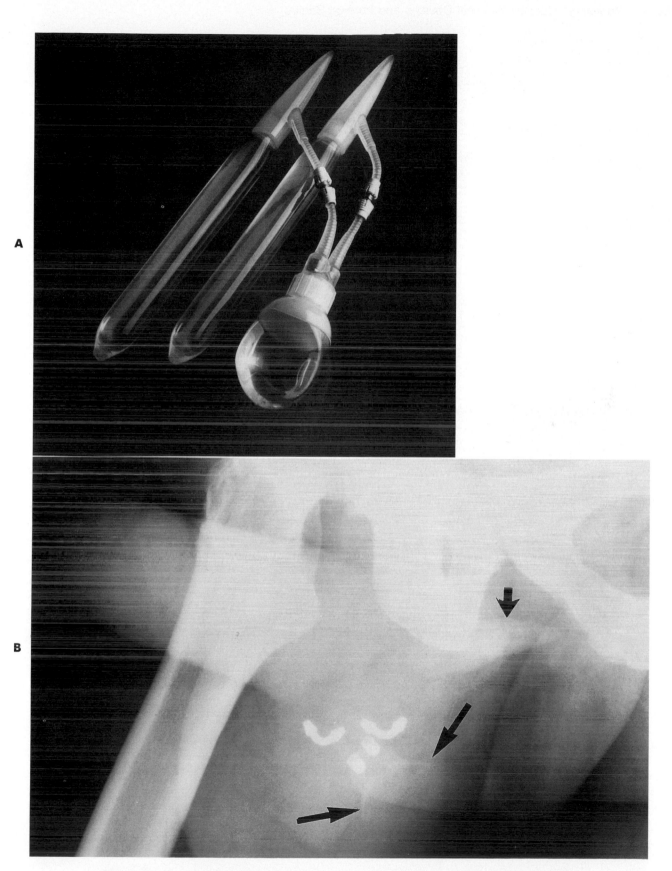

Fig. 8-40. Mentor GFS inflatable prosthesis. **A,** Photograph. **B,** Radiograph. The scrotal "Resipump" is faintly visible, *long arrows.* The cylindrical metal valves and curved tubing connectors are seen directly above. The conical crural tips of the corporal implants are also easily visible, *short arrow.* (**A,** Courtesy Mentor Corp., Goleta, Calif.; **B,** courtesy Dr. Richard L. Fein, N. Miami, Fla.)

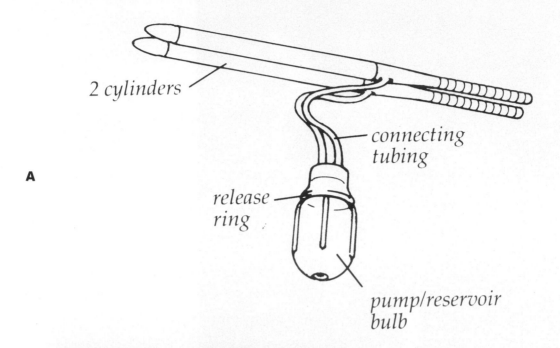

A

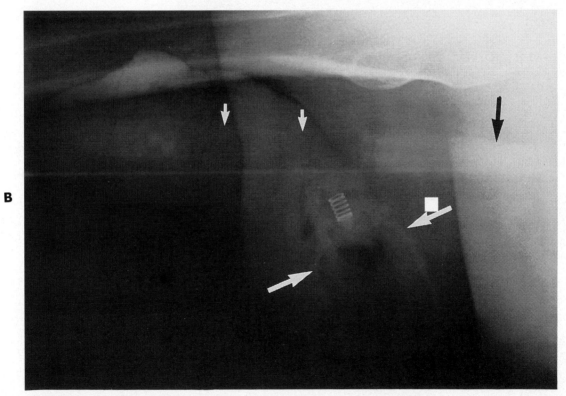

B

Fig. 8-41. Uni-Flate 1000 inflatable penile implant. **A,** Diagram. **B,** Radiograph. The combined reservoir-pump is clearly seen, *large white arrows.* The metallic spring in the release ring is part of the valve mechanism. The corporal cylinders are faintly visible, *small white arrows,* as are their denser crural ends, *black arrow.* (**A,** Courtesy Surgitek, Racine Wis.; **B,** courtesy Dr. Thomas H. Stanisic, Tucson.)

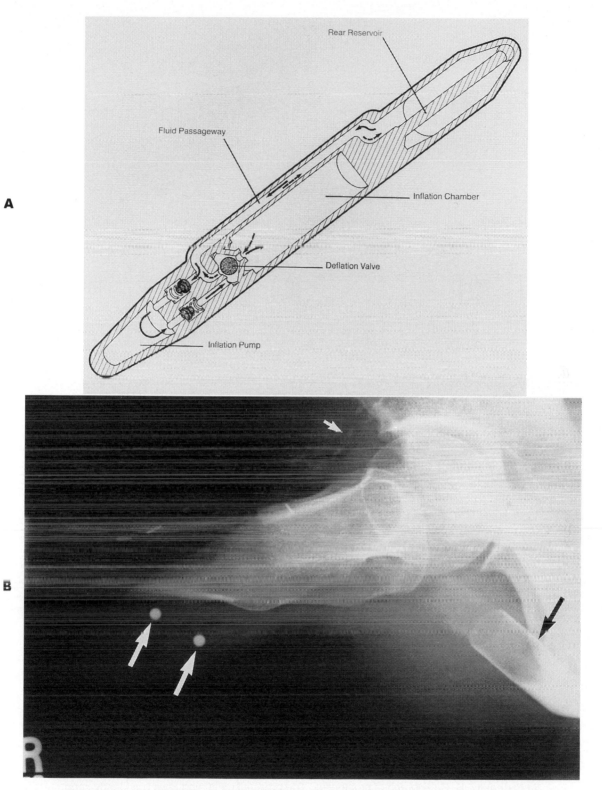

A

Rear Reservoir

Fluid Passageway

Inflation Chamber

Deflation Valve

Inflation Pump

B

R

Fig. 8-42. AMS Hydroflex self-contained penile prosthesis. **A,** Diagram. **B,** Radiograph. Only the distal ball valves, *large white arrows,* and the proximal metal caps, *black arrow,* can be seen. Notice calcification in the pudendal arteries, *small white arrow;* diabetic vascular disease is a primary cause of male impotence. (**A,** Courtesy American Medical Systems, Minnetonka, Minn.; **B,** courtesy Dr. Thomas H. Stanisic, Tucson.)

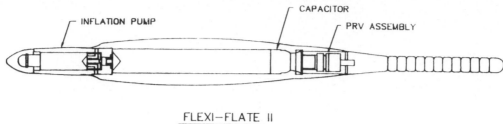

FLEXI—FLATE II

A

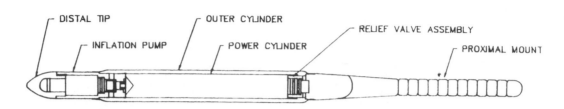

FLEXI—FLATE

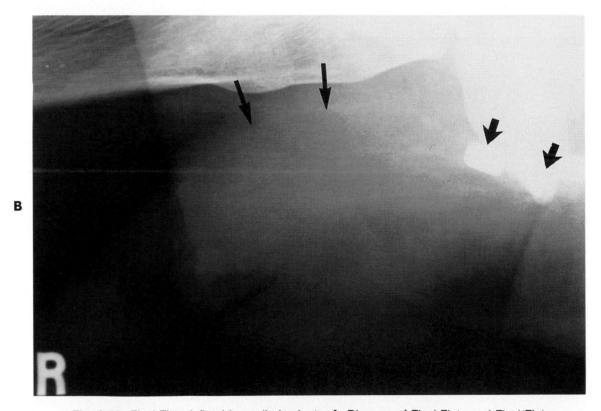

B

Fig. 8-43. Flexi-Flate inflatable penile implants. **A,** Diagram of Flexi-Flate and Flexi-Flate II prostheses. **B,** Radiograph of prostheses. The proximal metal end caps are clearly seen, *short arrows,* whereas the corporal cylinders are only faintly evident, *long arrows.*

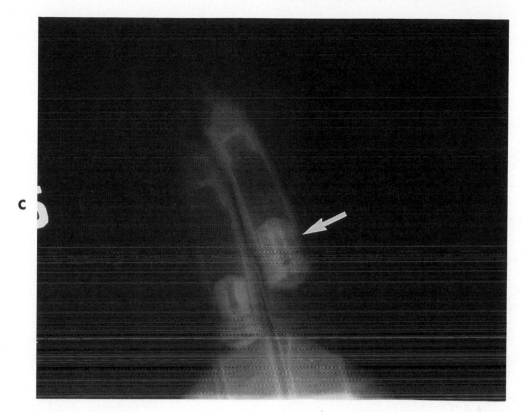

Fig. 8-43, cont'd. C, Radiograph using soft-tissue technique. The distal pumps are now well demonstrated, *arrow.*(**A,** Courtesy Medical Engineering Corp./Surgitek, Racine, Wis.; **B,** courtesy Dr. Thomas H. Stanisic, Tucson.)

helpful. Only those fluid-containing prostheses with added radiographic contrast can be easily evaluated for leakage. Tubing and connectors should be scrutinized for kinks or discontinuity. With the self-contained and semirigid implants, one must be alert for fracture of the silicone, central wire core, or tensioning cable.

Migration of the corporal implants or ancillary components can occur when a friction point develops and causes tissue erosion. It is important to keep in mind the anticipated location of each segment of a prosthetic system. Patient discomfort in the absence of infection should alert one to the possibility that migration may occur. Any prosthetic device may become infected, necessitating removal.* Often a rim of fibrosis remains and casts a radiographically visible silhouette of the prosthesis after its removal.

Artificial Urinary Sphincters

Urinary incontinence is a major problem for many patients. In selected individuals, a hydraulically operated artificial urinary sphincter (AUS) can restore urinary competence in someone with bladder outlet incontinence.[114-116] The sphincter device consists of an

intra-abdominal balloon reservoir to provide hydraulic pressure to maintain inflation of a cuff that closes the bladder neck or the bulbous urethra (Figs. 8-44 and 8-45). When the patient wishes to void, he or she activates a pump located in the scrotum or labia. The pump transfers fluid out of the cuff, which deflates and allows emptying of the bladder. The fluid passes through a control assembly into the balloon reservoir.

The patient can now void by active bladder emptying, by using the Valsalva maneuver, or by catheterization. The control assembly then will repressurize the urethral cuff by transferring fluid from the reservoir back to the cuff, thereby restoring patient continence.

All parts of the AUS are interconnected. Fluid loss from one part of the system will result in fluid loss from the entire system.[115] Most leaks are slow, and it is not possible to determine the site of the fluid loss. However, plain films are very useful for confirming fluid loss or malposition of system components in cases of AUS malfunction because the fluid is usually opacified with a dilute concentration of iodinated contrast medium[114-118] (Fig. 8-46). Sphincteric dysfunction results in either urinary incompetence or less commonly bladder-outlet obstruction.

AUS malfunction without fluid leak may be second-

---

*References 92, 93, 95, 96, 99, 102, 104, 106, 107.

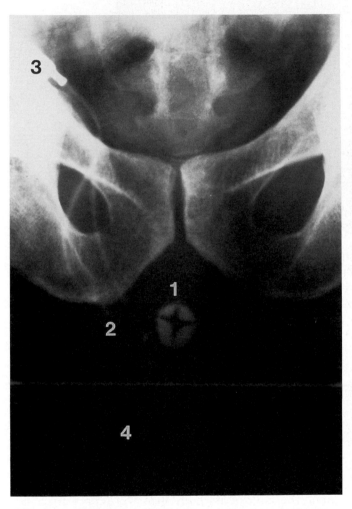

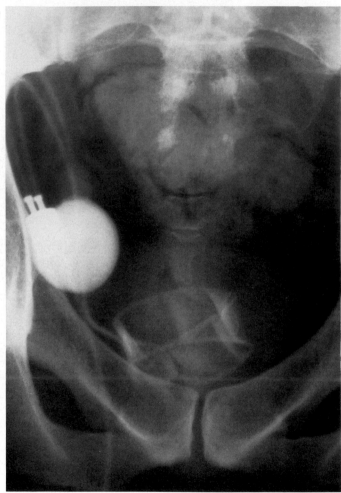

Fig. 8-44. AMS 791 artificial urinary sphincter. *1,* Inflatable cuff; *2,* connecting tube; *3,* control assembly; *4,* pump. (From Rose SC, Hansen ME, Webster GD, et al: *Radiology* 168:403-408, 1988.)

Fig. 8-45. AMS 800 artificial urinary sphincter in the normal, inflated continent state. (From Rose SC, Hansen ME, Webster GD, et al: *Radiology* 168:403-408, 1988.)

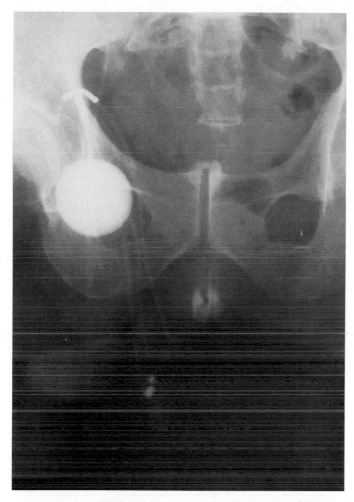

Fig. 8-46. Radiograph showing malposition of the balloon reservoir in an AMS 800 artificial urinary sphincter. There is inferior displacement of the balloon reservoir and the accompanying connecting tubes into the inguinal canal in this patient with an inguinal hernia that incorporated sphincter components. (From Rose SC, Hansen ME, Webster GD, et al: *Radiology* 168:403-408, 1988.)

ary to a kinked tube or, more commonly, failure of some component in the control system. Urodynamic measurements, cystourethroscopy, bladder catheterization to measure residual bladder volume and pressures, and inspection of the device at surgery may be required to ascertain the correct diagnosis.[115] Cuff erosion into the urethral mucosa can be a significant problem and is best diagnosed by cystourethroscopy.[115]

Prostatic hypertrophy and urethral strictures are common problems in men. In extreme cases they may cause acute urinary retention or chronic bladder distension with dribbling from overflow. Stents are now being explored for use in restoring reasonable urinary flow and continence in patients with these conditions. The stents are composed of a metallic mesh structure with the same basic design as those being used for vascular stenoses and malignant biliary stenoses (Fig. 8-47).

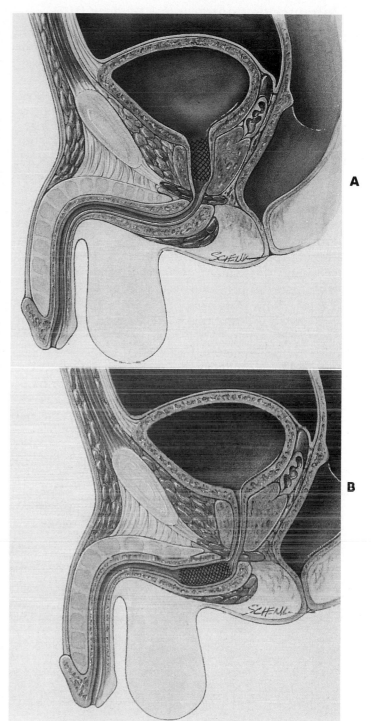

Fig. 8-47. UroLume Endourethral Wallstent Prosthesis. **A,** Prosthesis in the prostatic urethra. **B,** Prosthesis in the bulbous urethra. (**A** and **B,** Courtesy American Medical Systems, Minnetonka, Minn. In the USA the UroLume prosthesis is for investigational use only.)

Intrauterine Contraceptive Devices (IUD)

IUDs are a very popular form of contraception worldwide. The use of an intrauterine device for contraception was first described in 1909, and IUDs were available in the late 1920s and early 1930s in Japan and Germany, though there were little data at that time about their effectiveness or complications.[119] Their popular use began in the 1960s and continues to this day. More than 60 types of IUDs have been tested or marketed for contraception, and the People's Republic of China accounts for 75% of IUD usage in the world.[119]

Today the IUDs most commonly seen in patients are models of the TCu (Copper T) and the Cu-7 (G.D. Searle and Company, Skokie, Ill.), the Nova T (Leiras Pharmaceuticals, Turku, Finland), the Progestasert (Alza Corporation, Palo Alto, Calif.), the Multiload-250 (Organon International, Oss, The Netherlands), and the Lippes Loop (Ortho Pharmaceutical Corporation, Raritan, N.J.) (Figs. 8-48 to 8-52). There are also patients who probably have other older devices still in place.

Only the Progestasert (Fig. 8-48) and the Copper T380A are distributed in the United States. In 1985 Ortho Pharmaceutical Corporation discontinued distribution of the Lippes Loop. Similarly, in 1986 G.D. Searle and Company stopped the distribution of the Cu-7 and Copper T IUDs.[119]

Lippes Loop is still found in many women (Figs. 8-49 and 8-50). It is readily visible on plain radiographs because it is coated with barium sulfate. It is considered to be a "nonmedicated" IUD because its effectiveness does not depend on the addition of any drugs to its surface. The Cu-7, Copper T380A, TCu, Multiload, and Progestasert IUD are considered to be "medicated" because they rely on release of drugs or on the nature of their surface for their effectiveness. The Progestasert, for example, contains 38 mg of progesterone that is slowly released through its ethylene vinyl acetate copolymer stem over the approximate 18-month life of the IUD (Fig. 8-48). The effectiveness of the copper IUD is directly related to the amount of the exposed copper surfaces.[120] The use of copper or progesterone with an IUD appears to enhance its contraceptive ability.

Patients discontinue IUD usage for a variety of reasons, most frequently because they wish to become pregnant. Patients may also want to change their form of contraception, or they may be required to have their IUD removed because it is past its efficacy. Patients involuntarily discontinue IUD use because of pain, pelvic infection, expulsion of the IUD, irregular or increased menstrual bleeding, or pregnancy.

Patients with IUDs can be safely imaged with magnetic resonance. Moreover, MRI images of the pelvis are not significantly degraded by the presence of an IUD.[121]

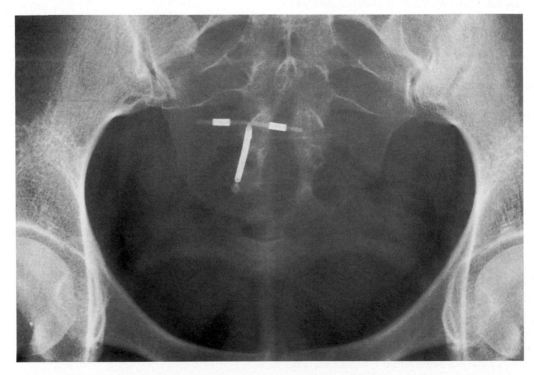

Fig. 8-48. Thirty-eight-year-old woman with a Progestasert IUD. (Courtesy Dr. George R. Barnes, Jr., Tucson.)

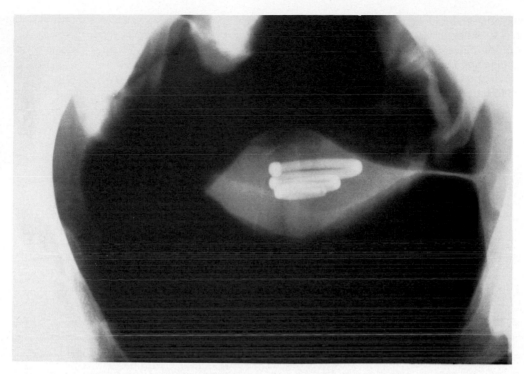

Fig. 8-49. Young woman with asymptomatic pneumoperitoneum after having a Lippes Loop IUD inserted. (Courtesy Dr. George R. Barnes, Jr., Tucson.)

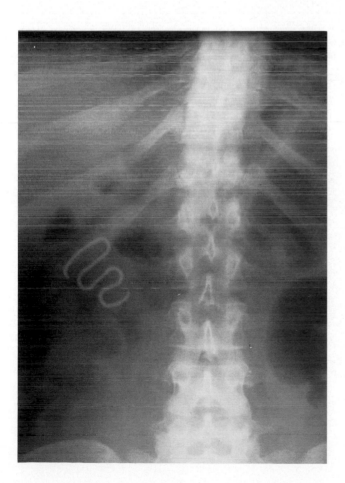

Fig. 8-50. Twenty-five-year-old woman whose IUD (Lippes Loop) had eroded through her uterus and became free in the peritoneum. She had no symptoms and had gone to her physician because she could no longer feel the string on the IUD. She was not treated and told to return if she had any problems. Three months later she suffered abdominal pain after an automobile accident. Surgical exploration of her abdomen revealed the IUD floating free in the left upper quadrant. There were no bowel or mesenteric abnormalities. (Courtesy Dr. George R. Barnes, Jr., Tucson.)

Fig. 8-51. Twenty-four-year-old woman with IUD and a 21-week gestation. **A,** Supine view of the abdomen. **B,** Magnified view of the pelvis. Arrows outline the fetal skull. She had vaginal bleeding from a placenta previa and delivered a stillborn 350-gram male infant. The IUD was found lodged on the maternal surface of the placenta.

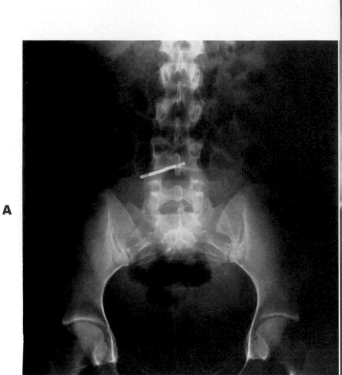

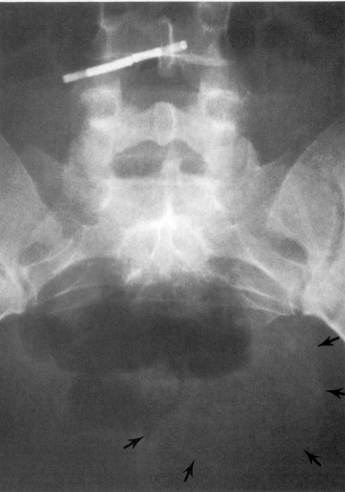

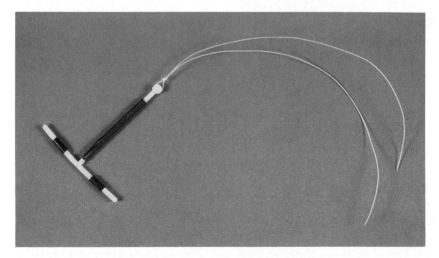

Fig. 8-52. Para-Gard Intrauterine Copper Contraceptive Model T.

There is no evidence that an IUD has sufficient torque to become displaced or injure body tissue during an MRI exam. It also does not heat up significantly to scar the endometrium.[121] There is no reason to screen patients for the presence of an IUD before one performs an MRI exam.

The most common problem associated with IUD use is a "missing" thread. Threads are attached to IUDs in order for the patient and her physician to be able to determine periodically if the IUD is still in place. It is not uncommon for these threads to break off and be lost or for them to migrate into the uterus and no longer be palpable. Ultrasound is usually highly accurate in determining the intrauterine location of an IUD. It is the initial imaging modality for determining the cause of a missing thread, though plain films and computed tomography may also prove useful.[121-131]

Uterine perforation by an IUD is uncommon (Fig. 8-50). It ranges from 1:350 to 1:2500 insertions.[123,128] When an IUD perforates the uterus, it usually produces a complete perforation leaving the IUD free in the peritoneum. Only 15% to 20% of perforations are partial with the IUD embedding deep in the uterine wall.[123,128] Patients with complete perforations are often asymptomatic, whereas those with partial perforations may have pain and abnormal bleeding. The decision as to whether to remove the perforated IUD surgically or to leave it alone depends on its location and the patient's clinical picture.[132] A perforating IUD does not necessarily have to be removed because many patients remain asymptomatic. Laparoscopy is useful for removal of a perforated IUD if it can be done safely.[132]

There seems to be no relationship between current or past IUD usage and an increased risk for having an ectopic pregnancy.[120,132] The progestin-only IUDs do appear to have a higher associated ectopic pregnancy rate in comparison to the copper IUDs.[120] However, most IUDs offer adequate protection against the development of an ectopic pregnancy.[119,120,133]

Intrauterine infection and endotoxic shock are possible complications in the rare patient who has both an IUD and an intrauterine pregnancy (Fig. 8-51), especially if there is a threatened abortion.[134] If the pregnancy is free of symptoms and progressing normally, the IUD should be left alone. There is no apparent association between an intrauterine pregnancy with an IUD in place and an increased incidence of fetal anomalies and malformations.[135]

Pessaries

Pessaries (Figs. 8-53 to 8-56), are simple mechanical devices for the treatment of vaginal and uterine prolapse. They have been used since the last century and are generally safe and relatively effective. There is even a case report of a pessary being in place for 57 years![136]

The modern treatment of prolapse is mainly surgical, but some believe there is still a place for the use of pessaries, especially as newer, plastic designs.[137] At one time rubber was used for pessary construction but was not as satisfactory as metal or plastic. Rubber pessaries carried relatively high risks of infection, ulceration, and possible later malignancy. Some of the problems related to pessary use probably result from neglect in which the pessary is overlooked and forgotten.[137]

The main indications for pessary use rather than surgery are a patient refusing surgery, failure of previous surgery to cure prolapse, preoperative healing of vaginal or cervical ulcerations in long-standing cases of uterine procidentia, uterine prolapse complicating pregnancy, and a patient who is a poor anesthesia risk because of cardiovascular or pulmonary disease.[137-141]

Various types of pessaries have been designed for different situations. Seven "common" types[139,140] are as follows:

1. Smith-Hodges. This is an elongated, curved ovoid used for symptomatic uterine retroflexion.
2. Gellhorn. The cervix sits on a disklike platform. A stem rests upon the perineum.

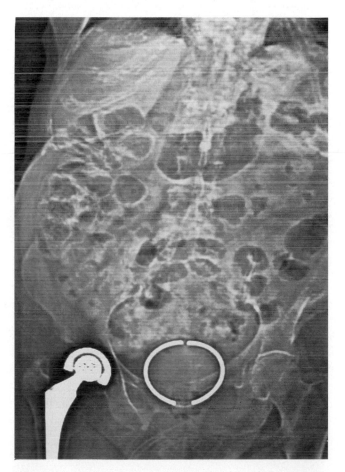

Fig. 8-53. Elderly lady with a pessary, possibly a Smith-Hodges type.

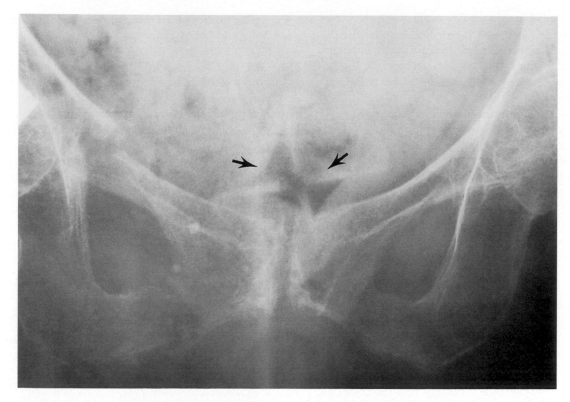

Fig. 8-54. Elderly lady with plastic "bee cell" pessary, *arrows*.

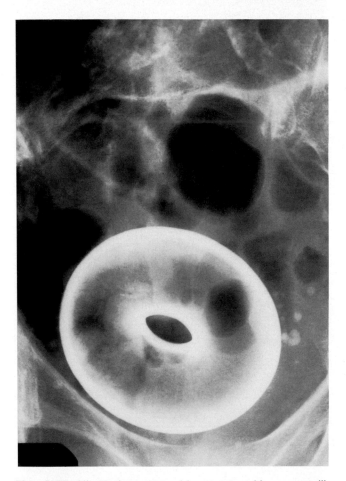

Fig. 8-55. Ninety-three-year-old woman with a metallic doughnut type of pessary.

3. Gehrung.
4. Ring (Figs. 8-55 and 8-56). This is a hard or soft doughnut design.
5. Bee-cell or ball (Fig. 8-54).
6. Napier. This is similar to the Gellhorn and is supported by a belt and is used in patients with an incompetent perineum.
7. Inflatable. It has a doughnut design with a valve to allow air inflation and deflation.

Pessaries should be removed periodically for cleaning. Although generally safe, neglected pessaries can cause ulceration, infection, perforation, and even fistula formation.[141,142] Sometimes they become incarcerated and encrusted.[139]

MISCELLANEOUS DEVICES AND MATERIALS

Odds and Ends

There is a large variety of incidental devices and materials that are sometimes seen lying within or on top of the lower chest, abdomen, and pelvis (Figs. 8-57 to 8-72). Occasionally, medications as well as interesting materials worn by patients are visible on radiographic studies and can confuse the inexperienced observer. These devices and materials include esophageal probes (to monitor esophageal pH, motility, and temperature), colon and rectum decompression tubes, operative cholangiography catheters, medications (such as enteric

Text continued on p. 292.

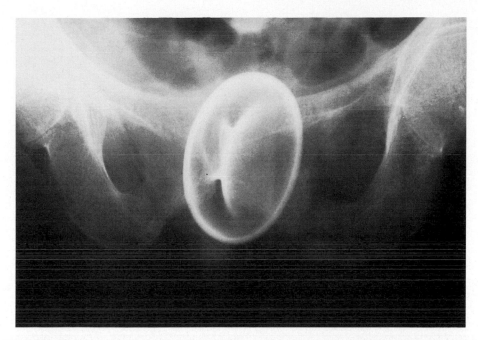

Fig. 8-56. Seventy-nine-year-old woman with a metallic doughnut pessary and severe uterine prolapse.

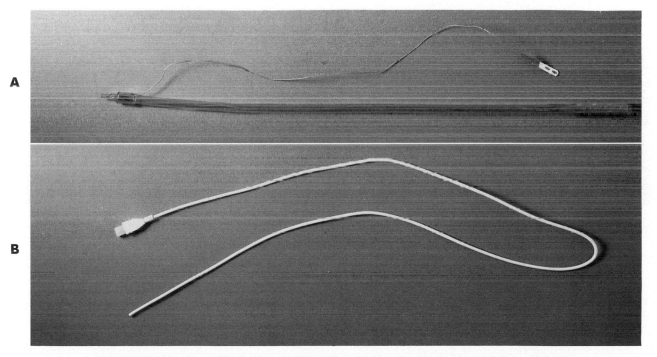

Fig. 8-57. A, Esophageal stethoscope with a temperature sensor (Mon-A-Therm). **B,** Esophageal/rectal temperature probe (Electromedics Inc.).

Continued.

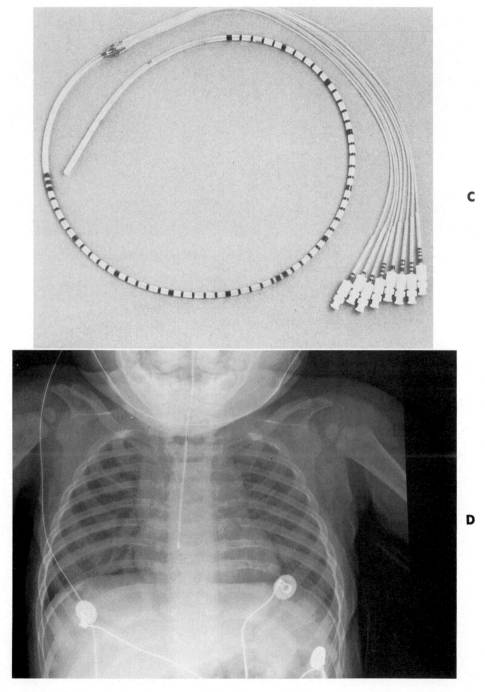

Fig. 8-57, cont'd. C, Esophageal motility catheter. **D,** Small child with esophageal pH monitor. (**C,** Courtesy Wilson-Cook, Winston-Salem, N.C.)

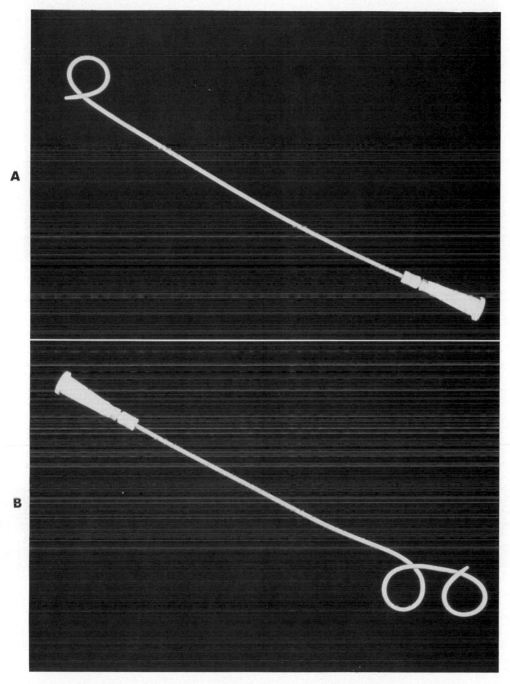

Fig. 8-58. One-loop, **A,** and two-loop, **B,** colon decompression catheters.
Continued.

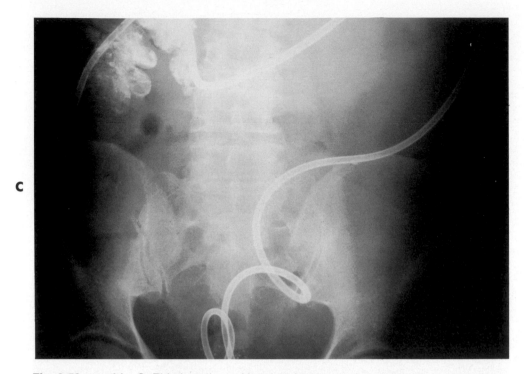

Fig. 8-58, cont'd. **C,** Elderly patient with colon decompression catheter extending all the way to the cecum. (**A** and **B,** Courtesy Wilson-Cook, Winston-Salem, N.C.)

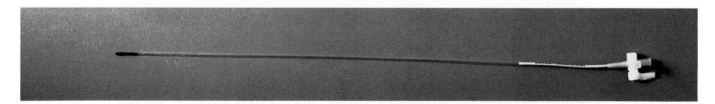

Fig. 8-59. Cholangiography catheter (Baxter, Deerfield, Ill.).

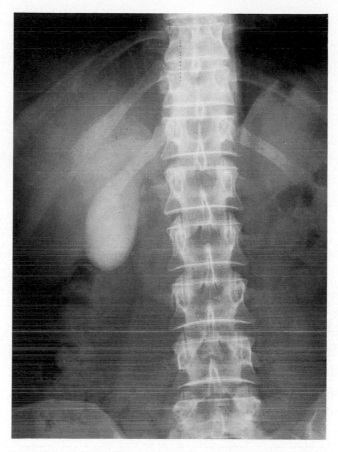

Fig. 8-60. Patient with a normal oral cholecystogram (OCG). Oral cholecystographic material has opacified the gallbladder and been excreted into the bowel.

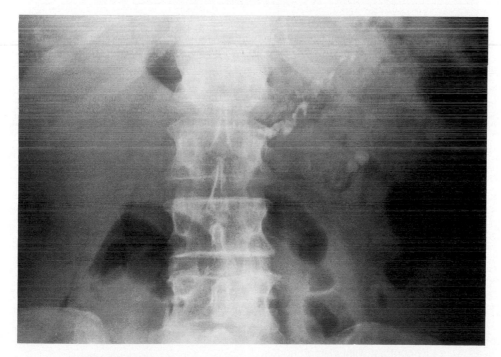

Fig. 8-61. Pepto-Bismol visible in the stomach and the jejunum.

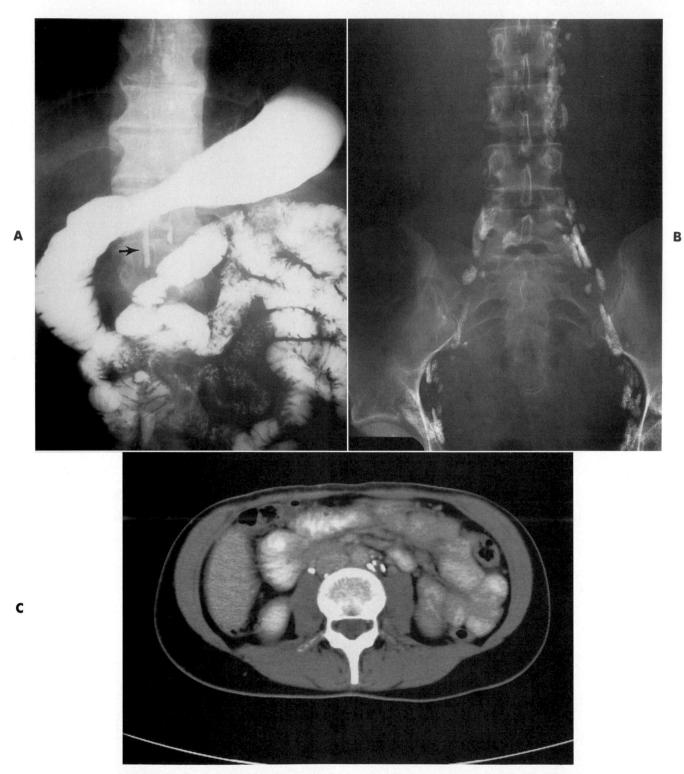

Fig. 8-62. A, Residual Pantopaque, *arrow,* is visible within the spinal canal on a patient who had undergone a myelogram many years before the upper gastrointestinal series. **B** and **C,** Patient with a normal lymphangiogram. Supine view of the abdomen, **B,** and CT scan, **C,** show contrast within lymph nodes.

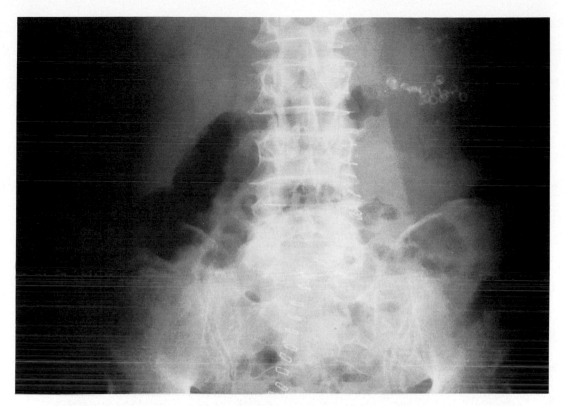

Fig. 8-63. Radiopaque markers are visible within the body of the stomach. They are used to assess gastric emptying and bowel motility.

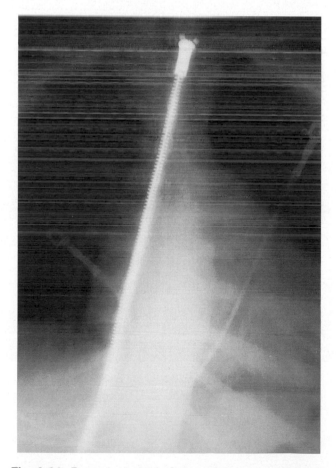

Fig. 8-64. Posey restraint jacket used to keep a patient in his bed. The zipper of the jacket is readily visible on plain radiographs.

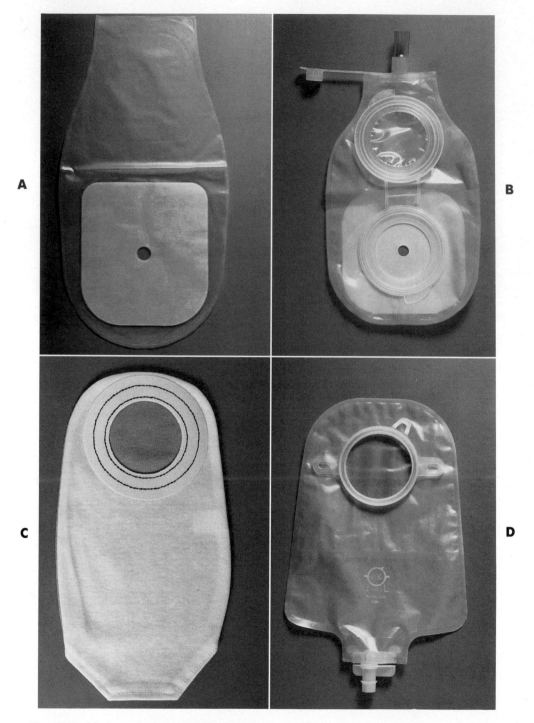

Fig. 8-65. Various drainage bags sometimes visible on patients' abdomen and pelvis. **A,** Ileostomy pouch. **B,** Uro pouch with flange. **C,** Urostomy pouch cover. **D,** Wound drainage collector (Hollister, Libertyville, Ill.).

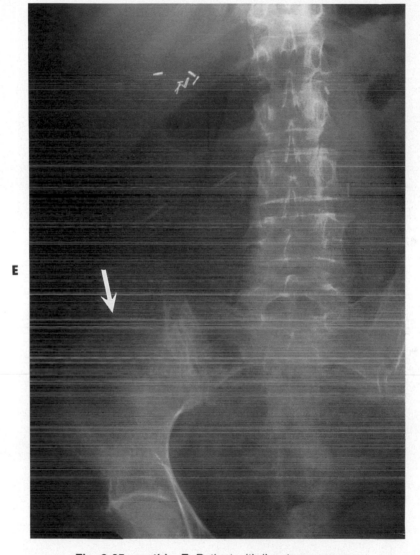

Fig. 8-65, cont'd.   E, Patient with ileostomy, *arrow.*

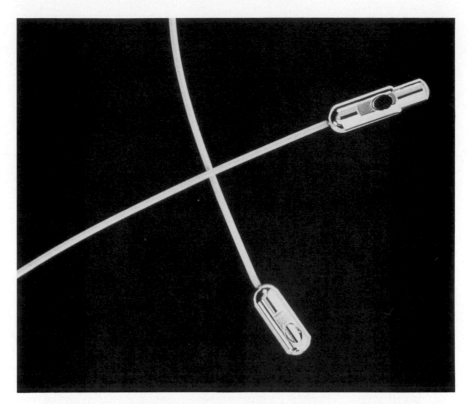

Fig. 8-66. Carey capsule (Wilson-Cook, Winston-Salem, N.C.). It is used for small-bowel biopsy.

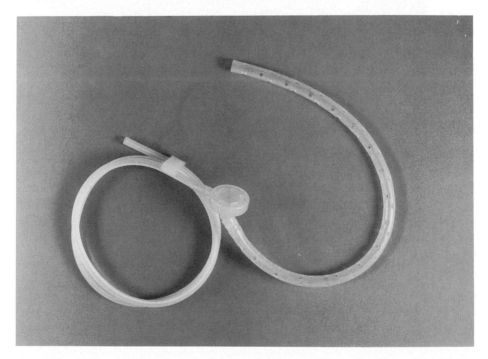

Fig. 8-67. LeVeen peritoneovenous shunt (Becton Dickinson, Franklin Lakes, N.J.).

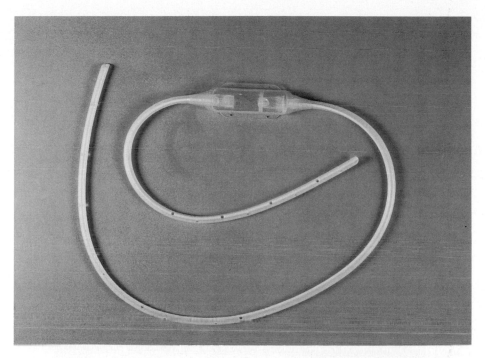

Fig. 8-68. Denver pleuroperitoneal shunt (Codman & Shurtleff, Randolph, Mass.)

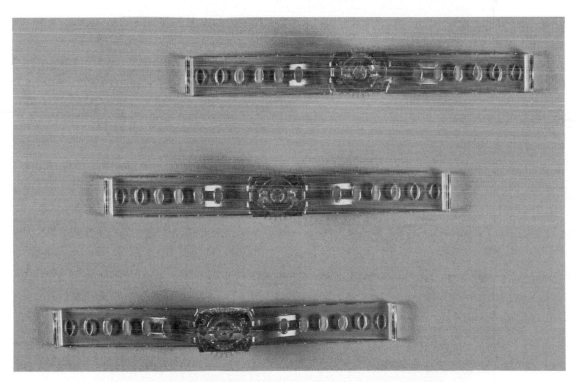

Fig. 8-69. Retention suture bridge (Ethicon, Somerville, N.J.).

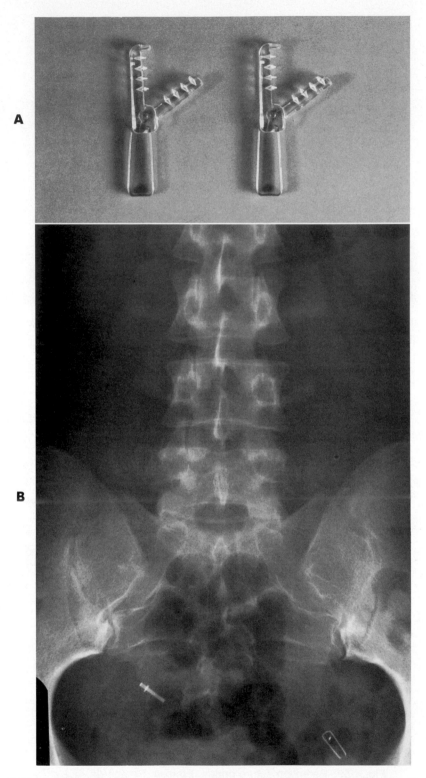

Fig. 8-70. A, Hulka clip (Richard Wolf, Knittlingen, Germany) for tubal ligation. **B,** Patient with tubal ligation clips.

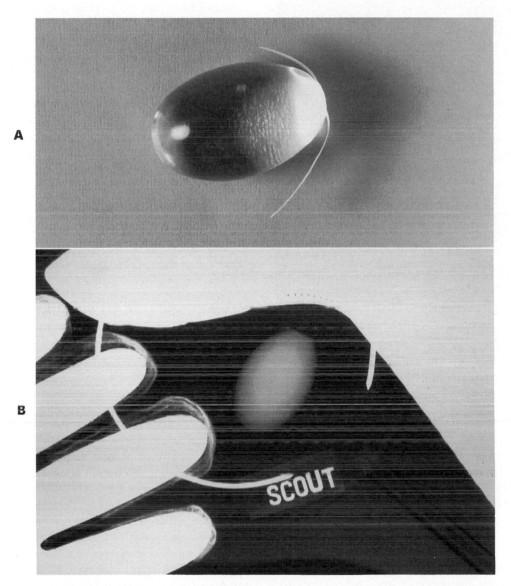

Fig. 8-71. A, Silicone testicular prosthesis. **B,** Radiograph. It is surrounded by objects commonly seen in everyday radiology, including lead markers and gloves, gonadal shield, and a compression paddle used for gastrointestinal studies. The rim of the compression balloon in the paddle is outlined by a metal ring.

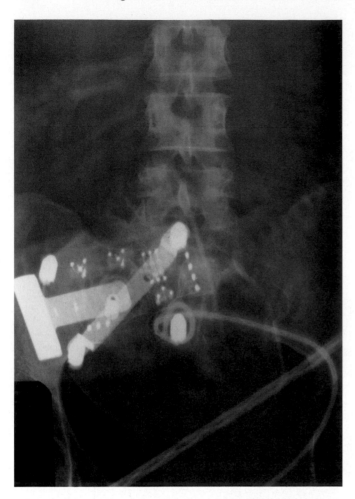

Fig. 8-72. Supine view of the abdomen obtained during late pregnancy. Notice the fetus and the fetal monitoring device.

coated prescription pills and tablets, Pepto-Bismol, Pantopaque), markers for assessment of gastric emptying and bowel motility, patient-restraint devices, bags or pouches to collect drainage fluids and stool, bowel biopsy devices, testicular prostheses, various apparatus used in everyday radiology, and even fetal monitoring equipment (Figs. 8-57 to 8-66, 8-71, and 8-72).

If an adequate history is not supplied, the radiologist may be unable to distinguish between the various catheters found overlying the abdomen and chest and to assess if their position and function are proper. A feeding tube might appear similar to a pH probe. The feeding tube should ideally be in the proximal small bowel, whereas the ideal location for an esophageal pH monitor is in the lower third of the esophagus just above the gastroesophageal junction (Fig. 8-57). Ostomy pouches and drainage bags of all types may produce confusing densities and not be easily recognized without experience and a proper history (Fig. 8-65).

Most medications are not radiopaque. However, enteric coated pills and medicines containing heavy metals or halogenated compounds, such as iodides, are often visible on radiographic exams (see also Chapter 3). Typical examples include potassium chloride pills, Pepto-Bismol, and the barium and iodine radiographic contrast agents (Figs. 8-60 and 8-61).

Pantopaque, an oil-based myelographic contrast agent, is not miscible with water.[143] It was the standard radiographic agent for myelography until the low osmolar water-soluble radiographic contrast agents were introduced. Pantopaque is not readily absorbed by the body, and traces of it can be visualized in the spinal canal, along nerve roots, and elsewhere in the body years after a patient has undergone a myelogram (Fig. 8-62). Ethiodol is an iodized oil used for lymphography (lymphangiography).[143,144] It is only slowly cleared from lymph nodes where it can be seen for months to a few years after a patient has undergone a lymphangiogram[144] (Fig. 8-62).

There is a large number of oral cholecystographic contrast agents, but they are rarely used because oral gallbladder exams (OCG) have been largely replaced by abdominal ultrasound and other studies.[143] Cholecystographic agents can occasionally be visualized in the bowel after they have been excreted from the biliary system or if they are absorbed incompletely (Fig. 8-60). The amount of gallbladder and bowel opacification produced by a given compound depends on a complex set of factors, including the status of the patient's liver, gallbladder, and pancreas, as well as the patient's diet.[145]

Peritoneal jugular shunts, commonly known as LeVeen shunts, are designed to drain fluid from the peritoneal cavity to the central venous system (Fig. 8-67). They are mainly used for intractable ascites and the hepatorenal syndrome.[146-148] Although they are quite effective in some patients, there are many potentially significant complications associated with their use including local wound infection, peritonitis, sepsis, venous thrombosis and embolism, bleeding, disseminated intravascular coagulation, bowel perforation, and fatal air embolism.[146-150] Their positioning and effectiveness are judged by the patient's clinical response and by plain films and shunt contrast studies. Sometimes, ultrasound or CT exams may provide useful information concerning their location and potential complications.

There are also pleuroperitoneal shunts (Denver shunt) for use in patients with intractable pleural effusions (Fig. 8-68). The proximal portion of the shunt consists of a fenestrated pleural catheter, the middle portion consists of a flexible pump chamber with two one-way valves, and the distal portion of the shunt consists of a fenestrated peritoneal catheter. The shunts are composed of silicone rubber. There is a barium stripe in the catheter walls to permit radiographic visualization of the shunt.

The Denver shunt is used in patients with chylothorax and for palliation in patients with intractable pleural effusion from primary or secondary intrathoracic neoplasms.[151-155] It can be used as an alternative to thoracentesis and sclerotherapy in selected patients. The pleuroperitoneal shunt has a potential risk for disseminating malignant neoplasm by shunting of fluid containing neoplastic cells. It is contraindicated in patients with infected pleural fluid or in patients with suspected intra-abdominal infections.

Large retention sutures and suture bridges may be used to close the abdominal wall. These are usually composed of rubber, plastic, or a combination of materials, such as plastic and metal (Fig. 8-69). Sometimes, large metal sutures may be used to close the abdominal wall without the use of a suture bridge. The choice of materials and the closure method are quite variable depending on the patient's condition and the surgeon's experience. Metal sutures are most commonly observed in the spine and sternum and less commonly seen in the abdomen.

Tubal ligation and vasectomy are common operations. They usually do not have any plain radiographic manifestations. The Hulka clip (Fig. 8-70) has been designed for tubal ligations, and occasionally this or another clip type may be seen in a patient with a tubal ligation.

Laparoscopic cholecystectomy is becoming a popular surgical procedure. The cholecystectomy is performed by laparoscopic vision through four ports in the anterior abdominal wall. There is no abdominal incision, and patients generally have considerably less postoperative discomfort and recover more quickly than with the more traditional type of cholecystectomy. Carbon dioxide is insufflated into the abdomen to facilitate visualization of the surgical field. Radiographic studies obtained during the procedure frequently show trocars, irrigators, clamps, forceps, and other pertinent surgical equipment in place.[156]

Tantalum Mesh

Tantalum is a noncorrosive, malleable metal found in some prosthetic devices. It has also been used for plates and disks to repair cranial defects and as a mesh for repairing abdominal wall defects (Fig. 8-73).

Thorotrast

Thorotrast, a 20% colloidal suspension of thorium dioxide, was a common contrast agent in the 1930s and 1940s.[157-164] Thorotrast produced excellent radiographic contrast because of thorium's high atomic number and the inert nature of thorium dioxide. However, thorium is radioactive with 11 radioactive isotopes, and Thorotrast was found to induce various neoplasms, particularly cholangiocarcinoma, hepatocellular carcinoma, and liver angiosarcoma.[159] In addition, Thoro-

trast can cause severe local and distant fibrosis, cirrhosis, and veno-occlusive disease. Therefore its use was stopped in the 1950s. Nevertheless, its effects on patients can still be seen, and physicians need to be aware of its appearance and potential for harm.

Because Thorotrast accumulates in the reticuloendothelial system and migrates to the lymphatics, these structures are often sufficiently radiopaque to be visible on plain films (Figs. 8-74 and 8-75). The liver may initially have a faint, diffuse increase in density or, later, a lacy reticular pattern as the Thorotrast migrates to the liver lymphatics.[157,162,165,166] The spleen typically becomes small and quite dense (Fig. 8-74) because of fibrosis and Thorotrast accumulation. Regional lymph nodes become opaque as they accumulate Thorotrast (Fig. 8-75). The peripancreatic, periportal, and perisplenic nodes are the ones most frequently visualized.[157]

Computed tomography may be especially helpful in diagnosing an hepatic neoplasm induced by Thorotrast.[157,165,167,168] Those patients with plain film findings of Thorotrast exposure probably should have periodic CT examinations to look for an induced neoplasm.

Thorotrast has also been documented to induce urinary tract malignancies, especially transitional cell carcinomas in patients who underwent retrograde pyelography.[169-171] As with other patients exposed to Thorotrast, these patients should be followed closely for the development of thorium-induced urinary tract neoplasms.[170]

Umbilical Catheters

Umbilical venous and arterial catheters have been in use since the late 1940s.[172-174] They are used routinely in premature infants for administration of fluids, parenteral nutrition, and antibiotic therapy. A properly placed umbilical venous catheter passes through the umbilicus, umbilical vein, left portal vein, and inferior vena cava into the right atrium.[174] A properly placed umbilical arterial catheter should pass through the umbilicus, umbilical artery, and common iliac artery into the aorta.[174] The tip of an umbilical artery catheter should be away from major vessel openings. Two positions fulfill this requirement: either a high position at the T6 to T10 level (Fig. 8-76) or a low position at the L3 to the L5 level.[174] The proper positioning of a catheter can be assessed by plain films, by contrast injection into the catheter, or by ultrasound evaluation of the abdomen.[173-179]

Umbilical catheters in the newborn are frequently life saving and usually without problems. One must be aware, however, of two main groups of complications associated with their use: vascular injuries and related sequelae and complications secondary to catheter malpositioning.[174]

Thromboembolic complications include thrombi

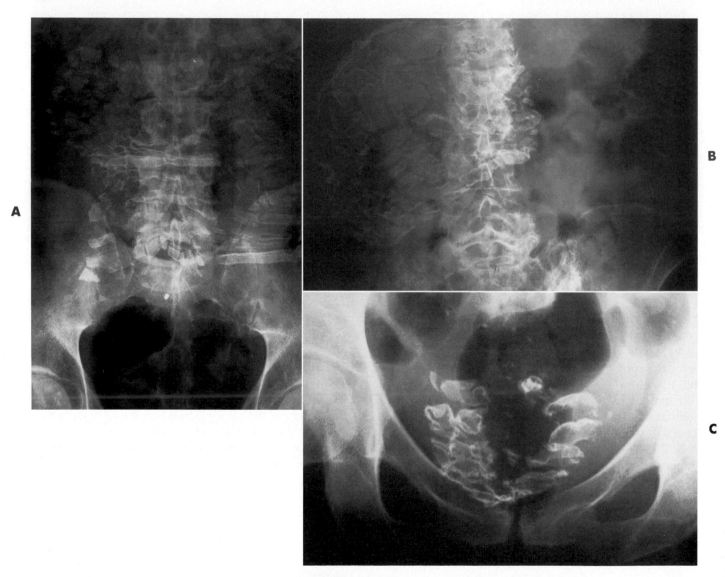

Fig. 8-73. Three patients with abdominal wall defects repaired with tantalum mesh.

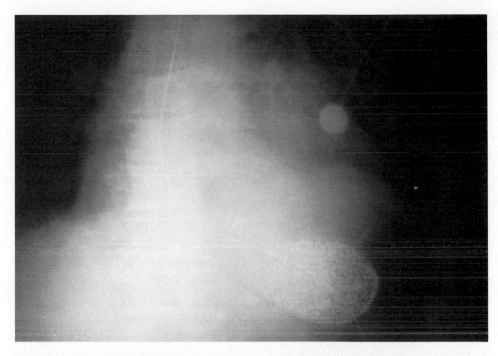

Fig. 8-74. Fifty-seven-year-old man with Thorotrast deposition in the spleen. (Courtesy George R. Barnes, Jr., Tucson.)

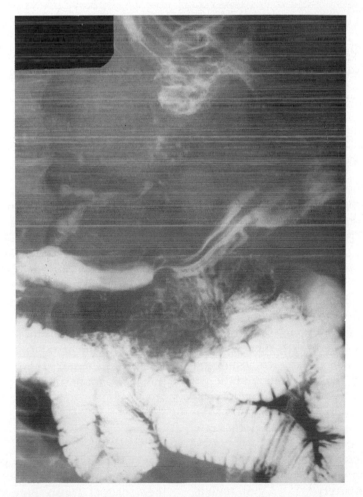

Fig. 8-75. Seventy-three-year-old man with Thorotrast deposition in the liver, spleen, and lymph nodes.

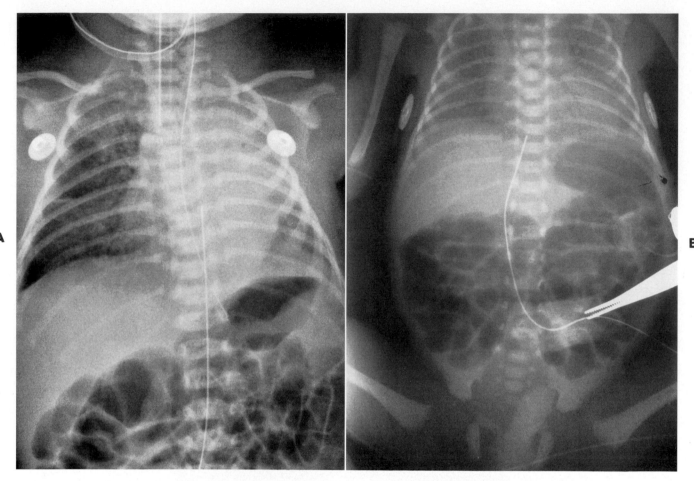

Fig. 8-76. A, One-day-old female with aspiration pneumonitis. Notice the good positioning of her umbilical artery catheter at the T8 to T9 level. Also notice the low position of her endotracheal tube at the carina and the high position of her feeding tube at the gastro-esophageal junction. **B,** Another child with proper positioning of umbilical venous catheter tip at the junction of the inferior vena cava and the right atrium.

in the aorta and pulmonary artery, occlusion of the hepatic artery, embolic phenomena, and aortic aneurysm formation.[177-185] Frequently, asymptomatic thrombus formation is seen with intra-aortic catheter use.[174,183] The majority of clots are self-limiting, but they may at times require fibrinolytic therapy or surgical removal.[174]

Umbilical catheter malposition is common. An umbilical venous catheter can enter the portal venous system, superior mesenteric vein, splenic vein, superior vena cava, or the jugular venous system, or it may even pass through a patent foramen ovale into the left atrium and beyond[184] (Figs. 8-77 and 8-78). Malposition of the venous catheter predisposes to venous thrombosis in small side vessels and injection of hyperosmolar solutions into the portal vein could lead to portal vein thrombosis or hepatic necrosis.[184]

An umbilical artery catheter can end up in the aortic arch, subclavian artery, the celiac artery, the renal artery, or the inferior gluteal artery.[174,177-184] An umbili-

cal catheter may perforate a vessel wall and become positioned in an abnormal location, such as the peritoneal, retroperitoneal, pleural, or pericardial spaces. This is life threatening because of possible severe hemorrhage or development of overwhelming sepsis.

If arterial perforation occurs, it is frequently where the umbilical artery joins the anterior abdominal wall or in the internal iliac artery just proximal to the umbilical artery branch.[184] Catheters can even fragment and embolize to distant sites.[174] Air embolism is not infrequent with umbilical catheterization. It is typically seen on the first film after umbilical venous catheterization. Air embolism usually causes no harm but is best avoided by meticulous technique during catheter insertion.[184]

Peritoneal Dialysis

Continuous ambulatory peritoneal dialysis (CAPD) is becoming more popular because it has a lower cost than hemodialysis. It also allows patients greater mobility and

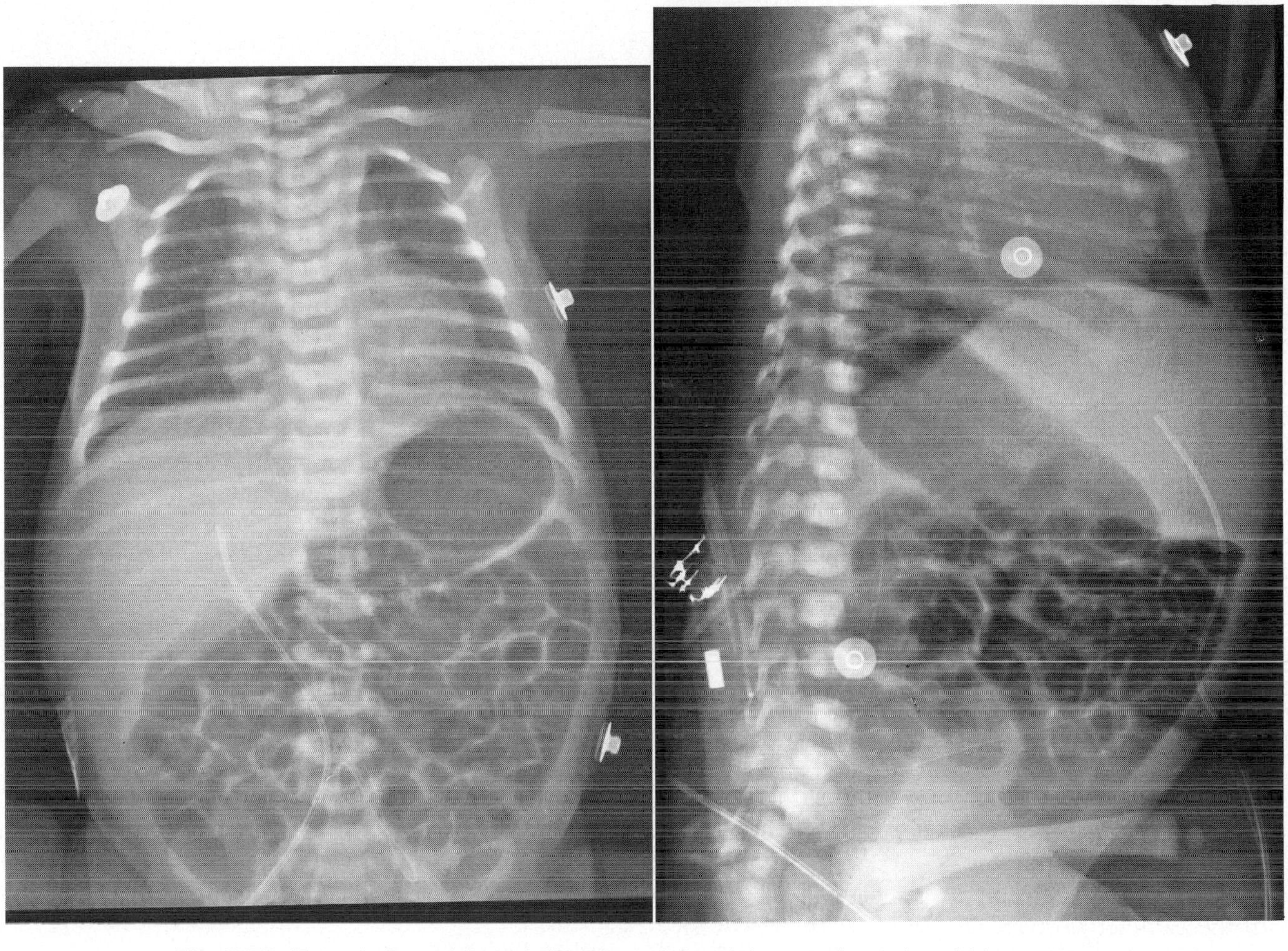

Fig. 8-77. Frontal, **A,** and lateral, **B,** views of the abdomen of a 1-day-old boy with an umbilical venous catheter lying in the left portal vein. It has not been advanced far enough and should ideally lie in the inferior vena cava or right atrium.

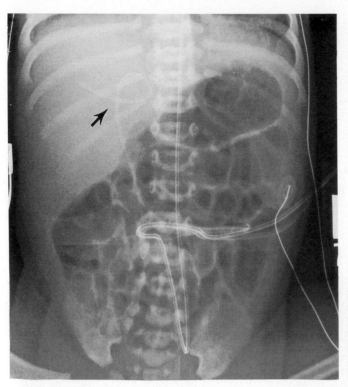

Fig. 8-78. Newborn girl with an umbilical venous catheter, *arrow*, curled in her right portal vein.

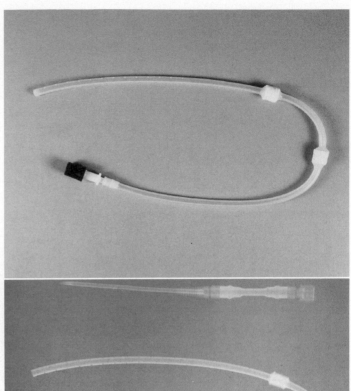

Fig. 8-79. A, Peritoneal dialysis catheter. There are multiple side holes and Dacron cuffs. **B,** Radiograph of a peritoneal dialysis catheter and a hemodialysis catheter.

requires fewer dietary restrictions.[186,187] Up to 25% of patients with end-stage renal disease could benefit from CAPD. The Tenckhoff catheter is the most frequently used peritoneal dialysis catheter. It and other similar peritoneal dialysis catheters are composed of silicone elastomer and contain multiple side holes (Fig. 8-79).

There are one or more Dacron felt cuffs near the end of the catheter. These are placed in the subcutaneous tissues to incite an inflammatory reaction to prevent retrograde infection. The catheters are surgically inserted with the catheter tip typically placed in the retrovesical space in men or in the pouch of Douglas in women (Fig. 8-80).

Peritoneal dialysis catheters are associated with many complications.[188-190] These include peritonitis, leakage, hernia formation at the catheter insertion site, wound infection, bowel perforation, adhesions, bowel obstruction, migration to an extraperitoneal location, and bleeding. These complications may occur in a high percentage of patients and necessitate eventual catheter removal. Some malfunctions, such as tube clotting and kinking and poor positioning within the peritoneal cavity, may be amenable to treatment by catheter manipulation. Other problems, such as extraperitoneal location of the catheter, require its removal.[190-193]

The position and functioning of the catheter can be assessed by plain films and injection of contrast material into the catheter in many cases.[190] Sometimes CT, ultrasound, or peritonography may be necessary to delineate loculated fluid collections or abscess formation.[194] Continuous-cycling peritoneal dialysis is often used in children with end-stage renal disease. For both CAPD and continuous-cycling peritoneal dialysis peritonitis is the most common complication.[195] A much feared complication of peritoneal dialysis is sclerosing peritonitis, which is an inflammatory process leading to the deposition of thick fibrous tissue throughout the peritoneal cavity with eventual small bowel obstruction and progression to patient death.[196-198] Fortunately, this complication is rare, and early diagnosis may possibly help reduce its grim prognosis.[198]

Ventriculoperitoneal Shunts

(See also Chapter 4.)

Ventriculoperitoneal (VP) shunting is a standard therapy for treatment of obstructive hydrocephalus. Although it was first performed by Kausch in 1905, it became the treatment of choice with the introduction of modern techniques by Ames in 1967.[199,200] VP shunts are often placed during infancy and early childhood and are expected to serve the individual for the rest of his or her life (Fig. 8-81). They are subject to a complication rate as high as 26%.[201] Because of this, radiologists and other physicians are frequently called upon to evaluate them.

Several different devices are available, but most of them consist of short proximal intracranial and long distal Silastic tubes connected to an intervening one-way valve. Among the types of valve systems in use are the Spitz-Holter, the Heyer Schulte, the Wade, and the Pudenz (Fig. 8-82). The latter differs significantly from the others because its valve is at the end of the distal catheter.[202]

Among the abdominal complications that can occur are the following: mechanical malfunction attributable to tube breakage, kinking, and disconnection;[203] intraperitoneal pseudocyst formation or loculation of fluid;[199,204] extraperitoneal migration of the catheter into locations such as the scrotum,[205] an umbilical her-

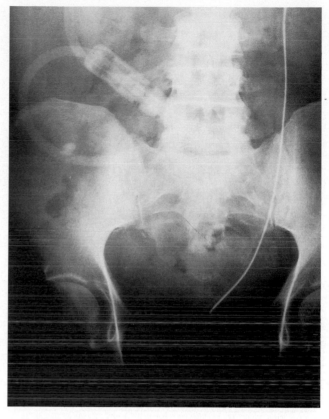

Fig. 8-80. Elderly man with a peritoneal dialysis catheter in the left side of the peritoneum. The catheter tip is in the retrovesical space. Overlying the right upper quadrant of the abdomen is a LaVeen peritoneovenous shunt.

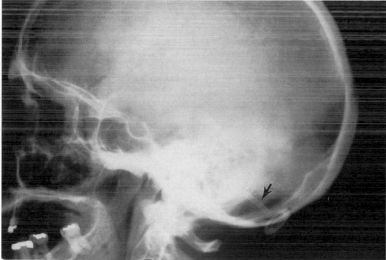

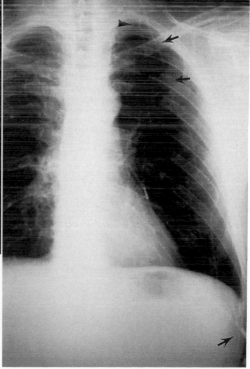

Fig. 8-81. Fifty-nine-year-old man with a ventriculoperitoneal shunt (*arrow* on each illustration) visible on skull (**A**), chest (**B** and **C**), and abdominal (**D**) radiographs. On **B** two opaque catheters can be seen overlying the neck and chest. The more medial catheter, *arrowhead,* represents an earlier shunt that failed and was replaced by the more laterally situated shunt.   *Continued.*

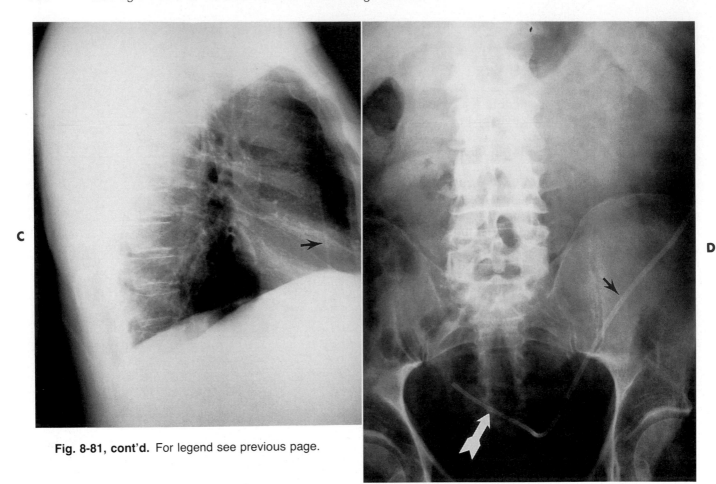

Fig. 8-81, cont'd. For legend see previous page.

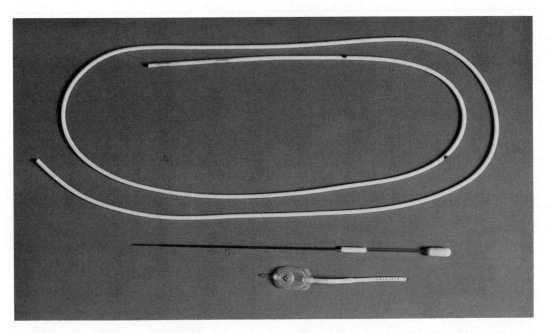

Fig. 8-82. CSF-Flow Control Shunt Kit (Pudenz-Schulte, Goleta, Calif.) ventriculoperitoneal shunt system.

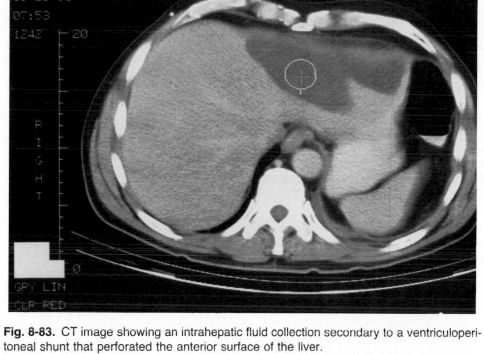

Fig. 8-83. CT image showing an intrahepatic fluid collection secondary to a ventriculoperitoneal shunt that perforated the anterior surface of the liver.

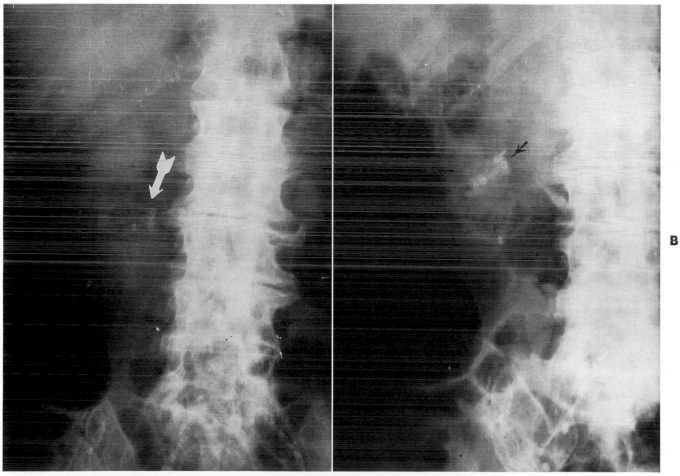

Fig. 8-84. Successive radiographs, **A** and **B,** taken several months apart show the progressive coiling of the end, *arrow,* of a ventriculoperitoneal shunt in an elderly patient.

nia,[206] and the subcutaneous fat;[207] perforation of the bowel including the rectum, usually without associated peritonitis,[208,209] and the stomach;[210] penetration of the liver with abscess formation;[211] penetration of the spleen with pseudocyst formation;[212] perforation of the urinary bladder, uterus, vagina, and gallbladder; intestinal obstruction attributable to adhesions, volvulus, or knotting of the catheter around the bowel; ascites; metastatic tumor spread through the tube; and intractable hiccup attributable to diaphragmatic irritation by the catheter[205,208] (Figs. 8-83 and 8-84). Should the catheter penetrate the diaphragm or be retracted into the chest, hydrothorax can result.[213]

When shunt malfunction is suspected, head CT for evaluation of ventricular size is usually the first imaging procedure performed. When symptoms indicate an abdominal complication, a plain abdominal film should be obtained first. This is particularly valuable to demonstrate tube shortening or disconnection or evidence of a mass or intestinal obstruction.[206,208] In the event that a mass is suspected, abdominal sonography is usually the method of choice to rule out a localized cerebrospinal fluid collection. If there is the possibility of an intestinal obstruction or if abdominal ultrasound is not helpful, abdominal CT is usually the imaging method of choice. For evaluation of shunt patency, radionuclide or contrast shuntography is the method of choice.[202,203,214]

REFERENCES

Esophageal Stents

1. Haynes JW, Miller PR, Steiger Z, et al: Celestin tube use: radiographic manifestations of associated complications, *Radiology* 150:41-44, 1984.
2. Jaffe MH, Fleischer D, Zeman RK, et al: Esophageal malignancy: imaging results and complications of combined endoscopic-radiologic palliation, *Radiology* 164:623-630, 1987.
3. Graham DY: Dilatation for the management of benign and malignant strictures of the esophagus. In Silvis S: *Therapeutic gastrointestinal endoscopy,* New York, 1985, Igaku-Shoin, pp 1-30.
4. Song H-Y, Choi K-C, Cho B-H, Ahn D-S, Kim K-S: Esophagogastric neoplasms: palliation with a modified Gianturco stent, *Radiology* 180:349-354, 1991.
5. Atkinson M: Endoscopic intubation of oesophageal malignant obstruction. In Bennett JR, Hunt RH, editors: *Therapeutic endoscopy and radiology of the gut,* ed 2, London, 1990, Williams & Wilkins, pp 53-64.

Long Intestinal Tubes; Gastrostomy Tubes

6. Morris HH III: Nasogastric intubation: a potentially knotty problem, *JAMA* 237:1432, 1977.
7. Hunter TB, Fon GT, Silverstein ME: Complications of intestinal tubes, *Am J Gastroenterol* 76:256-261, 1981.
8. Cohen OH, Silverstein ME: Unusual complication of Miller-Abbott intubation, *J Med Soc NJ* 49:435-437, 1952.
9. Hafner CD, Wylie JH, Brush BE: Complications of gastrointestinal intubation, *Arch Surg* 83:163-175, 1961.
10. Spiro RK: Intraluminal incarceration of long intestinal tubes, *Am J Gastroenterol* 66:160-166, 1976.
11. Rozanski J, Kleinfeld M: A complication of prolonged intestinal intubation: gaseous distention of the terminal balloon, *Am J Dig Dis* 20:1067-1070, 1975.
12. Coleman SL, Miller EW, Stroehlein JR, et al: Nonoperative retrieval of an impacted long intestinal tube, *Am J Dig Dis* 22:462-464, 1977.
13. Shub HA, Rubin RJ, Salvati EP: Intussusception complicating intestinal intubation with a long Cantor tube, *Dis Colon Rectum* 21:130-134, 1978.
14. Sower N, Wratten GP: Intussusception due to intestinal tubes: case reports and review of the literature, *Am J Surg* 110:441-444, 1965.
15. Bredfeldt JE, Moeller DD: Systemic mercury intoxication following rupture of a Miller-Abbott tube, *Am J Gastroenterol* 69:478-480, 1978.
16. Vas W, Tuttle RJ, Zylak CJ: Intravenous self-administration of metallic mercury, *Radiology* 137:313-315, 1980.
17. Peterson N, Warwick HS, Rohrmann CA Jr: Radiographic aspects of metallic mercury embolism, *AJR* 135:1079-1081, 1980.
18. Cassar-Pullicino VN, Taylor DN, Tech B, Fitz-Patrick JD: Multiple metallic mercury emboli, *Br J Radiol* 58:470-474, 1985.
19. Spizarny DL, Renzi P: Metallic mercury pulmonary emboli, *J Can Assoc Radiol* 38:60-61, 1987.
20. Cho SR, Messmer J, Bundrick T, Turner MA: Inadvertent inflation of the balloon: a rare but serious complication of Miller-Abbott intubation, *Br J Radiol* 60:547-551, 1987.
21. Ghahremani GG, Turner MA, Port RB: Iatrogenic intubation injuries of the upper gastrointestinal tract in adults, *Gastrointest Radiol* 5:1-10, 1980.
22. Wolff AP, Kessler S: Iatrogenic injury to the hypopharynx and cervical esophagus: an autopsy study, *Ann Otolaryngol* 82:778-783, 1973.
23. Price DB: Tubes in the alimentary and respiratory tracts: appearances on CT scans of the head and neck, *AJR* 156:1047-1051, 1991.
24. Vade A, Jafri SZH, Agha FP, et al: Radiologic evaluation of gastrostomy complications, *AJR* 141:325-330, 1983.
25. Hopens T, Schwesinger WH: Complications of tube gastrostomy: radiologic manifestations, *South Med J* 76:9-11, 1983.
26. Wolf EL, Frager D, Beneventano TC: Radiologic demonstration of important gastrostomy tube complications, *Gastrointest Radiol* 11:20-26, 1986.
27. Goodman P, Levine MS, Parkman HP: Extrusion of PEG tube from the stomach with fistula formation: an unusual complication of percutaneous endoscopic gastrostomy, *Gastrointest Radiol* 16:286-288, 1991.
28. Larson DE, Burton DD, Schroeder RW, DiMagno EP: Percutaneous endoscopic gastrostomy: indications, success, complications, and mortality in 314 consecutive patients, *Gastroenterology* 93:48-52, 1987.
29. Chung RS, Schertzer M: Pathogenesis of complications of percutaneous endoscopic gastrostomy: a lesson in surgical principles, *Am Surg* 56:134-137, 1990.
30. Kaplan DS, Fried MW: Migration of PEG tubes, *Am J Gastroenterol* 84:1590-1591, 1989.
31. Nelson AM: PEG feeding tube migration and erosion into the abdominal wall, *Gastrointest Endosc* 35:133, 1989.
32. Schwartz HI, Goldberg RI, Barkin JS, et al: PEG feeding tube migration impaction in the abdominal wall, *Gastrointest Endosc* 35:134, 1989.
33. Morrissey JF, Reichelderfer M: Gastrointestinal endoscopy, *N Engl J Med* 325:1142-1149, 1214-1222, 1991.
34. Ho CS, Yee ACN, McPherson R: Complications of surgical and percutaneous nonendoscopic gastrostomy: review of 233 patients, *Gastroenterology* 95:1206-1210, 1988.

Feeding Tubes

35. Balogh GJ, Adler SJ, VanderWoude J, et al: Pneumothorax as a complication of feeding tube placement, *AJR* 141:1275-1277, 1983.

36. Hand RW, Kempster M, Levy JH, et al: Inadvertent transbronchial insertion of narrow-bore feeding tubes in the pleural space, *JAMA* 251:2396-2397, 1984.

37. Stark P: Inadvertent nasogastric tube insertion into the tracheobronchial tree, *Radiology* 142:239-240, 1982.

38. Torrington KG, Bowman MA: Fatal hydrothorax and empyema complicating a malpositioned nasogastric tube, *Chest* 79:240-242, 1981.

39. Kiwak MG, Mcloud TC, Dedrick CG, Shepard JO: Entriflex feeding tube: need for care in using it, *AJR* 143:1341-1342, 1984.

40. Culpepper JA, Veremakis C, Guntupalli KK, Sladen A: Malpositioned nasogastric tube causing pneumothorax and bronchopleural fistula, *Chest* 81:389, 1982 (letter).

41. Scholten DJ, Wood TL, Thompson DR: Pneumothorax from nasoenteric feeding tube insertion, *Am Surg* 52:381-385, 1986.

42. Woodall BH, Winfield DF, Bisset GS III: Inadvertent tracheobronchial placement of feeding tubes, *Radiology* 165:727-729, 1987.

43. Wheeler PS: Feeding tubes that pierce the lung: a case study in risk prevention and quality assurance, *Radiology* 165:861, 1987.

44. Ghahremani GG, Gould RJ: Nasoenteric feeding tubes: radiographic detection of complications, *Dig Dis Sci* 31:574-585, 1986.

45. Ghahremani GG: Complications due to inadvertent tracheobronchial placement of feeding tubes, *Radiology* 167:875-876, 1988 (letter).

46. Miller KS, Tomlinson JR, Sahn SA: Pleuropulmonary complications of enteral tube feedings: two reports, review of the literature, and recommendations, *Chest* 88:230-233, 1985.

47. Woodall BH, Winfield DF, Bisset GS III: Complications due to inadvertent tracheobronchial placement of feeding tubes, *Radiology* 167:876, 1988 (reply).

48. McLean GK, Meranze SG, Burke DR: Enteric alimentation: a radiologic approach, *Radiology* 160:555-556, 1986.

49. Siegle RL, Rabinowitz JG, Sarasohn C: Intestinal perforation secondary to nasojejunal feeding tubes, *AJR* 126:1229-1232, 1976.

50. Ghahremani GG, Turner MA, Port RB: Iatrogenic intubation injuries of the upper gastrointestinal tract in adults, *Gastrointest Radiol* 5:1-10, 1980.

51. Gustke RF, Varma RR, Soergel KH: Gastric reflux during perfusion of the proximal small bowel, *Gastroenterology* 59:890-895, 1970.

52. Silk DBA, Rees RG, Keohane PP, Attrill H: Clinical efficacy and design changes of "fine bore" nasogastric feeding tubes: a seven-year-experience involving 809 intubations in 403 patients, *J Parenter Enteral Nutr* 11:378-383, 1987.

53. Ott DJ, Mattox HE, Gelfand DW, Chen MYM, Wu WC: Enteral feeding tubes: placement by using fluoroscopy and endoscopy, *AJR* 157:769-771, 1991.

54. Grant JP, Curtas MS, Kelvin FM: Fluoroscopic placement of nasojejunal feeding tubes with immediate feeding using a nonelemental diet, *J Parenter Enteral Nutr* 7:299-303, 1983.

55. Frederick PR, Miller MH, Morrison WJ: Feeding tube for fluoroscopic placement, *Radiology* 145:847, 1982.

56. Gutierrez ED, Balfe DM: Fluoroscopically guided nasoenteric feeding tube placement: results of a 1-year study, *Radiology* 178:759-762, 1991.

ERCP

57. Cotton PB, Williams CB: *Practical gastrointestinal endoscopy,* Oxford, 1990, Blackwell Scientific.

58. Bellon EM: *Radiologic interpretation of ERCP: a clinical atlas,* New Hyde Park, NY, 1983, Medical Examination Publishing Co.

59. Pott G, Schrameyer B: *ERCP atlas,* Toronto, 1989, B.C. Decker, Inc. (Mosby-Year Book, St. Louis).

Urinary Stents

60. Lang EK: Antegrade ureteral stenting for dehiscence, strictures, and fistulae, *AJR* 143:795-801, 1984.

61. Mitty HA, Train JS, Dan SJ: Antegrade ureteral stenting in the management of fistulas, strictures, and calculi, *Radiology* 149:433-438, 1983.

62. Mardis HK, Kroeger RM, Hepperlin TW, et al: Polyethylene double-pigtail ureteral stents, *Urol Clin North Am* 9:95-101, 1982.

63. Mitty HA, Rackson ME, Dan SJ, Train JS: Experience with a new ureteral stent made of a biocompatible copolymer, *Radiology* 168:557-559, 1988.

64. Rackson ME, Mitty HA, Lossef SV, et al: Biocompatible copolymer ureteral stent: maintenance of patency beyond six months, *AJR* 153:783-784, 1989.

65. Kahn RI: Percutaneous antegrade indwelling silicone stent, *Urology (Urotech),* pp 22-24, May 1988.

66. Cardella JF, Castaneda-Zuniga WR, Hunter DW, et al: Urine-compatible polymer for long-term ureteral stenting, *Radiology* 161:313-318, 1986.

67. LeRoy AJ, Williams HJ, Segura JW, et al: Indwelling ureteral stents: percutaneous management of complications, *Radiology* 158:219-222, 1986.

68. Mitty HA, Dan SJ, Train JS: Antegrade ureteral stents: technical and catheter-related problems with polyethylene and polyurethane, *Radiology* 165:439-443, 1987.

69. Druy EM: A dilating introducer-sheath for the antegrade insertion of ureteral stents, *AJR* 145:1274-1276, 1985.

70. Rozenblit G, Tarasov E, Srur MF, et al: Druy ureteral stent set: clinical experience in 25 patients, *Radiology* 160:737-740, 1986.

71. Smith AD: Percutaneous ureteral surgery and stenting, *Urology* 23(suppl):37-42, 1984.

72. Rackson ME, Mitty HA, Dan SJ, Train JS: Elevated bladder pressure: a cause of apparent ureteral stent failure, *AJR* 151:335-336, 1988.

73. Jennifer JD, Rickards D, Milroy EJG: Stricture disease: radiology of urethral stents, *Radiology* 180:447-450, 1991.

74. Rousseau H, Puel J, Joffre F, et al: Self-expanding endovascular prosthesis: an experimental study, *Radiology* 164:709-714, 1987.

75. Dick R, Gillams A, Dooley JS, Hobbs FF: Stainless steel mesh stents for biliary strictures, *J Intervent Radiol* 4:95-98, 1989.

76. Putnam JS, Uchida BT, Antonovic R, Rosch J: Superior vena cava syndrome associated with massive thrombosis: treatment with expandable wire stents, *Radiology* 167:727-728, 1988.

77. Gunther RW, Vorwerk D, Bohndorf K, et al: Venous stenosis in dialysis shunts: treatment with self-expanding metallic stents, *Radiology* 170:401-405, 1989.

78. Chapple CR, Milroy EJG, Rickards D: Permanently implanted urethral stent for prostatic obstruction in the unfit patient: preliminary report, *Br J Urol* 66:58-65, 1990.

79. Shaw PJR, Milroy EJG, Timoney AG, et al: Permanent external striated sphincter stents in patients with spinal injuries, *Br J Urol* 66:297-302, 1990.

80. McInerney PD, Vanner TF, Harris SAB, Stephenson TP: Permanent urethral stents for detrusor sphincter dyssynergia, *Br J Urol* 67:291-294, 1991.

Suprapubic Cystostomy

81. Hodgkinson CP, Hodari AA: Trocar suprapubic cystostomy for postoperative bladder drainage in the female, *Am J Obstet Gynecol* 96:773-781, 1966.

82. Cook JB, Smith PH: Percutaneous suprapubic cystostomy after spinal cord injury, *Br J Urol* 48:119-121, 1976.

83. Morehouse DD: Emergency management of urethral trauma, *Urol Clin North Am* 9:251-254, 1982.

84. Retik AB, Perlmutter AD: Temporary urinary diversion in infants and young children. In Walsh PC, Gittes RF, Perlmutter AD, Stamey TA, editors: *Campbell's urology,* ed 5, Philadelphia, 1986, Saunders, pp 2116-2136.

85. Papanicolaou N, Pfister RC, Nocks BN: Percutaneous, large-bore, suprapubic cystostomy: technique and results, *AJR* 152:303-306, 1989.

86. Lieber MM, Utz DC: Open bladder surgery. In Walsh PC, Gittes RF, Perlmutter AD, Stamey TA, editors: *Campbell's urology,* ed 5, Philadelphia, 1986, Saunders, pp 2640-2641.

87. Perkash I: Problems of decatheterization in long-term spinal cord injury patients, *J Urol* 124:249-253, 1980.

88. Noll F, Russe O, Kling E, et al: Intermittent catheterization versus percutaneous suprapubic cystostomy in the early management of traumatic spinal cord lesions, *Paraplegia* 26:4-9, 1988.

89. Ingram JM: Suprapubic cystostomy by trocar catheter: a preliminary report, *Am J Obstet Gynecol* 113:1108-1112, 1972.

Foley Catheters

90. Walters NA, Kilbey J, Rickards D: Technical note: a technique for the removal of retained balloon bladder catheters, *Br J Radiol* 61:320-321, 1988.

91. Garrett JP: Technical note: methods for deflating retained urinary catheters, *Clin Radiol* 40:319, 1989.

Penile Prostheses

92. Ahlberg B, Brattberg A, Norlen BJ: Eight years of clinical experience with inflatable and semirigid penile implants, *Scand J Urol Nephrol* 20:241-244, 1986.

93. Benson RC Jr, Patterson DE, Barrett DM: Long-term results with the Jonas malleable penile prosthesis, *J Urol* 134:899-901, 1985.

94. Benson RC Jr: Penile prostheses: semirigid rod penile prostheses, *Semin Urol* 2:152-157, 1984.

95. Brooks MB: 42 months of experience with the Mentor inflatable penile prosthesis, *J Urol* 139:48-49, 1988.

96. Engel RM, Smolev JK, Hackler R: Experience with the Mentor inflatable penile prostheses, *J Urol* 135:1181-1182, 1986.

97. Fallon B, Rosenberg S, Culp DA: Long-term followup in patients with an inflatable penile prosthesis, *J Urol* 132:270-271, 1984.

98. Finney RP: Finney flexirod prosthesis, *Urology* 23(5 Spec No.):79-82, 1984.

99. Fishman IJ, Scott FB, Light JK: Experience with inflatable penile prosthesis, *Urology* 23(5 Spec No.):86-92, 1984.

100. Gregory JG, Purcell MH: Penile prosthesis: review of current models, mechanical reliability, and product cost, *Urology* 29:150-152, 1987.

101. Jonas U: Letter to the editor, *J Urol* 134:901, 1985.

102. Kabalin JN, Kessler R: Five-year followup of the Scott inflatable penile prosthesis and comparison with semirigid penile prosthesis, *J Urol* 140:1428-1430, 1988.

103. Krane RJ: Omniphase penile prosthesis, *Semin Urol* 4:247-251, 1986.

104. Merrill DC: Clinical experience with the Mentor inflatable penile prosthesis in 301 patients, *J Urol* 140:1424-1427, 1988.

105. Merrill DC, Javaheri P: Mentor inflatable penile prosthesis: preliminary clinical results in 30 patients, *Urology* 23(5 Spec No.):72-74, 1984.

106. Montague DK: Experience with Jonas malleable prosthesis, *Urology* 23(5 Spec No.):83-85, 1984.

107. Mulcahy JJ: Use of CX cylinders in association with AMS 700 inflatable penile prosthesis, *J Urol* 140:1420-1421, 1988.

108. Mulcahy JJ: The Hydroflex self-contained inflatable prosthesis: experience in 100 patients, *J Urol* 140:1422-1423, 1988.

109. Product literature. Dacomed Corp., 1701 E. 79th St., Minneapolis, MN 55420.

110. Product literature. Medical Engineering Corp./Surgitek, 3037 Mt. Pleasant St., Racine, WI 53404.

111. Scott FB, Bradley WE, Timm GW: Management of erectile impotence: use of implantable inflatable prosthesis, *Urology* 2:80-82, 1973.

112. Sidi AA, Koleilat N, Fraley EE: Evaluation and treatment of organic impotence, *Invest Radiol* 23:778-789, 1988.

113. Tawil EA, Gregory JG: Failure of the Jonas prosthesis, *J Urol* 135:702-703, 1986.

Artificial Urinary Sphincters

114. Lorentzen T, Dorph S, Hald T: Artificial urinary sphincters: radiographic evaluation, *Acta Radiol* 28:63-66, 1987.

115. Rose SC, Hansen ME, Webster GD, et al: Artificial urinary sphincters: plain radiography of malfunction and complications, *Radiology* 168:403-408, 1988.

116. Scott FB, Bradley WE, Timm GW: Treatment of urinary incontinence by implantable prosthetic sphincter, *Urology* 1:252-259, 1973.

117. Pagani JJ, Cochran ST, Bruskewitz R, et al: Radiographic evaluation of an artificial urinary sphincter (AMS 742) *Radiology* 134:361-365, 1980.

118. Taylor GA, Lebowitz RL: Artificial urinary sphincters in children: radiographic evaluation, *Radiology* 155:91-97, 1985.

Intrauterine Contraceptive Devices (IUD)

119. Edelman DA, Zatuchni GI, Goldsmith A: In Webster JG, editor-in-chief: *Encyclopedia of medical devices and instrumentation,* New York, 1988, Wiley, pp 880-882.

120. Sivin I: Dose- and age-dependent ectopic pregnancy risks with intrauterine contraception, *Obstet Gynecol Surg* 78:291-298, 1991.

121. Mark AS, Hricak H: Intrauterine contraceptive devices: MR imaging, *Radiology* 162:311-314, 1987.

122. Callen PW, Filly RA, Munyer TP: Intrauterine contraceptive devices: evaluation by sonography, *AJR* 135:797-800, 1980.

123. Zakin D, Stern WZ, Rosenblatt R: Complete and partial uterine perforation and embedding following insertion of intrauterine devices, parts I and II, *Obstet Gynecol Surg* 36:335-353, 401-417, 1981.

124. Cochrane WJ: The value of ultrasound in the management of intrauterine devices: ultrasound and the intrauterine device. In Sanders RC, James AE, editors: Ultrasonography in obstetrics and gynecology, Norwalk, Conn., 1985, Appleton-Century-Crofts.

125. Gross BH, Callen PW: Ultrasonography in the detection of intrauterine contraceptive devices. In Callen PW, editor: Ultrasonography in obstetrics and gynecology, Philadelphia, 1983, Saunders, pp 349-358.

126. Shimkin PM, Siegel HA, Seaman WB: Radiographic aspects of perforated intrauterine contraceptive devices, *Radiology* 92:353-358, 1969.

127. Zakin D, Stern WZ, Rosenblatt R: Perforated and embedded intrauterine devices, *JAMA* 247:2144-2146, 1982.

128. Rosenblatt R, Zakin D, Stern WZ, Kutcher R: Uterine perforation and embedding by intrauterine device: evaluation by US and hysterography, *Radiology* 157:765-770, 1985.

129. Richardson ML, Kinard RE, Watters DH: Location of intrauterine devices: evaluation by computed tomography, *Radiology* 142:690, 1982.

130. Najarian KE, Kurtz AB: New observations in the sonographic evaluation of intrauterine contraceptive devices, *J Ultrasound Med* 5:205-210, 1986.

131. Hederström E, Ahlgren M, Salminen H: Computed tomography for localization of intra-abdominally dislocated intrauterine devices, *Acta Radiol* 30:531-534, 1989.

132. Adoni A, Chetrit AB: The management of intrauterine devices following uterine perforation, *Contraception* 43:77-81, 1991.

133. Edelman DA, Porter CW: The intrauterine device and ectopic pregnancy, *Contraception* 36:85-97, 1987.

134. Calderone MS: *Manual of family planning and contraceptive practice,* Baltimore, 1970, Williams & Wilkins, pp 331-349.

135. Reid DE, Christian CD: *Controversy in obstetrics and gynecology II,* 1974, Philadelphia, Saunders, p 341.

Pessaries

136. Summers JL, Ford ML: The forgotten pessary: a medical oddity, *Am J Obstet Gynecol* 111:307-308, 1971.

137. Willims B: The modern pessary treatment of vaginal prolapse, *Practitioner* 201:782-783, 1968.

138. Hill PS: Uterine prolapse complicating pregnancy, *J Reprod Med* 29:631-633, 1984.

139. Poma PA: Management of incarcerated vaginal pessaries, *J Am Geriatr Soc* 29:325-327, 1981.

140. Benson RC: *Current obstetric and gynecologic diagnosis and treatment,* ed 2, Los Altos, Calif., 1978, Lange, pp 253-256.

141. Goldstein I, Wise GJ, Tancer LM: A vesicovaginal fistula and intravesical foreign body, *Am J Obstet Gynecol* 163:589-591, 1990.

142. Russell JK: The dangerous vaginal pessary, *Br Med J* 2:1595-1597, 1961.

Odds and Ends

143. Hunter TB, Fajardo LL: Outline of radiographic contrast agents, *Appl Radiol* 16(11):137-158, 1987.

144. North TB, Lindell MM, Bao-Shan J, Wallace S: Current use of lymphography for staging lymphomas and genital tumors, *AJR* 158:725-728, 1992.

145. Fon GT, Hunter TB, Berk RN, Capp MP: The effect of diet and fasting on gallbladder opacification during oral cholecystography in dogs as measured by computed tomography, *Radiology* 136:585-592, 1980.

146. Epstein M: Peritoneovenous shunt in the management of ascites and the hepatorenal syndrome, *Gastroenterology* 82:790, 1982.

147. Greenlee HB, Stanley MM, Reinhardt GF: Intractable ascites treated with peritoneovenous shunts (LeVeen): a 24- to 64-month follow-up of results in 53 alcoholic cirrhotics, *Arch Surg* 116:518-524, 1981.

148. Kudak SK, Fabian TC, Minton JP: LeVeen shunts in patients with intractable malignant ascites, *J Surg Oncol* 13:61-66, 1980.

149. Kozarek RA, Sanowski RA, Cintora I: Laparoscopy in a patient with LeVeen shunt: prevention of air embolism, *Gastrointest Endosc* 30:193-195, 1984.

150. Greig PD, Langer B, Blendis LM, et al: Complications after peritoneovenous shunting for ascites, *Am J Surg* 139:125-131, 1980.

151. Little AG, Ferguson MK, Golomb HM, et al: Pleuroperitoneal shunting for malignant pleural effusions, *Cancer* 58:2740-2743, 1986.

152. Hussain SA: Pleuroperitoneal shunt in recurrent pleural effusions, *Ann Thorac Surg* 41:609-611, 1986.

153. Cummings SP, Wyatt DA, Baker JW, et al: Successful treatment of postoperative chylothorax using an external pleuroperitoneal shunt, *Ann Thorac Surg* 54(2):276-278, 1992.

154. Pass HI, Roth JA: Treatment of chylothorax, *J Thorac Cardiovasc Surg* 90:451-452, 1985 (letter).

155. Milsom JW, Kron IL, Rheuban KS, Rodgers BM: Chylothorax: an assessment of current surgical practice, *J Thorac Cardiovasc Surg* 89:221-227, 1985.

156. Balachandran S, Goodman P, Saydjari R, et al: Operative cholangiography in patients undergoing laparoscopic cholecystectomy: unique radiographic findings, *AJR* 159:65-67, 1992.

Thorotrast

157. Levy DW, Rindsberg S, Friedman AC, et al: Thorotrast-induced hepatosplenic neoplasia: CT identification, *AJR* 146:997-1004, 1986.

158. Lightfoote JB, Heitz CJ Jr, Smolin MF: CT appearance of reticuloendothelial Thorotrast deposition with hepatic angiosarcoma, *CT Clin Symp* 7:1-5, 1984.

159. MacMahon HE, Murphy AS, Bates MI: Endothelial-cell sarcoma of liver following Thorotrast injections, *Am J Pathol* 23:585-611, 1947.

160. Janower ML, Miettinen OS, Flynn MJ: Effects of long-term Thorotrast exposure, *Radiology* 103:13-20, 1972.

161. Kaul A, Noffz W: Tissue dose in Thorotrast patients, *Health Phys* 35:113-121, 1978.

162. Looney WB: An investigation of the late clinical findings following Thorotrast (thorium dioxide) administration, *AJR* 83:163-185, 1960.

163. Kato Y, Mori T, Kumatori T: Estimated absorbed dose in tissues and radiation effects in Japanese Thorotrast patients, *Health Phys* 44:273-279, 1983.

164. Christensen P, Madsen MR, Jensen OM: Latency of Thorotrast-induced renal tumors, *Scand J Urol Nephrol* 17:127-130, 1983.

165. Silverman PM, Ram PC, Korobkin M: CT appearance of abdominal Thorotrast deposition and Thorotrast-induced angiosarcoma of the liver, *J Comput Assist Tomogr* 4:655-658, 1983.

166. Gondos B: Late clinical roentgen observations following Thorotrast administration, *Clin Radiol* 24:195-203, 1973.

167. Findley A, Childress MH: Computed tomography of thorotrastosis, *J Comput Assist Tomogr* 11:188-189, 1987.

168. Rao BK, Brodell GK, Haaga JR, et al: Visceral CT findings associated with Thorotrast, *J Comput Assist Tomogr* 10:57-61, 1986.

169. Kauzlaric D, Barmeir E, Luscieti P, et al: Renal carcinoma after retrograde pyelography with Thorotrast, *AJR* 148:897-898, 1987.

170. Oyen RH, Gielen JL, Van Poppel HP, et al: Renal thorium deposition associated with transitional cell carcinoma: radiologic demonstration in two patients, *Radiology* 169:705-707, 1988.

171. Reiner M, Siebenthal J: Late effects of Thorotrast in man, *Helv Med Acta* 34:351-364, 1968.

Umbilical Catheters

172. Diamond LK: Erythroblastosis foetalis or haemolytic disease of newborn, *Proc R Soc Med* 40:546-550, 1947.

173. Baker DH, Berdon WE, James SL: Proper localization of umbilical arterial and venous catheters by lateral roentgenograms, *Pediatrics* 43:34-39, 1969.

174. Das Narla L, Hom M, Lofland GK, Moskowitz WB: Evaluation of umbilical catheter and tube placement in premature infants, *RadioGraphics* 11:849-863, 1991.

175. Rosen MS, Reich SB: Umbilical venous catheterization in the newborn: identification of correct positioning, *Radiology* 95:335-340, 1970.

176. Campbell RE: Roentgenologic features of umbilical vascular catheterization in the newborn, *AJR* 112:68-76, 1971.

177. Weber AL, DeLuca S, Shannon DC: Normal and abnormal position of the umbilical artery and venous catheter on the roentgenogram and review of complications, *AJR* 120:361-367, 1974.

178. Oppenheimer DA, Carroll BA, Garth KE, Parker BR: Sonographic localization of neonatal umbilical catheters, *AJR* 138:1025-1032, 1982.

179. Oppenheimer DA, Carroll BA, Garth KE: Ultrasonic detection of complications following umbilical arterial catheterization in the neonate, *Radiology* 145:667-672, 1982.
180. Tooley WH: What is the risk of an umbilical artery catheter? *Pediatrics* 50:1-2, 1972.
181. Tyson JE, DeSa DJ, Moore S: Thromboatheromatous complications of umbilical arterial catheterization in the newborn period: clinicopathological study, *Arch Dis Child* 51:744-754, 1976.
182. Wigger HJ, Bransilver BR, Blanc WA: Thromboses due to catheterization in infants and children, *J Pediatr* 76:1-11, 1970.
183. Neal WA, Reynolds JW, Jarvis CM, et al: Umbilical artery catheterization: demonstration of arterial thrombosis by aortography, *Pediatrics* 50:6-12, 1972.
184. Lester PD, Jung AL: Complications of intubation and catheterization in the neonatal intensive care unit, *RadioGraphics* 1:35-60, 1981.
185. Williams HJ, Jarvis CW, Neal WA, Reynolds JW: Vascular thromboembolism complicating umbilical artery catheterization, *AJR* 116:475-486, 1972.

Peritoneal Dialysis

186. Tenckhoff H: Peritoneal dialysis today: a new look, *Nephron* 12:420-436, 1974.
187. Tenckhoff H, Schechter H: A bacteriologically safe peritoneal access device, *Trans Am Soc Artif Intern Organs* 14:181-186, 1968.
188. Fleisher AG, Kimmelstiel FM, Lattes CG, Miller RE: Surgical complications of peritoneal dialysis catheters, *Am J Surg* 149:726-729, 1985.
189. Olcott C, Feldman CA, Coplon NS, et al: Continuous ambulatory peritoneal dialysis: technique of catheter insertion and management of associated surgical complications, *Am J Surg* 146:98-102, 1983.
190. Perlmutt LM, Braun SD, Cohan RH, Dunnick NR: Extraperitoneal placement of Tenckhoff catheters: a cause of immediate malfunction, *AJR* 148:1211-1212, 1987.
191. Degesys GE, Miller GA, Ford KK, Dunnick NR: Tenckhoff peritoneal dialysis catheters: the use of fluoroscopy in management, *Radiology* 154:819-820, 1985.
192. Jaques P, Richey W, Mandel S: Tenckhoff peritoneal dialysis catheter: cannulography and manipulation, *AJR* 135:83-86, 1980.
193. Davis R, Young J, Diamond D, Bourke E: Management of chronic peritoneal catheter malfunction, *Am J Nephrol* 2:85-90, 1982.
194. Magill HL, Roy S III, Stapleton FB: CT peritoneography in evaluation of pediatric dialysis complications, *AJR* 147:325-328, 1986.
195. Warady BA, Campoy SF, Gross SP, et al: Peritonitis with continous ambulatory peritoneal dialysis and continous cycling peritoneal dialysis, *J Pediatr* 105:726-730, 1984.
196. Gandhi VC, Humayun HM, Ing JS, et al: Sclerotic thickening of the peritoneal membrane in maintenance peritoneal dialysis patients, *Arch Intern Med* 140:1201-1203, 1980.
197. Holland P: Sclerosing encapsulating peritonitis in chronic ambulatory peritoneal dialysis, *Clin Radiol* 41:19-23, 1990.
198. Hollman AS, McMillan MA, Briggs JD, et al: Ultrasound changes in sclerosing peritonitis following continous ambulatory peritoneal dialysis, *Clin Radiol* 43:176-179, 1991.

Ventriculoperitoneal Shunts

199. Gaskill SJ, Marlin AE: Pseudocysts of the abdomen associated with ventriculoperitoneal shunts: a report of twelve cases and a review of the literature, *Pediatr Neurosci* 15:23-27, 1989.
200. Ames RH: Ventriculoperitoneal shunts in the management of hydrocephalus, *J Neurosurg* 27:525-529, 1967.
201. Agha FP, Amendola MA, Shirazi KK, et al: Abdominal complications of ventriculo-peritoneal shunts with emphasis on the role of imaging methods, *Surg Gynecol Obstet* 156:473-478, 1983.
202. Sweeney LE, Thomas PS: Contrast examination of cerebrospinal fluid shunt malfunction in infancy and childhood, *Pediatr Radiol* 17:177-183, 1987.
203. Blair K, AuCoin R, Kloiber R, Molnar CP: The complementary role of plain radiographs and radionuclide shuntography in evaluating CSF-VP shunts, *Clin Nucl Med* 14:121-123, 1989.
204. Eschelman DJ, Lee VW: Lesser sac cerebrospinal fluid collection of a ventriculoperitoneal shunt, *Clin Nucl Med* 15:415-417, 1990.
205. Albala DM, Danaher JW, Huntsman WT: Ventriculoperitoneal shunt migration into the scrotum, *Am Surg* 55:685-688, 1989.
206. Murtagh FR, Quencer RM, Poole CA: Extracranial complications of cerebrospinal fluid shunt function in childhood hydrocephalus, *AJR* 135:763-766, 1980.
207. Chow CC, Haney P: Abdominal wall cyst: a complication of ventriculoperitoneal shunting, *Pediatr Radiol* 21:305-306, 1991.
208. Bryant MS, Bremer AM, Tepas JJ III, et al: Abdominal complications of ventriculoperitoneal shunts, *Am Surg* 54:50-55, 1988.
209. Jamjoom AB, Rawlinson JN, Kirkpatrick JN: Passage of tube per rectum: an unusual complication of a ventriculoperitoneal shunt, *Br J Clin Pract* 44:525-526, 1990.
210. Oi S, Shose Y, Asano N, Oshio T, Matsumoto S: Intragastric migration of a ventriculoperitoneal shunt catheter, *Neurosurgery* 21:255-257, 1987.
211. Paone RF, Mercer LC: Hepatic abscess caused by a ventriculoperitoneal shunt, *Pediatr Infect Dis J* 10:338-339, 1991.
212. Mata J, Alegret X, Llauger J: Splenic pseudocyst as a complication of ventriculoperitoneal shunt: CT features, *J Comput Assist Tomogr* 10:341-342, 1986.
213. Dickman CA, Gilbertson D, Pittman HW, et al: Tension hydrothorax from intrapleural migration of a ventriculoperitoneal shunt, *Pediatr Neurosci* 15:313-316, 1989.
214. Lecklitner ML, Brady MB: Scintigraphic evaluation of cerebrospinal fluid diversionary shunt: complications of the proximal limb, *Semin Nucl Med* 15:395-396, 1985.

9

Medical Devices and Foreign Bodies Associated with Surgery

David G. Bragg
Tim B. Hunter
James A. Warneke

In postoperative patients, surgical apparatus can normally be found lying on or contained within the body as a consequence of their recent surgery. These include such devices as large rubber abdominal retention sutures, wire sutures, surgical drains, and abdominal wound gauze packs and bandages. Other devices, such as retained abdominal sponges and needles, are abnormal and have usually been accidently left behind after surgery. Retained surgical devices, fortunately, are rare but may be difficult to detect because of nonspecific patient symptoms and findings. Such retained objects unfortunately can cause long-term patient morbidity or even patient death. Their radiographic appearance is usually characteristic, though often subtle, and frequently overlooked by surgeons, radiologists, and other physicians.

The problem of retained surgical equipment is best solved by eternal vigilance on the part of all medical personnel both during and after surgery. By being familiar with the expected radiographic appearance of common pieces of surgical equipment, the radiologist, surgeon, and referring physician are more likely to recognize them on a radiographic study. This leads to more prompt patient treatment and a more favorable result for the patient.

SURGICAL SPONGES

The retained surgical sponge is an infrequent event, heralded either by the report of a misplaced sponge from the operating room, or the delayed presentation, months to years subsequent to surgery. The term "gossypiboma" ('cotton-tumor' with an epenthetic -b-) is used to describe the cotton matrix found as the nidus of the foreign-body reaction when a surgical sponge is left within a body cavity. The cotton material, being inert, does not undergo degeneration or appear to be involved in any biochemical reaction but forms the nidus for an inflammatory reaction with surrounding fibrosis, retraction, and the development of a foreign-body granuloma.[1]

It is estimated that the incidence of retained surgical foreign bodies is one per 1000 to 1500 laparotomies.[2] A large number of patients with retained surgical sponges may go unnoticed for years after surgery. In one article it was reported that nearly 50% were discovered 5 years or longer after surgery.[3] It is estimated that approximately one third of patients remain asymptomatic with the foreign body incidentally detected radiographically.[2]

The clinical presentation of a retained surgical foreign body in the abdomen is variable, ranging from an incidental discovery on a radiograph of the abdomen to an intense inflammatory reaction with obstruction or perforation. Occasionally, fistulization can occur. An unusual presentation as a pancreatic pseudocyst has also been reported.[2]

Radiopaque markers for surgical sponges have been used for years, even though there have been variations in these markers with time (Figs. 9-1 to 9-3). An article was published in 1955,[4] and a further review of the commonly used surgical sponges and opaque radiographic markers was published in 1978.[5] Some changes with sponge identification were noted in the more re-

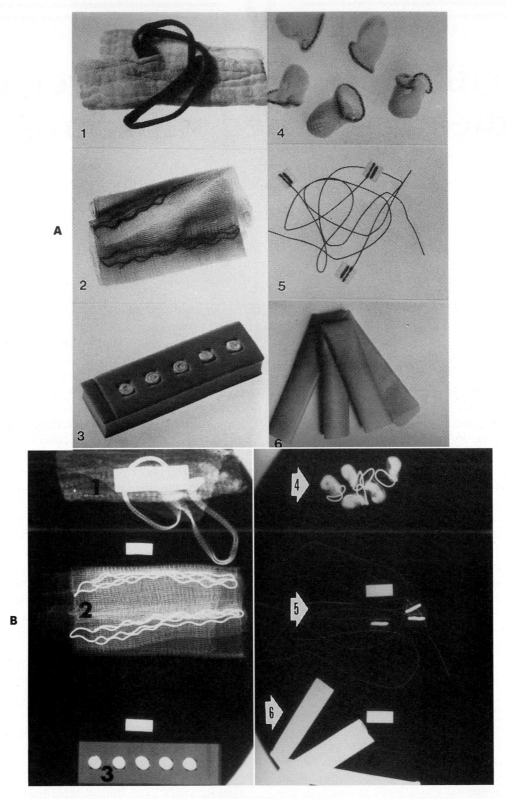

Fig. 9-1. A, Photographs and, **B,** specimen radiographs of commonly used surgical sponges and their corresponding opaque markers found in hospital usage in 1978. *1,* Laparotomy sponge; *2,* 4 × 4 sponge; *3,* Kittner sponge; *4,* peanut sponge; *5,* neuro sponges; *6,* Penrose drain. (From Williams RG, Bragg DG, Nelson JA: *Radiology* 129:323-326, 1978.)

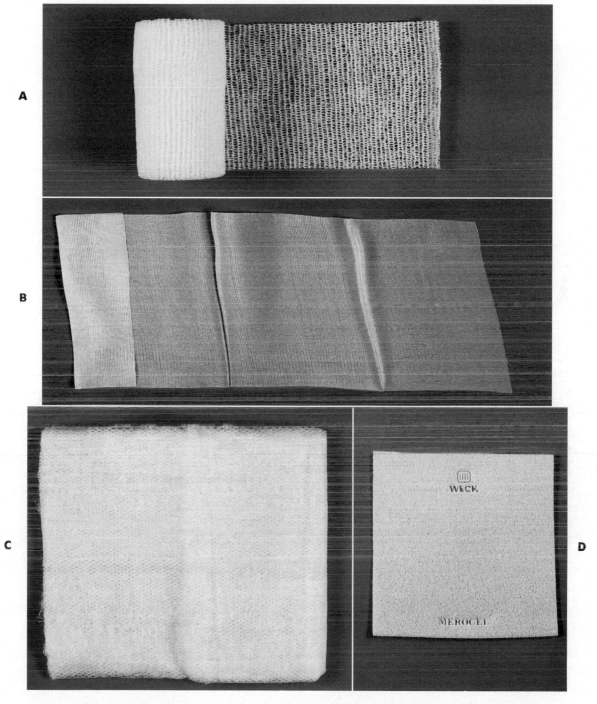

Fig. 9-2. Close-up views of various surgical sponges, dressings, and ties. **A,** Conforming dressing. **B,** Surgical dressing. **C,** Combine dressing. **D,** Weck-Wipe. *Continued.*

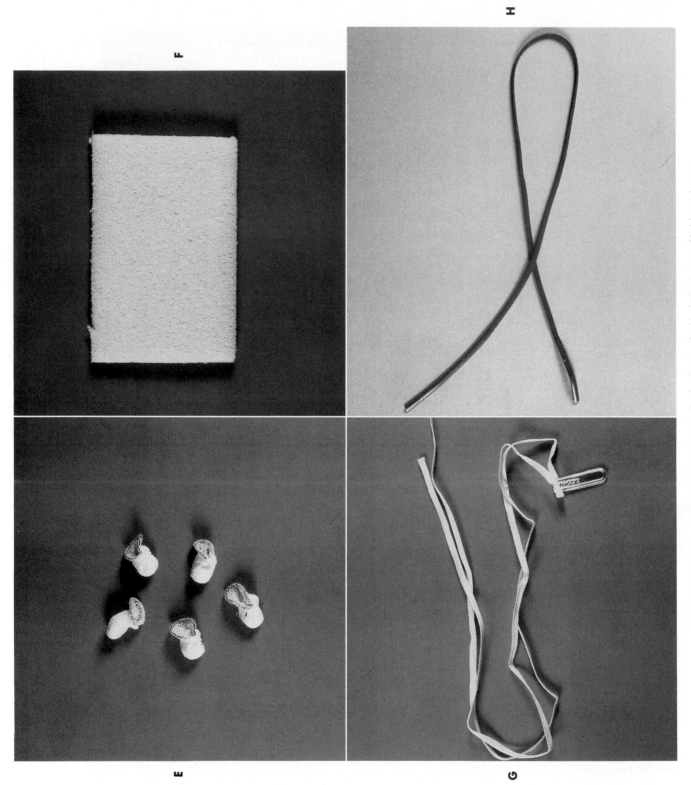

Fig. 9-2, cont'd. E, Peanut dissectors. **F,** Gelfoam. **G,** Umbilical tape. **H,** Vessel tape.

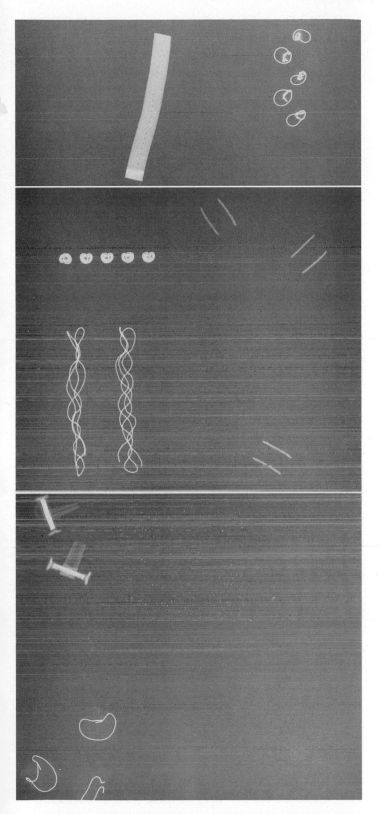

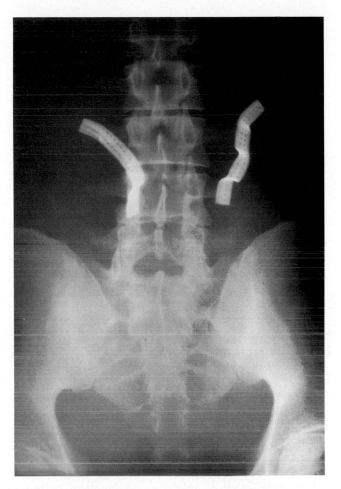

Fig. 9-4. Laparotomy sponges. The clearly identified lucent needle holes traverse the crenated opaque markers found incidentally in the abdomen of a patient without corresponding symptoms.

Fig. 9-3. Radiographs of some items comparable to those in Fig. 9-2. **A,** Laparotomy sponge and peanut dissectors. **B,** Five Kittner dissectors, one 4 × 4, 16-ply sponge, and three surgical patties. **C,** Two spring clips, one Weck-Wipe (speckled densities), 2-inch dental roll (faint parallel densities), large Gelfoam pad (not radiographically visible), and three tonsil sponges. (Radiographic technique: 47 kVp, 4 mAs, Quanta 3 film and screen.)

cent study.[4] The identifying opaque markers are common to sponges used in North America; however, there appears to be less uniformity in other countries. A recent article from Korea mentioned the absence of radiopaque markers in surgical sponges in that country.[6]

The most common retained surgical foreign body is the laparotomy sponge (Fig. 9-4). This rectangular cotton sponge is used to pack the corners of the exposed body cavity. This sponge absorbs blood and other fluids and quickly becomes camouflaged. Its ribbonlike marker is characteristic and easily identified on plain films of the abdomen, even though the strip often appears crenated. The laparotomy sponge should not be present outside of an operating room environment unless an open wound has been packed with such material, an event that should be well-known to the doctors and nurses caring for the patient. With that exception, surgical markers identifying sponges should not be evident on plain films outside of the operating room environment. A ready reference should be available to identify such sponges and indicate their presence to the referring physician (see Figs. 9-1, 9-10, and 9-11).

The neurosurgical sponges used in spinal operative procedures are smaller, with correspondingly smaller opaque markers, and are difficult to visualize radiographically.[5] The most common neurosurgical sponges and cottonoids used in the operating room should all contain visible radiopaque markers (see Figs. 9-1 to 9-3). Cottonoids are the more commonly misplaced or retained sponges in such neurosurgical events.[7]

Detection

The detection of the retained surgical sponge or other abnormal apparatus usually begins with the plain radiographic film (Figs. 9-4 to 9-9, 9-16, and 9-17). Any identified foreign body should be viewed with the suspicion that it may represent a retained surgical sponge, particularly when found within the chest or abdomen. Not infrequently, these opaque clues are ignored, with the radiologist presuming they represent external artifacts from clothing, cutaneous foreign bodies, and so forth.

Recently, ultrasound, computed tomography (CT),

and magnetic resonance imaging (MRI) have been used as a more sophisticated means to identify these foreign bodies.[6-10]

On ultrasound, the appearance of the retained surgical sponge has been described as "a clear-cut acoustic shadow with no echoes within."[8] In another review, ultrasound showed a "reniform mass with an ectogenic center and hypoechoic rim."[6] These authors believed that the primary ultrasound differential diagnosis was with an abscess, which may be found in addition to the foreign body.

On CT, the surgical foreign body is usually found to exhibit a sharply defined mass with enhancing walls after contrast administration (Fig. 9-9, *B* and *C*). Mixed densities may be seen within the center of the lesion.[6] The appearance of retained gelatin-sponge material may mimic an ovarian teratoma on MRI scanning.[10] The gelatin material is used as a hemostatic agent, which normally is absorbed in 2 to 4 weeks but may remain visible longer.

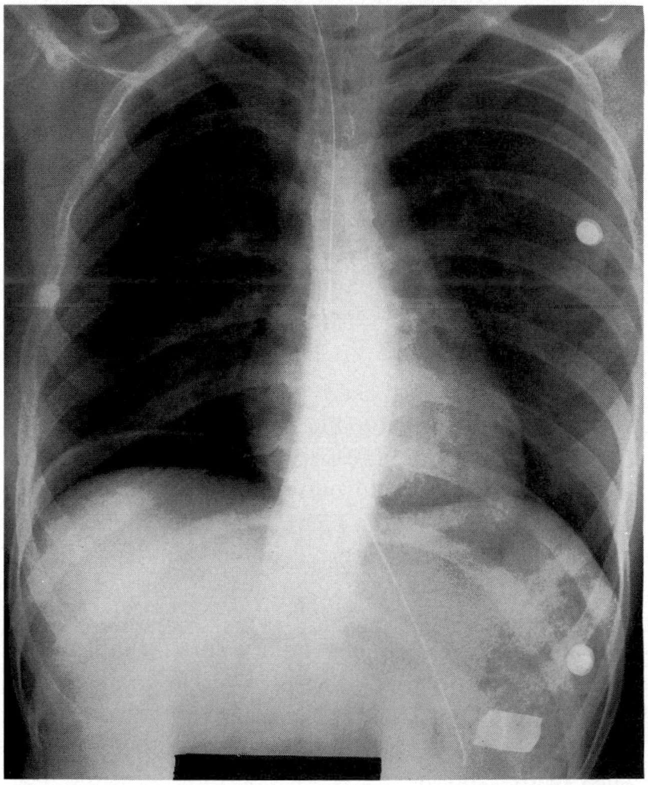

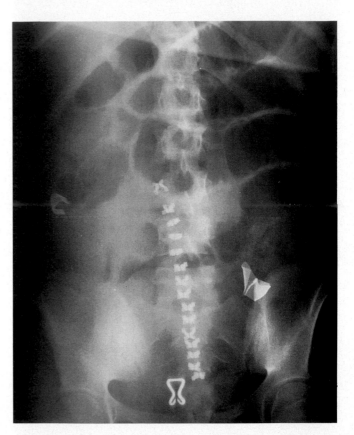

Fig. 9-6. This 15-year-old girl had undergone an uncomplicated cesarean section. Approximately 6 days postoperatively she developed symptoms of intestinal obstruction, and this radiograph showing the dilated loops of small bowel and two laparotomy sponges was obtained. She was reexplored, and the sponges were removed without further incident. (From Williams RG, Bragg DG, Nelson JA: *Radiology* 129:323-326, 1978.)

Fig. 9-5. This 22-year-old woman had previously undergone an emergency splenectomy for a ruptured spleen secondary to blunt trauma. The postoperative chest radiograph demonstrated the retained left upper quadrant laparotomy sponge. (From Williams RG, Bragg DG, Nelson JA: *Radiology* 129:323-326, 1978.)

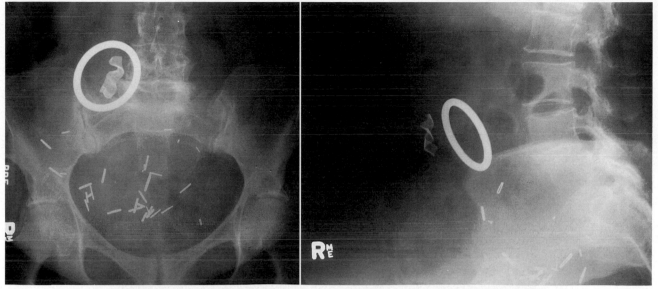

Fig. 9-7. This 60-year-old white woman had undergone an exploratory laparotomy 3 months earlier, at which time a leiomyosarcoma was discovered. The opaque foreign body in both illustrations represents a ring laparotomy sponge instead of the usual cloth strap. The sponge markers can be seen on the anteroposterior and lateral views of the abdomen obtained before an intravenous pyelogram. (From Williams RG, Bragg DG, Nelson JA: *Radiology* 129:323-326, 1978.)

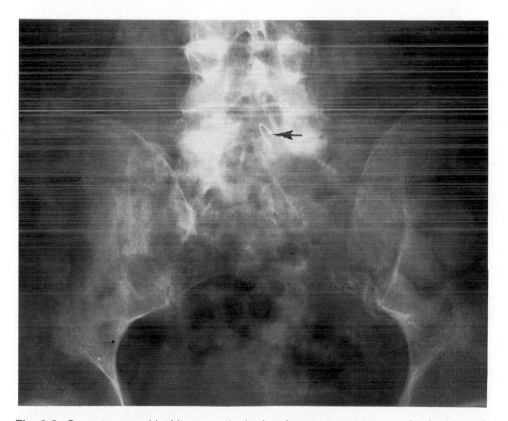

Fig. 9-8. Seventy-year-old white man who had undergone an emergency laminectomy for decompression of a herniated lumbar disk. The postoperative film shows the laminectomy defect with curvilinear metallic marker, *arrow,* indicating a retained peanut sponge. (From Williams RG, Bragg DG, Nelson JA: *Radiology* 129:323-326, 1978.)

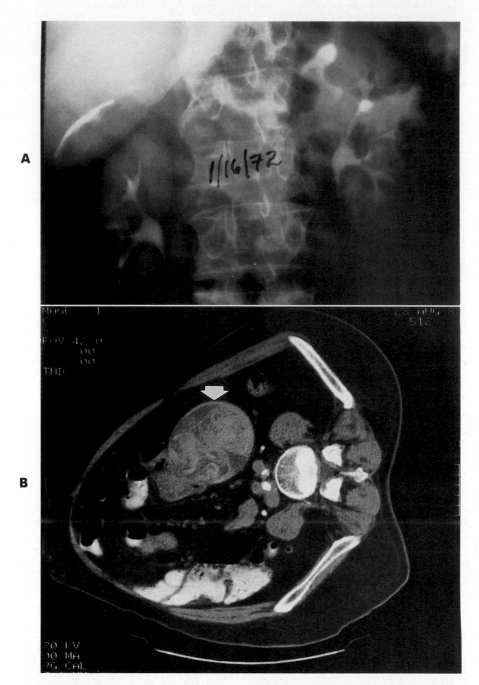

Fig. 9-9. A, Seventy-three-year-old white man was found to have linear calcifications in the right upper quadrant at the time of an intravenous pyelogram. He had undergone a partial gastrectomy 13 years previous to that time. He, however, showed no symptoms referable to this calcification. Autopsy findings subsequently revealed a chronic abscess in the right upper quadrant with calcifications found around a retained surgical sponge, which contained no opaque marker. **B** and **C,** CT study of an elderly man with a retained surgical sponge (gossypiboma) in the left lower quadrant of the abdomen. **B,** Non−contrast enhanced right lateral decubitus view. Notice the large mass, *arrow,* simulating a tumor or loop of distended bowel. **C,** Contrast-enhanced scan showing a well-defined 7.8 cm mass, *arrow,* with mixed densities in its interior. (**A** from Williams RG, Bragg DG, Nelson JA: *Radiology* 129:323-326, 1978; **B** and **C,** courtesy Dr. Robert E. Stejskal, Phoenix, Ariz.)

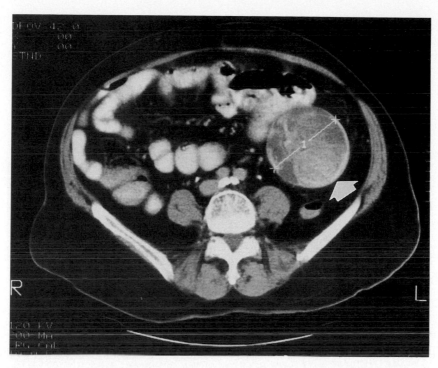

Fig. 9-9, cont'd. For legend see opposite page.

The infrequent challenge presented by the retained surgical sponge is usually discovered incidentally on routine radiographs of the chest or abdomen in a patient with symptoms or occasionally in an individual without symptoms. The common radiopaque markers should be the clue to diagnosis. More complex, cross-sectional imaging techniques may exhibit common patterns suggestive of a retained surgical sponge, but these appearances may be confused with other diagnoses. Familiarity with the radiopaque marker systems seen on plain radiographs should enable one to arrive at an appropriate, correct diagnosis.

SURGICAL NEEDLES, STAPLES, AND OTHER MISCELLANEOUS EQUIPMENT

There are many varieties of surgical needles, staples, sutures, ties, drains, and other devices. Individual variations occur from medical center to medical center. Nevertheless, these surgical devices have a somewhat standard appearance and function. It is a good idea to become familiar with those items used at one's own medical center (Figs. 9-10 to 9-15). This will increase the likelihood of recognizing an inappropriate surgical foreign body when it appears on a radiographic exam.

It should be noted that some of the surgical needles, such as those used for fine-detail plastic surgery and ophthalmology, may be only a few millimeters in size and not be readily recognizable because of their small size (Figs. 9-10 and 9-11). Surgical ties are indistinct radiographically. Hemostatic clips and skin staples may have a similar appearance (Fig. 9-12). Small surgical staples have an appearance similar to skin staples, except for their small size.

The decision regarding the size of the needles to be used, the placement of hemostatic clips, and the use of surgical staples versus surgical sutures is an individual one with a given surgeon. Some surgeons never use surgical staples, preferring suturing to stapling. Other surgeons use staples extensively.

Surgical clips are used almost exclusively to control bleeding vessels. In the majority of operations, the resulting clip placement has no significance except to show where there were significant bleeding points. Surgical clips are traditionally used to mark the site of the vagus nerve in vagotomy procedures, and clips may also be used to mark tumor margins in cases where later radiation therapy will be applied to the tumor bed. Surgical clips may also occasionally mark the site of lymph nodes removed during tumor-staging procedures.

The detection of a retained piece of surgical equipment is important but made difficult because of the poor radiopacity, small size of the object, or the physician's unfamiliarity with its appearance. Even an obvious retained needle (Fig. 9-16) may be overlooked, or an object may be assumed to lie on top of the patient rather than being retained within the patient. Surprisingly large objects may be mistakenly left behind in a patient (Fig. 9-17). This is especially true during emergency surgical procedures.

Text continued on page 322.

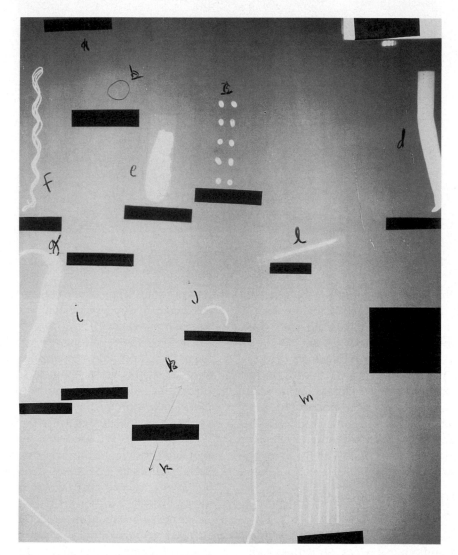

Fig. 9-10. Radiograph used by on-call radiology residents at the University Medical Center, Tucson, Arizona. It illustrates the common surgical devices they might encounter on call, when they are asked by a referring physician if something has been inadvertently abandoned in the patient after surgery. *a,* Peanut sponge; *b,* small needle; *c,* clamp tips; *d,* large sponge; *e,* umbilical tape; *f,* small sponge; *g,* sternum needle; *h,* surgical blade; *i,* suture needle; *j,* suture needle; *k,* small sponges (patties); *l,* IV needle; *m,* vessel ties.

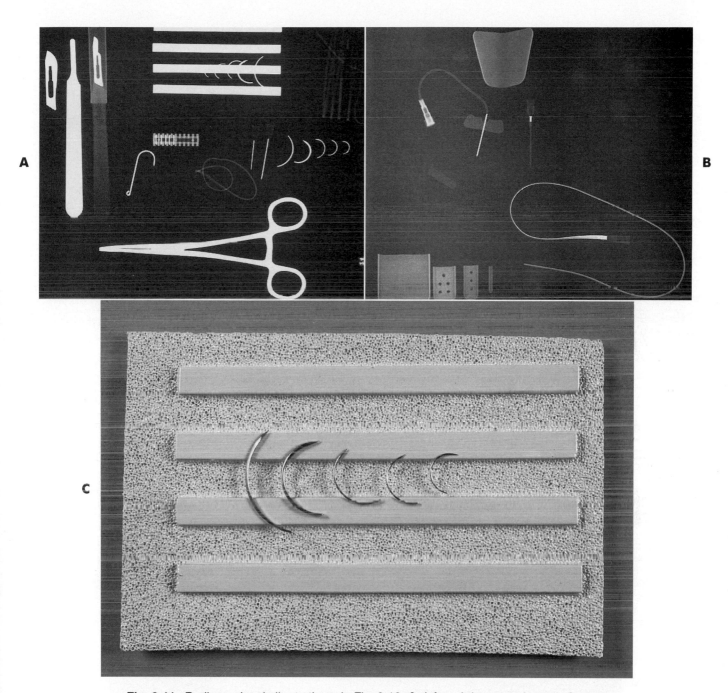

Fig. 9-11. Radiographs similar to those in Fig. 9-10. **A,** *left to right, top to bottom,* Scalpel blades and scalpel, needles resting on a magnetic needle mat, vessel ties, hemostatic clips, surgical needles, Derma Hook, vessel tie (suture), and hemostat. **B,** *left to right, top to bottom,* Nasal splint, 21-gauge scalp vein needle, 18-gauge Jelco catheter, umbilical tape (barely visible), sentinel line catheter, and clamp tips. **C,** Photograph of magnetic needle mat used to hold and organize needles during surgery. Some needles may be quite tiny, only a few millimeters long. (Radiographic technique for **A** and **B:** 47 kVp, 4 mAs, Quanta 3 film and screen.)

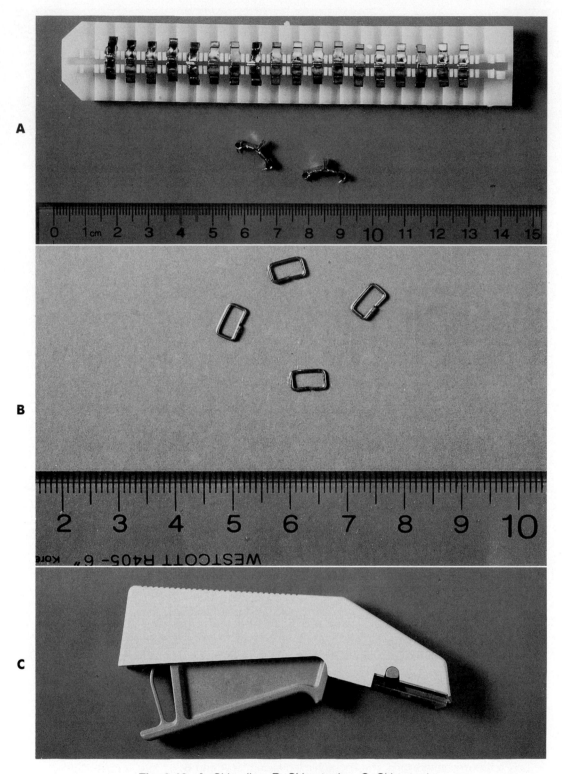

Fig. 9-12. A, Skin clips. **B,** Skin staples. **C,** Skin stapler.

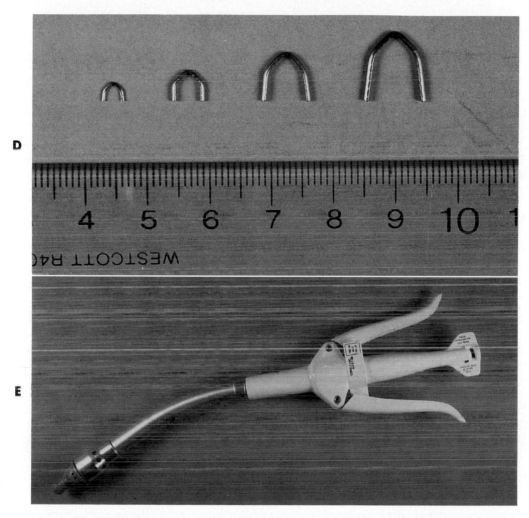

Fig. 9-12, cont'd. D, Tantalum hemoclips (small, medium, large). **E,** Disposable surgical stapler (United States Surgical Corp.).

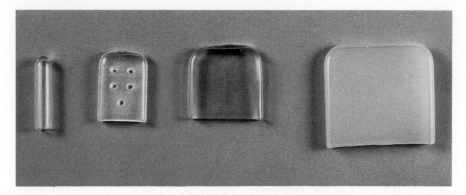

Fig. 9-13. Clamp tips are used to cover the tips of various surgical clamps. They help minimize tissue damage, but they can come off the clamp and be lost in the surgical field.

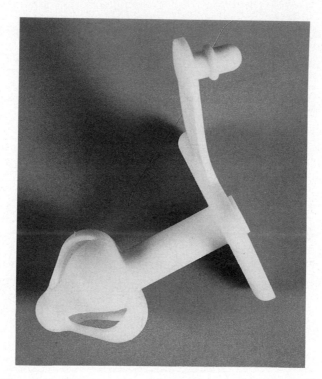

Fig. 9-14. Percutaneous endoscopic gastrostomy (PEG) button. Once a gastrostomy tract has matured after many weeks of a PEG tube being in place, the PEG tube can be pulled out and the PEG button placed. The button sits in the anterior abdominal wall with the rounded, acornlike end fastened in the stomach and the capped end available on the abdominal wall for the administration of feedings, insertion of tubes for suctioning, and so on.

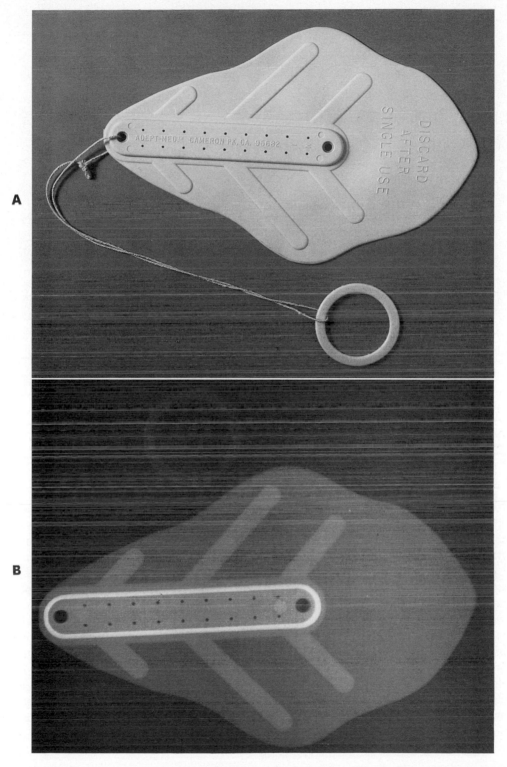

Fig. 9-15. Fish viscera retainer. Photograph, **A,** and radiograph, **B.** This retainer is used to hold viscera in place during surgery, substituting as an artificial abdominal wall. This device should be removed at the completion of surgery.

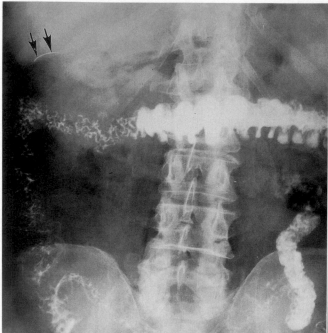

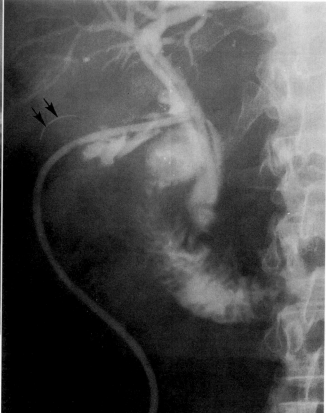

B

Fig. 9-16. A, Incidentally noted in this postevacuation film taken after a barium enema was a curvilinear needle in the right upper quadrant, *arrows.* **B,** At the time of an earlier T-tube cholecystectomy examination the needle was overlooked, *arrows.* The needle was a consequence of a cholecystectomy performed 2 weeks before the cholecystogram. The patient had no symptoms referable to this foreign body. (From Williams RG, Bragg DG, Nelson JA: *Radiology* 129:323-326, 1978.)

SURGICAL DRAINS

Surgical drains are used in all parts of the body to drain extracellular fluid and facilitate wound healing. Drains are designed to remove fluid collections that could otherwise lead to infection, abscess formation, and wound breakdown. The use of drains for a particular procedure and the type of drain employed is subject to the experience of the individual operating physician; it is often a matter of considerable debate among various physicians.

Currently, most drains are radiopaque for convenient radiographic localization. There are three general types of abdominal drains:

1. Closed wound suction drains
2. Gravity drains
3. Sump drains

Closed-Wound Suction Drains

These drains offer a constant level of suction, sometimes with a choice of suction pressures. Usually, there is an internal drainage catheter hooked to an evacuator bottle or collector. The purpose, as with all drainage systems, is to reduce fluid collections and improve tissue approximation. Suction drain design variations include the size and evacuation pressure of the fluid collector, the use of an antireflux valve to prevent reflux of materials back into the patient, and differing configurations of the collector for easy and safe emptying of the collected fluids.

Closed-wound suction systems often use soft, inert silicone drains (Fig. 9-18). The drains come in round and flat designs and are of different lengths, hole patterns, and sizes for varying surgical needs. Sometimes the appearance of a retained surgical sponge and a flat silicone drain may be similar and cause confusion.[11] Adequate patient history and familiarity with this possibility may help prevent misdiagnosing the radiopaque portion of flat silicone drain with a retained sponge.

Gravity Drains

Gravity drains rely on gravity and fluid tension dynamics to drain fluids away from surgical beds and help tissue approximation and wound healing. Traditional gravity drains include the Penrose and T-tube designs

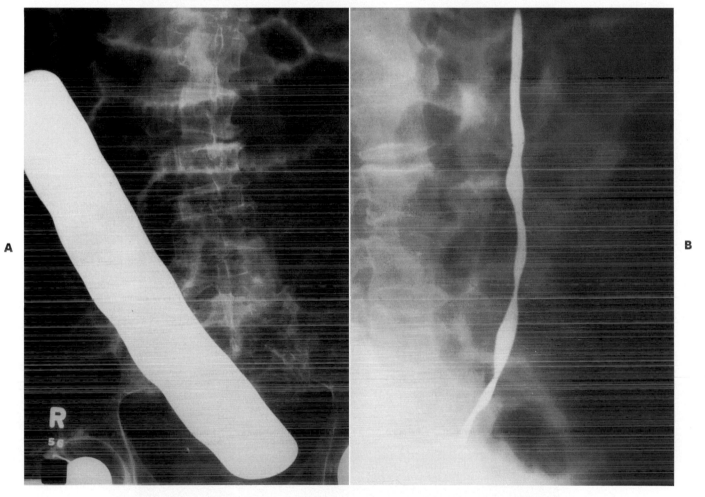

Fig. 9-17. This elderly patient had frontal, **A,** and lateral, **B,** radiographs of the abdomen, obtained 9 days after an emergency pyloroplasty and vagotomy for ulcer disease. These radiographs reveal a malleable retractor left behind after that surgical procedure. There was no point of obstruction, merely a postoperative ileus despite this large retained opaque metallic foreign body.

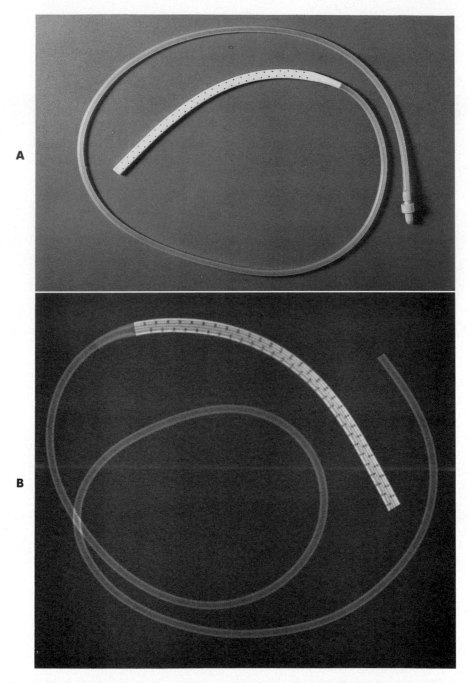

Fig. 9-18. A, ReliaVac Hubless Silicone Flat Drain (Davol). **B,** Radiograph of a similar drain. (Technique: 47 kVp, 4 mAs, Quanta 3 film and screen.) **C,** Flat drains, *arrows,* in a patient after multiple abdominal and pelvis surgeries. Notice also the retention sutures and contrast material in a colonic mucus fistula.

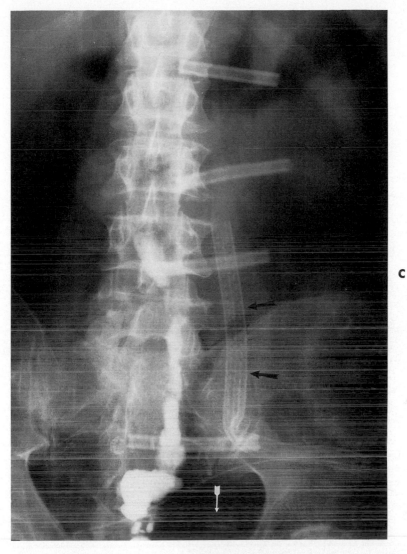

C

Fig. 9-18, cont'd. For legend see opposite page.

Fig. 9-19. A, Penrose Tubing (Smith & Nephew Perry). **B,** Radiograph of similar tubing (radiographic technique same as for Fig. 9-18).

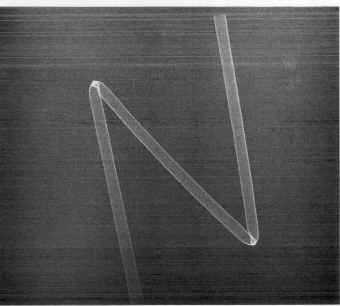

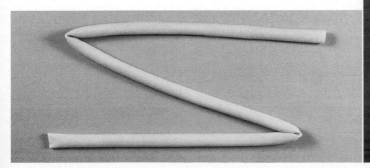

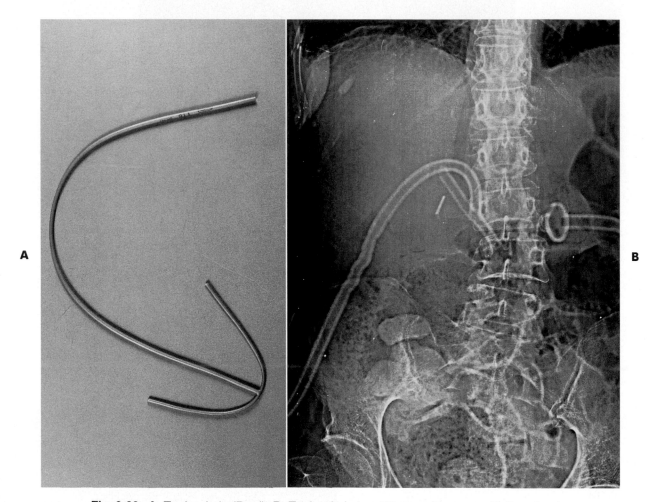

Fig. 9-20. A, T-tube drain (Bard). **B,** T-tube drain in a 56-year-old woman. Notice also the nephrostomy tube on the left.

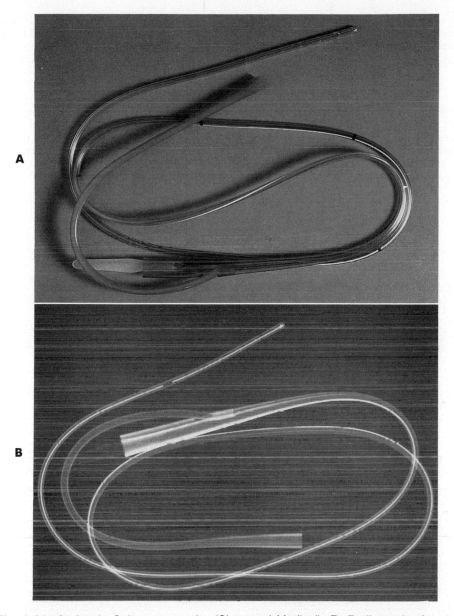

Fig. 9-21. A, Argyle Salem sump tube (Sherwood Medical). **B,** Radiograph of a similar drain. (Technique: 47 kVp, 4 mAs, Quanta 3 film and screen.)

(Figs. 9-19 and 9-20). Penrose drains vary in their length and width. These drains are also convenient for use as tourniquets. T-tube drains vary in the length and width of their stems and crossbars. Penrose drains are often made out of soft, latex rubber to lessen wound irritation. T-tubes are most often used for bile duct drainage (Fig. 9-20). Latex is frequently used because its presence over time stimulates fibrous tract development, which will facilitate later percutaneous stone removal.

Sump Drains

Sump drains enhance wound fluid flow at a low level of suction. Modern designs often incorporate a triple-lumen configuration (Fig. 9-21). There is a large central lumen for maximum fluid removal. A second lumen is used for suction of air into the drain site to maintain pressure for forcing the fluid out of the surgical bed or abscess cavity. The air intake is usually filtered to prevent bacterial contamination of the wound site. There may also be a suture tab for ease of suturing the drainage tube in place. The third lumen is for irrigation of the drain site and instillation of medication.

REFERENCES

1. Sturdy JH, Baird RM, Gerein AN: Surgical sponges: a cause of granuloma and adhesion formation, *Ann Surg* 165:128-134, 1967.

2. Rappaport W, Haynes K: The retained surgical sponge following intra-abdominal surgery, *Arch Surg* 125:405-407, 1990.

3. Chorvat G, Kahn J, Camelot G, et al: Clinical course following retention of sponges left in the abdomen, *Ann Chir* 30:643-646, 1976.

4. Olnick HM, Weens HS, Rogers JV Jr, et al: Radiological diagnosis of retained surgical sponges, *JAMA* 159:1525-1527, 1955.

5. Williams RG, Bragg DG, Nelson JA: Gossypiboma—the problem of the retained surgical sponge, *Radiology* 129:323-326, 1978.

6. Choi BI, Kim SH, Uyu ES, et al: Retained surgical sponge: diagnosis with CT and sonography, *AJR* 150:1047-1050, 1988.

7. Nabors MW, McCrary ME, Clemente RJ, et al: Identification of a retained surgical sponge using magnetic resonance imaging, *Neurosurgery* 18:496-498, 1986.

8. Barriga P, Garcia C: Ultrasonography in the detection of intra-abdominal retained surgical sponge, *J Ultrasound Med* 3:173-176, 1984.

9. Apter S, Hertz M, Rubinstein ZJ, Zissin R: Gossypiboma in the early post-operative period: a diagnostic problem, *Clin Radiol* 42:128-129, 1990.

10. Hoeffner EG, Soulen RL, Christensen CW: Gelatin sponge mimicking a pelvic neoplasm on MR imaging, *AJR* 157:1227-1228, 1991.

11. Herbetko J, Burhenne HJ: Silicone drain mimicking a surgical sponge, *Radiology* 182:572-573, 1992.

10

Common Surgical Procedures

· ·

James A. Warneke
Tim B. Hunter

This brief chapter is intended to illustrate some of the common surgical procedures. Radiologists and other physicians frequently see patients who have had one or more of these operations. We hope to illustrate with drawings and radiographs the basic purpose of the procedures and the relevant anatomy. This chapter is not intended to illustrate or discuss the actual surgical techniques. There is often no absolute way to perform an operation. Our intention is to illustrate one generally accepted way to perform a given type of procedure. For many of these operations, there may be multiple other techniques to accomplish the same result for the patient.

RADICAL NECK SURGERY

Radical neck surgery is designed to remove metastatic spread of carcinoma to the cervical lymph nodes. The sternocleidomastoid muscle, jugular vein, and occasionally the eleventh cranial, or accessory, nerve are removed (Fig. 10-1). A wide variety of different incisions may be used.

LUNG RESECTION

An incision along the lateral chest wall is performed, sometimes with removal of a portion of the thoracic cage. The nature and extent of the surgical procedure vary with the pleuropulmonary abnormality from a simple staple line for a biopsy or wedge resection to a pneumonectomy. When an entire lung is removed, the hilar vein, artery, and bronchus are transected and ligated (Fig. 10-2). There is often an accompanying lymph node dissection.

CORONARY ARTERY BYPASS

Surgical approaches to coronary occlusive disease are increasingly being performed by endovascular techniques. Few imaging studies are useful in the management of this technique, other than the assessment of complications and guidance during the procedure.

Coronary artery bypass surgery was first performed at the Cleveland Clinic in 1967, utilizing a reversed segment of the saphenous vein, with an anastomosis between the aorta and the portion of the coronary artery distal to the occlusion or stenosis. Markers were occasionally used to identify the site of the graft for subsequent angiographic evaluation (Fig. 10-3). Vascular clips are also hallmarks of the procedure, which is approached through a midline sternotomy incision.

In most centers at the present time, internal mammary artery grafts are used for the bypass. This approach obviates the need for limb/vein salvage and takes advantage of a similar-caliber vessel with a higher patency rate. The imaging hallmark of the internal mammary bypass graft are unilateral vascular clips anteriorly originating from the site of the harvest procedure.

CARDIAC TRANSPLANTATION

The diseased recipient heart is resected, with the posterior atrial walls being left on each side. The donor heart is anastomosed to the remaining portions of the right and left atria, the aorta, and the pulmonary artery (Fig. 10-4). The dorsal portions of the recipient heart atria are left in place to simplify the surgery. This obviates the need for anastomosis of the inferior and superior vena cava and the pulmonary veins.

329

Fig. 10-1. Radical neck surgery. **A,** Drawing of surgical procedure. **B,** Chest radiograph of a patient having a recent radical neck resection. Notice the surgical drains, skin clips, and nasogastric tube.

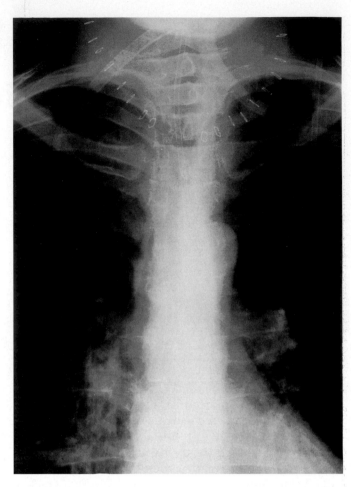

B

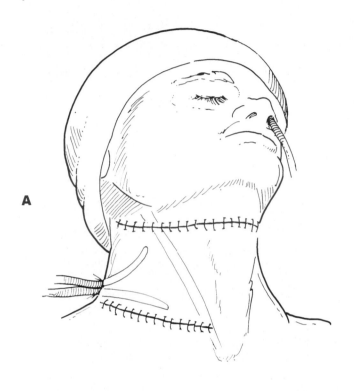

A

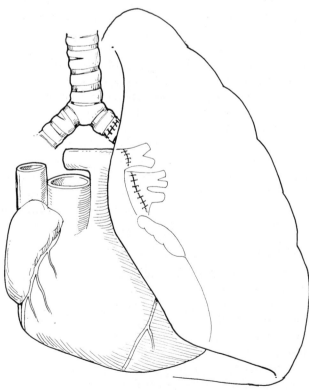

Fig. 10-2. Lung resection. Usually, plain chest radiographs show only a faintly visualized surgical staple line near the hilum.

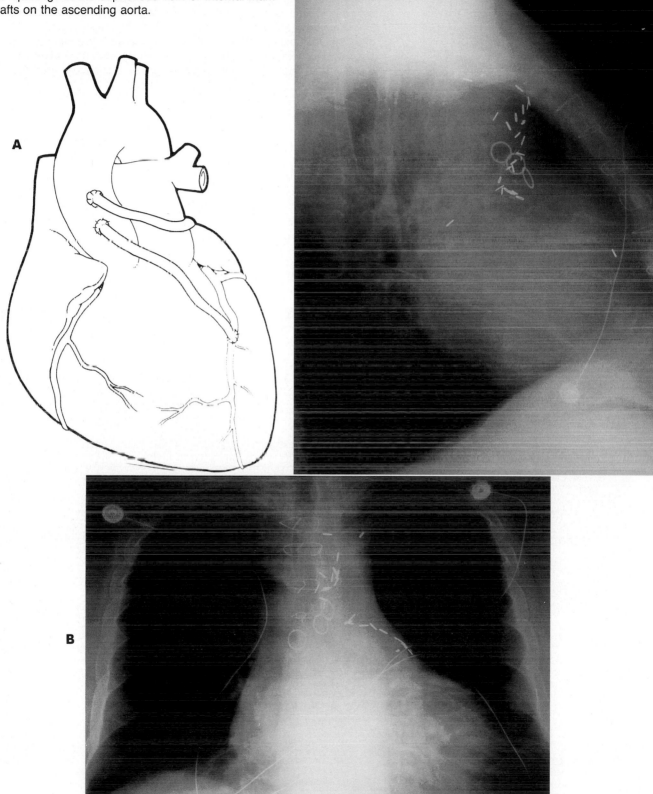

Fig. 10-3. Drawing, **A,** and chest radiograph frontal, **B,** and lateral views, **C,** of a patient who has undergone a coronary artery bypass procedure. Notice the metallic rings used to mark the openings of the saphenous vein or internal mammary grafts on the ascending aorta.

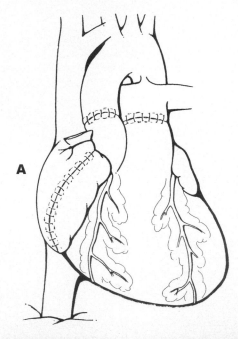

Fig. 10-4. A, Drawing of a heart transplant. Frontal, **B,** and lateral, **C,** views of a patient with a heart lung transplant. There are sternal sutures, hemoclips in the mediastinum, and surgical staples for the lung anastomoses. Notice also the Port-A-Cath infusion device. Very often the postoperative chest radiographs in heart transplant patients are indistinguishable from those of patients undergoing routine cardiac surgery, such as a valve replacement or a coronary artery bypass graft.

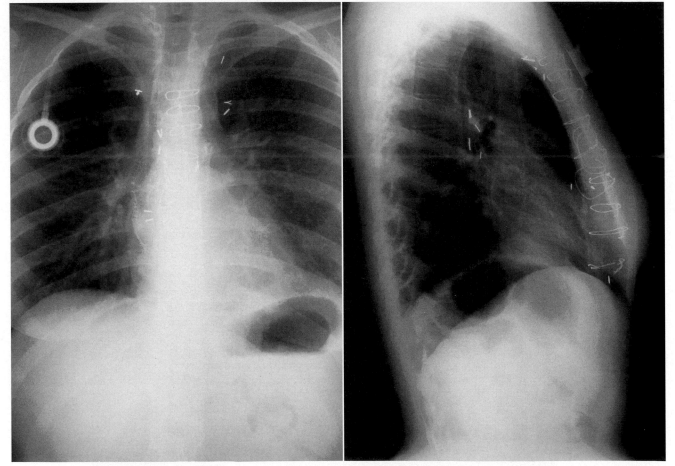

BREAST OPERATIONS

Radical Mastectomy

Radical mastectomy was the standard treatment for breast cancer until the 1970s. It has since been replaced by less aggressive procedures. The entire breast, pectoralis major muscle, pectoralis minor muscle, and the axillary contents are removed, leaving only the skin lying against the chest wall (Fig. 10-5, *A*).

Modified Radical Mastectomy

A modified radical mastectomy is the removal of the entire breast and the axillary contents. Unlike the radical mastectomy, it leaves the pectoralis muscles in place.

Simple Mastectomy

A simple mastectomy is the complete removal of the breast, including the nipple, and may be accompanied by an axillary node dissection (Fig. 10-5, *B*).

GASTRIC PULL-THROUGH (ESOPHAGOGASTRECTOMY)

Gastric pull-through is performed after resection of the thoracic esophagus, usually for cancer or benign strictures. After resection of the mediastinal esophagus, the stomach is brought through the mediastinum and anastomosed to the cervical esophagus above the left thoracic supraclavicular inlet (Fig. 10-6). A pyloroplasty is also performed to allow better gastric emptying. The repositioned gastric outlet is usually at the level of the diaphragm.

HIATUS HERNIA AND GASTROESOPHAGEAL REFLUX OPERATIONS

Nissen Fundoplication

In the Nissen fundoplication the short gastric vessels are transected, and the proximal greater curvature of the stomach is wrapped around the gastroesophageal junction (Fig. 10-7). The esophageal hiatus is narrowed to prevent herniation of the stomach into the mediastinum. Either an abdominal or left lateral thoracic incision is used for the surgery.

Angelchik Prosthesis

The Angelchik prosthesis is a donut-shaped device designed to fit around the gastroesophageal junction to prevent gastroesophageal reflux. The prosthesis is composed of silicone rubber and contains a metal ring to make it radiographically visible (Fig. 10-8).

GASTRIC OPERATIONS

Vagotomy and Pyloroplasty

In vagotomy and pyloroplasty the vagal trunks are divided because they parallel the distal esophagus and are often marked with hemoclips (Fig. 10-9). Vagotomy greatly reduces gastric secretion, but it also significantly slows gastric motility. Therefore, to facilitate gastric emptying a pyloroplasty is often performed to obliterate the pyloric sphincter.

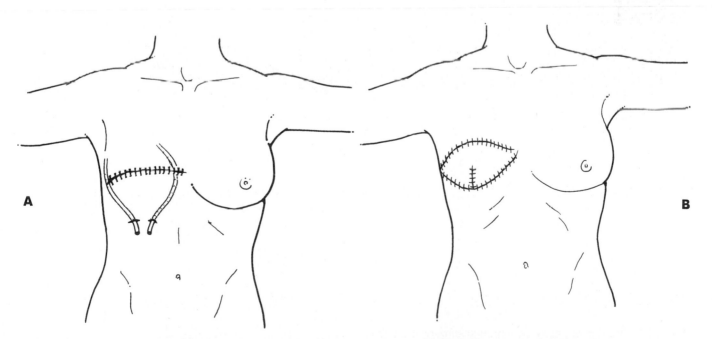

Fig. 10-5. Drawings of a radical mastectomy, **A,** and simple mastectomy, **B.**

Continued.

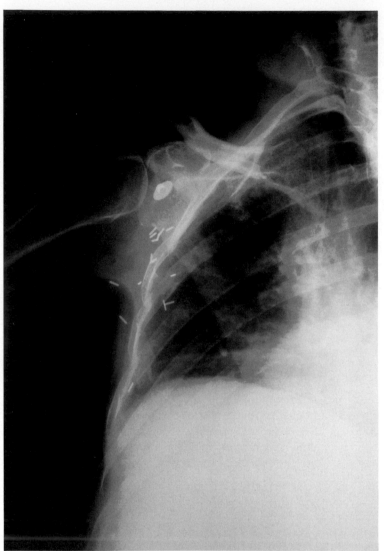

C

Fig. 10-5, cont'd. C, Radiograph of a patient who has undergone a right radical mastectomy. The right breast is absent, and surgical clips are in the right axilla.

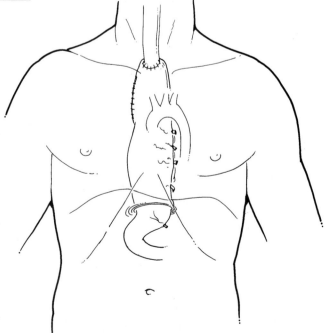

Fig. 10-6. Drawing of gastric pull-through surgery for esophageal carcinoma. The stomach now resides in the chest.

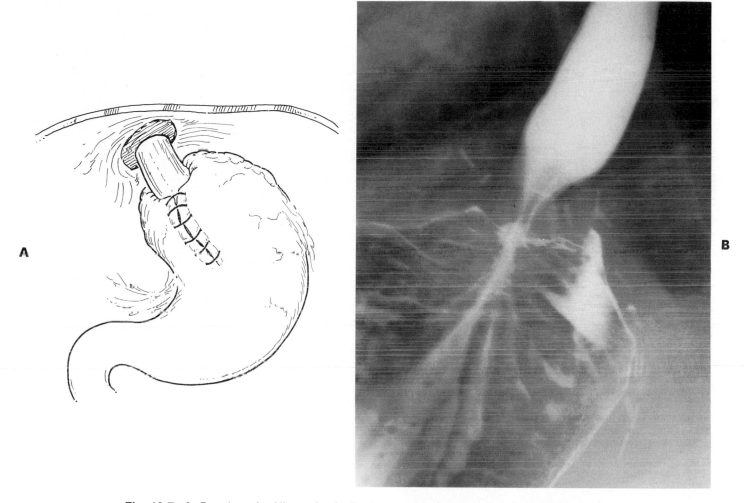

Fig. 10-7. A, Drawing of a Nissen fundoplication surgery for gastroesophageal reflux. **B,** Upper gastrointestinal series showing the deformity produced at the gastroesophageal junction by a Nissen procedure.

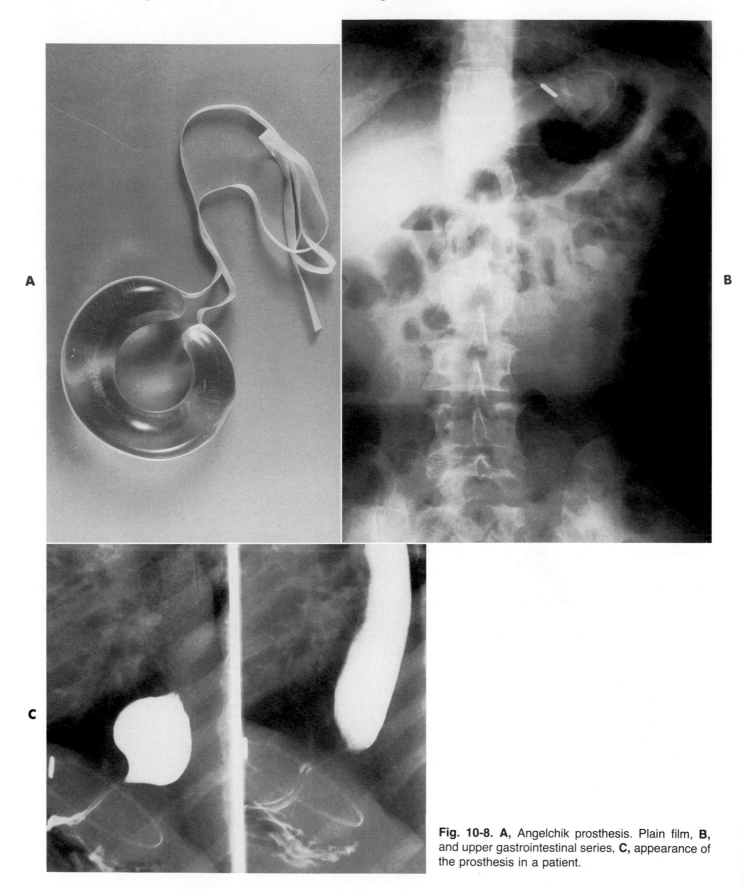

Fig. 10-8. A, Angelchik prosthesis. Plain film, **B,** and upper gastrointestinal series, **C,** appearance of the prosthesis in a patient.

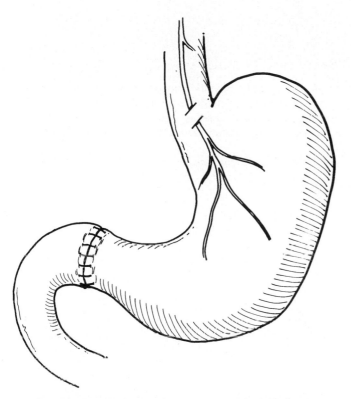

Fig. 10-9. Drawing of a vagotomy and pyloroplasty.

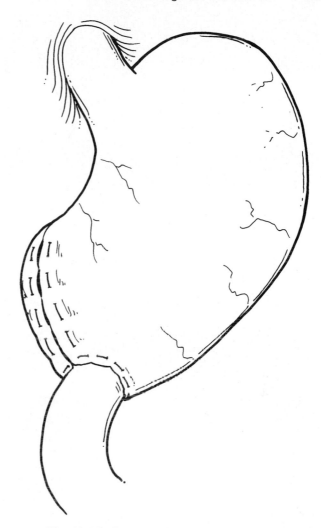

Fig. 10-10. Drawing of a Billroth I procedure.

Billroth I

An antrectomy (40% distal gastrectomy) is performed to remove the gastric secretory cells, and the duodenum is anastomosed to the gastric remnant (Fig. 10-10).

Billroth II

After the gastric antrum is resected, the duodenum is oversown to close its open proximal end. The open end of the stomach is narrowed, and the stomach is anastomosed to the proximal jejunum (Fig. 10-11).

Gastroenterostomy

Gastroenterostomy is usually a palliative operation for establishing gastrointestinal tract continuity and proper transit. It can be used to bypass strictures in the distal area of the stomach or in the duodenum from such conditions as peptic ulcer disease, stenosing Crohn's disease, and nonresectable malignant obstructions of the distal area of the stomach and of the duodenum. There are three general types of gastroenterostomies: the inferior antecolic gastroenterostomy, the anterior antecolic gastroenterostomy, and the posterior retrocolic gastroenterostomy (Fig. 10-12). A gastroenterostomy may also be combined with a vagotomy in the case of peptic acid disease.

Gastric Bypass

Gastric bypass surgery is designed for weight reduction. It is based on the observation that distal partial gastrectomy surgery for ulcer disease is often associated with weight loss and on the concept that a small gastric pouch for receiving feedings should produce early patient satiety and thereby reduce patient caloric intake. The gastric bypass procedure creates a small fundic pouch utilizing either a horizontal or a diagonal row of staples to alter the gastric lumen. A small stoma created by a gastrojejunotomy is used to drain the stomach (Fig. 10-13).

ROUX-EN-Y ANASTOMOSIS

The Roux-en-Y anastomosis is a diverting drainage procedure for abnormalities such as a pancreatic pseudocyst and obstruction of the biliary system or the stomach (Fig. 10-14). It provides the surgeon a free limb

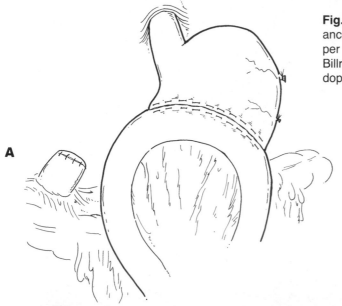

A

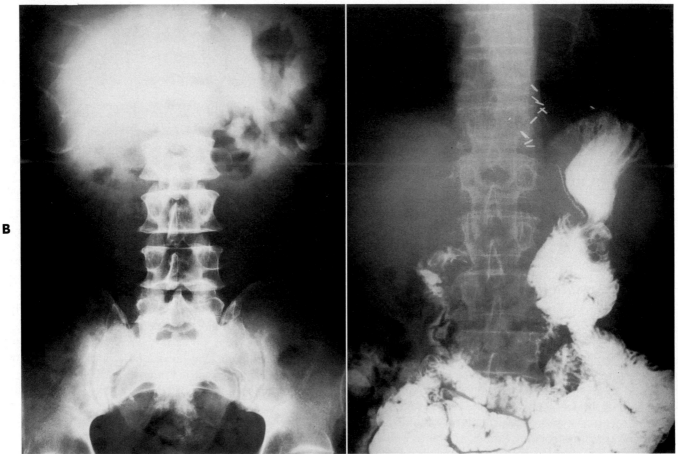

Fig. 10-11. A, Drawing of a Billroth II procedure. **B,** Plain film appearance of a patient who has undergone a Billroth II procedure. **C,** Upper gastrointestinal series in another patient who has undergone a Billroth II procedure. This patient has also undergone a Nissen fundoplication.

B

C

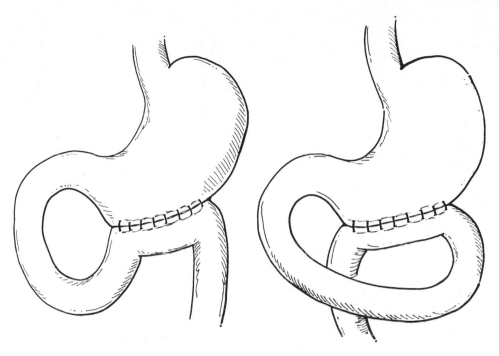

Fig. 10-12. Drawing of a gastroenterostomy.

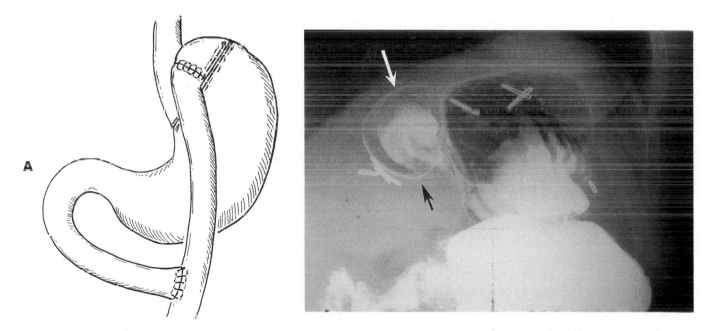

Fig. 10-13. A, Drawing of gastric bypass surgery. There are many variations in how the small gastric pouch is drained. **B,** Upper gastrointestinal series on a patient having a gastric bypass. Notice the small gastric pouch, *arrows.*

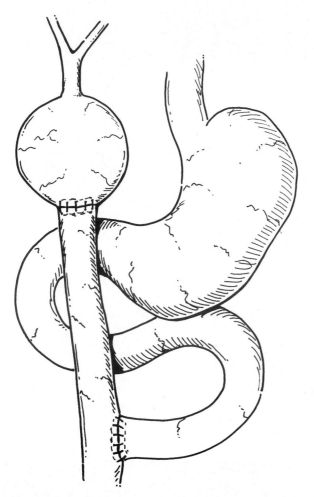

Fig. 10-14. Drawing of a Roux-en-Y procedure. In this case the Roux-en-Y is draining a choledochal cyst.

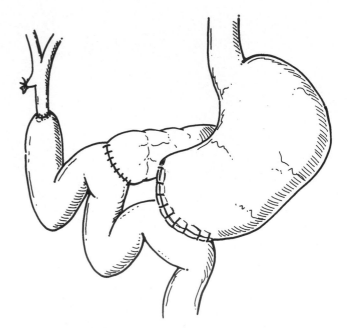

Fig. 10-15. Drawing of a Whipple procedure.

for drainage, and its configuration varies greatly with the surgical circumstances. Most of the time, a roux-en-Y is not completely visualized on radiographic studies, though barium and air may sometimes undergo reflux into the diverting limb.

WHIPPLE PROCEDURE

The Whipple procedure is used for patients with a carcinoma involving the head of the pancreas. It is basically a pancreaticoduodenectomy with reconstruction of the bile duct and drainage of the stomach, usually with a splenectomy (Fig. 10-15).

COLON RESECTION

Segmental colon resection is usually performed for cancer with or without a regional lymph node dissection. A total colectomy is most frequently performed for inflammatory bowel disease. A segment of colon is removed, and the open ends are placed together in a variety of configurations depending on the surgeon's preference. Typical configurations are end to end or end to

side (Fig. 10-16). Either sutures or staples may be used to approximate the bowel loops, depending on the preference of the surgeon.

HARTMAN POUCH

The sigmoid colon is resected, usually for a sigmoid or high rectal carcinoma. The rectum is closed at its open end where it was connected to the sigmoid portion of the colon. This now leaves a blind rectal pouch in place. The proximal portion of the colon is then approximated to the anterior abdominal wall as a colostomy (Fig. 10-17).

BLADDER RESECTION AND ILEAL CONDUIT

Bladder resection is usually performed in patients with cancer. However, it may be performed for functional or infectious abnormalities. One performs a urinary diversion after a bladder resection is done by isolating a segment of small bowel from the remainder of the intestinal tract. The ureters are connected to the isolated ileum, and this ileal loop is brought out to the abdominal wall as an ostomy (Fig. 10-18).

RIGHT HEPATIC RESECTION

Hepatic resection is usually performed in patients with primary or focal hepatic metastatic neoplasms. Resection of the right lobe of the liver is accomplished when one divides the right branches of the portal vein, hepatic artery, and hepatic duct. The liver is resected along a line from the gallbladder fossa to the vena cava (Fig. 10-19). Within approximately 2 weeks the liver regenerates to approximately its original size and shape.

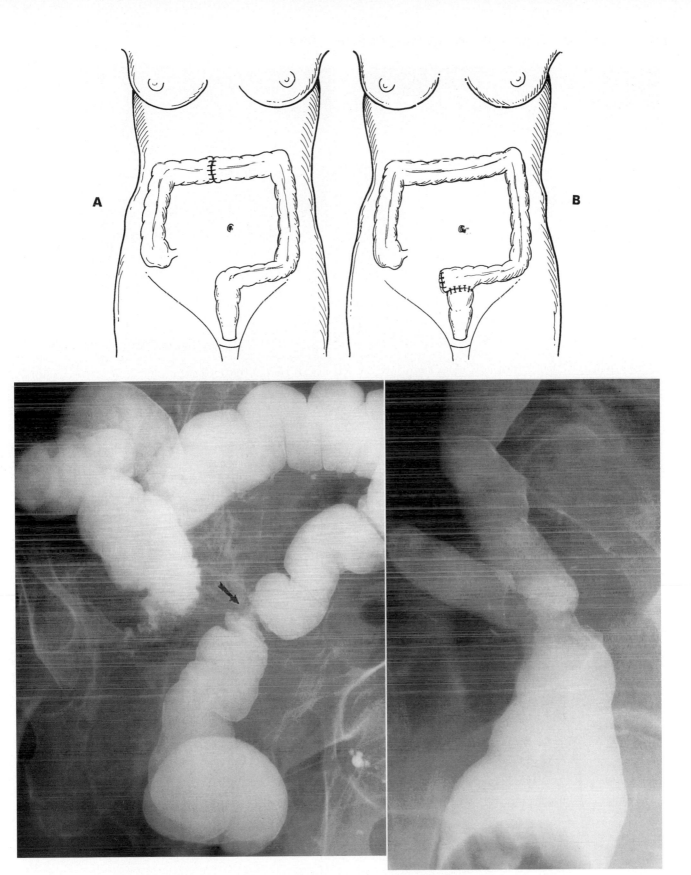

Fig. 10-16. Drawings of side-to-side, **A,** and end-to-side, **B,** bowel resections. These anastomoses may be used for either small bowel or colon surgery. **C,** Barium enema on a patient who has undergone an end-to-end sigmoid colon resection for a carcinoma. Notice the area of narrowing at the anastomosis, *arrow.* This proved to be a benign stricture. **D** and **E,** Complex end-to-side anastomoses in patients undergoing colon resection for carcinoma. **F,** Surgical staples in the right lower quadrant of a patient show where he has undergone small bowel resection for Crohn's disease. *Continued.*

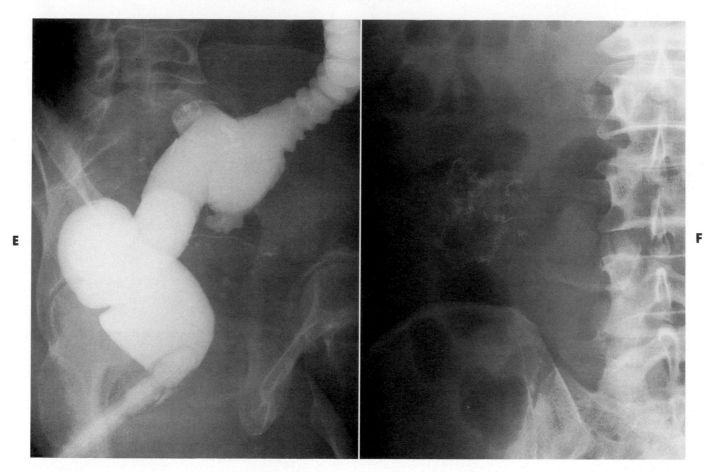

E   F

Fig. 10-16, cont'd. For legend see previous page.

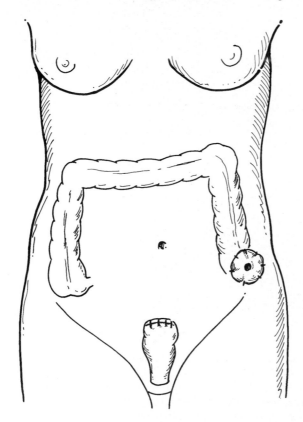

Fig. 10-17. Drawing of a Hartman pouch.

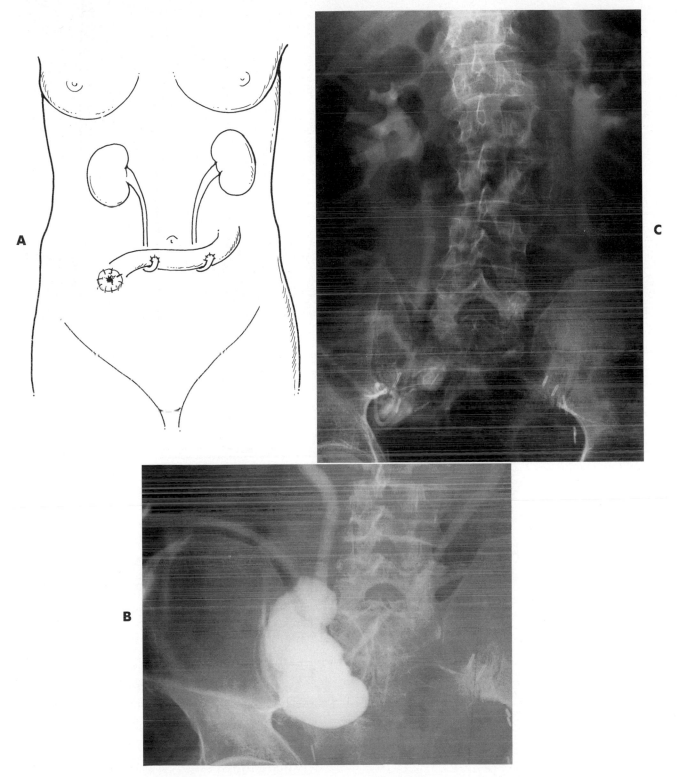

Fig. 10-18. A, Drawing of a bladder resection and ileal conduit. **B,** Contrast injection into an ileal loop (conduit). Notice the contrast reflux into both ureters. **C,** Supine view of the abdomen in the same patient shows contrast has refluxed into both kidneys.

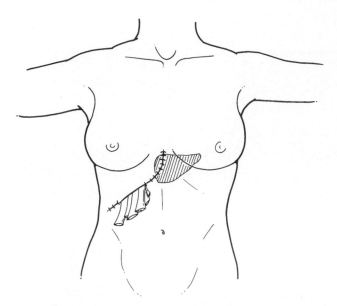

Fig. 10-19. Drawing showing resection of the right lobe of the liver.

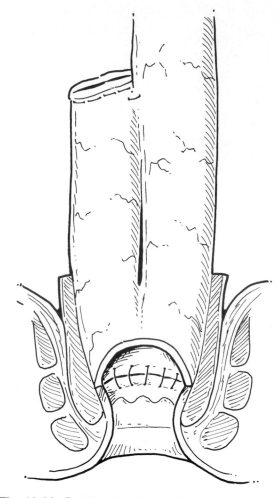

Fig. 10-20. Drawing showing an ileoanal pull-through.

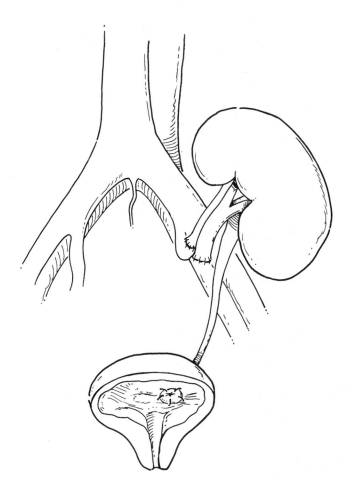

Fig. 10-21. Drawing showing the typical anatomy for a renal transplantation.

ILEOANAL PULL-THROUGH

An ileoanal pull-through is performed after total colectomy to provide a fecal reservoir and preserve continence. A total colectomy is performed with stripping of the rectal mucosa to preserve the anal sphincters. The ileum is then connected to the anus to make a pouch with the ileum serving as a reservoir (Fig. 10-20).

RENAL TRANSPLANTATION

The donor kidney is placed in the iliac fossa of the pelvis with the renal vessels connected to the iliac vessels and the ureter sewn into the bladder (Fig. 10-21).

AORTOFEMORAL (ILIAC) BYPASS

Arterial bypass surgery is performed for either occlusive or aneurysmal disease. A synthetic graft is usually bridged from the infrarenal aorta to the iliac or femoral arteries (Fig. 10-22). For aneurysms, this graft may extend only to the distal aorta at the bifurcation. There are many different techniques used for arterial anasto-

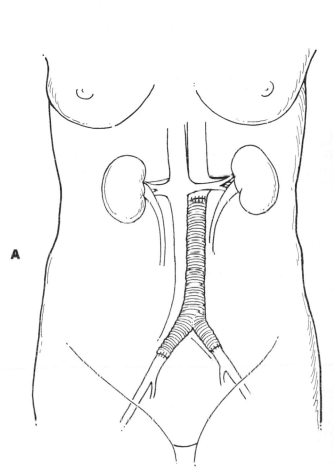

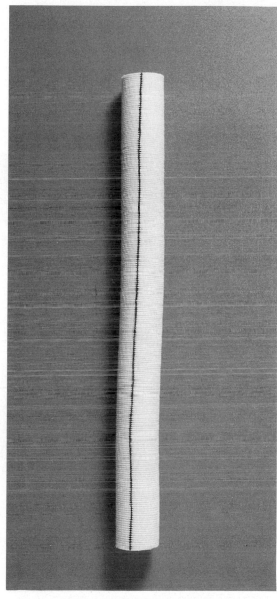

A

B

Fig. 10-22. A, Drawing showing a typical aortoiliac bypass graft. Sometimes the native aorta is wrapped around the graft. There are many different types of surgical connections that are used to bypass areas of narrowing or aneurysm formation. **B,** Photograph of a woven Dacron graft (Meadox Medicals).

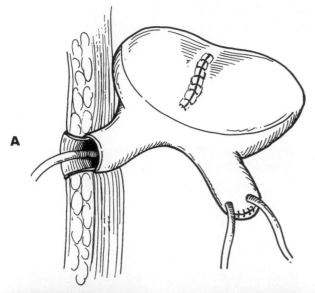

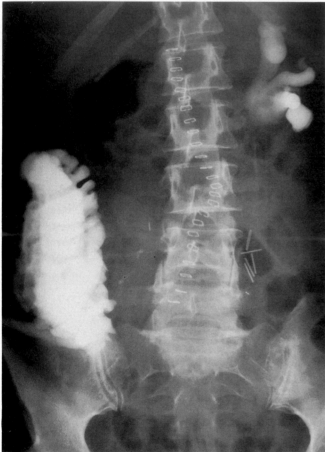

Fig. 10-23. A, Drawing of a Koch type of urinary reservoir. There are several different types of reservoir designs. **B,** Contrast study outlining Indiana reservoir in a patient.

mosis of the native and synthetic vessels, and the anatomy may become quite confusing. In cases of abdominal aortic aneurysms, the native vessel is often wrapped around the graft.

URINARY RESERVOIRS

An excluded portion of either the small bowel or the colon can be harvested to create a urinary reservoir, providing continence to a patient whose bladder has been resected (Fig. 10-23). The reservoir may be periodically catheterized through an ostomy opening. There are many different forms of urinary reservoirs with differing surgical anatomies.

FURTHER READINGS

General Texts

Schwartz SI (editor in chief), Shires GT, Spencer FC, Storer EH (associate editors): *Principles of surgery,* ed 4, New York, 1984, McGraw-Hill.

Sabiston DC Jr, editor: *Textbook of surgery: the biological basis of modern surgical practice,* ed 14, Philadelphia, 1991, Saunders.

Davis JH, Foster RS Jr, Gamelli RL: *Essentials of clinical surgery,* St. Louis, 1991, Mosby.

Nyhaus LM, Baker RJ, editors: *Mastery of surgery,* vol I and II, Boston, 1984, Little, Brown, & Co.

Teplick JG, Haskin ME, editors: *Surgical radiology,* vol I-III, Philadelphia, 1981, Saunders.

Burkitt HG, Quick CRG, Gatt D, Deakin PJ: *Essential surgery: problems, diagnosis, and management,* Edinburgh, 1990, Churchill Livingstone.

Bland KI, Copeland EM III, editors: *The breast: comprehensive management of benign and malignant diseases,* Philadelphia, 1991, Saunders.

Caine R, Pollard SG: *Operative surgery,* New York, 1992, Gower Medical Publishing.

Pulmonary and Cardiac Surgery

Spirn PW, Gross GW, Wechsler RJ, Steiner RM: Radiology of the chest after thoracic surgery, *Semin Roentgenol* 23:9-31, 1988.

McGovern EM, Trastek VF, Pairolero PC, Payne S: Completion pneumonectomy: indications, complications, and results, *Ann Thorac Surg* 46:141-146, 1988.

Landay MJ, Mootz AR, Estrera AS: Apparatus seen on chest radiographs after cardiac surgery in adults, *Radiology* 174:477-482, 1990.

Carter AR, Sostman HD, Curtis AM, Swett HA: Thoracic alterations after cardiac surgery, *AJR* 140:475-481, 1983.

Katzberg RW, Whitehouse GH, deWeese JA: The early radiologic findings in the adult chest after cardiopulmonary bypass surgery, *Cardiovasc Radiol* 1:205-215, 1978.

Goodman LR: Postoperative chest radiograph. II. Alterations after major intrathoracic surgery, *AJR* 134:803-810, 1980.

Hiatus Hernia; Gastroesophageal Reflux

Richter JE: Surgery for reflux disease—reflections of a gastroenterologist, *N Engl J Med* 326:825-827, 1992.

Spechler SJ: Department of Veterans Affairs Gastroesophageal Reflux Disease Study Group: comparison of medical and surgical therapy for complicated gastroesophageal reflux disease in veterans, *N Engl J Med* 326:786-792, 1992.

Zalev AH, Henderson RD, Marryatt GV: The total fundoplication gastroplasty: surgical procedure and radiologic appearance, *J Can Assoc Radiol* 40:12-17, 1989.

Angelchik Prosthesis

Starling JR, Reichelderfer MO, Pellett JR, Belzer FO: Treatment of symptomatic gastroesophageal reflux using the Angelchik prosthesis, *Ann Surg* 195:686-690, 1982.

Curtis DJ, Benjamin SB, Kerr R, Castell DO: Angelchik antireflux device: radiographic appearance of complications, *Radiology* 151:311-313, 1984.

Moussa SE, Tunuguntla K, Chan CH, et al: Endoscopic removal of an intact anti-reflux prosthesis 6 years after implantation, *Gastrointest Endosc* 36:525-527, 1990.

Ritchie PD, Milkins R, Fleming EL, Nott D: The Angelchik prosthesis results and complications, *Aust NZ J Surg* 57:621-625, 1987.

Jamieson GG: The Angelchik prosthesis— results and complications, *Aust NZ J Surg* 57:591, 1987.

Gastric Pull-Through (Esophagogastrectomy)

Owen JW, Balfe DM, Koehler RE, et al: Radiologic evaluation of complications after esophagogastrectomy, *AJR* 140:1163-1169, 1983.

Agha FP, Orringer MB, Amendol MA: Gastric interposition following transhiatal esophagectomy: radiographic evaluation, *Gastrointest Radiol* 10:17-24, 1985.

Reichle RL, Fishman EK, Nixon MS, et al: Evaluation of the postsurgical esophagus after partial esophagogastrectomy, *Invest Radiol* 28:247-257, 1993.

Gastric Bypass Surgery

Poulos A, Peat K, Lorman JG, et al: Gastric operation for the morbidly obese, *AJR* 136:867-870, 1981.

Smith C, Gardiner R, Kubicka RA, Dieschbourg JJ: Gastric restrictive surgery for obesity: early radiologic evaluation, *Radiology* 153:321-327, 1984.

Mishkin JD, Meranze SG, Burke DR, et al: Interventional radiologic treatment of complications following gastric bypass surgery for morbid obesity, *Gastrointest Radiol* 13:9-14, 1988.

Renal Transplantation

Dodd GD III, Tublin ME, Shah A, Zajko AB: Review: imaging of vascular complications associated with renal transplants, *AJR* 157:449-459, 1991.

Hanto DW, Simmons RL: Renal transplantation: clinical considerations, *Radiol Clin North Am* 25:239-248, 1987.

Kirchner PT, Rosenthall L: Renal transplant evaluation, *Semin Nucl Med* 12:370-378, 1982.

Kaude JV, Hawkins IF: Renal transplantation. In Abrams HL, editor: *Abrams angiography: vascular and interventional radiology,* Boston, 1983, Little, Brown & Co, pp 1365-1391.

Aortic Aneurysms

LaRoy LL, Cormier PJ, Matalon TAS, et al: Imaging of abdominal aortic aneurysms, *AJR* 152:785-792, 1989.

Thompson JE, Garrett WV, Patman RD, et al: Surgery for abdominal aortic aneurysms. In Bergan J, Yao J, editors: *Aneurysms: diagnosis and treatment,* New York, 1982, Grune & Stratton, pp 287-299.

Ramchandani P, Ball D: Abdominal aortic aneurysms: diagnosis, measurement and treatment, *Postgrad Radiol* 6:259-278, 1986.

Hilton S, Megibow AJ, Naidich DP, Bosniak MA: Computed tomography of the postoperative abdominal aorta, *Radiology* 145:403-407, 1982.

Urinary Reservoirs

Kenney PJ, Hamrick KM, Samuels LJ, et al: Radiologic evaluation of continent urinary reservoirs, *RadioGraphics* 10:455-466, 1990.

Amis ES Jr, Newhouse JH, Olsson CA: Continent urinary diversions: review of current surgical procedures and radiologic imaging, *Radiology* 168:395-401, 1988.

11

Orthopedic Devices

James B. Benjamin
Pamela J. Lund

Informed and pertinent radiographic interpretation of orthopedic devices can be frustrating. Orthopedists use a bewildering array of implants, which change almost daily. In addition, there is a plethora of bone and soft-tissue procedures, which most surgeons modify to suit the particular needs of any given case. There are many articles written for the radiologist in an attempt to identify implants,[1-4] and it is not the intention of this chapter to generate an all-inclusive list. Although exact identification of an implant may be of historic or intellectual interest, the more important considerations include its location, position, and the host response to the implant. The focus of this chapter is directed toward the rationale for the use of different implants and important radiographic findings associated with their use. Techniques for optimizing CT and MRI evaluation of these devices are also explored.

IMPLANT MATERIALS

(See also Chapter 1.)

Orthopedic surgery often involves the implantation of foreign material, the composition of which can be divided into several categories.

Metals

The metals used in orthopedic surgery are chosen for their mechanical and physical properties, biocompatibility, and cost. Characteristics such as elasticity and ductility are important when one is using implants for fracture fixation, whereas materials with higher fatigue strength are more appropriate for prostheses that will be subjected to repetitive stresses over time. Biocom-

patibility is also an important issue in terms of the initial host response to the implant as well as the long-term effects of metal-ion leaching into surrounding tissues and host organs. Finally, cost is currently and will become an increasingly important issue in determining metallic implant design and composition.

Metal implants are easily imaged radiographically but extremely difficult to evaluate by newer modalities such as computed tomography and magnetic resonance imaging. Their presence also creates problems with imaging of surrounding bone and soft tissue because of the metallic artifacts they produce (see also Chapters 15 to 17).

Stainless steel is used extensively in fracture fixation devices. It has good fatigue strength, is inexpensive, and has excellent machinability. Most pins, plates, intramedullary nails, screws, and wires are manufactured from this material. Cobalt-chromium alloys are corrosion resistant and have mechanical properties that make them ideal for use in fabricating prostheses. Both commercially pure titanium and titanium alloys offer excellent biocompatibility and mechanical properties, making them highly suitable for prosthetic fabrication. Titanium has poor wear characteristics and is not suitable for use as an articulating surface.[5] More recently, titanium has been used for fracture fixation devices such as rods, plates, and screws.

Plastics and Polymers

Ultrahigh molecular weight polyethylene (UHMWPE) has been used for approximately 30 years as the bearing interface in total joint arthroplasty. Initially, tibial, patellar, and acetabular components were made entirely of UHMWPE and included wire markers to allow for radiographic visualization. Because of problems of late deformation and breakage of unsupported polyethylene, most of these components were metal backed in the 1970s and 1980s. Polyethylene is also used in other settings, as in the fabrication of intramedullary plugs for cement restriction in total hip arthroplasty.

Silicone elastomer (Silastic) has been used to fabricate implants for arthroplasty of the small joints in the hands and feet (Fig. 11-1). These flexible implants act as spacers in the carpus, metacarpophalangeal (MCP), metatarsophalangeal (MTP), and interphalangeal (IP) joints. Unfortunately they have poor wear properties resulting in problems of breakage and fragmentation, which lead to an inflammatory osteolytic response. This has resulted in changes in fabrication and the use of metal grommets in an attempt to minimize this problem (Fig. 11-1).

Poly(methyl methacrylate), or PMME, has been used for over 30 years to anchor orthopedic implants to the skeleton. Although radiolucent by itself, all commercially available PMME used for orthopedic implantation now contains barium to allow radiographic visualization. Powdered methacrylate is mixed with a liquid monomer to form a workable dough that has a polymerization time of 10 to 15 minutes. PMME is also often used as a bulk spacer in tumor and joint excision surgery. Antibiotics can be added to PMME, which provides an ideal method of prolonged local delivery as the antibiotics elute over a period of weeks into surrounding tissues.[6] When used in this fashion, the PMME is usually made into "beads" and implanted into an infected area (Fig. 11-2).

Miscellaneous

Ceramics are metal oxides that have extremely low coefficients of friction, making them ideal in certain settings for articular bearing surfaces. Ceramics used in orthopedics, aluminum oxide and zirconium oxide, are radiodense and are currently used in the fabrication of femoral heads in total hip replacements (Fig. 11-3). Some prosthetic hip systems of European design use ceramic acetabular components as well.

Polytetrafluoroethylene (Gore-Tex, Teflon) is best known for its use in sport wear, but Gore-Tex has also been utilized in the production of a synthetic ligament. This braided multifilament ligament is used for reconstruction of the anterior cruciate ligament.[7] Although the material itself is radiolucent, the metal grommets at the anchoring points are easily visualized (Fig. 11-4).

Carbon fiber has also been used in fabricating synthetic ligaments. It is radiolucent. Biologic implants (bone, osteochondral composites, and ligaments) are routinely implanted in reconstructive surgery. This material can be obtained either from the patient in whom it is used (autograft) or from cadaver donors (allograft). Autologous bone grafting is done in a wide variety of situations, including fractures, arthrodesis, joint reconstruction, and tumor surgery. Although autologous grafting represents the ideal in terms of histocompatibility and osteogenic stimulation, it does have some drawbacks. Obtaining the graft routinely requires an additional surgical procedure, and the amount of graft that can be harvested from any individual is finite.

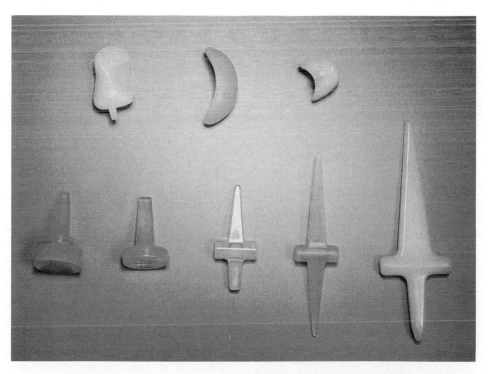

Fig. 11-1. Various types of Silastic (silicone elastomer) implants.

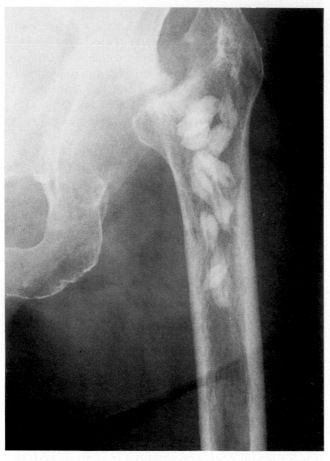

Fig. 11-2. Methyl methacrylate antibiotic "beads" inserted into proximal femur after removal of infected total hip arthroplasty joint.

Homologous bone grafting allows much more latitude in terms of the amount of bone available and enables the surgeon to place large structural or intercalary grafts in salvage procedures where there is significant loss of bone stock. Radiographic evaluation should focus on complications, such as delayed or nonunion, fracture, or resorption, which may be attributable to infection or an autoimmune response.[8] Osteochondral articular grafting is performed much less frequently and often only in centers with special interest in these procedures.[9] Tendon and ligament grafting is routinely performed to reconstruct structures such as the anterior cruciate ligament and lateral ankle ligaments. These procedures are most commonly done with autografts, but some centers routinely use allografts.

FRACTURE FIXATION

The wide variety of devices used in fracture fixation can be grouped into several general categories: pins, wires, screws, plates, intramedullary rods, and external fixators. Most of these implants are fabricated from stainless steel, although more recently, some screws, plates, and rods have been made from titanium. Fracture fixation devices are often used with one another to obtain the most desirable biomechanical construct.

Pins

Steinman pins and Kirschner wires are commonly used for temporary fixation of fracture fragments during fracture reduction and are also used to attach skeletal traction. The pins are both smooth and threaded

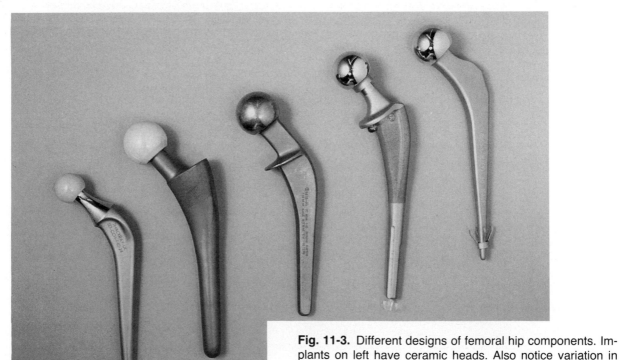

Fig. 11-3. Different designs of femoral hip components. Implants on left have ceramic heads. Also notice variation in head diameter.

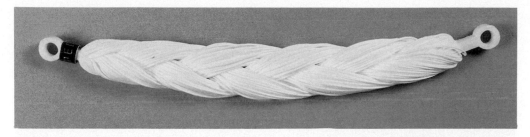

Fig. 11-4. Woven Gore-Tex anterior cruciate ligament substitute.

and come in a variety of diameters. Pins are also used extensively in cannulated screw systems to allow accurate placement of larger screws into bone. In certain settings pins are used for definitive fixation of fracture fragments and can be left percutaneously, for ease of removal, or buried deep beneath skin and subcutaneous tissue (Fig. 11-5).

Pins used for definitive fixation should be followed closely for migration, a significant problem when pins are used around the shoulder, because reports of migration into the chest, mediastinum, and neck are not uncommon. Pins can also be used with wires to create tension-band fixation, which is a dynamic form of fracture fixation creating compression at the site of fracture (Fig. 11-6).[10]

Wires

Wires of various diameters and, more recently, braided cables are used most commonly with other modalities in fracture fixation and to reattach osteotomized bone fragments. These osteotomies are most commonly done at the greater trochanter (Fig. 11-7) and olecranon to provide surgical exposure but can be performed at any site of muscle or ligament attachment. As described above, wires can be used with pins or screws to create a tension band, which uses distractive muscular forces to create compression at the fracture site.

In conjunction with intramedullary fixation, circumferential wires are also commonly used to stabilize long bone fractures. These wires work in the same manner as barrel stays and are called "cerclage wires" (Fig. 11-8). A potential complication of cerclage wiring is the interruption of the periosteal blood supply with subsequent bone necrosis or failure of fracture union, a complication seen more frequently with the use of bands designed for the same purpose.

Wires are also used for suturing bone and soft tissue. The most common complication seen with wires is breakage. Although this should be noted, it is usually of little significance unless it leads to loss of position of bone fragments or migration of wire fragments.

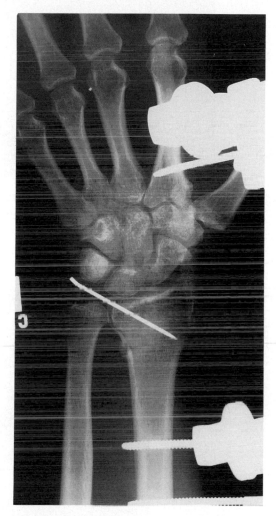

Fig. 11-5. External fixator used to treat distal radius fracture with percutaneous pin. Notice the unilateral threaded pins in radius and in index metacarpal bone.

Screws

There are several basic terms used in describing screws. These terms are related to the screw design and function (Fig. 11-9). The screw head is the bulbous end of the screw that engages the screwdriver. The shank or core of the screw is the solid central portion of the

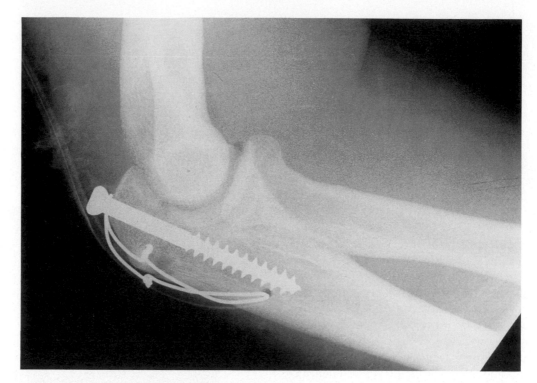

Fig. 11-6. Tension band fixation of an olecranon fracture using a cancellous screw. The looped wire transforms the distractive pull of the triceps into compression at the fracture site.

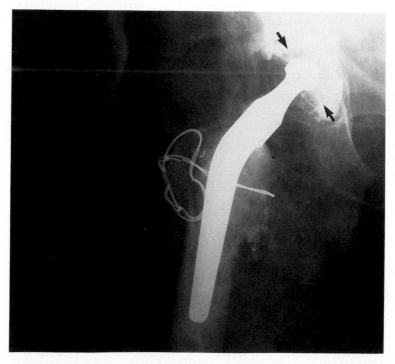

Fig. 11-7. A cemented total hip arthroplasty joint done using a trochanteric osteotomy that has been fixed with wires. The wire is broken laterally and there is evidence of polyethylene wear in the acetabulum, *arrows,* revealed by the asymmetric position of the prosthetic femoral head.

screw, which can be of variable diameter between the threaded and nonthreaded portion of the screw. A screw can be partially or completely threaded, and the distance between the threads is called the "pitch." Screws have a wide variety of sizes and lengths to facilitate their use in different locations.

Screw designs can also vary depending on their intended use. Cancellous screws have larger thread diameter and pitch and are often partially threaded. In contrast, cortical screws commonly have smaller thread diameter and pitch and are fully threaded.[10] Screws are commonly used with plates and washers, which allow soft-tissue anchorage and increase the surface area of the screw head to maximize the holding power of the screw.

A screw that crosses a fracture line is called an "interfragmentary, or lag, screw." When properly applied, this screw provides compression between fracture fragments, which enhances stability and promotes healing. A syndesmotic screw is one that is placed across the distal tibiofibular joint parallel to and 1 to 2 cm proximal to the ankle joint (Fig. 11-10). This screw is intended to stabilize the ankle mortise in cases where the syndesmotic ligaments have been disrupted.[11]

From a radiographic standpoint, minor variations in screw design, screw size, or number of screws is not of major concern. Screw breakage, loosening, or change in position are important observations.

The wide variety of specialty screws have design considerations to allow their use in selected settings. Hip pins used to stabilize intracapsular hip fractures are actually modified screws that are threaded distally and have a nut on the proximal end rather than a head. Cannulated screws have the same appearance as standard screws except that the shank is hollow (Fig. 11-11), a feature that allows the screws to be placed over a guide pin for more exact placement. The guide pin placement is usually confirmed radiographically before screw placement and is routinely removed once the screw is placed.

A Herbert screw is a modified screw that was developed for fixation of scaphoid fractures.[12] The screw has threads of different pitch on each end and an unthreaded central shank (Figs. 11-11 and 11-12). The Herbert screw lacks a head and is designed to be countersunk in the scaphoid. The original screw is small to allow its use in the carpus, and this design has also proved efficacious for fixation of osteochondral fractures in larger joints. Subsequently, larger screws of the same design have been developed. A Kurosaka screw is a short, broad, headless screw designed to anchor ante-

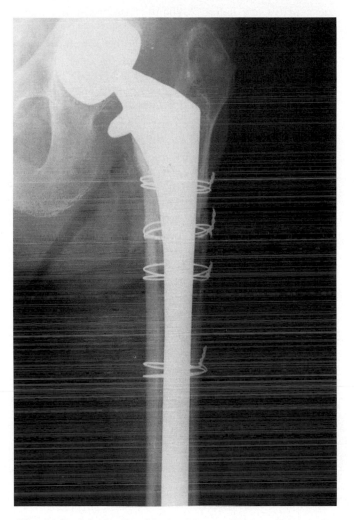

Fig. 11-8. A long-stem bipolar hip prosthesis with cerclage wires in the diaphysis of the femur.

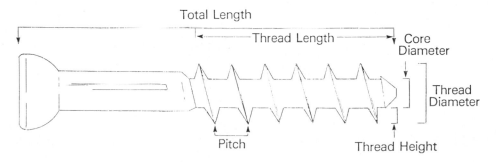

Fig. 11-9. Screw anatomy.

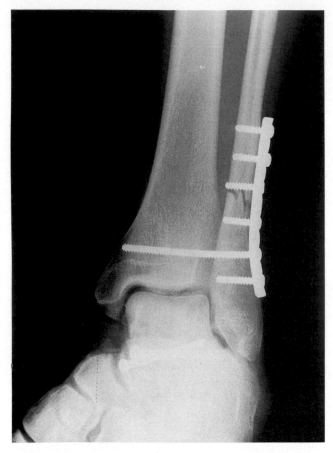

Fig. 11-10. Ankle fracture fixed with a six-hole dynamic compression plate and syndesmotic screw.

rior cruciate grafts in the metaphysis of the tibia and femur[13] (Fig. 11-13).

Plates

Plates come in a wide variety of sizes and shapes and have round or oval holes for screw fixation. The oval holes are designed to provide compression of the fracture as eccentrically placed screws are tightened on either side of the fracture line.[10] Because of this feature, these plates are called "dynamic compression plates" (DCP).

Other plate designs include one-third tubular plates, reconstruction plates, and blade plates (Fig. 11-14). One-third tubular plates are thinner than the DCPs, have a similar radiographic appearance, and are commonly used in treating distal fibular fractures. Reconstruction plates are notched between the holes, and this feature allows them to be bent or contoured in three planes. These plates are commonly used to accommodate the complex anatomy of pelvis fractures (Fig. 11-15).

Blade plates have a sharply angled extension at the end of the plate so that it can be placed into the metaphysis for fixation (Fig. 11-16). Used in the proximal and distal femur, they have a wide range of angles to accommodate different situations. There is also a host of other plate shapes that are designed to accommodate variances in anatomy in the metaphysis of different bones. A recent modification of DCP design is the low contact DCP (LC-DCP), developed to minimize periosteal compression in an attempt to facilitate fracture healing.[10]

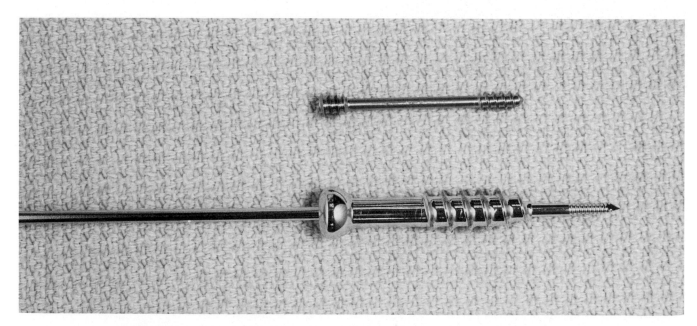

Fig. 11-11. Cannulated screw with threaded-tipped guide pin and Herbert screw.

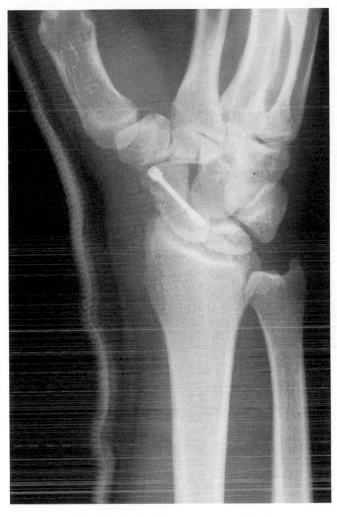

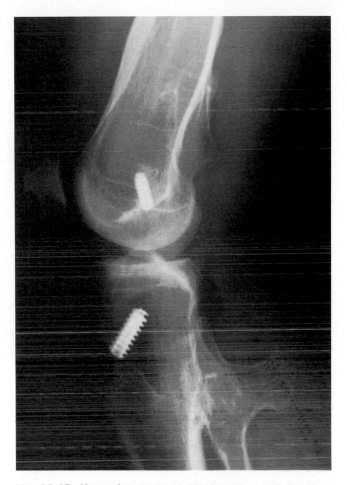

Fig. 11-13. Kurosaka screws used to anchor anterior cruciate graft in femoral and tibial metaphysis. Notice the multiple osteochondromas.

Fig. 11-12. Herbert screw transfixing a scaphoid fracture.

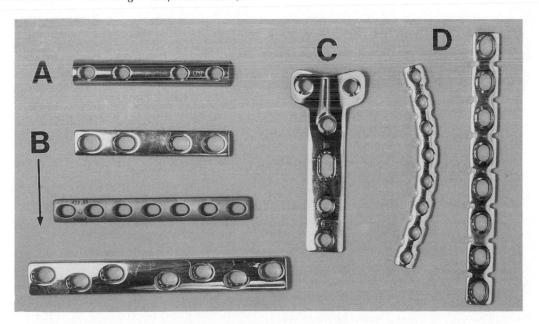

Fig. 11-14. Internal fixation plates. **A,** One-third tubular plate. **B,** Dynamic compression plates. **C,** T-plate. **D,** Reconstruction plates.

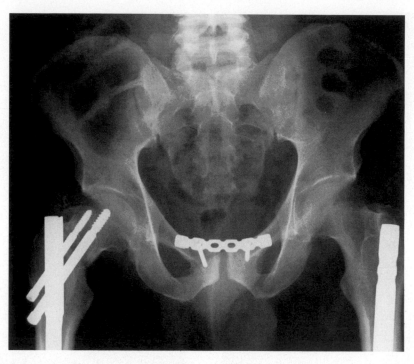

Fig. 11-15. Reconstruction rod fixing ipsilateral femoral neck and femoral shaft fracture (not visible) on right. Reconstruction plate on pelvis and unlocked intramedullary rod in left femur.

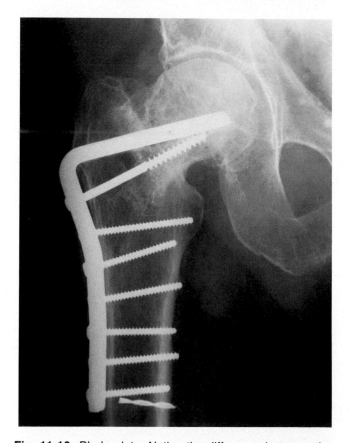

Fig. 11-16. Blade plate. Notice the difference between the cancellous screw proximally and the remaining six cortical screws. Also of note is the broken drill bit distally.

Plates can also be used to anchor fixation devices, usually large screws, in the treatment of intertrochanteric and supracondylar femur fractures. These devices are called "compression screws and side plates" because the end of the plate has a barrel that engages the large lag screw and allows it to slide to compensate for compression or collapse at the fracture site. The fracture can also be compressed dynamically by the use of a smaller screw, which engages the large lag screw (Fig. 11-17).

Some terms that are commonly used with fracture plating are "compression plating" and "neutralization plating." Compression plating takes advantage of the DCP design to apply compression to the fracture ends. In cases with comminution, bone loss, or anatomic considerations that prevent compression, the plate is applied in a neutral mode, in that the plate is intended solely to hold fracture fragments in place during healing. It is important to recognize that the same type of plate can be used in either fashion and the radiographic appearance may not differ.

Often, not all the screw holes in a plate are filled. This is done intentionally when fracture patterns do not allow adequate screw purchase or when additional screws do not improve the strength or rigidity of fixation. A general rule of thumb used when plating diaphyseal fractures in long bones is that a minimum of six cortices should be engaged by screws on each side of the fracture except for the femur, which requires eight. Although most commonly used for fracture fixation in

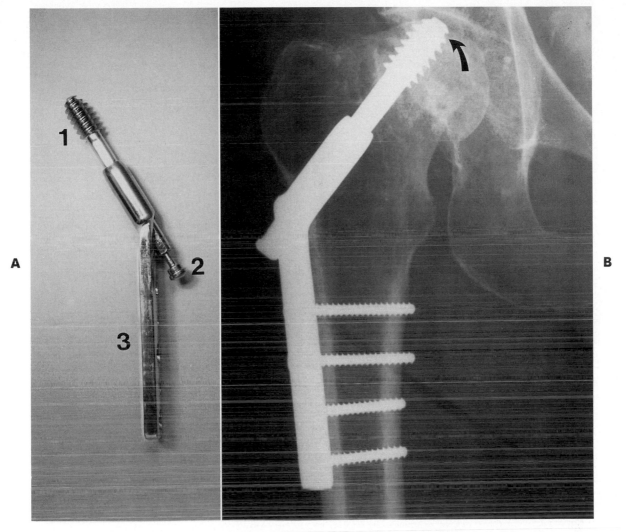

Fig. 11-17. Compression hip screw. **A,** This device is composed of three parts: *1,* lag screw; *2,* compression screw; *3,* barrel and side plate. **B,** Compression hip screw. The lag screw has slid distally in the barrel, allowing the fracture site to become compressed. However, this did not prevent the screw from cutting out of the femoral head, *curved arrow.*

long bones, plates are also used in the lumbar and cervical spine to stabilize spinal segments.

The actual size, shape, and number of holes in a plate are not of critical importance in the radiographic evaluation of plate fixation. Of more important consideration is the location of the plate, that is, whether it symmetrically spans the fracture and the fracture reduction. Plates should not impinge on joint motion, and neither the plate nor any of the associated screws should violate articular surfaces. Plate breakage, changes in position of a plate, or loosening of screws usually indicates failure of fixation and should be noted.

Intramedullary Rods

Gerhard Kuntscher is credited with popularizing intramedullary nailing of long bone fractures beginning in 1940.[14] Intramedullary nailing revolutionized the treatment of femur fractures and is currently the treatment of choice for femur, tibia, and humerus fractures. Most intramedullary nailings are done "closed" in that the fracture itself is not exposed, rather the rod is inserted either in an antegrade or retrograde fashion through a limited exposure at the end of the bone. In the femur and tibia this is done from the proximal end. After exposure, the metaphyseal portion is opened with an awl and a guide wire is passed through the proximal fragment, across the fracture, and into the distal fragment. Flexible reamers are used to enlarge the intramedullary canal, and a rod of appropriate dimensions is then passed over the guide wire. The availability of high-quality portable fluoroscopic imaging equipment was critical for the development of this technique.

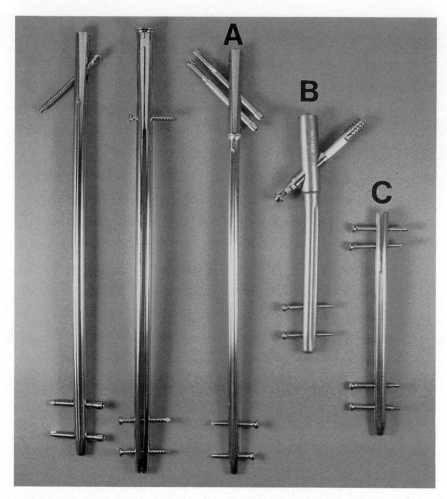

Fig. 11-18. Locking femoral intramedullary rods. **A,** Reconstruction rods. **B,** Intramedullary hip screw. **C,** Supracondylar rod.

Intramedullary rods provide excellent stability against bending forces in long bones but do not control rotation or compressive forces in situations where the bone itself cannot contribute to the stability. Intramedullary rods of contemporary design used for femur fractures are all curved to accommodate the anterior bow of the femur. For the most part, they are cannulated to allow them to be inserted over a guide wire. Although they vary in design, all have screw holes both proximally and distally (visible on the lateral projection) to allow interlocking screws to be used (Fig. 11-18).

The interlocking screws provide rotational control as well as preventing collapse or shortening of the fracture. The single proximal locking screw is usually placed obliquely from superior and lateral in the intertrochanteric area. In some rod designs the proximal screw is placed perpendicularly to the bone in the subtrochanteric area (Fig. 11-18). Distal locking screws, usually two in number, are inserted, from lateral to medial, perpendicularly to the long axis of the rod.

When a rod is locked both proximally and distally it is said to be "statically locked" in that all planes of motion are controlled or static. When a rod is locked at only one end, it is said to "dynamically locked" because compression at the fracture site can occur. Interlocking of intramedullary rods has greatly expanded the utilization of this technique because fractures with significant comminution or bone loss can be managed definitively.

Rods of older design do not have screw holes and can be used only in a dynamic mode. The original Kuntscher rods were straight and employed three-point intramedullary contact to enhance fixation. Reconstruction rods are used to treat femoral fractures with ipsilateral femoral neck, intertrochanteric fractures, or subtrochanteric fractures and have the proximal locking holes oriented to allow screws to be placed into the femoral neck and head (Figs. 11-15 and 11-18).

Tibial nails possess the same basic characteristics as femoral nails in terms of design and application. In most contemporary tibial rod designs there are usually two

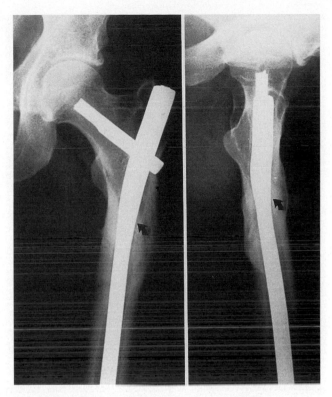

Fig. 11-20. Zickle nail. The sharp bend in the rod seen in the subtrochanteric area, *arrow,* often resulted in refracture when the rod was removed.

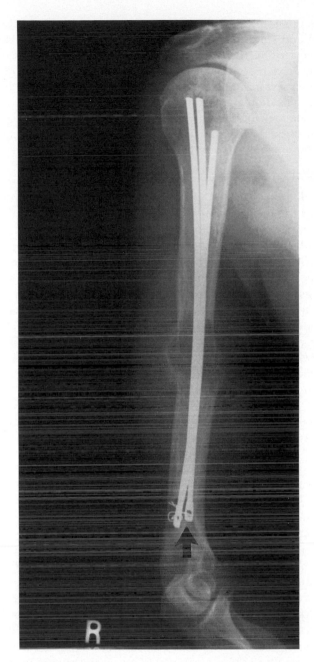

Fig. 11-19. Flexible intramedullary rods used to treat a humerus fracture. The wire in the eyelets distally, *arrow,* prevents the rods from backing out of the insertion portal.

proximal and two distal locking screw holes. Screws are the most commonly used method for locking rods, though some systems utilize distal fins, wires, or techniques that expand the fluted distal end of the rod. Rods that are used to treat tibia and femur fractures and that allow for locking range in diameter from 8 to 16 mm.

There is a host of other intramedullary nail designs that differ significantly from the description above. The first group consists of smaller-diameter, solid rods that can be bent to accommodate variations in anatomy of different bones. Their stability is imparted by the use of multiple rods stacked in the intramedullary canal. The use of multiple insertion portals and divergence of the ends of the rods in the metaphyseal area provides some axial and rotational stability (Fig. 11-19).

In bones of smaller diameter a single rod can be bent to give contact at several areas on the endosteal cortex, thus providing stable fixation. The Rush pin with its sled runner tip and hooked end is the prototype for this group of nails, which includes Enders nails and chondrocephalic nails. The Zickle nail, consisting of a solid intramedullary nail with a triphalanged pin inserted into the femoral head, was originally developed to treat subtrochanteric fractures, but because of problems of refracture during removal and with the advent of newer designs, the Zickle is no longer extensively used (Fig. 11-20).

Some rod designs employ a short intramedullary rod with multiple transverse or oblique interlocking screws. These devices are designed to be used in diaphyseal-metaphyseal fractures, which often have extension into the adjacent joint (see Fig. 11-18). Another unique rod design often used in children with osteogenesis imperfecta who require multiple osteotomies to correct long bone deformities employs a two-part telescoping rod, which allows the rod to lengthen as the child grows.[15]

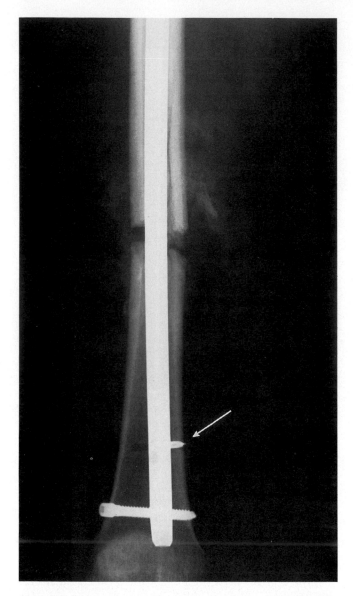

Fig. 11-21. Residual lengthening of a femur fracture after static nailing. Only one screw hole distally is filled, and a broken drill bit, *arrow*, can be seen adjacent to the more proximal locking hole.

As with plates and screws, identification of the rod manufacturer is not an important radiographic consideration. Fracture alignment and implant position are most important. Interlocking rods are technically difficult to properly insert, and a host of complications are associated with their use. Change in bone length is common especially with statically locked rods (Fig. 11-21). Also, distraction at the fracture site may occur if intraoperative traction is not released before distal locking. Although fracture union is unaffected, a leg-length discrepancy may result.

Distal screw targeting can be the most difficult aspect of inserting locked rods, and a potential complication

is missing the holes with the interlocking screws. The lateral view should confirm that the locking screws do engage the rod. Biomechanically, the locking holes in the rod represent weakened areas, and rod or screw breakage may occur at these sites.[16] As with other fracture fixation, neither the rods nor the screws should violate articular surfaces. Some rods are designed to be inserted through the joint; however, they should remain countersunk so as not to impinge on joint motion.

External Fixation

External skeletal fixation is utilized in many settings for the management of orthopedic conditions. In open fractures with significant soft-tissue injury requiring vascular procedures, fasciotomy, tissue flaps, or multiple débridements, external fixators provide an excellent means of fracture immobilization while still allowing access to the surrounding soft tissues. Threaded pins of varying diameters are placed percutaneously into the bone above and below the level of the fracture and are connected by an external frame to allow rigid immobilization (Figs. 11-5 and 11-22). Many external frames are now fabricated from radiolucent materials, such as carbon fiber, which facilitate radiographic evaluation.

When threaded pins are used, they are placed through the subcutaneous border of the bone in a unilateral fashion. The threaded end of the pin penetrates the near cortex and medullary canal to engage the far cortex without penetrating the muscle compartments; thus the risk of injury to neurovascular structures is avoided.

External fixators are also commonly used in the treatment of pelvic fractures. In this setting the pins are placed in the wing or anterior aspect of the ilium. Although fixators are good at stabilizing some pelvic disruptions, such as "open-book" type of fractures, they provide little control over posterior instability. Because of these limitations, open reduction and internal fixation are becoming more common in the treatment of displaced pelvic fractures, and external frames are being used less for definitive treatment.

Another common site for frame application is in distal radius fractures. In this setting pins are placed in the radius and in the index metacarpal, and distraction is placed across the carpus. This technique utilizes the surrounding soft tissues, or ligamentotaxis, to obtain an indirect reduction of the fracture (see Fig. 11-5).

A relatively new modification of external fixation, developed by the Russian surgeon Ilizarov, has gained great popularity in recent years. This technique employs the use of small-diameter smooth wires that transfix the extremity and are connected by a circumferential frame. The Ilizarov technique is used most often in reconstructive settings to lengthen limbs, transport bone segments, and correct angular deformities (Fig. 11-23). The indications for its use continue to expand, and the better

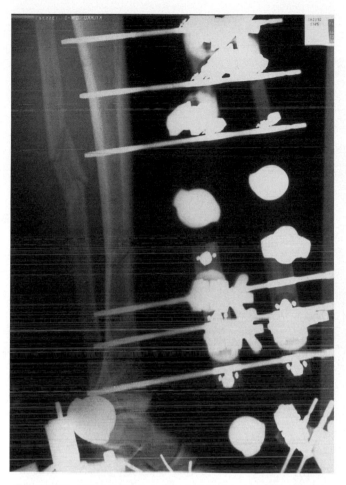

Fig. 11-22. Tibia fracture treated with an external fixator. Notice the unilateral pins, which just penetrate the far cortex, and the radiolucent connecting rods.

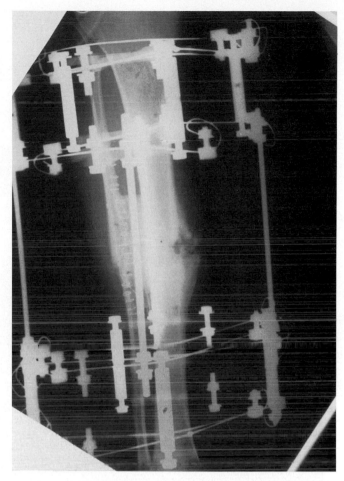

Fig. 11-23. Ilizarov device. The pins are smooth and of smaller diameter than that of standard fixators and transfix the extremity.

understanding of bone and soft-tissue physiology allow its application in almost any part of the extremity.

External fixators can be placed across joints to help prevent contractures or control position and are also used for immobilization in arthrodesis and osteotomy procedures. The location of the pins and limb alignment are important radiographic considerations, as is evidence of pin loosening, breakage, or infection. Limited radiographic visualization attributable to the external frame may require special views or fluoroscopic positioning for optimal assessment of bone anatomy.[17]

Computed tomography and ultrasonography have been used successfully to allow more accurate and sensitive evaluation of new bone formation within corticotomy and osteotomy intervals in patients undergoing treatment in Ilizarov frames.[18] Complications including soft-tissue interposition, pseudarthrosis, and cyst formation can also be identified with these modalities (Fig. 11-24). The use of magnetic resonance imaging is currently limited by the ferromagnetic construction of these devices.

Casts

External immobilization of extremities with casts and splints is an everyday occurrence with orthopedic patients. Casts and splints may be made from many different materials, including plaster of paris, synthetic casting material, and metal (Fig. 11-25). Plaster of paris is the material most frequently used to fabricate splints and casts because it possesses properties that make it ideal for this purpose. It is inexpensive, easy to mold, "breathable," and absorbent. Synthetic casting materials are lighter and stronger but more expensive and non-absorbent.

Casts and splints can be used either for temporary immobilization of an extremity or for definitive treatment of fractures. They may be used with internal fixation to provide additional support or protection of an extremity. Braces are also used to limit the range of motion of a joint after a surgical procedure or trauma. In some settings, percutaneous pins are combined with a plaster cast to achieve a construct similar to an external fixator. This technique is commonly referred to as "pins in plaster."

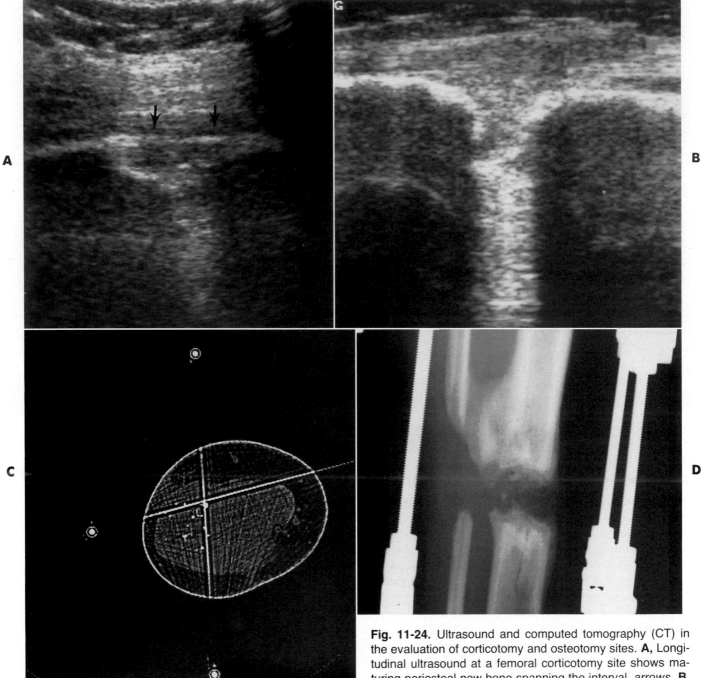

Fig. 11-24. Ultrasound and computed tomography (CT) in the evaluation of corticotomy and osteotomy sites. **A,** Longitudinal ultrasound at a femoral corticotomy site shows maturing periosteal new bone spanning the interval, *arrows.* **B,** Longitudinal image in different patient without adequate periosteal new bone demonstrates lack of linear periosteal echo, with prominent posterior through-transmission. **C,** Axial CT image at the corticotomy site confirms lack of new bone. Notice prominent metallic artifact from the Ilizarov frame. **D,** Anteroposterior radiograph obtained at the time of the CT and ultrasonography shows little new bone formation.

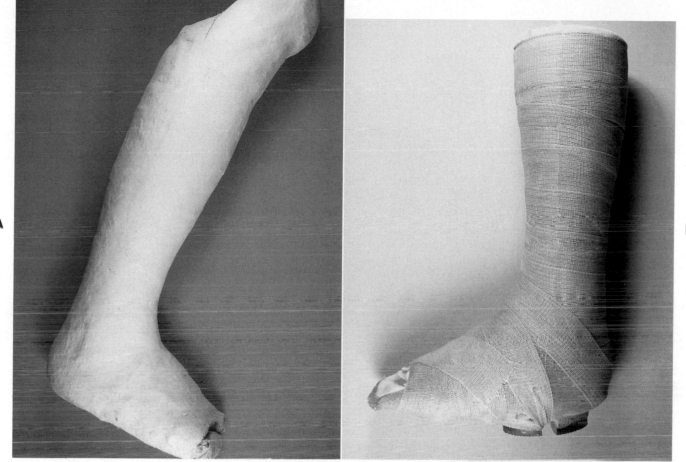

Fig. 11-25. A, Plaster cast. **B,** Fiberglass cast.

All current materials used for casting and bracing are radiopaque. Their presence decreases the detail seen on plain radiographic studies. Synthetic casting materials interfere least with the x-ray beam penetration. Plaster of paris absorbs more of the x-ray beam than synthetic materials do, and wet plaster is even more radiopaque than dry plaster. The most radiopaque material for casts is metal. CT and MRI studies are not degraded by the presence of these materials with the exception of metal casts and braces. Because the radiographic detail can be significantly diminished in the presence of a cast or splint, the interpretation of these studies should focus attention on the overall position and alignment of bones or implants rather than on fine bone detail.

JOINT ARTHROPLASTY

Although joint implantation surgery has been performed for many years, John Carnley, a British surgeon, is considered the father of modern joint replacement surgery. His pioneering work in the late 1950s and early 1960s revolutionized orthopedic surgery and resulted in his being knighted for his contribution to medicine.[19]

Sir Charnley developed an articulated hip replacement consisting of a stemmed metal ball and a polyethylene cup that were anchored to the skeleton with the use of methyl methacrylate. Although there have been numerous technologic advancements in the ensuing three decades, the basic principles developed by Charnley have stood the test of time.

During the late 1960s and early 1970s there was a proliferation of this technology and designs for replacement of almost every major joint in the body were developed. Although early results were satisfactory, problems with implant loosening and osteolysis at the methyl methacrylate–bone interface became apparent in the second decade. It was believed that if the cement could be eliminated the problem of late aseptic loosening could be avoided. This premise triggered a wave of intensive research and development into alternative forms of implant fixation with an emphasis on "biologic" fixation.

Two forms of biologic fixation resulted from these efforts. Bone ingrowth employs implants with porous surfaces that allow bone and other tissue to form in the

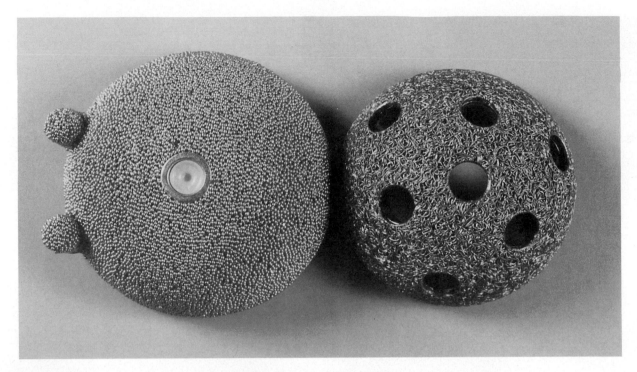

Fig. 11-26. Two types of porous-coated acetabular components.

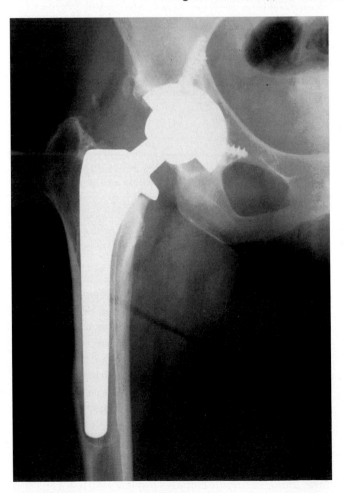

Fig. 11-27. Osteolysis associated with a noncemented total hip arthroplasty. There is a radiolucency around the entire femoral stem with a sclerotic margin. There is also noticeable thinning of the lateral cortex.

interstices and provide a microinterlock[20] (Fig. 11-26). Osseointegration denotes actual chemical bonding between living bone and an implant. Scandinavian researchers found that threaded implants fabricated from pure titanium could actually form a chemical bond with living bone.[21] More recently, surface coatings of hydroxyapatite (HA) on metal have demonstrated this same phenomenon and actually appear to stimulate bone formation.[22,23]

Unfortunately, these alternative forms of fixation have failed to resolve all of the problems that were formerly attributed to methyl methacrylate. Osteolysis still occurs around noncemented implants, and it is now recognized that this biologic response occurs with any type of wear debris and can be seen with methyl methacrylate, polyethylene, or metal particles[24,25] (Fig. 11-27).

The generation of microscopic wear debris appears to be a key issue in determining the longevity of joint implants. Recent efforts have been directed toward reducing joint interface friction and wear, and the use of ceramic bearing surfaces and polyethylene modification have been developed as a result. At the present time most artificial joints still employ a metal-on-polyethylene bearing surface and utilize a combination of cemented and noncemented fixation, which has been termed "hybrid fixation."

Hip Arthroplasty

Hip arthroplasty encompasses a wide range of implants. Hip-resurfacing procedures were done as some of the earliest forms of hip arthroplasty. The Smith

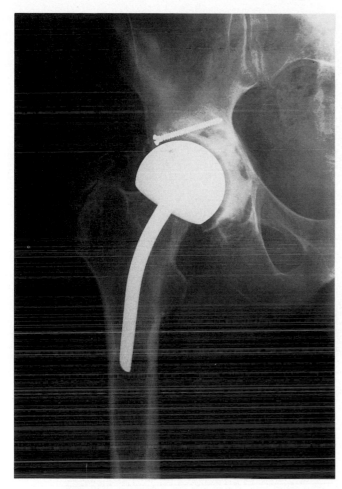

Fig. 11-28. Resurfacing hip arthroplasty. The all-polyethylene acetabular component is radiolucent. There is osteolysis at the tip of the stem seen as thinning of the cortex.

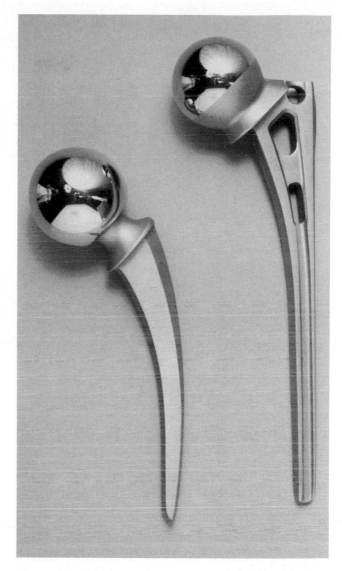

Fig. 11-29. Endoprostheses are single-piece devices that can be used with cement, *left,* or are cementless, *right.* The head diameters match those of the femoral head, which they replace.

Peterson cup employed a metal cap that was placed on the reamed femoral head. In this procedure the acetabulum was also reamed but used no formal acetabular component, instead relying on the "plasticity" of the acetabulum to form new articular surface. The ability of this procedure to provide reliable pain relief and function was limited.

The successor of the Smith Peterson cup was a more formal resurfacing procedure in which the acetabulum was also addressed[26] (Fig. 11-28). Although some centers reported good long-term results with this type of procedure, it is not routinely performed at the present time.

An endoprosthesis consists of single piece, a press-fit stem with a ball that matches the diameter of the acetabulum. With this type of prosthesis the ball articulates with the hyaline cartilage of the acetabulum (Fig. 11-29). Newer designs are modular with separate ball and stem, and although the stem is usually press fit into the

femoral canal, some prostheses are designed to be cemented. These implants are routinely used in the treatment of intracapsular hip fractures.

Bipolar prostheses were developed to address some of the problems seen with endoprostheses, that is, wear of the acetabular cartilage leading to protrusio acetabuli. A bipolar prosthesis consists of a stem and a small-diameter head with a separate acetabular component consisting of a metal shell lined with high-density polyethylene (HDPE). Once the properly sized acetabular component is selected the two snap together as an articulating unit. The external diameter of the cap matches that of the acetabulum, and the internal bearing surface articulates with the small-diameter head. Mo-

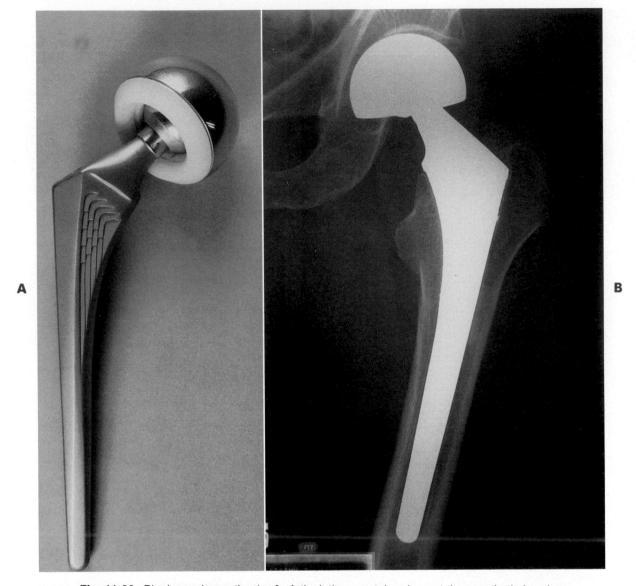

Fig. 11-30. Bipolar endoprosthesis. **A,** Articulation can take place at the prosthetic head–polyethylene interface and at the metal surface–articular cartilage interface. **B,** Bipolar prosthesis demonstrating bone remodeling. There has been rounding off of the proximal medial cortex and subtle cortical thickening at the stem tip. There is also evidence of bead shedding adjacent to the stem in the area of the greater trochanter.

tion can take place at the inner bearing surface or at the metal acetabular surface (Fig. 11-30). The bipolar prosthesis has also been used, with mixed results, as a salvage procedure for failed acetabular components in total hip arthroplasty.

Traditional total hip arthroplasty designs consist of a stemmed femoral component with a small-diameter head, ranging from 22 to 32 mm in diameter, and a hemispherical HDPE acetabular component. The acetabular component may be metal backed, and any or all of the components may be cemented (Fig. 11-31). To-tal hip arthroplasty is at the present time the most com-

monly performed joint replacement, with approximately 150,000 a year being done in the United States alone.

Historically, hip arthroplasty designs have varied considerably, and design variations should not be a primary concern when one is evaluating hip prostheses radiographically. Initial considerations after implantation should concentrate on the position of the implant. Our preference is an anteroposterior view with the hip in neutral rotation and a Johnson cross-table lateral view to include the entire acetabulum and femoral component. Although the cross-table lateral view does not pro-

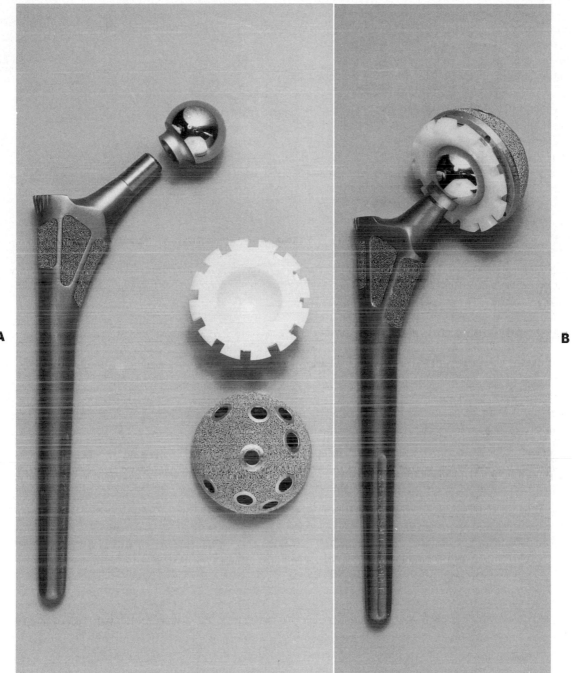

Fig. 11-31. Modular noncemented total hip prosthesis. **A,** Implants consist of a proximally porous-coated stem and prosthetic head and a porous-coated metal acetabular component with a polyethylene liner. **B,** Assembled implant.

vide the detail of a frog-leg lateral view, it is much safer in terms of hip positioning in the initial postoperative period and does provide a lateral view of the acetabulum.

Ideal cup position should be 40 to 50 degrees of abduction from the horizontal and 20 to 30 degrees anteverted from the coronal plane. Although abduction is easy to determine, anteversion is often difficult to evaluate, even in the cross-table lateral projection.[27] The goal of joint replacement is to reconstruct the normal biomechanical anatomy of the hip and place the center of rotation of the prostheses at the point of the normal hip. Cup position relative to the tear figure is often the best indicator of its superoinferior position. Individual pelvic anatomy will ultimately determine the optimal position, and some variation in cup orientation is certainly acceptable. However, any large variation should be noted.

The ideal position of the femoral component should demonstrate that the stem is centered in the femoral canal on the anteroposterior view. Valgus position of the stem is preferable to varus, and obviously the stem should not project outside of the cortex on any view. A general rule of thumb is that the center of the femoral head should be at the same level as the tip of the greater trochanter. Some surgical approaches utilize an osteotomy of the greater trochanter to gain exposure to the hip. Although usually returned to an anatomic position, the trochanter may be advanced distally.

Another concern in the immediate postoperative setting is whether the hip is dislocated (Fig. 11-32). The type of fixation used to anchor a hip prosthesis should also be noted. Cement is easily visible on both the acetabular and femoral side and should be contained within the prepared femoral and acetabular beds. Cement extruded outside the cortex of the femur into the pelvis or into the area of the obturator foramen implies that there was a bone or soft-tissue defect that was not occluded before cementing was done.

Noncemented fixation is any type that does not utilize PMMA. Porous coating is often visible radiographically, but hydroxyapatite coating is not.[23] Component manufacturer, variations in component design, or relative size of the components is not of great significance. Any additional hardware associated with the implant should be noted, especially in revision cases where bone grafting or fracture fixation is commonly seen.

Late radiographic considerations in total hip arthroplasty should focus predominantly on the bone-implant interface.[28] Although the goal of hip arthroplasty is to recreate a normal biomechanical function of the hip, the placement of a large, stiff metal implant in the proximal area of the femur can drastically change the forces transmitted to the host bone. As a living tissue, bone reacts to changes in stress by remodeling according to Wolf's

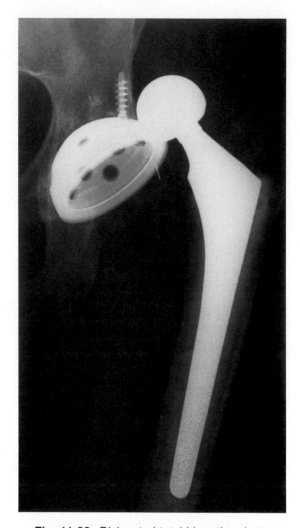

Fig. 11-32. Dislocated total hip arthroplasty.

law; bone mass is increased in areas of compression and resorbed at sites that are not stressed or mechanically loaded.

Common bone changes seen in long-term follow-up study of hip arthroplasty include bone resorption in the area of the proximal medial cortex because of stress shielding and hypertrophy of the cortex at the tip of the stem because of increased stress transfer at this area (see Fig. 11-30, *B*). Endosteal widening seen with aging also occurs in the presence of total hip arthroplasty. Predominant acetabular changes include superior or medial migration of the cup.

The bone-implant interface represents perhaps the most critical area of radiographic concern; this interface reflects the relative fixation of an implant and ultimately the clinical success. The bone-implant interface at the acetabulum has been divided into three zones on the anteroposterior projection, with zone 1 representing the superior lateral third, zone 2 the middle third, and zone 3 the inferior medial third (Fig. 11-33). In an ideal

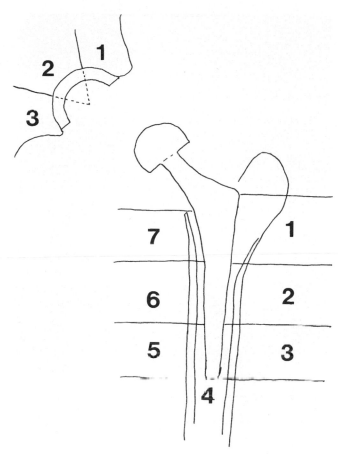

Fig. 11-33. Radiographic zones for acetabular and femoral prostheses.

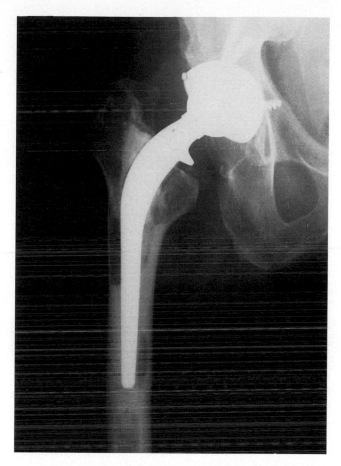

Fig. 11-34. Cemented total hip arthroplasty with focal osteolysis about the stem in zones 2, 5, and 7.

cemented acetabular component there should be an indistinct area of transition between the cement and bone. Evidence of acetabular component loosening includes a continuous radiolucency of greater than 1 mm in all three zones, radiolucency of greater than 2 mm in any one zone, migration of the cup superiorly or medially, or rotation of the cup when compared to the immediate postoperative radiographs. Often with superior migration there is no radiolucency in zone 1 because the cancellous bone is compressed and resorbed in front of the migrating cup. One should also check for migration of the prosthetic femoral head within the acetabular component because late polyethylene wear is also a concern (see Fig. 11-7).

The femoral bone–implant interface has also been divided into zones for radiographic analysis.[29] There are seven zones in both the anteroposterior and lateral projection. Zones 1 to 3 in the anteroposterior projection run from superior lateral to inferior lateral, with zone 4 representing the interface at the tip of the stem. Zones 5 to 7 run from inferior medial to superior medial. In the lateral projection zones 1 to 3 represent the anterior interface from proximal to distal, with zone 4 again

representing the tip of the stem. Zones 5 to 7 represent the posterior interface from distal to proximal (Fig. 11-33). Although this system seems cumbersome, it is very helpful in identifying changes at the bone-implant interface, which often are very localized.

Changes worthy of note in long-term follow-up study of hip arthroplasty include progressive radiolucencies at the bone-cement or bone-implant interface, bone resorption or hypertrophy, or sclerotic endosteal lines around implants. Although focal zones of implant bone lucency are quite specific for identification of loosening, sensitivity can be improved with the use of technetium bone scintigraphy.[30,31] Arthrography is associated with a significant number of false-negative results and is rarely used to diagnose implant loosening.[32] Fracture of the cement mantle, fracture or migration of implants, or osteolysis around implants should also be noted on follow-up radiographs (Fig. 11-34).

Focal osteolysis, initially termed "cement disease," can be seen surrounding cemented and noncemented implants and is triggered by generation of wear particles, cement, polyethylene, or metal. In porous-coated ingrowth prostheses, dissociation of beads or fiber pads

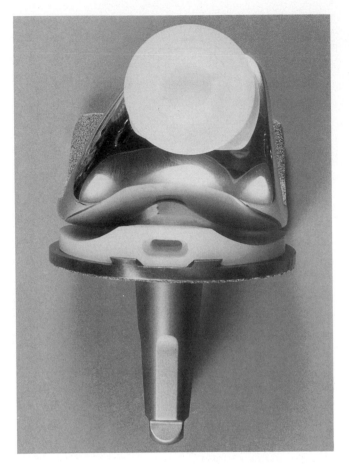

Fig. 11-35. Contemporary total knee arthroplasty. Patellar component and tibial insert are ultrahigh molecular weight polyethylene.

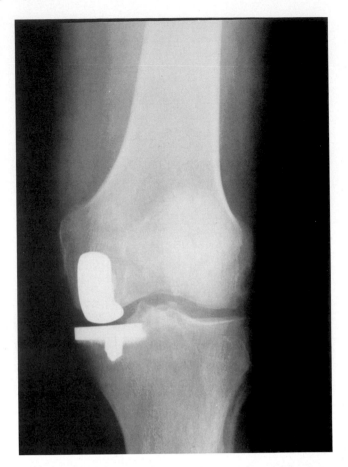

Fig. 11-36. Medial unicompartmental knee prosthesis.

can be seen both acutely and with long-term follow-up study. Acute dissociation of a small number of beads can occur during insertion and is of little consequence. Progressive dissociation of beads implies less than satisfactory fixation of the implant and should be noted. Fibrous ingrowth into porous implants is often associated with a stable, narrow radiolucency bordered by a sclerotic margin adjacent to the porous-coated areas of the implant.[33]

Knee Arthroplasty

Modern tricompartmental knee arthroplasty involves a multiradius metal femoral component that resurfaces both condyles and the trochlear notch. The tibial component consists of a metal-backed polyethylene tray that articulates with the femoral component. The patella is often resurfaced with a HDPE component, which may be metal backed (Fig. 11-35). This design has evolved over the last three decades from single condylar designs used in tandem, hinged prostheses, and mold arthroplasty similar to the cup arthroplasty seen in the hip. Components may be stemmed, cemented, or screw anchored and can vary considerably in design. Critical to

the function of total knee arthroplasty are an intact quadriceps mechanism and medial collateral ligament. The anterior cruciate ligament, if present at the time of arthroplasty, has to be removed.

There remains some controversy on the importance of an intact posterior cruciate ligament, but most knee designs allow for at least its partial retention. Unicompartmental knee arthroplasty is the resurfacing of a single condyle, usually medial, and its corresponding tibial articulation (Fig. 11-36). It is used when an arthrosis is confined to a single compartment. Isolated patellofemoral resurfacing has also been developed but is no longer routinely performed because of poor long-term results.

Initial radiographic evaluation of knee arthroplasty should concentrate on position and alignment.[34] Postoperative evaluation should include all components on anteroposterior and lateral views centered at the joint. Standing anteroposterior and Merchant view of both knees as well as supine anteroposterior and lateral views should be obtained in the early postoperative follow-up examination. On the anteroposterior view the tibial component should be oriented at 90 degrees to the long axis of the tibia. Some knees are designed to be placed in 1 to 2 degrees of varus; however, more than 5 degrees of varus or valgus alignment is abnormal.

In the lateral projection the tibial component should be at 90 degrees to the long axis of the tibia or sloped several degrees posteriorly. Anterior slope or excessive posterior slope greater than 7 degrees should be avoided. The tibial component should be centered on the tibia on both the anteroposterior and lateral projection and should cover most of the proximal area of the tibia without overhang. The femoral component size should closely match the original contour of the femur unless there is significant bone deformity preoperatively. On the anteroposterior projection the femoral component should be oriented in 5 to 7 degrees of valgus relative to the long axis of the femur. Varus orientation or excessive valgus orientation of the femoral component should be avoided. On the lateral projection the femoral component should be aligned so that the posterior aspect of the anterior flange is parallel to and flush with the anterior cortex of the femur.

Notching of the anterior femur creates a stress riser, which may result in a supracondylar fracture.[35,36] Accurate visualization of the orientation of knee components is often difficult because of the metal obscuring the bone-prosthesis interface. True anteroposterior and lateral views with the x-ray beam parallel to the interfaces are required to make accurate assessments. Alignment of the knee is also difficult to assess with non-weight bearing views and requires standing anteroposterior views of the knees for confirmation. More detailed information on alignment requires standing whole-leg views, which include the femoral head, knee, and ankle joint to allow evaluation of the mechanical axis of the lower extremity.

The patellar component is best evaluated on the lateral and Merchant views of the knee. On the lateral projection the patellar resection should be symmetric, and the thickness of the bone-prosthesis construct should approximate that of the original patella. The Merchant view should document that the patella is seated symmetrically in the trochlear groove of the femoral component.

Evaluation of knee implants at long-term-follow-up study, as with hip arthroplasty, should focus on the bone-implant interface.[34] There are similar systems that divide the undersurface of the tibial component into zones to identify areas of radiolucency.[37] In noncemented tibial components, a common mode of failure is subsidence or settling of the anterior portion of the tibial tray into the metaphyseal bone (Fig. 11-37). Tibial component failure is unusual but more common than failure of the femoral component. Because of the large metal prosthesis that encompasses the end of the femur, it is difficult to consistently evaluate the interface on the

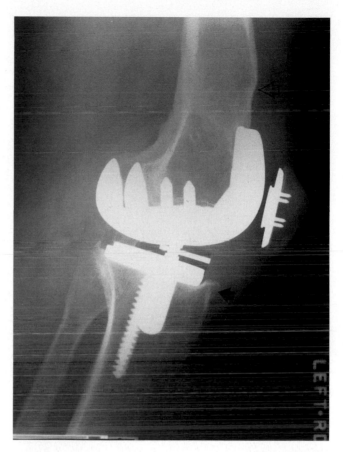

Fig. 11-37. Noncemented total knee arthroplasty. The anterior cortex of the femur has been notched, *open arrow,* and the tibial component has subsided, *closed arrow.* The patellar component is metal backed.

femoral side, even with a well-aligned lateral view.

Patellar problems include subluxation, dislocation, and loosening. Dissociation of an all-polyethylene patellar component can be difficult to recognize, but the displaced component can often be seen as a relative intra-articular radiolucency. Metal-backed patellar components can fail in two ways. Failure at the bone-prosthesis interface is usually evident and accompanied by broken pegs, loose beads, or displacement of the implant. Another method of failure is dissociation of the polyethylene from the metal backing. This mode of failure has been common enough to cause many surgeons to abandon this design.[38] Although easily diagnosed clinically, the polyethylene dissociation can be difficult to detect radiographically. This phenomenon results in metal-on-metal articulation between the femoral and patellar prosthesis leading to an intense metallic synovitis. In chronic cases a metallic outline of the synovial cavity can be seen.[39]

Foot and Ankle Arthroplasty

Ankle arthroplasty employs very similar metal on polyethylene designs seen in other joints. This proce-

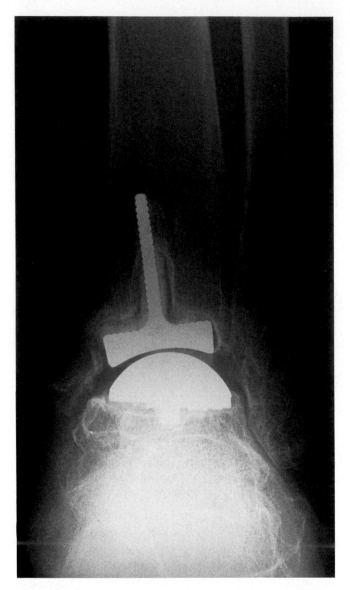

Fig. 11-38. Total ankle arthroplasty. The tibial component has subsided into the distal tibia and is surrounded by a significant radiolucent line.

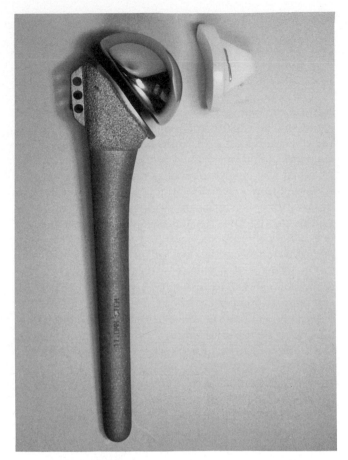

Fig. 11-39. Total shoulder prosthesis.

sult of the relative structural weakness of the metaphyseal bone in this area (Fig. 11-38).

Metatarsophalangeal joints can be replaced with silicone elastomer (Silastic) and polyethylene spacers especially at the hallux. Because of problems of breakage and fragmentation of the implants leading to synovitis and bone resorption, these types of implants are less commonly performed.[40] More commonly seen procedures in the toes are resection arthroplasty and arthrodesis.

Upper Extremity Arthroplasty

Shoulder arthroplasty is used for primary treatment of complex proximal humeral fractures as well as arthritic conditions of the shoulder.[41] As with hip arthroplasty, the shoulder replacement employs a stemmed ball that is anchored in the proximal humerus. The glenoid component is polyethylene and can be metal backed (Fig. 11-39). Because the shoulder implant is much less constrained than the hip, it relies to a great degree on the competency of the rotator cuff for stability.

Initial radiographic evaluation should include anteroposterior views in internal and external rotation as well

dure is done on a limited basis because of the excellent results seen with ankle arthrodesis. Its use is currently limited to rheumatoid arthritis patients with diffuse joint involvement in the foot who are unable to compensate for motion loss accompanying arthrodesis. As with other forms of arthroplasty, alignment of the implant should be evaluated initially. The tibial component, which is often stemmed, should have its articulating surface perpendicular to the long axis of the tibia. There should be no residual bone or cement debris left in the posterior recess of the ankle because this may lead to impingement with plantar flexion. The most common late change seen radiographically is the migration of the tibial component into the metaphysis, a re-as an axial view. Complete radiographic evaluation may be delayed until the patient's rehabilitation has progressed to the point where sufficient range of motion is regained to allow all these studies. The stem should be contained within the humerus, and the prosthetic humeral head should reconstruct the size and position of the original. Shortening of the humeral neck can occur especially in fracture reconstruction and should be avoided because it creates an imbalance in the shoulder musculature, which compromises function. The glenoid and humeral components should articulate without any significant subluxation either superiorly or inferiorly.

Late changes that should be noted are loosening of either component. Radiolucencies are often seen in the immediate postoperative period surrounding cemented glenoid components, probably attributable to difficulty in pressure injecting cement in this area. Certainly, any progressive radiolucencies should be noted.

Elbow arthroplasty remains one of the biggest challenges in joint reconstruction.[42] The forces transmitted across the elbow because of the long lever arm of the forearm and the limited bone stock available at the elbow to anchor the prosthesis make the long-term success of elbow arthroplasty a formidable proposition. Elbow designs range from resurfacing procedures that require minimal bone resection to stemmed implants anchored in the humerus and ulna. Although the articulating interface is metal on polyethylene, the actual design can vary from minimally constrained to a fixed hinge (Fig. 11-40). Alignment and subluxation are considerations with less constrained implants but are not an issue with hinged designs.

Late changes at the bone-implant interface remain the important issue in the radiographic evaluation of these devices. The humeral component is the most common site of failure, and special attention should be given to anterior migration of the proximal end of the humeral stem. Considerable reactive bone remodeling may also occur at this site.

Wrist arthroplasty remains divided between the use of metal on polyethylene and Silastic spacer implants. As in the ankle, arthrodesis is a reliable first choice for treatment of isolated wrist arthrosis. However, in patients with diffuse arthritic involvement of the upper extremity preservation of wrist motion can be critical to overall function. Motor balance around the carpus is imperative to the success of wrist arthroplasty, and often the soft-tissue reconstruction is the most important part of the procedure. Regardless of which type of implant is used, reconstitution of carpal height and alignment is an essential part of the procedure and should be noted on the postoperative radiographs.

The long finger metacarpal is often used to locate the center of rotation in the coronal plane, and stemmed

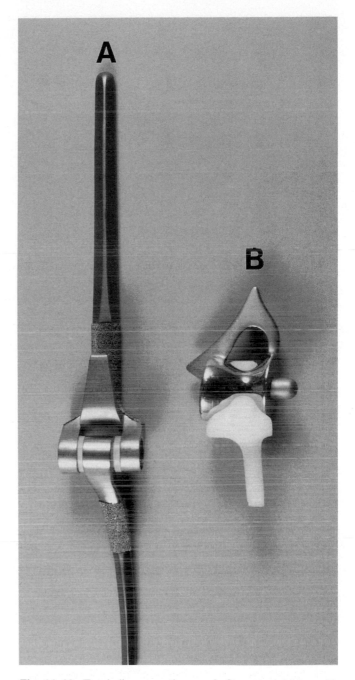

Fig. 11-40. Total elbow prostheses. **A,** Stemmed design with hinged articulation. **B,** Resurfacing design with nonconstrained interface.

implants are usually inserted into this bone. In the lateral projection the carpal alignment should be restored to a neutral alignment in relationship to the long axis of the radius, though dorsiflexion and palmar flexion through the implant is certainly acceptable.

Long-term evaluation of wrist arthroplasty should continue to concentrate on alignment because dynamic motor imbalance around the wrist can recur, especially in inflammatory arthropathies. Silastic wrist implants

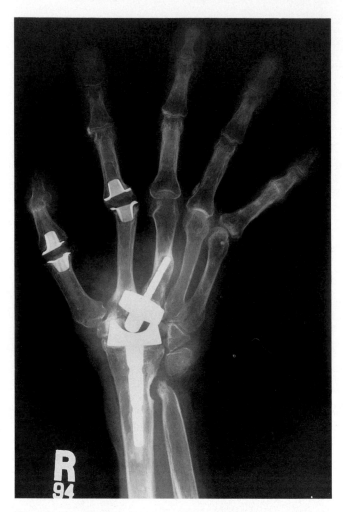

Fig. 11-41. Total wrist arthroplasty and Silastic (silicone elastomer) metacarpophalangeal implants. The wrist is malaligned in ulnar deviation, and there has been remodeling around the long finger metacarpal implant. Metal grommets have been used with the Silastic implants, and a narrow sclerotic margin can be seen around the index finger prosthesis.

should be followed closely for evidence of breakage or osteolysis in the surrounding bone. A sclerotic margin often develops around these types of implants because they do not rely on fixation to the skeleton to function (Fig. 11-41). This reaction should not be interpreted as a pathologic change. Evidence of loosening around cemented or noncemented metal wrist implants should be noted in follow-up radiographic studies. Migration of stems out of the radius or metacarpal canals can be seen with implant loosening (Fig. 11-41).

Limited arthroplasty in the carpus using Silastic or metal implants to replace individual carpal bones can also be performed (see Fig. 11-1). These implants show mixed results because of the difficulty in maintaining the intricate carpal balance that relies not only on bone anatomy but also on a complex system of intercarpal

and radiocarpal ligaments. Obviously, carpal alignment and evidence of carpal instability are important issues in radiographic evaluation of these implants. Osteolysis secondary to wear particles is also commonly seen with these prostheses.

Arthroplasty of the carpometacarpal joint of the thumb, metacarpophalangeal, and interphalangeal joints of the fingers are routinely performed in patients with inflammatory arthropathies. Silastic implants are the most commonly used for these procedures, but there is a host of other designs manufactured for the same purpose. The parameters for radiographic evaluation are the same as for other implants of this design.

Infection of total joint arthroplasties can occur acutely as a result of bacterial contamination at the time of surgery or later as a result of hematogenous or contiguous spread from another site. These prostheses are predisposed to infection because they provide large sites for bacterial proliferation that cannot be effectively defended by the body's immune system. There is some evidence that methyl methacrylate may actually inhibit the immune response.[43] In the acute setting radiographs may not demonstrate any abnormality. Established infections demonstrate implant loosening and often a prominent periosteal reaction.[34] Sequential scintigraphy with technetium and gallium in the presence of infection demonstrate discordant areas of uptake whereas concordant areas of uptake are seen in many settings, and this finding is nonspecific.[31]

SPINAL IMPLANTS

Spinal implants can be roughly divided into two groups: anteriorly placed implants and posteriorly placed implants. Spinal instrumentation is performed for a variety of reasons, including correction of deformity and stabilization of a spine after either fracture or surgical decompression of neural elements, and is routinely done with fusion of the segments involved. There has been an intense resurgence of interest in spine surgery, which has corresponded with advances in spinal imaging and a proliferation of spinal implant devices.

Posterior Instrumentation

Posterior spinal instrumentation is more commonly performed because it allows easier decompression and visualization of neural elements and the surgical approach is much simpler than anterior approaches through the neck, chest, or abdomen. Posterior instrumentation in the cervical spine is usually limited to combinations of wires and bone graft. Because of the limited space available and the size of the vertebrae, the more substantial implants used in the thoracic and lumbar regions are not applicable in this area. Wiring techniques in the cervical spine use the lamina and spinous processes as anchor points for stabilization (Fig. 11-42).

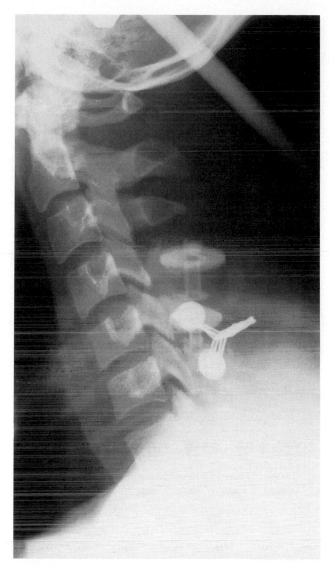

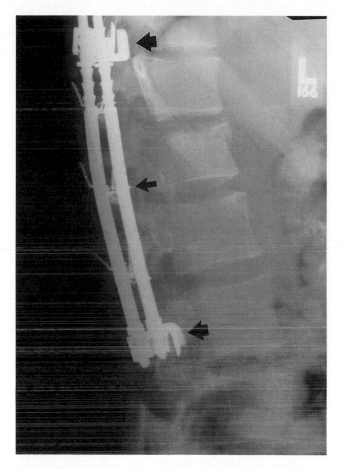

Fig. 11-43. Harrington rodding of the thoracolumbar junction. Hooks, *large arrows,* are used to anchor the rod ends in the posterior spinal elements. Segmental wires, *small arrow,* have been used to augment fixation.

Fig. 11-42. Posterior cervical wiring of C5-6. The spinous processes have been used to anchor the wires.

Radiographic evaluation of cervical spine surgery should involve noting the levels involved, including the occiput, and how the vertebrae are stabilized. The position of the vertebrae in relation to each other and fracture or facet reduction, if applicable, should also be mentioned. Late findings should involve noting the integrity of fixation devices, bone graft and fusion, and spinal alignment. Evaluation of stability should include lateral radiographs in flexion and extension.

The biomechanics of the thoracic and lumbar spine differ considerably, and implants used in these areas are correspondingly structurally diverse. Most implants utilize the posterior bony elements as sites of attachment in the thoracic and lumbar areas of the spine. Harrington rods use hooks in the lamina of the thoracic spine and in the facet joints of the lumbar spine to connect rods

at the superior and inferior anchoring points (Fig. 11-43).

Segmental posterior stabilization of the thoracic and lumbar spine can be achieved in several ways. Luque pioneered this method of fixation by using sublaminar wires to anchor rods[44] (Fig. 11-44). Although this method provided very secure fixation, it was associated with neurologic complications because the wires required "blind" passage under the lamina. This technique has for the most part been replaced with segmental wires passed through the base of the spinous process, which is technically easier and avoids risk to the neural elements.[45] Segmental fixation can also be achieved with the use of screws placed through the pedicles into the vertebral body. The pedicular screws can be connected with plates or rods[46] (Fig. 11-45).

These rigid methods of spinal stabilization have allowed surgeons to perform aggressive neurologic decompression by resecting the posterior bone elements including the facet joints. They also allow the reduction of spinal deformities including scoliosis and spondylolis-

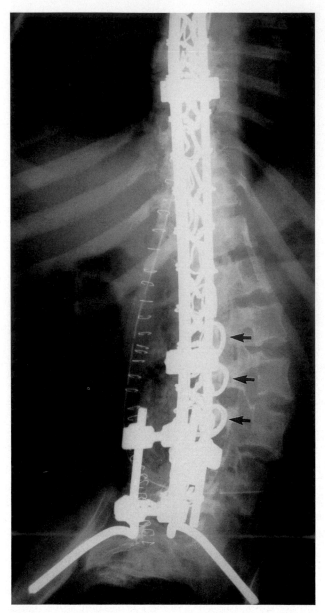

Fig. 11-44. Segmental spinal fixation using Luque sublaminar wires to treat scoliosis. Although difficult to visualize because of the overlying rods, several of the looped wires can be seen, *arrows*. Notice that the rods are coupled to sacral bars inferiorly.

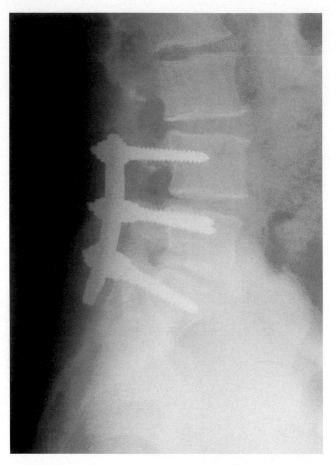

Fig. 11-45. Segmental fixation utilizing pedicular screws. The screws are linked, in this case, to Steffe plates posteriorly.

thesis. There are currently clinical trials utilizing artificial ligaments to stabilize the spine. These radiolucent devices will undoubtedly be used in conjunction with bony fusion, though their specific applications have yet to be elucidated.

The bulk of metal used in spinal instrumentation often obscures the underlying bone anatomy. Radiography is limited in its ability to image the details of spinal instrumentation, though evaluation should include the levels spanned by the fixation devices and the type and position of anchoring devices. Levels of bone decompression and correction of deformity should be noted. Late radiographic evaluation should involve noting the maintenance of spinal alignment and the integrity of the fixation, specifically the integrity of wires, rods, hooks, and screws. Evidence of bone fusion or pseudoarthrosis at involved spinal segments should be addressed.

Instability at levels above and below the fixation is a major concern with long-term follow-up study. Rigid fixation of spinal segments significantly alters the biomechanics of the spine and concentration of motion and stress occurs at the transitional vertebra at the ends of the immobilized segments. This can result in late degenerative changes and instability at these levels. Radiographic evaluation including lateral views in neutral, flexion, and extension is most useful to detect significant instability.

Computed tomographic evaluation of metallic spinal implants is limited by artifacts but can be diagnostic if optimized as described below. Magnetic resonance is also degraded by the presence of the large implants, though the use of nonferromagnetic materials in the future may alleviate this problem.

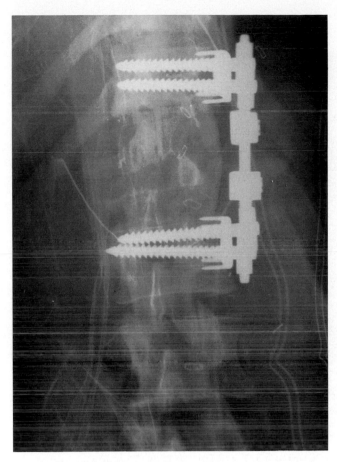

Fig. 11-46. Anterior spinal fixation utilizing screws placed into the vertebral bodies and linked with a unilateral rod.

Anterior Instrumentation

Anterior spinal instrumentation does not vary considerably from the types of devices used posteriorly. The use of plates in the cervical spine is becoming more common, anchored with screws extending into the vertebral body. Anterior thoracic and lumbar implants may also be anchored to the vertebral body. Forces of distraction applied to the concave side of a deformity, or compression applied to the convex side can be used to correct and stabilize spinal deformity. The attachment of spinal implants can be at each vertebral body, that is, segmental, or it can span segments with anchoring points at each end[47-49] (Fig. 11-46).

There is currently a variety of artificial disk replacements undergoing clinical trials.[50] These implants are intended to replace interbody fusion as a means of correcting degenerated, unstable disks, and their designs range from traditional metal-on-polyethylene to radiolucent composite materials.

Radiographic evaluation of anterior instrumentation should initially concentrate on the location of the implants and levels instrumented. Correction of deformity

and bony decompression can also be evaluated radiographically. Fixation devices should not violate neural foramina or the spinal canal. With screw-anchored devices placed from anterior to posterior, careful attention should be given to screw-tip position relative to the posterior cortex of the vertebral body and neural structures. As with other implants, in late follow-up study one should note the integrity of the fixation devices and the maintenance of alignment.

IMAGING TECHNIQUES

Radiography

Standard radiography continues to be the mainstay for evaluation of orthopedic devices. Although radiographic evaluation of patients who have undergone implantation of orthopedic hardware is similar to routine examination, attention to a few details will yield more consistent examinations. The use of manual technical settings are ideal; phototimed images of metallic devices are usually overpenetrated with low contrast in the soft tissue and bony areas. Soft-tissue thickness should determine the kilovolt peak (kVp) and milliampere (mA) settings in patients with metal implants. Careful, standardized patient positioning and beam centering will facilitate comparative, sequential evaluation of implants for position change, fractures, and changes at the host-implant interface. To this end, the entire implant must be included in the study and prior radiographs should be evaluated with each new study.

Special radiographic techniques for evaluating implants will be dictated by the clinical presentation. Dynamic evaluation with videofluoroscopy may be useful in patients with implant pain or instability induced by specific movements or positions. Complex motion tomography is often helpful in confirming subtle abnormalities seen on routine radiographic examinations. Linear tomography is limited by the relatively thick focal zone (5 mm), which reduces resolution.

Computed Tomography

Cross-sectional and multiplanar imaging of orthopedic devices can be important adjuncts in the evaluation of patients with orthopedic implants. However, substantial limitations are encountered with the use of computed tomography (CT) and magnetic resonance (MR) when these devices are evaluated. Standard transaxial CT images are degraded by metallic artifact seen as starburst-pattern streaks emanating from the center of the implant, which can obscure both the device itself and the surrounding structures (see also Chapter 15). As the x-ray beam passes through a stationary metallic structure, its energy is almost completely attenuated, resulting in missing projection data and pronounced degradation of the reconstructed image. Scatter and partial

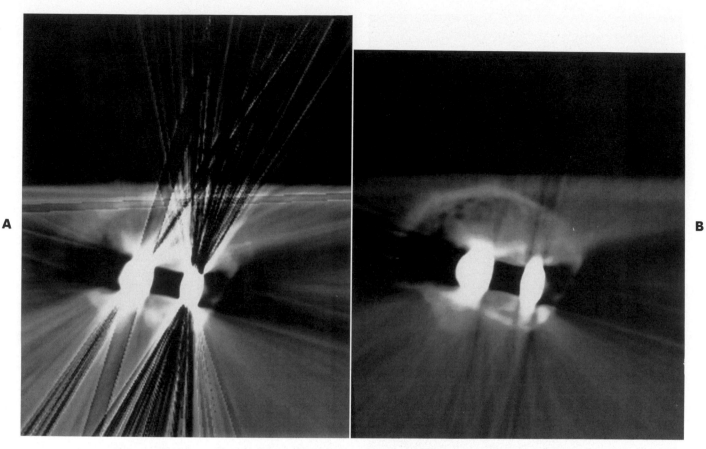

Fig. 11-47. Effects of decreasing slice thickness on metallic CT artifacts. **A,** Axial CT of a femoral phantom, with metallic endoprosthesis, at 10 mm slice thickness. Excessive starburst-pattern metallic artifact is seen. **B,** Metallic artifact is reduced at 5 mm slice thickness with improved visualization of surrounding bone. Very thin sections (<2 mm) may actually increase artifact as effective penetration is reduced.

volume averaging also can interfere with accurate reconstruction. Artifacts from moving metallic devices such as heart valves and surgical clips are, for the most part, related to motion and aliasing, which contribute little to stationary device artifacts.[51]

The reduction of artifacts from orthopedic implants may be achieved in several ways. The simplest technique involves reducing attenuation by decreasing slice thickness and increasing beam energy (Figs. 11-47 and 11-48). Reformatting images in new orthogonal oblique planes using commercially available software[52] has been, in our hands, less productive. Reconstruction planes may be altered to optimize volume averaging of the missing data, which can also be artificially replaced before reconstruction.[53] However, generating artificial replacement data for the missing projections requires special computer software and large memory with no documented improvement in diagnostic accuracy. Recognition that certain materials, such as plastics and polymers, will result in less image attenuation allows patient selection to yield optimal imaging results.

Magnetic Resonance

The tissue contrast, spatial resolution, and multiplanar capabilities of magnetic resonance imaging have propelled it to the forefront of musculoskeletal imaging. Unfortunately, MR images of metallic devices are often nondiagnostic because of magnetic susceptibility artifact (see also Chapters 16 and 17). These artifacts are attributable primarily to inhomogeneities of the local magnetic field and radiofrequency amplitude caused by the presence of ferromagnetic materials. In an inhomogeneous magnetic field, spinning protons decay rapidly, producing a local signal void and distorting coordinates used in Fourier imaging. The true magnetic properties of the metal and surrounding structures are obscured, and a characteristic signal void associated with alternating bright and dark bands is seen.[54]

Alloy composition is an important determinant of the extent of artifact degradation. Several authors have demonstrated that intravascular devices composed of titanium alloys produce substantially less artifact when compared to stainless steel and cobalt-chromium al-

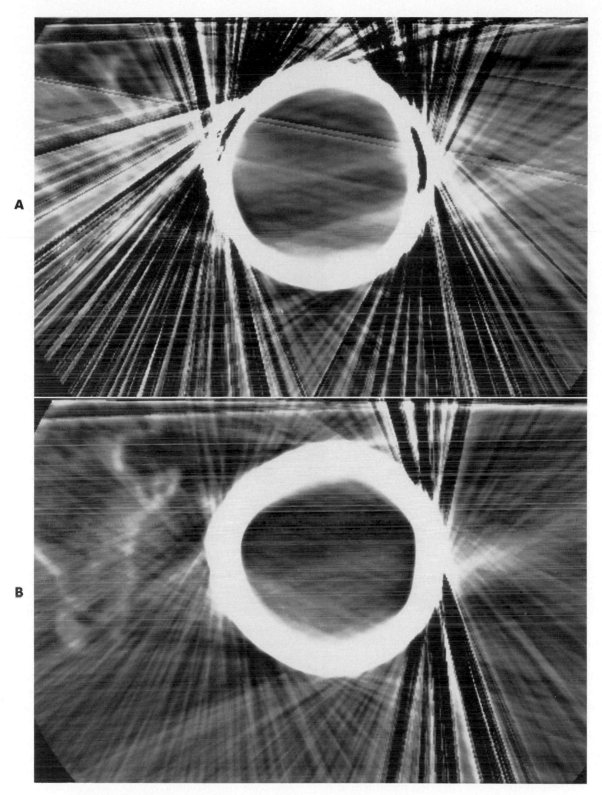

Fig. 11-48. Effects of increasing energy on metallic CT artifacts. **A,** Axial CT of the femoral endoprosthesis phantom at 150 mA. **B,** Equivalent level image at 200 mA demonstrates considerable reduction in metallic artifact. The morphology of the greater trochanter can now be identified.

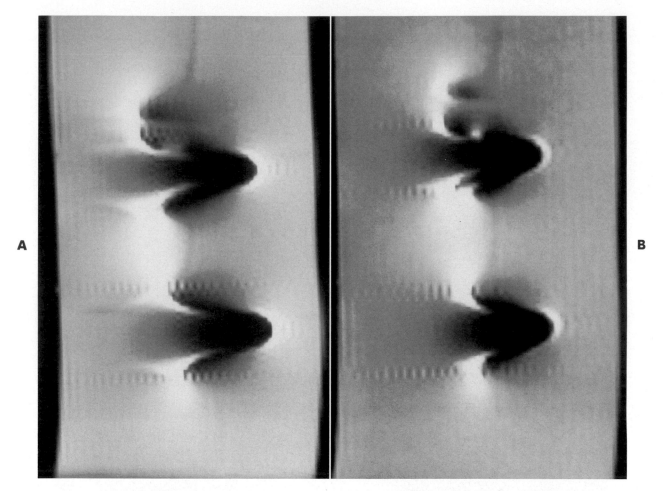

Fig. 11-49. Effect of changing bandwidth on metallic magnetic resonance artifacts at TR 2000/TE 20. **A,** Cobalt-chromium prostheses suspended in gel shows characteristic signal void surrounded by high signal "blossom" characteristic for ferromagnetic materials (bandwidth 20 kHz). **B,** At bandwidth of 41 kHz, signal void and surrounding high signal are substantially reduced.

loys.[55,56] We have imaged commonly used alloys in phantoms and cadavers at various spin-echo (SE) and gradient-echo (GRE) pulse sequences at 0.5 and 1.5 teslas (T) using narrow and wide band-width techniques. Reduced metallic artifact was seen at lower field strength and wide band width as shown in Fig. 11-49. Spin-echo sequences that incorporate shorter sampling times were superior to gradient-echo sequences. As expected, titanium-based alloy images were superior to cobalt-chromium or stainless steel regardless of MR parameters (Fig. 11-50).

Because metallic artifacts are projected predominantly along the frequency-encoded axis, displaying the region of interest in the phase-encoded plane will also optimize diagnostic information (Fig. 11-51). Using wide band-width SE imaging, we were able to diagnose osteonecrosis in a patient with a stainless steel hip implant that could not be seen on routine narrow band-width sequences (Fig. 11-52).

SUMMARY

Radiographic evaluation of implants used in orthopedic surgery can be challenging. Understanding the intended purpose of the implant is critical to provide accurate information concerning its status at any given point in time. There is often too much concern given to variations in implant design at the expense of how the implant is functioning. There are a limited number of things that can change about an implant when followed over time. It can break, move, become infected, or trigger a host response. In some settings the response is favorable, such as the formation of bone or collagen deposition in a ligament graft. In other settings the host response can be unfavorable, as seen with osteolysis around a loose implant or a bone graft. Special attention to radiographic details such as patient and implant positioning, and technical parameters affecting visualization of metallic devices with CT and MR will yield optimal images in this diverse and expanding group of patients.

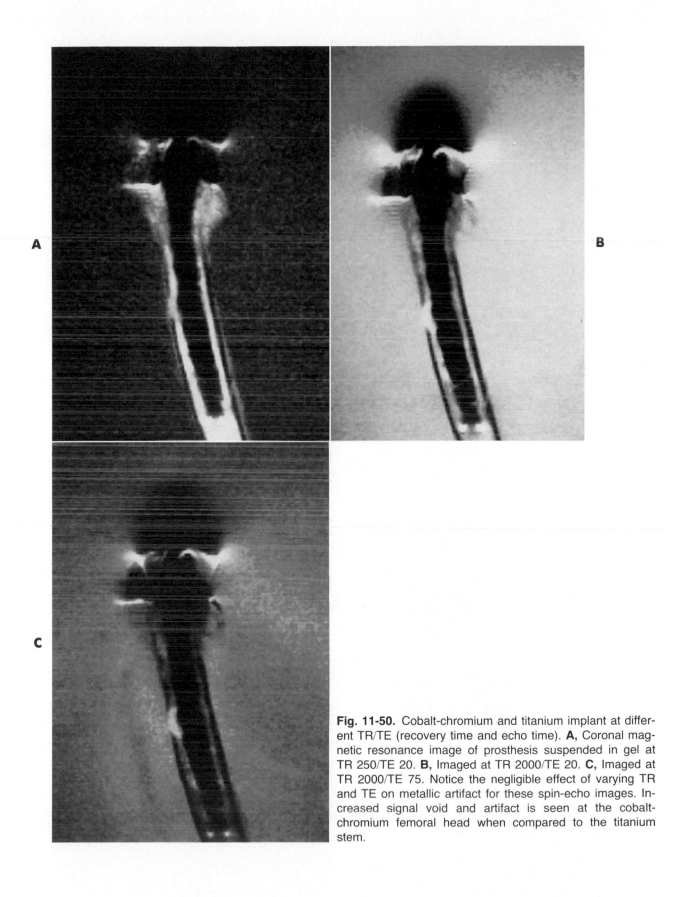

Fig. 11-50. Cobalt-chromium and titanium implant at different TR/TE (recovery time and echo time). **A,** Coronal magnetic resonance image of prosthesis suspended in gel at TR 250/TE 20. **B,** Imaged at TR 2000/TE 20. **C,** Imaged at TR 2000/TE 75. Notice the negligible effect of varying TR and TE on metallic artifact for these spin-echo images. Increased signal void and artifact is seen at the cobalt-chromium femoral head when compared to the titanium stem.

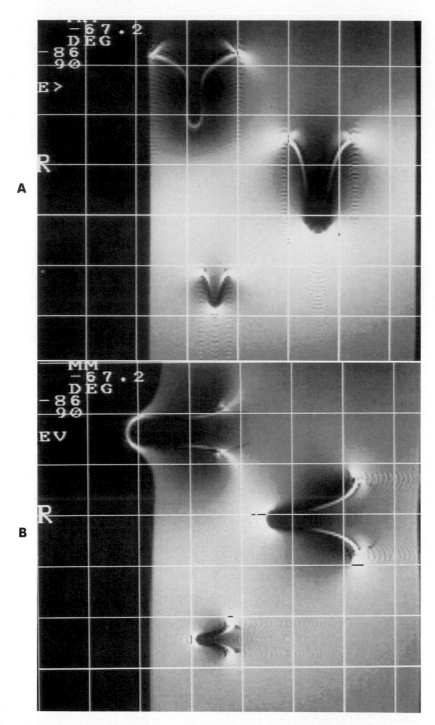

Fig. 11-51. Phase and frequency axis effects on magnetic resonance artifacts. Clockwise from the top are identically sized metallic cylinders embedded in gel composed of cobalt-chromium, stainless steel, and titanium alloys, respectively. **A,** Frequency-encoded axis in *y* plane creates the largest artifact from top to bottom of image. **B,** Phase and frequency axis transposed showing maximum artifact from side to side. Notice that the smallest total artifact is produced by the minimally ferromagnetic titanium alloy.

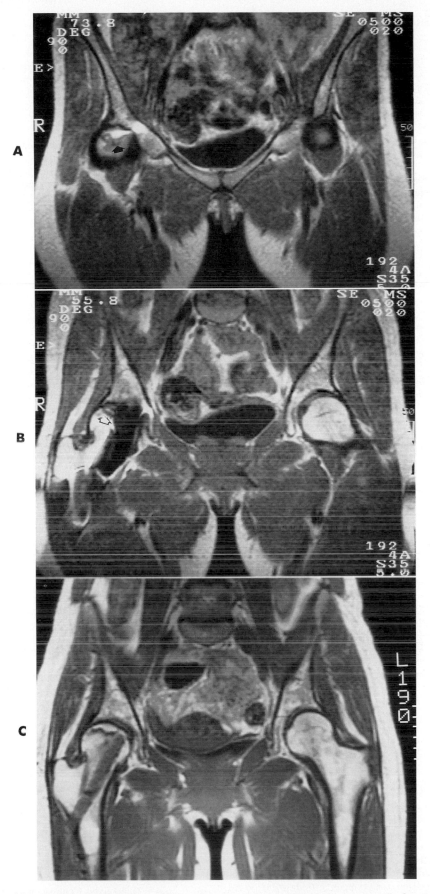

Fig. 11-52. Femoral head osteonecrosis in a patient after dynamic hip screw placement. **A,** Coronal T1 (TR 500/TE 20) images at the anterior hip using wide bandwidth technique. Linear low signal at interface of necrotic and viable bone, *arrow,* with small metallic artifact. **B,** Coronal T1 image at tear figure and metallic-implant level. Metallic artifact is more prominent, though the focus of osteonecrosis can be seen, *arrow.* Frequency is encoded in the *y* axis, minimizing mediolateral image degradation. **C,** Coronal T1 image at midacetabulum after removal of hip screw. Osteonecrosis and hardware tract are evident. The initial routine narrow bandwidth images were nondiagnostic in this patient.

REFERENCES

1. Felson B, Wiot JF, editor: Orthopedic prosthetic procedures, *Semin Roentgenol* 21(1), Jan 1986.
2. Rabin DN, Smith C, Kubicka RA, et al: Problem prostheses: the radiographic evaluation of total joint replacement, *RadioGraphics* 7(6):1107-1128, 1987.
3. Richardson ML, Kilcoyne RF, Mayo KA, et al: Radiographic evaluation of modern orthopedic fixation devices, *RadioGraphics* 7(4):685-702, 1987.
4. Staple TW, editor: Symposium on Orthopedic Radiology, *Radiol Clin North Am* 13(1), April 1975.
5. Rostlund T, Albrektsson B, Albrektsson T: Wear of ion-implanted pure titanium against UHMWPE, *Biomaterials* 10:176-181, 1989.
6. Trippel SB: Current concepts review: antibiotic impregnated cement in total joint arthroplasty, *J Bone Joint Surg* 68A:1297-1302, 1986.
7. Woods GA, Indelicato PA, Prevot TJ: The Gore-Tex anterior cruciate ligament prosthesis: two versus three year results, *Am J Sports Med* 19(1):48-55, 1991.
8. Kattapuram SV, Phillips WC, Mankin HJ: Intercalary bone allografts: radiographic evaluation, *Radiology* 170:137-141, 1989.
9. Meyers MH, Akeson W, Convery FR: Resurfacing of the knee with fresh osteochondral allograft, *J Bone Joint Surg* 71A(5):704-713, 1989.
10. Müller ME, Allgöwer M, Schneider R, Willenegger H: *Manual of internal fixation: techniques recommended by the AO-ASIF Group,* ed 3, Berlin, 1991, Springer-Verlag.
11. Solari J, Benjamin J, Wilson J, et al: Ankle mortise stability. In Weber C: Fractures: indications for syndesmotic fixation, *J Orthop Trauma* 5(2):190-195, 1991.
12. Herbert TJ, Fisher WE: Management of the fractured scaphoid using a new bone screw, *J Bone Joint Surg* 66B:114-123, 1984.
13. Kurosaka M, Yoshiya S, Andrish JT: A biomechanical comparison of different surgical techniques of graft fixation in anterior cruciate ligament reconstruction, *Am J Sports Med* 15:225-229, 1987.
14. Kuntscher G: Die Marknagelung von Knochenbrüchen, *Arch Klin Chir* 200:443, 1940.
15. Bailey RW, Dubow HI: Evolution of the concept of an extensible nail accommodating to normal longitudinal bone growth: clinical considerations and implications, *Clin Orthop* 159:157-170, 1981.
16. Bucholz RW, Ross SE, Lawrence KL: Fatigue fractures of the interlocking nail in the treatment of fractures of the distal part of the femoral shaft, *J Bone Joint Surg* 69A(9):1391-1399, 1987.
17. Vade A, Eissenstat R: Radiographic features of bone lengthening procedures, *Radiology* 174:531-537, 1990.
18. Young JW, Kostrubiak IS, Resnik CS, Paley D: Sonographic evaluation of bone production at the distraction site in Ilizarov limb-lengthening procedures, *AJR* 154:125-128, 1990.
19. Charnley J: Low friction arthroplasty of the hip: theory and practice, Berlin, New York, 1979, Springer-Verlag.
20. Bobyn JD, Pilliar RM, Cameron HU, Weatherly GC: Osteogenic phenomena across endosteal bone–implant spaces with porous surfaced intramedullary implants, *Acta Orthop Scand* 52:145-153, 1981.
21. Brånemark PI, Hansson BO, Adell R, et al: Osseointegrated implants in the treatment of the edentulous jaw: experience from a 10 year period, *Scand J Plast Reconstr Surg* 11:Suppl 16, 1977.
22. Furlong RJ, Osborn JF: Fixation of hip protheses by hydroxyapatite ceramic coatings, *J Bone Joint Surg* 73B:741-745, 1991.
23. Szivek JA: Bioceramic coatings for artificial joint fixation, *Invest Radiol* 27(7):553-558, 1992.
24. Brown IW, Ring PA: Osteolytic changes in the upper femoral shaft following porous-coated hip replacement, *J Bone Joint Surg* 67B:218-221, 1985.
25. Goldring SR, Schiller AL, Roelke M, et al: The synovial like membrane at the bone-cement interface in loose total hip replacements and its proposed role in bone lysis, *J Bone Joint Surg* 65A:575-584, 1983.
26. Amstutz HC, Graff-Radford A, Mai LL, Thomas BJ: Surface replacement of the hip with the Tharies system: two to five year results, *J Bone Joint Surg* 63A:1069-1077, 1981.
27. Ghelman B: Three methods for determining anteversion and retroversion of a total hip prosthesis, *AJR* 133:1127-1134, 1979.
28. Johnston RC, Fitzgerald RH, Harris WH, et al: Clinical and radiographic evaluation of total hip replacement: a standard system of terminology for reporting results, *J Bone Joint Surg* 72A(2):161-168, 1990.
29. Gruen TA, McNeice GM, Amstutz HC: "Modes of failure" of cemented stem-type femoral components: a radiographic analysis of loosening, *Clin Orthop* 141:17-27, 1979.
30. Aliabadi P, Tumeh SS, Weissman BN, McNeil BJ: Cemented total hip prosthesis: radiographic and scintigraphic evaluation, *Radiology* 173:203-206, 1989.
31. Rosenthall L, Lisbona R, Hernandez M, Hadjipavlou A: Tc-PP and Ga imaging following insertion of orthopaedic devices, *Radiology* 133:717-721, 1979.
32. Gelman MI, Coleman RE, Stevens PM, Davey BW: Radiography, radionuclide imaging and arthrography in the evaluation of total hip and knee replacement, *Radiology* 128:677-682, 1978.
33. Kaplan PA, Montesi SA, Jardon OM, Gregory PR: Bone ingrowth hip prostheses in asymptomatic patients: radiographic features, *Radiology* 169:221-227, 1988.
34. Schneider R, Hood RW, Ranawat CS: Radiologic evaluation of knee arthroplasty, *Orthop Clin North Am* 13(1):225-244, 1982.
35. Aaron RK, Scott R: Supracondylar fracture of the femur after total knee arthroplasty, *Clin Orthop* 219:136-139, 1987.
36. Ritter MA, Faris PM, Keating EM: Anterior femoral notching and ipsilateral supracondylar femur fracture in total knee arthroplasty, *J Arthroplasty* 3(2):185-188, 1988.
37. Ranawat CS, Boachie-Adjei O: Survivorship analysis and results of total condylar knee arthroplasty, *Clin Orthop* 226:6-13, 1988.
38. Bayley JC, Scott RD, Ewald FC, Holmes GB: Failure of the metal-backed patellar component after total knee replacement, *J Bone Joint Surg* 70A:668-674, 1988.
39. Weissman BN, Scott RD, Brick GW, Corson JM: Radiographic detection of metal induced synovitis as a complication of arthroplasty of the knee, *J Bone Joint Surg* 73A(7):1002-1007, 1991.
40. Granberry WM, Noble PC, Bishop JO, Tullos HS: Use of a hinged silicone prosthesis for replacement arthroplasty of the first metatarsophalangeal joint, *J Bone Joint Surg* 73A(10):1453-1459, 1991.
41. Neer CS, Watson KC, Stanton FJ: Recent experience in total shoulder replacement, *J Bone Joint Surg* 64A:319-337, 1982.
42. Inglis AE, Pellicci PM: Total elbow replacement, *J Bone Joint Surg* 62A:1252-1258, 1980.
43. Brause BD: Infected total knee replacement: diagnostic, therapeutic and prophylactic considerations, *Orthop Clin North Am* 13(1):245-249, 1982.
44. Luque ER: Segmental spinal instrumentation for correction of scoliosis, *Clin Orthop* 163:192-198, 1982.
45. Drummond DS: Harrington instrumentation with spinous process wiring for idiopathic scoliosis, *Orthop Clin North Am* 19(2):281-289, 1988.
46. Steffee AD, Biscup RS, Sitkowski DJ: Segmental spine plates with pedicle screw fixation: a new internal fixation device for disorders of the lumbar and thoracolumbar spine, *Clin Orthop* 203:45-53, 1986.
47. Cotrel Y, Dubeousset J, Guillaumat M: New universal instrumentation in spinal surgery, *Clin Orthop* 227:10-23, 1988.

48. Dwyer AF: Experience of anterior correction of scoliosis, *Clin Orthop* 191-206, 1973.
49. Kaneda K, Abumi K, Fujiya M: Burst fractures with neurologic deficits of the thoracolumbar-lumbar spine: results of anterior decompression and stabilization with anterior instrumentation, *Spine* 9(8):788-795, 1984.
50. Lee CK, Langrana NA, Parsons JR, Zimmerman MC: Development of a prosthetic intervertebral disc, *Spine* 16(6):253-255, 1991.
51. Robertson DD, Weiss PJ, Fishmen EK, et al: Evaluation of CT techniques for reducing artifacts in the presence of metallic orthopedic implants, *J Comput Assist Tomogr* 12(2):236-241, 1988.
52. Fishman EK, Magid D, Robertson DD, et al: Metallic hip implants: CT with multiplanar reconstruction, *Radiology* 160:675-681, 1986.
53. Kalender WA, Hebel R, Ebersberger J: Reduction of CT artifacts caused by metallic implants, *Radiology* 164:576-577, 1987.
54. Augustiny N, Von Schulthess GK, Dieter M, Bosiger P: Magnetic resonance imaging of large nonferromagnetic metallic implants at 1.5 T, *J Comput Assist Tomogr* 11(4):678-683, 1987.
55. Teitelbaum GP, Bradley WG, Klein BD: MR imaging artifacts, ferromagnetism and magnetic torque of intravascular filters, stents and coils, *Radiology* 166:657-664, 1988.
56. Teitelbaum GP, Ortega HV, Vinitski S, et al: Low artifact intravascular devices: MR imaging evaluation, *Radiology* 168:713-719, 1988.

12

Devices Associated with Interventional Radiology

Stephen H. Smyth
Gerald D. Pond

ANGIOGRAPHY AND INTERVENTIONAL DEVICES

Vascular and interventional radiology has progressed rapidly during the last 20 years. Formerly "angiographers" performed strictly diagnostic procedures. Now therapeutic procedures comprise a large percentage, if not the majority, of work performed by angiographer/interventionalists. The rapid improvement in techniques and equipment in this field have caused many treatments that were the exclusive purview of surgeons to fall into the category of routine cases for interventional radiologists.

The devices discussed in this chapter represent only those more commonly utilized in current practice. A multitude of devices have been introduced and then rapidly replaced by safer, faster, or otherwise technically superior devices. Some devices may enjoy regional popularity and may be representative only of local experience, or they may be devices designed for less common disorders and therefore rarely seen. This chapter does not endeavor to be encyclopedic. For a comprehensive review of interventional radiology and its associated equipment, refer to one of several texts dedicated to this subject.[4,20]

PERCUTANEOUS DRAINAGE OF ABSCESSES AND FLUID COLLECTIONS

The accepted method of abscess treatment has always been surgical drainage; however, there is now recogni-

tion of the important role for percutaneous management in many cases.[42] Factors affecting this change have included recognition of decreased mortality with percutaneous drainage as opposed to operative treatment, a high success rate, and wide availability of imaging identification of abscesses allowing for radiologic procedures to be performed with moderate ease.[4,20] Percutaneous abscess drainage is associated with high technical success rates and low morbidity and mortality.

The indications for percutaneous abscess drainage vary among institutions. The typical indications for percutaneous abscess drainage include the development of an abscess complicating prior surgery or development of an abscess in a patient considered a surgical risk. Contraindications to percutaneous drainage include an uncontrollable coagulopathy and lack of safe access to the abscess.

A large variety of catheters are now available for abscess drainage procedures (Fig. 12-1). The essential features of such catheters are multiple side holes and a lumen size adequate for the viscosity of the drainage fluid. Today most catheters are either a single-lumen drain or a sump drain. The sump drain has two lumens allowing for continous irrigation, whereas the single-lumen catheter allows for intermittent irrigation. The advantage of the sump drain is an increased drainage efficiency of approximately two to four times that of a nonsump system.[4] In addition, the sump drain allows for simultaneous drainage and cavity irrigation with various fluids and medications.

Most drainage catheters are equipped with a pigtail, "tulip," or "accordion" configuration that can be locked in this configuration when tension is placed on a string

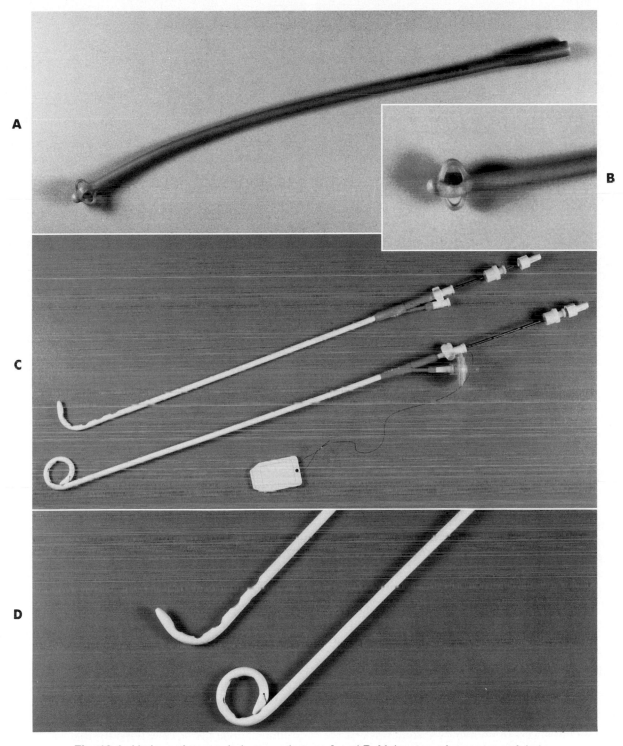

Fig. 12-1. Various abscess drainage catheters. **A** and **B,** Malecot mushroom type of drainage catheter (Bard Urological). **C** and **D,** Van Sonnenberg sump drainage catheter with Cope loop open and closed (Medi-tech).

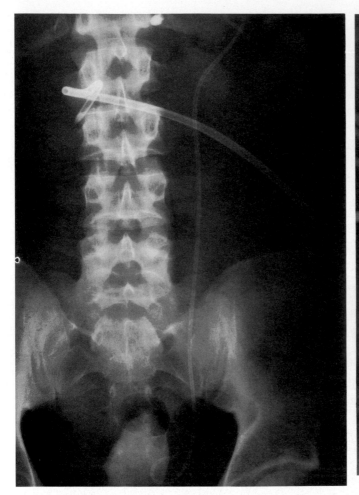

Fig. 12-2. Elderly man with a left ureteral stent and a single-lumen large locking pigtail abscess drainage catheter.

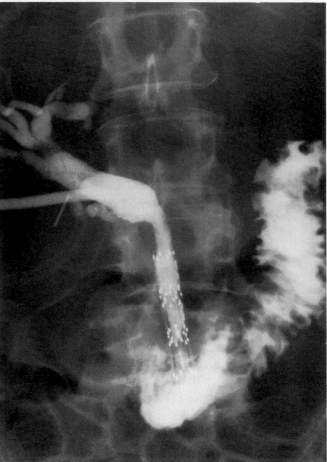

Fig. 12-3. Cholangiogram performed through exteriorized hepatic drain in 60-year-old female with bile duct stricture. The drain is a locking (Cope loop) pigtail drain located in the common hepatic duct. In the common bile duct two Gianturco-Rosch double-body Z-stents have been placed with overlap of one segment of each two-part stent. The more dense welds can be seen at the apex of each Z turn of the stent.

utilized for fixation. These self-retaining devices (that is, Cope loop, Hawkin's accordion, Malecot tip), once locked into place, help to prevent catheter migration or accidental withdrawal (Figs. 12-1 and 12-2).

The decision for removal of an abscess drainage catheter follows the same surgical principles used for removal of a surgically placed drain. The factors in the decision include the amount of daily drainage, the character of the drainage, the size of the abscess cavity as visualized on CT exams, sinograms, or ultrasound studies, and the patient's clinical course.[4,20]

BILIARY INTERVENTIONAL DEVICES

Percutaneous access to the biliary system was first reported as gallbladder puncture with contrast instillation in 1921.[2] In 1937, intraductal injection of contrast into hepatic ducts was performed.[4] Using access tubes placed either percutaneously or surgically, treatment of biliary calculi followed. In 1956 Remolar[35] described external retrograde biliary drainage. Percutaneous

transhepatic antegrade drainage was first described in 1974 by Molnar,[30] and since then biliary intervention has become accepted therapy for obstructive jaundice. Endoscopic access to the biliary tract has also been pursued with successful retrograde placement of a nasobiliary catheter in 1976 and endoprostheses in 1979.[4]

Typical indications for percutaneous biliary drainage include obstructive jaundice with pruritus, septicemia caused by obstruction, preoperative decompression, and palliation of unresectable malignancy.[4,20,44] Contraindications are a coagulopathy that cannot be corrected and gross ascites. Before the procedure is performed patients are given antibiotics to reduce the incidence of sepsis and atropine to prevent vagal episodes. The most common approach used for access is by the right midaxillary route, though a subxiphoid approach is employed for left-sided access.[4,20]

Devices for biliary drainage can be classified as those providing internal-external drainage, those providing retrograde drainage only (external drainage), and those that have no external components after placement and provide only antegrade (internal) drainage.[4]

Although almost any catheter can be utilized to provide internal-external drainage, several specialized catheters that have self-retaining devices have been developed. A self-retaining accordion catheter has been developed by Hawkins.[17] It is a 6.5 French Teflon catheter that assumes a Z configuration after the self-retaining device has been engaged. A second type of self-retaining catheter is one with a Cope loop that holds the distal end of the catheter in a pigtail configuration. This fixed loop prevents migration and unintentional removal[6] (Figs. 12-3 and 12-4). The self-retaining portion of these catheters is usually placed in the duodenum. If it is not possible to traverse the biliary duct stricture or occlusion, the self-retaining portion may be locked in an obstructed, dilated duct.

Internal drainage catheters of biocompatible plastic differ considerably. These stents consist of a relatively short drainage catheter, long enough to traverse the area of obstruction. The stent is tethered with a nylon string secured to a subcutaneous silicone elastomer (Silastic) button. Although some patients prefer this invisible device and no routine maintenance is necessary, it has a propensity for obstruction within 12 months, and the requirement for complete revision of failed stents make it attractive only to a minority of terminally ill patients.

A superior option in the view of most interventionalists is an internal stent placed either by retrograde endoscopy alone, or with the assistance of a percutaneously placed guide wire in the duodenum, a combined radiology/gastroenterology procedure (Fig. 12-5). These internal stents are not only invisible, but also they can be readily exchanged endoscopically when they become occluded.

Although metal endoprostheses were originally designed for intravascular use, in 1985 the first use of a metal stent in the biliary system of an animal was described.[3] At least five different metallic stents have been developed.[23] The Gianturco-Rosch Z-stent is made of round stainless steel wire in a Z configuration. This device is self-expanding (Figs. 12-6 and 12-7). The Wallstent is a self-expanding wire mesh tube available in two different lengths up to 68 mm. There are 24 wires

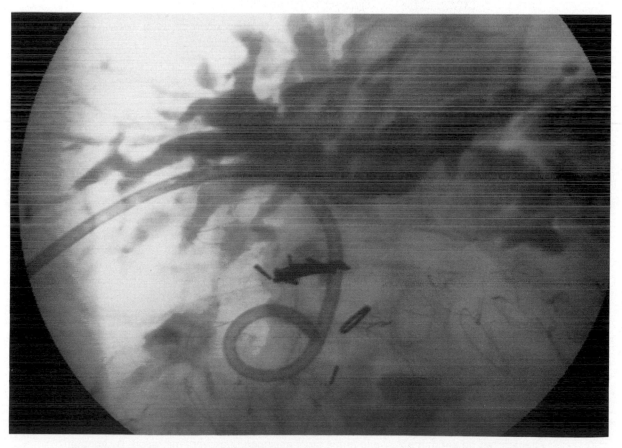

Fig. 12-4. Elderly woman with gallbladder carcinoma obstructing the common bile duct. A percutaneous biliary drain has been placed.

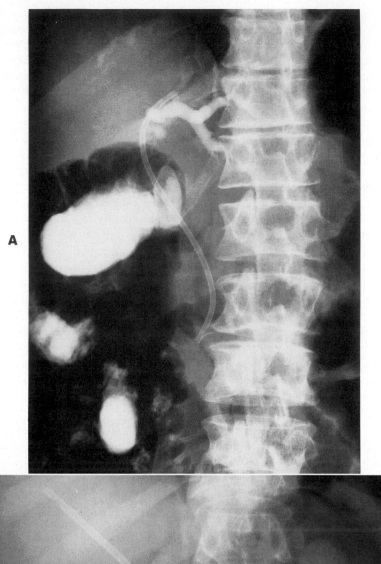

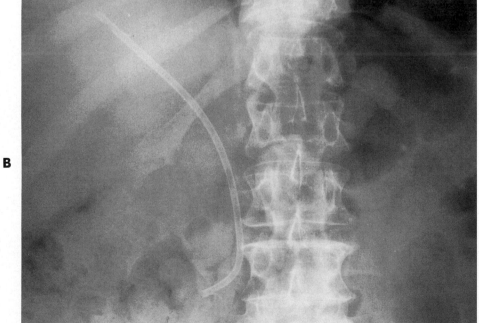

Fig. 12-5. A, Abdominal radiograph of a 58-year-old man with cholangiocarcinoma and biliary stenosis. Endoscopic retrograde placement of a biliary stent has been performed. Flanges can be seen at either end of the stent designed to prevent migration. **B,** Another patient with an internal biliary stent. This stent has only a slight flaring at its ends to prevent migration.

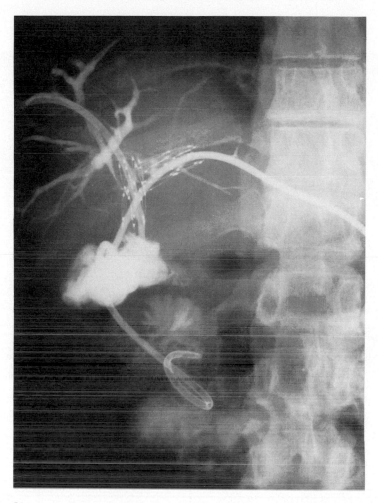

Fig. 12-6. Gianturco-Rosch Z-stents in a middle-aged man with biliary strictures. Notice also that right and left biliary direct drains are still present with Cope loop locking pigtail catheters.

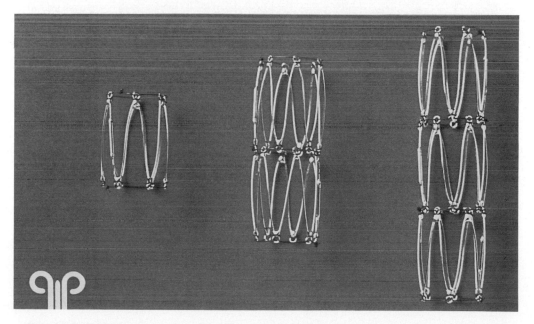

Fig. 12-7. Z-stent can be used to open an area of stenosis or tumor to allow drainage of the biliary system. (Courtesy Wilson-Cook, Winston-Salem, N.C.)

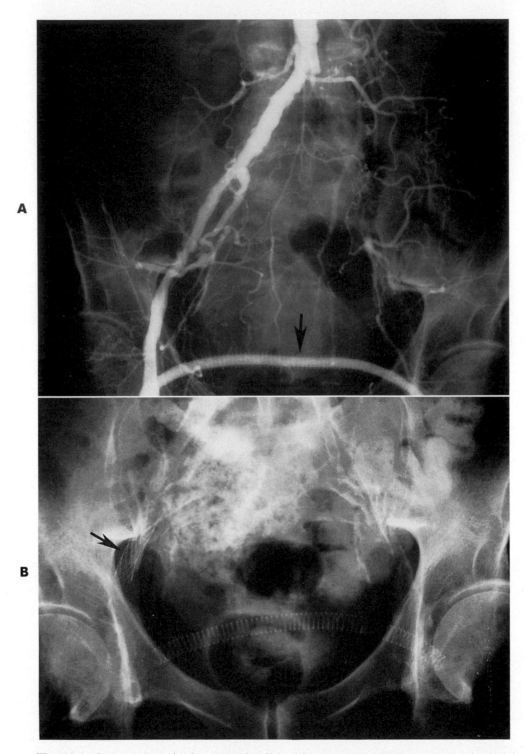

Fig. 12-8. Palmaz stent. In the example shown the stent was used in a case of arterial stenosis. The Palmaz stent can also be used in cases of bile duct obstruction. **A,** Aortogram demonstrates an occluded left common iliac artery and a ringed Gore-Tex right-to-left femoral-femoral graft, *arrow*. The right external iliac artery has an eccentric inflow stenosis. **B,** View of the pelvis showing both the Gore-Tex graft and a Palmaz stent that has now been placed across the right external iliac artery stenosis.

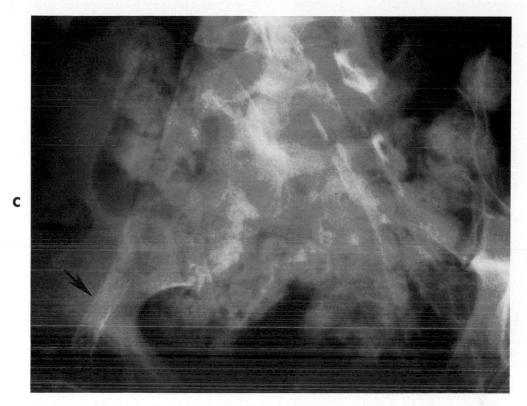

Fig. 12-8, cont'd. C, Close-up view of the Palmaz stent. Notice the "diamond-lattice" appearance of the stent.

braided together to form the stent, which is deliverable through a 7 French catheter. The Palmaz stent requires a balloon for expansion. It is also made of stainless steel. In its unexpanded configuration it has the appearance of a narrow tube with lattice type of slots, which upon expansion assume a diamond configuration (Fig. 12-8).

PERCUTANEOUS NEPHROSTOMY AND URETERAL STENTS

Percutaneous drainage of obstructed renal collecting structures was first accomplished in 1955.[12] Since that time, computed tomography, ultrasound, or fluoroscopically guided placement of drainage catheters into the renal collecting systems has become a common procedure, replacing surgical nephrostomy in most patients. Large-bore stoma access for endosurgery may still require the enlargement of nephrostomies during surgery, though initial access is usually provided by the radiologist.

Usual indications for percutaneous nephrostomy are for provision of external drainage of renal collecting systems, or access for ureteral stenting, stone extraction, stricture dilatation, and management of complications such as fistulas or leaks of the urinary tract.[4,20,21,44]

Several devices have been utilized to perform percutaneous nephrostomy including simple angiographic catheters, polyethylene pigtail catheters, and self-retaining catheters. Although Malecot (mushroom or tulip) type of catheters (Fig. 12-9) have been popular in the past, catheters with a Cope loop self-retaining device are now more common (Fig. 12-10).

When nephrostomy catheters are used alone, drainage is external. When a ureteral stent has also been placed, percutaneous nephrostomy tubes are left in as a precaution and are removed after 1 to 3 days, when adequate function of the ureteral stent is assured. Ureteral stents are placed for relief of ureteral obstruction by providing internal drainage. Very frequently, antegrade percutaneous placement is required after failed attempts at retrograde placement. The obstructions most commonly treated with ureteral stents are attributable to malignancy; ureteral stents are also used for strictures, to facilitate ureteral healing after injury, to facilitate passage or lithotripsy of stones, and to identify the ureters during major abdominal and pelvic surgery in order to protect them from inadvertent injury.[4,20,21,44]

The original ureteral stents utilized and placed percutaneously were Silastic, double-pigtail stents with side holes along their entire length. These are soft biocompatible devices, which cause a minimum of bladder irritation. However, they must be placed through peel-away polyethylene sheaths, requiring liberal use of mineral oil to overcome friction. Placement can become extremely tedious and may be impossible, especially in

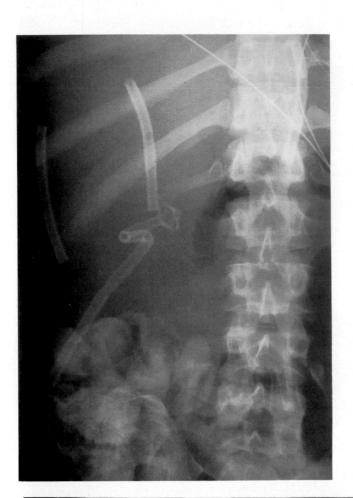

Fig. 12-9. A Malecot (mushroom) catheter has been placed in the right renal pelvis after pyelolithotomy. Notice also the large abdominal retention sutures.

Fig. 12-10. Eight-year-old girl with chronic urinary tract infections and right ureteral implant for ureteral vesical junction obstruction. **A,** Percutaneously placed ureteral stents and locking pigtail nephrostomy drains are present bilaterally. **B,** Contrast injection into the right nephrostomy tube shows there is good contrast drainage into the bladder but some reflux into the distal aspect of the left ureter.

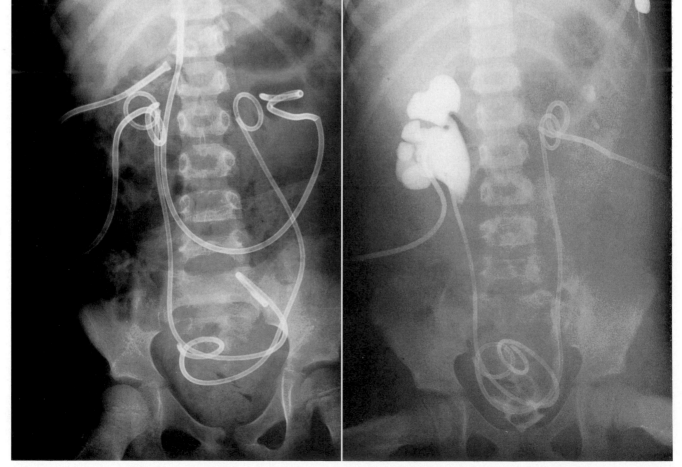

A

B

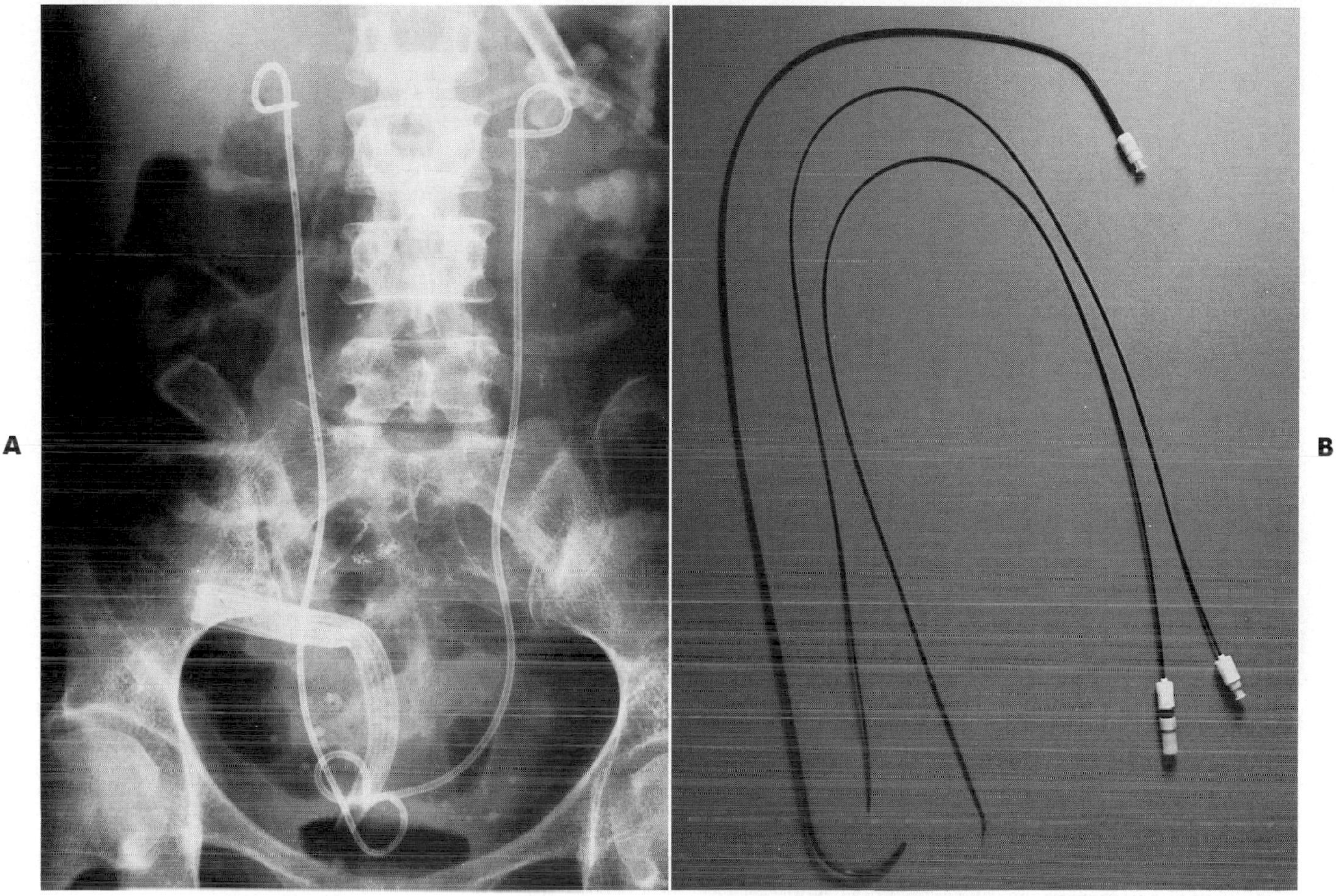

Fig. 12-11. A, Sixty-one-year-old woman with bilateral ureteral stents. The left ureteral stent has been placed in an antegrade direction (the tapered end is in the bladder) and the right ureteral stent was placed in a retrograde direction (the tapered end is in the renal pelvis). There is also a surgically placed gastrostomy tube with a Malecot tip, a Jackson-Pratt drain in the pelvis, and an ostomy ring from a colostomy in the right lateral area of the abdomen. **B,** Retrograde nephrostomy set was typically inserted during cystoscopy. Notice the tapered ends of the different-sized catheters.

tortuous ureters. More recently, biocompatible materials with improved "pushability" have been introduced. They are stiffer than Silastic catheters but are well tolerated by most patients. Once positioned, these stents may become encrusted and fail within 3 months to a year. They must then be exchanged. Fortunately, percutaneous access does not need to be repeated, since the exchange usually can be done cystoscopically.

Today's internal stents use double pigtails to prevent migration and decrease bladder irritation, commonly seen in earlier single-pigtail stents.[4] Antegrade stents can be differentiated from retrograde stents by a tapered end in the bladder. The tapered end represents the end that was first advanced into the collecting system from the percutaneous approach (Fig. 12-11).

PERCUTANEOUS GASTROSTOMY AND GASTROJEJUNOSTOMY

Before the introduction of percutaneous endoscopic gastrostomy (PEG) in 1980, surgery was the only means of placement of feeding gastrostomies. Although a percutaneous approach was first described in 1967, clinical use began in 1981.[9,19,34] In 1983 percutaneous placement of a feeding gastrostomy was performed using the Seldinger technique.[18] This allowed placement in patients who couldn't undergo surgery.

Indications for gastrostomy placement are the same as for surgical placement: nutritional support in the debilitated patient with insufficient oral intake, metabolic abnormalities of gastric or small bowel motility, and diseases of the stomach and small bowel.[20,44] Contraindi-

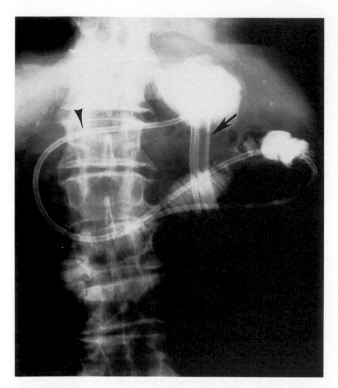

Fig. 12-12. Upper abdomen after percutaneous placement of a gastrojejunostomy in a patient with esophageal carcinoma. Although a gastrostomy tube, *arrow,* had been placed endoscopically, development of esophageal occlusion from the carcinoma and development of extensive portal-pancreatic adenopathy required placement of a gastrojejunostomy tube, *arrowhead,* because of gastric retention. The Cope loop is in the stomach next to the gastrostomy tube tip and is hidden by overlying contrast material.

cations to the procedure are uncorrectable coagulopathy, lack of a satisfactory route to the stomach, presence of a ventriculoperitoneal shunt, massive ascites, gastric varices, and involvement of the stomach wall with malignancy.

Almost any locking catheter can be used for gastrostomy or gastrojejunostomy (Figs. 12-12 and 12-13). Most come with a Cope loop. Cook, Inc., has designed a tube with a Cope loop in the proximal portion of the catheter to prevent accidental withdrawal of the catheter. The long distal end can be placed into the duodenum or jejunum preventing or minimizing reflux of feedings into the stomach and esophagus (Fig. 12-12).

Complications occur in 4% to 16% of these patients, with approximately 3% requiring laparotomy.[44] The complications include peritonitis, hemorrhage, subcutaneous emphysema, aspiration, and leakage about the puncture site.[20,44]

EMBOLOTHERAPY

Transcatheter embolotherapy is a technique frequently employed by the interventional radiologist. The indications for embolization therapy have expanded dramatically. It is basically used to interrupt harmful forms of vascular supply. Interruption of vessels supplying ateriovenous malformations (AVM), AV fistulas, and sites of active hemorrhage are frequent targets.[4,20,21,44] Trauma patients can be treated by embolization to quickly arrest blood loss, particularly after significant

Fig. 12-13. Elderly male with percutaneously placed gastrojejunostomy tube.

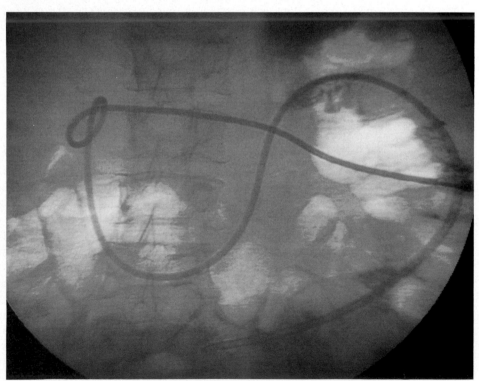

pelvic injury. Lesions previously treatable only by surgical ligation can be dealt with more easily by embolization. Embolization is also used for ablating or devascularizing tumors before surgery and for palliating tumors.[4,20,21,44] The only significant contraindication is inability to safely place the embolic agent into the offending vessel.

The list of embolic materials and devices is long (Figs. 12-14 to 12-17). The first material reported was paraffin, used to embolize a carotid artery in 1904.[4] Contemporary agents include two groups, those that are visible on plain radiographs and those that are not. Those not visible on conventional radiographs include cyanoacrylates, autologous blood clot, silicone spheres, Gelfoam (Upjohn) powder and plugs, pre-sized fragments of PVA (polyvinyl alcohol), absolute ethanol, collagen, heated contrast medium, hypertonic dextrose, thrombin, and chemical irritants that produce intimal damage and secondary thrombosis. Plain radiographs in these patients usually reveal nothing unless organ infarction occurs, in which case nitrogen comes out of solution from blood and accumulates within the viscus. This may simulate a gas-producing infection (Fig. 12-14). Embolic agents visible on plain radiographs include particulate metals, especially barium and tantalum, oil-based contrast agents, such as Ethiodol (ethiodized oil), and devices of larger size, such as stainless steel coils, metallic plugs, and detachable balloons. These are readily indentifiable on follow-up radiographs in most patients (Figs. 12-15 to 12-17).

The decision as to which embolic material to use depends on the desired level of blockade (peripheral versus central occlusion), the desired duration of occlusion (permanent or temporary), the specific vascular anatomy involved, and very often the clinical circumstances (emergency versus elective).

INFERIOR VENA CAVA FILTERS

Pulmonary embolism is believed to occur in over 500,000 patients in the United States annually, resulting in 300,000 hospitalizations and between 50,000 and 100,000 deaths.[7] In patients who have failed heparin therapy or have a contraindication to anticoagulation, inferior vena cava (IVC) ligation or plication was the procedure of choice until the introduction of the Mobin-Uddin (M-U) umbrella in 1970.[*] The M-U umbrella consists of a skeleton of six cobalt-chromium spokes and a weblike silicone rubber cover (Figs. 12-18

*References 1, 5, 13-15, 25-29, 31-33, 40, 41.

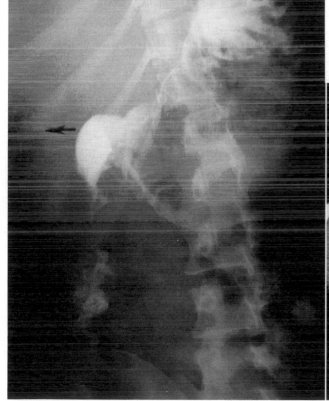

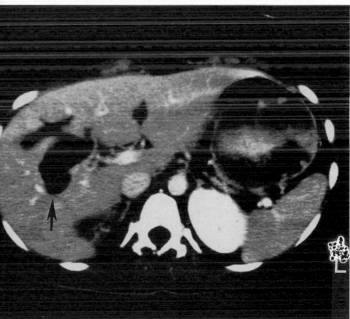

Fig. 12-14. Gelfoam (Upjohn) was used to embolize a hepatic arterial bleeder in a trauma patient. Notice the lucency, *arrow,* in the right upper quadrant of the abdomen on an upper gastrointestinal series radiograph, **A,** and a CT scan, **B,** caused by a localized area of apparent liver infarction.

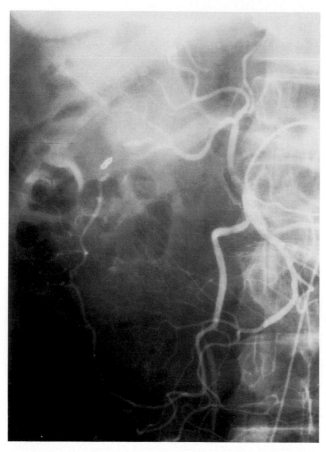

Fig. 12-15. Arteriogram of a 67-year-old male with bleeding from the right colon. A microcoil (Tracker) has been placed in the distal middle colic artery branch of the superior mesenteric artery.

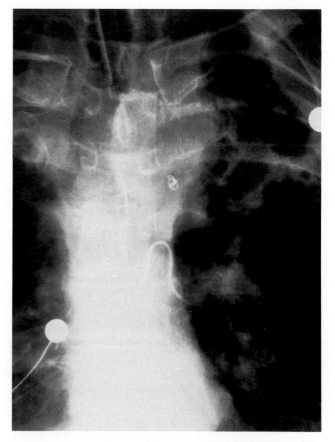

Fig. 12-16. Bronchial artery embolization performed in a patient with hemoptysis. The coils can be seen to the left of the fifth thoracic vertebral body.

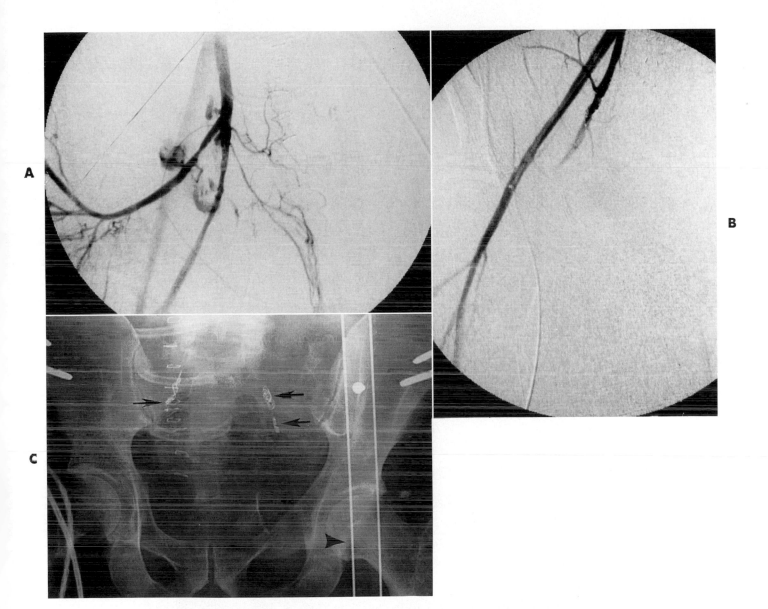

Fig. 12-17. Motor vehicle accident victim with hypotension from internal bleeding. **A,** Digital arteriogram showing active hemorrhage from the right internal iliac artery. **B,** Hemorrhage has stopped after coil embolization. **C,** Plain radiograph of the pelvis showing embolized coils, *arrows,* bilaterally in the internal iliac distribution. Notice also the presence of sacral and pelvic fractures, large abdominal retention sutures, skin staples, and the prominent linear density, *arrowhead,* produced by the patient lying on a trauma board.

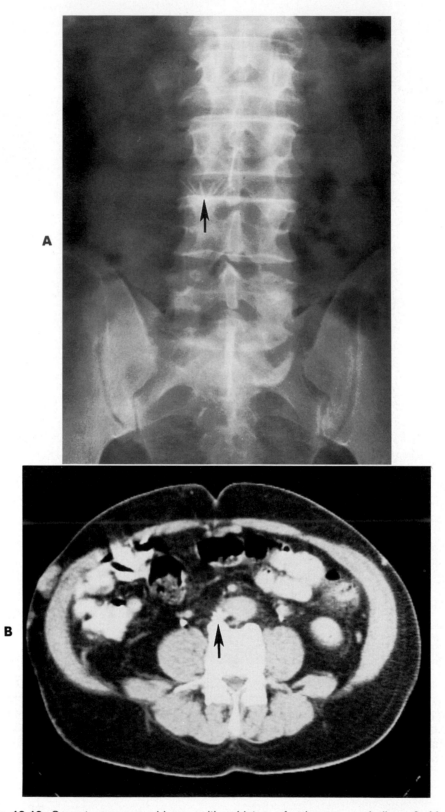

Fig. 12-18. Seventy-one-year-old man with a history of pulmonary embolism. **A,** Mobin-Uddin umbrella, *arrow,* in the inferior vena cava is seen at the L3-4 disk level. **B,** A CT study of the abdomen demonstrates a "star" pattern formed by the Mobin-Uddin umbrella.

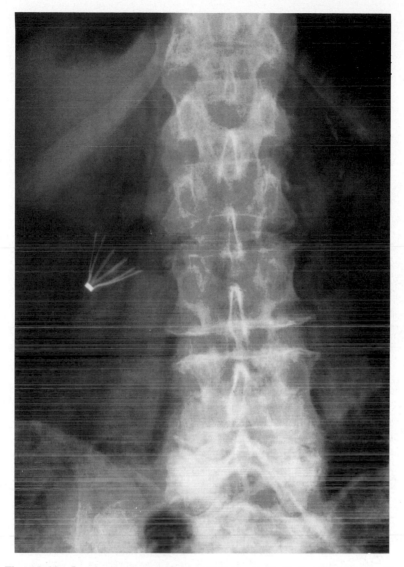

Fig. 12-19. Surgically placed Mobin-Uddin umbrella in the right renal vein.

and 12-19). Deployed, it has a flattened conelike configuration, with the spokes directed cranially on the periphery and caudally at the apex.

Unfortunately, the M-U device was associated with a high incidence (>60%) of vena cava thrombosis, with the same result as vena cava ligation.[25] Furthermore, rapid development of large retroperitoneal collaterals occurs after IVC occlusion, often providing large conduits through which recurrent embolism occurred (10% to 20%) with either vena cava ligation or the placement of a Mobin-Udin umbrella.

Because of this, the inferior vena cava filter was introduced in 1973 as a superior alternative. It interrupts the transit of clots from the lower extremity to the lungs and maintains inferior vena cava patency (92% to 97%).[13,24] It manages this by presenting an enormous surface area for transit of normal blood compared to the M-U device. The Kimray-Greenfield (K-G) filter (Medi-

tech, Inc.) was the first FDA-approved filter with these attributes of good filtration with preservation of vena cava patency.[13] The original design was a 4.6 cm device with a cone-shaped apex and six radiating stainless-steel legs, each terminating in a recurved hook, which fixes the device to the walls of the inferior vena cava[11] (Fig. 12-20).

At first, both the M-U and the K-G filters were placed using a cutdown by surgeons. Later and with increasing frequency, radiologists placed these filters using percutaneous access, despite the large venotomy defects created by the introducers.[15,33] Typically the filters are positioned in an infrarenal location, though if a thrombus has extended above that level a suprarenal location may also be employed (Figs. 12-21 and 12-22).

There are several problems that may occur with the Kinray-Greenfield filter. These include malpositioning, failure to deploy, migration, penetration of the inferior

Fig. 12-20. A, Original-design stainless-steel Kimray-Greenfield inferior vena cava filter. The filter was placed intraoperatively and is located near the level of the renal veins. **B,** Surgically placed 24 French Greenfield filter. It is partially entering the right renal vein.

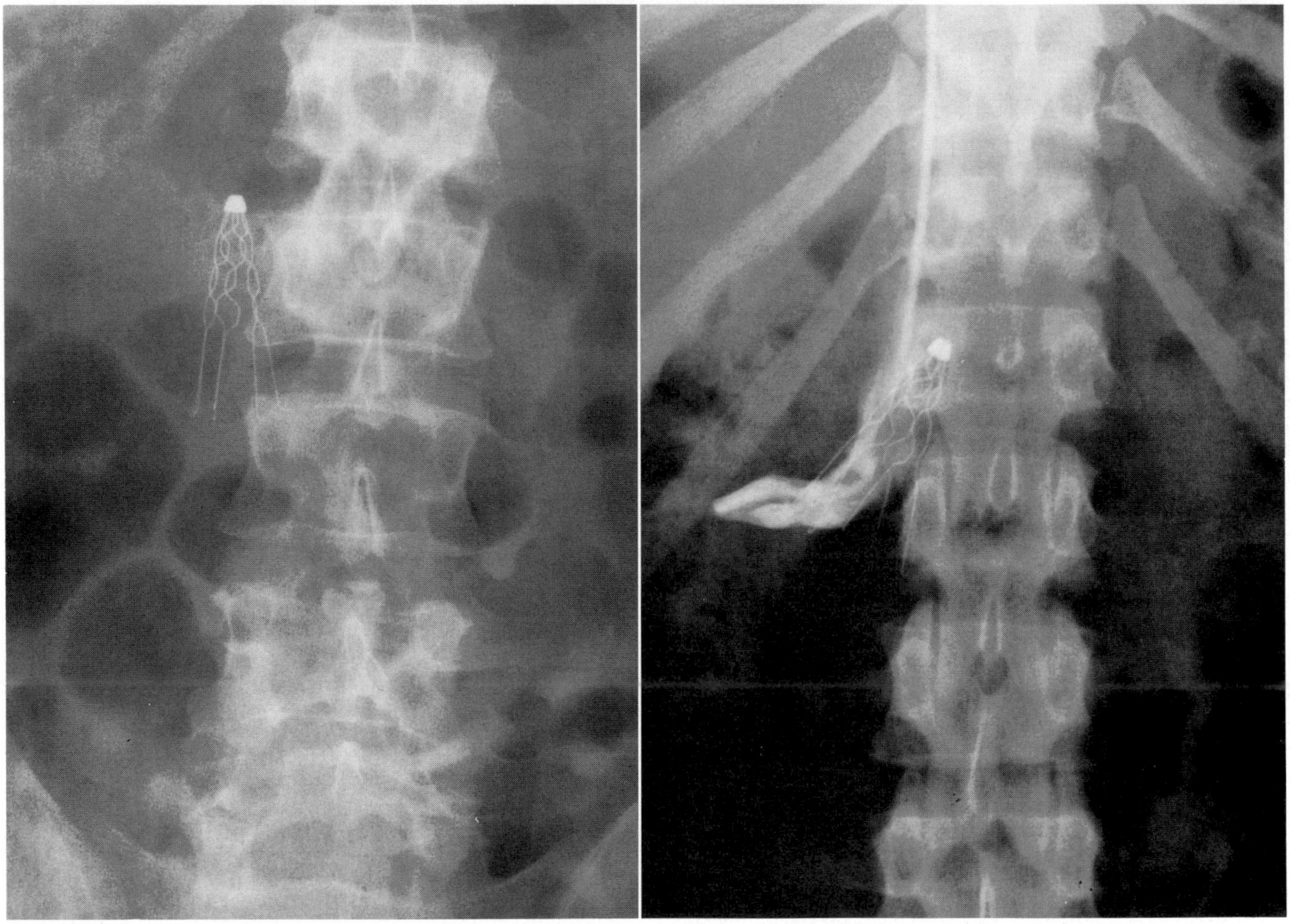

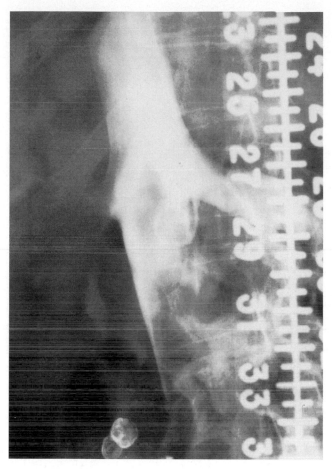

Fig 12-21 Venacavogram performed via the right internal jugular vein demonstrates a clot in the inferior vena cava extending near the renal vein level.

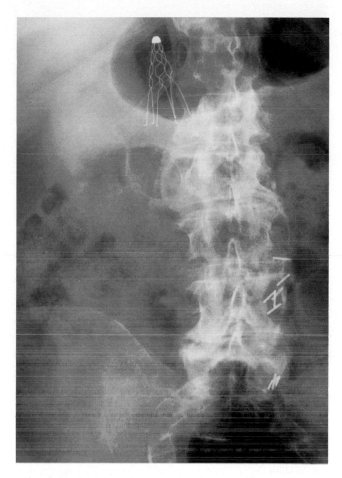

Fig 12-22 Patient with thrombus in the inferior vena cava superior to the renal vein level. Suprarenal placement of a stainless-steel Kimray-Greenfield filter was performed.

vena cava, aorta, vertebral bodies, or even the ureter, intestinal tract, and the liver.[15,22,33,43,45]

The original version of the K-G filter required a 30 French (1 cm) tract through which a 24 French introducer is passed.[11] A newer K-G filter requires only a 14 French sheath. The filter is not stainless steel but is made from a titanium alloy. Its appearance has changed slightly with the new modifications (Fig. 12-23). The apex of the filter is smaller. The hook includes a loop, which provides a source of resistance to perforation of the inferior vena cava.

Continued filter development has led to two other filters available for general use, the bird's nest filter (Cook, Inc., Bloomington, Indiana) and the Vena Tech filter[10,37,38] (Figs. 12-24 to 12-27). The bird's nest filter is percutaneously introduced through a 12 French catheter. It is composed of four 25 cm long stainless-steel 0.18 mm wires that are attached to two V-shaped struts. These struts provide the proximal and distal fixation for the filter and the containment of the "bird's nest" formed by the tangle of wires formed in the IVC (Figs.

12-26 and 12-27). Radiographically demonstrable problems with the bird's nest filter include bending of the supporting struts and prolapse of the wires beyond the field of containment defined by the struts (Fig. 12-26).

The Vena Tech filter introduced in the late 1980s is made of stainless-steel alloy.[11,36] Its basic structure has similarities to the Kimray-Greenfield filters because of its cone shape (Figs. 12-24 and 12-25). However, instead of hooks at the caudal tip of the spokes, hinged struts are pushed against the wall of the IVC by the central spokes. These struts are barbed to anchor the device. Migration of the filter has occurred in as much as 26% of cases.[36] Another difficulty with this filter has been frequent failure of the filter struts to fully deploy (Fig. 12-27).

Another device occasionally used is the Simon nitinol filter, a thermal alloy that has "petals" and struts to secure it when it deploys after being warmed by the blood (Fig. 12-28). It uses the smaller introducer sheath (10 French) of all FDA-approved filters.[39] Use of other filters, such as the cloverleaf, the Gunther, and the Am-

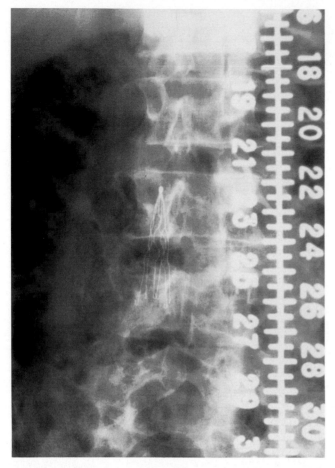

Fig. 12-23. Percutaneously placed titanium Greenfield filter.

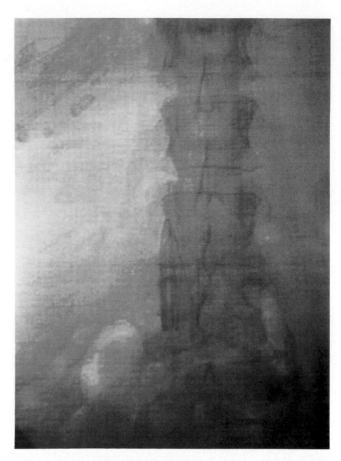

Fig. 12-24. Abdominal radiograph of 71-year-old woman after placement of Vena-Tech inferior vena cava filter. The filter has asymmetric deployment with the cone of the filter being tipped to the right with respect to the side rails.

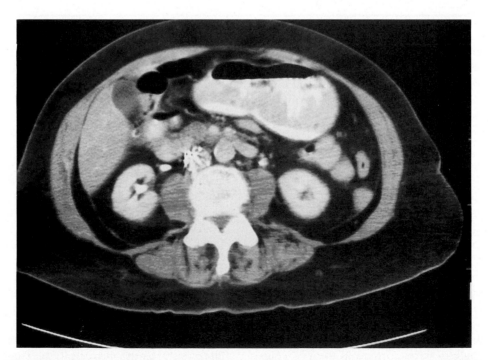

Fig. 12-25. CT image of the same patient described in Fig. 12-24. The Vena-Tech filter side rails can be seen deployed against the walls of the inferior vena cava. The cone portion of the filter is tipped to the right side of the inferior vena cava.

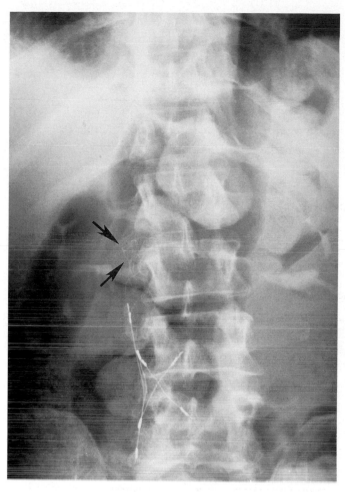

Fig. 12-26. Bird's nest filter located in the inferior vena cava. There is protrusion of the wires, *arrows,* cephalad to the filter's superior strut. A bend in the medial limb of the inferior strut is present.

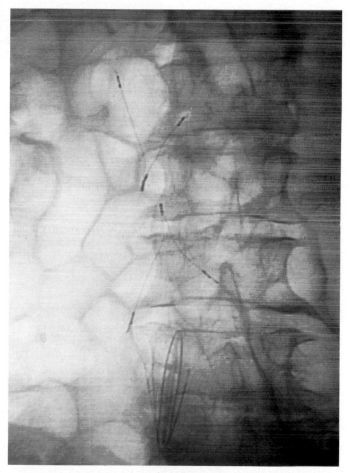

Fig. 12-27. Seventy-four-year-old man with iliac deep venous thrombosis. A jugular approach was utilized to place a Vena-Tech filter in the lower inferior vena cava. Because of difficulties in rapid deployment, the inferior portions of the side rails failed to deploy. After attempts at manipulation after deployment failed to deploy the stent fully, a second filter (Bird's nest) was placed superior to the first.

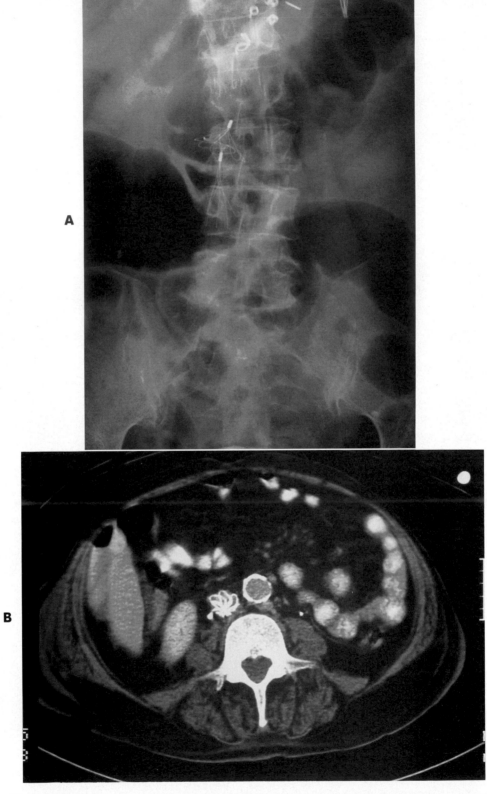

Fig. 12-28. Simon nitinol filter. **A,** Plain radiograph of the abdomen shows a filter in the inferior vena cava. **B,** CT scan of a different patient shows a Simon nitinol filter in the inferior vena cava.

platz has been limited because they are in clinical trials and are not yet FDA approved.[8,16]

REFERENCES

1. Adams JT, DeWeese JA: Partial interruption of the inferior vena cava with a new plastic clip, *Surg Gynecol Obstet* 123:1087-1088, 1966.
2. Burhenne HJ: The history of interventional radiology of the biliary tract, *Radiol Clin North Am* 28:1139-1144, 1990.
3. Carrasco CH, Wallace S, Charnsangavej CH, et al: Expandable biliary endoprostheses: an experimental study, *AJR* 145:1279-1281, 1985.
4. Castaneda-Zuniga WR, Tadavarthy SM: Interventional radiology (Golden's diagnostic radiology), Baltimore, 1988, Williams & Wilkins.
5. Cimochowski GE, Evans RH, et al: Greenfield filter versus Mobin-Uddin umbrella: the continuing quest for the ideal method of vena caval interruption, *J Thorac Cardiovasc Surg* 79:358-365, 1980.
6. Cope C: Improved anchoring of nephrostomy catheters: hook technique, *AJR* 135:402-403, 1980.
7. Dalen JE, Alpert JS: Natural history of pulmonary embolism, *Prog Cardiovasc Dis* 17:259-269, 1975.
8. Epstein DH, Darcy MD, et al: Experience with the Amplatz retrievable vena cava filter, *Radiology* 172:105-110, 1989.
9. Gauderer MWL, Ponsky JL, Izant RJ: Gastrostomy without laparotomy: a percutaneous endoscopic technique, *J Pediatr Surg* 15:872-875, 1980.
10. Gianturco C, Anderson JH, et al: A new vena cava filter: experimental animal evaluation, *Radiology* 137:835-837, 1980.
11. Gómez GA, Cutler BS, et al: Transvenous interruption of the inferior vena cava, *Surgery* 93:612-619, 1983.
12. Goodwin WE, Casey WC, Woolf W: Percutaneous trocar (needle) nephrostomy in hydronephrosis, *JAMA* 157:891-894, 1955.
13. Greenfield LJ, McCurdy JR, Brown PP, et al: A new intracaval filter permitting continued flow and resolution of emboli, *Surgery* 73:599-606, 1973.
14. Greenfield LJ: Current indications for and results of Greenfield filter placement, *J Vasc Surg* 1:502-504, 1984.
15. Greenfield LJ, Michna BA: Twelve-year clinical experience with the Greenfield vena cava filter, *Surgery* 104:706-712, 1988.
16. Gunther RW, Schild H, et al: First clinical results with a new caval filter, *Cardiovasc Intervent Radiol* 10:104-108, 1987.
17. Hawkins IF Jr: Single-step placement of a self-retaining accordion catheter, *Semin Intervent Radiol* 1:15-18, 1984.
18. Ho CS: Percutaneous gastrostomy for jejunal feeding, *Radiology* 149:595-596, 1983.
19. Jascalevich ME: Experimental trocar gastrostomy, *Surgery* 62:452-453, 1967.
20. Kadir S: *Current practice of interventional radiology,* St. Louis, 1991, Mosby.
21. Kandarpa K: *Handbook of cardiovascular and interventional radiologic procedures,* Boston, 1989, Little, Brown & Co.
22. Kim D, Porter DH, et al: Perforation of the inferior vena cava with aortic and vertebral penetration by a suprarenal Greenfield filter, *Radiology* 172:721-723, 1989.
23. Lammer J, Flueckiger F, Hausegger KA, et al: Biliary expandable metal stents, *Semin Intervent Radiol* 8:233-241, 1991.
24. Maroney TP: Venography and vena cava filters, *Curr Opin Radiol* 3:175-180, 1991.
25. McIntyre AB, McCready RA, et al: A ten year follow-up study of the Mobin-Uddin filter for vena cava interruption, *Surg Gynecol Obstet* 158:513-516, 1984.
26. Miles RM, Chappell F, et al: A partially occluding vena caval clip for the prevention of pulmonary embolism, *Am Surg* 30:40-47, 1964.
27. Mobin-Uddin K, et al: A vena caval filter for prevention of pulmonary embolus, *Surg Forum* 18:209-211, 1967.
28. Mobin-Uddin K, Jude JR, et al: A new catheter technique of interruption of the inferior vena cava for prevention of pulmonary embolism, *Am Surg* 35:889-894, 1969.
29. Mobin-Uddin K, McLean R, et al: Caval interruption for prevention of pulmonary embolism: long term results of a new method, *Arch Surg* 99:711-715, 1969.
30. Molnar W, Stockum AE: Relief of obstructive jaundice through percutaneous transhepatic catheter: a new therapeutic method, *AJR* 122:356-367, 1974.
31. Moretz WH, Still JM Jr, et al: Partial occlusion of the inferior vena cava with a smooth Teflon clip: analysis of long term results, *Surgery* 71:710-719, 1972.
32. Ochsner A, Ochsner JL, et al: Prevention of pulmonary embolism by caval ligation, *Ann Surg* 171:923-936, 1970.
33. Paris SO, Tobin KD: Percutaneous insertion of the Greenfield filter, *AJR* 152:933-938, 1989.
34. Preshaw RM: A percutaneous method for inserting a feeding gastrostomy tube, *Surg Gynecol Obstet* 152:659-660, 1981.
35. Remolar J, Katz S, Rybak B, et al: Percutaneous transhepatic cholangiography, *Gastroenterology* 31:39-46, 1956.
36. Ricco JB, Crochet D, et al: Percutaneous transvenous caval interruption with the "LGM" filter: early results of a multicenter trial, *Ann Vasc Surg* 3:242, 1988.
37. Roehm JOF Jr: The bird's nest filter: a new percutaneous transcatheter inferior vena cava filter, *J Vasc Surg* 1:498-501, 1984.
38. Roehm JOF Jr, Gianturco C, et al: Percutaneous transcatheter filter for the inferior vena cava: a new device for treatment of patients with pulmonary embolism, *Radiology* 150:255-257, 1984.
39. Simon M, Athanasoulis CA, et al: Simon nitinol inferior vena cava filter: initial clinical experience, work in progress, *Radiology* 172:99-103, 1989.
40. Spencer FC, Quattlebaum JK, et al: Plication of the inferior vena cava for pulmonary embolism: a report of 20 cases, *Ann Surg* 155:827-837, 1962.
41. Stansel HC: Vena cava interruption: three points of view, *Cont Surg* 20:43-68, 1982.
42. van Sonnenberg E, D'Agostino HB, Casola G, et al: Percutaneous abscess drainage: current concepts, *Radiology* 181:617, 1991.
43. Wingerd M, Bernhard VM, et al: Comparison of caval filters in the management of venous thrombolism, *Arch Surg* 113:1264-1271, 1978.
44. Wojtowycz MM: *Interventional radiology and angiography* (Handbooks in Radiology), St. Louis, 1990, Mosby–Year Book.
45. Yune HY: Inferior vena cava filter: search for an ideal device, *Radiology* 172:15-16, 1989.

13

Artifacts in Computed Radiography

· ·

Steven L. Solomon

This chapter illustrates many of the artifacts encountered that are specific to computed (or computerized) radiography, some of which can simulate pathologic lesions. Computed radiographic systems that use photostimulable storage phosphors have been introduced into radiology departments throughout the world since the mid-1980s. By 1991 more than 50 systems were in operation in the United States and approximately 500 systems had been installed in Japan.[1]

Computed radiography has great potential clinical usefulness in chest, pediatric, genitourinary, gastrointestinal, vascular, and neuroradiology imaging.[2-7] In general, computed radiography devices are reliable with excellent image quality, but, on occasion, puzzling artifacts can be encountered, some of which have the potential to mimic true disease. Artifacts that are not unique to computed radiography (fogging, double exposure, foreign bodies) may have their severity or appearance modified by computed radiography.

LIGHT-BULB EFFECT

The lower, outer portions of a film occasionally appear darkened relative to the remainder of the image (Fig. 13-1). This artifactual darkening, referred to as the light-bulb effect by Fuji Medical Systems U.S.A. (Stamford, Conn.), is caused by backscattered radiation entering the photostimulable phosphor imaging plate from the patient's bed. This artifact is seen most frequently when the exposure is increased for obese patients or when the x-ray beam has not been collimated to the region of interest. The wide dynamic range and high sensitivity of the imaging plate makes computed radiography more susceptible to this artifact than conventional film-screen portable examinations.

With chest radiography, the artifact could be misconstrued as representing a pneumothorax or pneumoperitoneum in a supine patient; in addition, it can alter the contrast and brightness of the affected portions of the image, potentially obscuring abnormalities. Reducing backscatter by lowering the kilovoltage or by more precise collimation will limit the prevalence and influence of this artifact. A lead backing applied to the cassette has been proposed as a possible solution.[1]

FOGGING

The wide dynamic range and high sensitivity of the imaging plate used in computed radiography result in a greater susceptibility to fogging (Fig. 13-2). Because the imaging plates have such a high sensitivity, extra precautions should be taken so that they are not exposed to extraneous radiation.

DOUBLE EXPOSURE

With conventional film-screen techniques, most double exposures result in a darkened, unreadable image. The wide dynamic range of the imaging plate used in computed radiography allows an image similar in den-

Much of the material for this chapter was previously published in Solomon SL, Jost RG, Glazer HS, Sagel SS, Anderson DJ, Molina PL: Artifacts in computed radiography, *AJR* 157:181-185, 1991, and is reprinted here with permission of authors and publisher.

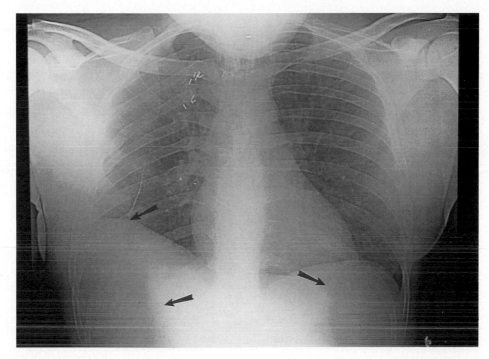

Fig. 13-1. Light-bulb effect. Lower, outer portions of this computed radiograph, *arrows,* are darkened because of back-scattered radiation from the patient's bed. Wide dynamic range and high sensitivity of photostimulable phosphor imaging plate makes computed radiography much more susceptible to this artifact than conventional portable film-screen radiographs.

sity to a single exposure to result from most inadvertent double exposures (Fig. 13-3). If the relative exposure of both examinations is comparable, they will be equally well seen on the output image, and the nature of the problem should be readily apparent. If one exposure is significantly less than the other, the artifact may be subtle and simulate abnormalities. A related and visually indistinguishable situation can occur if a latent image on the imaging plate has not been completely erased.

Computed radiography systems are capable of erasing an imaging plate that has received up to five times the normal exposure. If an exposure greater than this has occurred, the imaging plate is transported to a special unerased plate tray after it has been read. If this imaging plate is inadvertently used for another examination, a double-exposure artifact may result. Incompletely erased imaging plates should be carefully erased in the "imaging plate erasure mode."

QUANTUM MOTTLE

The wide dynamic range of the imaging plate can create an image when underexposure or overexposure would result in an unreadable image using conventional film-screen methods. In the case of considerable underexposure, the image will appear grainy because of quantum mottle (Fig. 13-4). Such images, which one can readily identify by noting a high sensitivity number in the parameter display area, must be interpreted with caution, because subtle findings may not be apparent because of the reduced signal-to-noise ratio.

SIMULATED DIAPHRAGMATIC CALCIFICATION, PNEUMOTHORAX, OR PNEUMOMEDIASTINUM

The normal computed radiography output consists of two images, one processed to resemble a normal film screen radiograph and one processed with an unsharp masking algorithm that results in a degree of edge enhancement and widened latitude. The unsharp masking algorithm can result in artifactual black and white bands at the interface of structures with greatly disparate densities. This can result in the appearance of diaphragmatic calcification (Fig. 13-5). The erroneous diagnosis of asbestos exposure could result. Alternatively, as has been suggested by Oestmann et al.,[8] the corresponding black band may be misinterpreted as a pneumothorax or pneumomediastinum. This artifact is always much less apparent on the non−edge enhanced image, an important differential point. Comparison to prior radiographs, if available, or a follow-up conventional radiograph is helpful in ambiguous cases. If this artifact is problematic, the spatial frequency-processing parameters can be modified to lessen the effect.

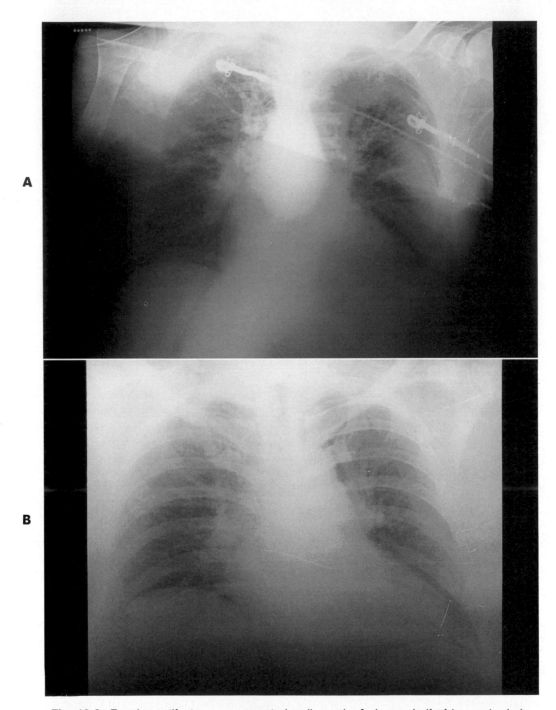

Fig. 13-2. Fogging artifacts on a computed radiograph. **A,** Lower half of image is darkened by exposure to extraneous radiation. High sensitivity of imaging plates requires that extra precautions be taken to prevent inadvertent radiation exposure. **B,** Fogging in lower portion of image is caused by radium implants placed in the pelvis to treat cervical cancer. We have not seen this artifact to the same degree with conventional film-screen techniques.

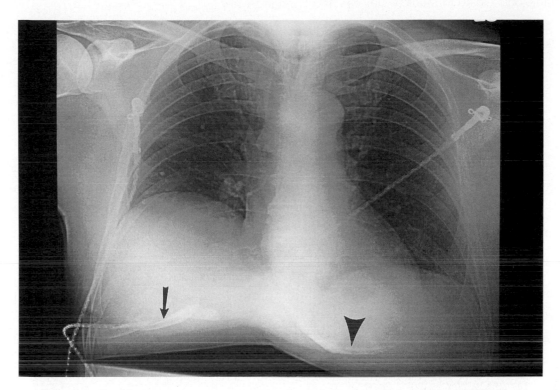

Fig. 13-3. Double exposures on computed radiograph. Horizontally oriented abdominal examination is seen overlying dominant chest study. Portions of right ribs, *arrow,* and right iliac crest, *arrowhead,* are apparent.

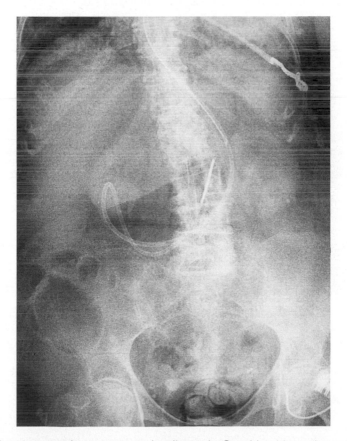

Fig. 13-4. Quantum mottle on computed radiograph. Considerable underexposure of this abdominal examination still results in an interpretable, albeit grainy and suboptimal, image because of the wide dynamic range of the imaging plate.

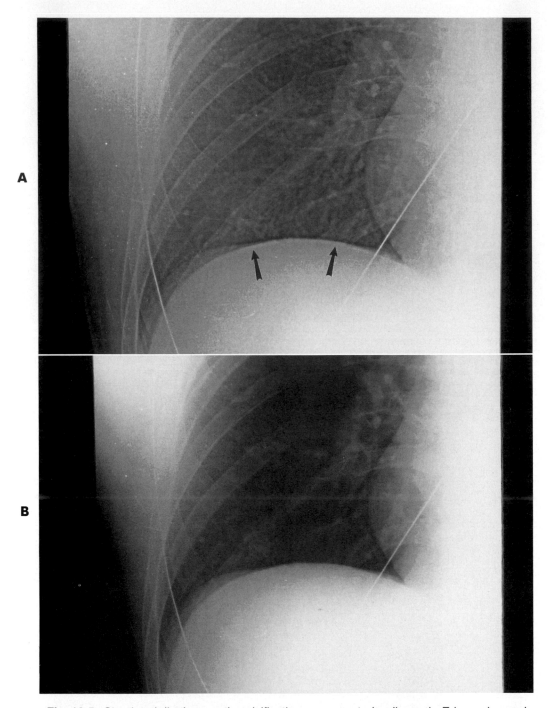

Fig. 13-5. Simulated diaphragmatic calcification on computed radiograph. Edge-enhanced image, **A,** shows apparent calcification of right hemidiaphragm, *arrows,* that is not seen on unenhanced image, **B,** an important differential point. This artifact almost always involves right hemidiaphragm, probably because of heart and pericardial fat overlying left hemidiaphragm, which reduce abrupt changes in tissue density at this site. Alternatively, the overlying black band may simulate a basilar pneumothorax. A similar artifact is also seen frequently at edges of both breasts.

ALTERATIONS IN IMAGE CONTRAST AND DENSITY

A contrast resolution of 10 bits per pixel (1024 shades of gray) was chosen in the design of the currently used computed radiography systems. The imaging plate on the other hand has a dynamic range exceeding 10^4. The image information contained on the imaging plate must be mapped onto these relatively few shades of gray. As part of this mapping process, the imaging plate is scanned twice. The first scan is performed with a high-speed low-intensity laser, and histogram analysis is performed upon the light emission from portions of the image. The portions of the image plate examined are determined by the algorithm chosen for the image. The result of this analysis determines the density and contrast parameters used in the final reading of the imaging plate and creation of the output image.

The algorithms designed for each body part make certain assumptions about the expected useful density range contained in the image. If the expected density range is exceeded, information can be lost (Fig. 13-6). For example, the chest algorithm does not guarantee the preservation of image information from the skin. Fortunately, most of these instances will occur outside of the regions of interest for the examination. If an algorithm for the wrong body part is chosen, the density and contrast settings will not be optimal for the body part imaged (Fig. 13-7).

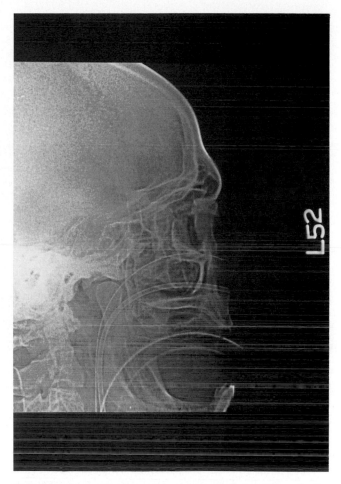

Fig. 13-6. Loss of information on computed radiograph. External portions of nasogastric, feeding, and endotracheal tubes are not visualized because expected useful density range for a skull examination has been exceeded at these sites.

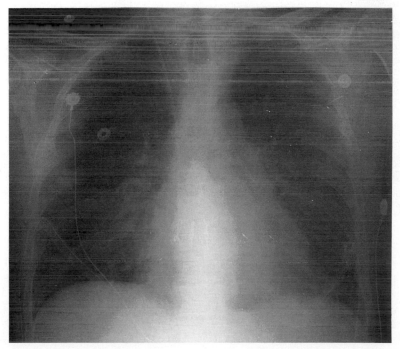

Fig. 13-7. Altered contrast parameters on computed radiograph. This chest image was inadvertently printed using an algorithm designed for the mandible. Result is a darkened image with suboptimal contrast.

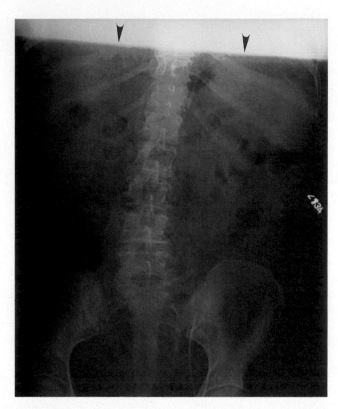

Fig. 13-8. Poor collimation on computed radiograph. First generation of computed radiography software relies on collimation margins, *arrowheads,* being less than 3 degrees from parallel to edge of imaging plate when automatic modes are used. If this angle is exceeded, as has occurred in this image, the area of collimation will not be recognized as such and the display algorithm will include this area in its determination of image density and contrast. Result will be overall darkening of the region of interest.

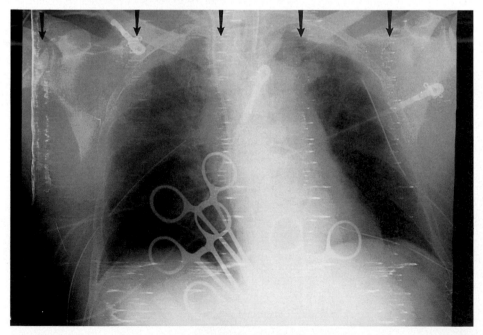

Fig. 13-9. Foreign substances on a computed radiograph. A liquid, possibly blood, was spilled on the imaging plate during this intraoperative examination. Because of rollers used in early computerized radiography equipment, this manifests as an artifact, *arrows,* seen all across image at constant intervals.

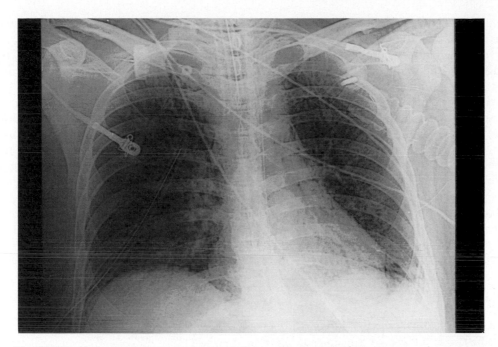

Fig. 13-10. Abnormal edge enhancement. Edge-enhancement image-processing parameters have been altered on this computed radiograph, resulting in dramatic augmentation of edge enhancement. This artifact is probably attributable to noise from electrical power supply and should be corrected by turning off and restarting the computed radiography device.

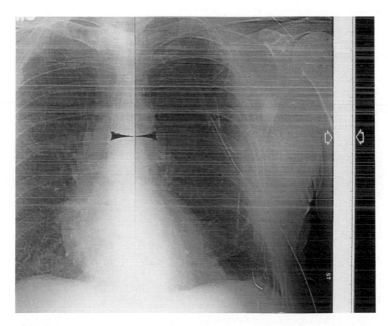

Fig. 13-11. Zipper artifact. Information from central portion of this computed radiograph, *arrowheads,* is missing, with apparent absence of a portion of the vertebral bodies. Amount of information lost is reflected by width of a white vertical band at right side of image, *arrows.* This artifact is caused by temporary interruption of image plate reading while image plate continues to be transported through reading device. Cause is probably a sudden drop in the power-supply voltage.

The automatic modes use the entire image for histogram analysis as opposed to the semiautomatic modes, which perform histogram analysis only on selected portions of the image data. The shape of collimation is critically important in the automatic modes on computed radiography devices using first-generation software. If a collimation border is greater than 3 degrees from parallel to the edge of the imaging plate, the area of collimation will not be recognized as such and will be included in the subsequent determination of image density and contrast. This can result in considerable image darkening in the region of interest (Fig. 13-8).

The edge-enhancement and widened latitude present on the unsharp masked output image result in a loss of area contrast. This has been reported to reduce the conspicuity of structures without discrete margins, such as pulmonary infiltrates and some bone lesions.[8,9]

FOREIGN BODIES

As with conventional film-screen systems, foreign bodies, such as dust, can adhere to the imaging plate and result in artifacts simulating calcifications. Spillage of a liquid on the imaging plate before its processing by the computed radiography device is shown in Fig. 13-9. The repetitive nature of the artifact is attributable to the rollers used in the plate-transport mechanism. Newer computed radiography systems use belts to transport the plates and therefore would not propagate the artifact.

EQUIPMENT MALFUNCTION

On occasion, images in which the edge enhancement has been dramatically augmented have been observed (Fig. 13-10). This is probably the result of an alteration of the image-processing parameters stored in memory because of noise from the electrical power supply.[10] This artifact has been seen only on edge-enhanced images, a potential clue to its presence in more subtle cases. One should correct the problem by turning off and restarting the computed radiography device. The power-supply noise and variance may need to be checked if the problem is recurrent.

Rarely, images are seen in which multiple vertical scan lines are missing with apparent narrowing of the affected portion of the image (Fig. 13-11), referred to by us as the "zipper" artifact. The exact amount of missing information is reflected by the width of a lucent vertical band at the right side of the image. This artifact results when the reading process is temporarily discontinued while the imaging plate continues to move through the reading device. The cause is probably a sudden drop in the power-supply voltage.[10]

Occasional misalignment of the laser used to print the output image has been described.[8] This is best seen with artificial structures such as lead letters but can produce irregular bone margins simulating disease.

REFERENCES

1. Armstrong D: Personal communication, Fuji Medical Systems U.S.A., Inc., Stamford, Conn.
2. Fajardo LL, Hillman BJ, Hunter TB, et al: Excretory urography using computed radiography, *Radiology* 162:345-351, 1987.
3. Kangarloo H, Boechat MI, Barbaric Z, et al: Two-year clinical experience with a computed radiography system, *AJR* 151:605-608, 1988.
4. Kogutt MS, Jones JP, Perkins DD: Low-dose digital computed radiography in pediatric chest imaging, *AJR* 151:775-779, 1988.
5. Sagel SS, Jost RG, Glazer HS, et al: Digital mobile radiography, *J Thorac Imaging* 5(1):36-48, 1990.
6. Tateno Y, Iinuma T, Takano M, editors: *Computed radiography,* Tokyo, 1987, Springer-Verlag.
7. Yang PJ, Seeley GW, Carmody RF, et al: Conventional vs computed radiography: evaluation of myelography, *AJNR* 9:165-168, 1988.
8. Oestmann JW, Prokop M, Schaefer CM, Galanski M: Hardware and software artifacts in storage phosphor radiography, *RadioGraphics* 11:795-805, 1991.
9. Prokop M, Galanski M, Oestmann JW, et al: Storage phosphor versus screen-film radiography: effect of varying exposure parameters and unsharp mask filtering on detectability of cortical bone defects, *Radiology* 177:109-113, 1990.
10. Hishinuma K: Personal communication, Fuji Medical Systems Japan, Inc., Tokyo, Japan.

14

Ultrasound Imaging: Artifacts and Medical Devices

· ·

Kathleen A. Scanlan
K. Rebecca Hunt

Ultrasound is a unique technology using high-frequency sound waves to view body structures. The resultant images frequently do not display anatomy and pathologic conditions as distinctly as other radiologic modalities, such as plain radiography, computed tomography, and magnetic resonance imaging. Therefore medical devices and foreign objects may not be as easily recognized by those inexperienced in ultrasound interpretation. Moreover, various artifacts are unique to ultrasound. If they are unappreciated by the interpreter, they may cause significant image degradation and even lead to misdiagnosis. Therefore it is important for the radiologist and referring physician to be familiar with not only the appearance of medical devices and foreign bodies on ultrasound imaging, but also the appearance of common ultrasound artifacts.

ULTRASOUND ARTIFACTS AND THEIR ORIGINS*

Artifacts are encountered daily in clinical ultrasound imaging. Artifactual images may be generated in B-mode gray-scale imaging, spectral pulsed Doppler imaging, and color Doppler imaging. Most of these distortions can be understood at a basic level by an appreciation

of three major factors: the form of the focused sound beam, the interaction of sound with tissue, and the assumptions made in the spatial assignment of reflected echoes.

Ultrasound systems assign depth based on the time interval of round-trip echo travel and are assumed to have a straight line and singular path from transducer to reflector and reflector to transducer. The same speed of sound is assumed in all tissues for the purpose of spatial assignment.

Some inherent acoustic artifacts are used reflexively to characterize tissue. Strong acoustic enhancement behind an anechoic structure confirms the diagnosis of a cyst. Clean acoustic shadowing distal to an echogenic focus in the gallbladder leads us to the diagnosis of gallstones. However, if unrecognized, acoustic artifacts can cause serious misdiagnosis. For example, an unsuspected mirror artifact in the pelvis may mimic a cystic mass and lead to an erroneous diagnosis of pelvic abscess.

Recognition of ultrasound artifacts is essential for accurate diagnosis. Several commonly encountered artifacts are illustrated accompanied by a basic physical explanation of the occurrence.

B-Mode Gray Scale

Reverberation

When a sound beam is perpendicular to an interface, the amount of reflected sound depends on the amplitude of the incident beam and the acoustic impedance difference between the two media. With large differences the reflection of sound is maximized, and sound transmission through the interface is very poor. This

*Much of the material for this section is reprinted with permission from Scanlan KA: Sonographic artifacts and their origins, *AJR* 156:1267-1272, 1991.

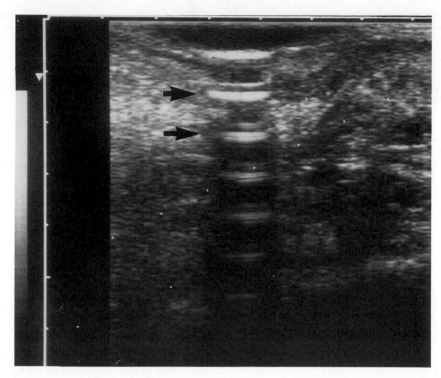

Fig. 14-1. Endorectal prostate sonogram, sagittal view. An air bubble trapped within the fluid-filled condom causes repeated reverberation bands, *arrows*. The artifact completely obscures the image. If the air bubble cannot be eliminated, one can improve the image by tipping the bubble to the end of the condom. (From Scanlan KA: *AJR* 156:1267-1272, 1991.)

phenomenon tends to occur at soft-tissue/gas and fluid/gas interfaces. Sound reflected from such an interface will strike the transducer and reenter the patient. When this echo again returns to the transducer, it will receive a spatial assignment twice as deep as the original reflector. This "round trip" of the sound may be repeated several times.[1]

Reverberation bands

Reverberation artifact is usually seen as bright parallel lines occurring at regular intervals (Fig. 14-1). Echoes that have taken more time to return to the transducer are electronically boosted by the equipment. This is done to compensate for the tissue attenuation of returning deep echoes in the normal imaging situation and serves to enhance the reverberation artifact.

Reverberation pseudomass

Another form of reverberation artifact is created by returned echoes from a gas-filled or fluid-filled structure located deep to the transducer, usually in the pelvis. The near "wall" of the pseudomass results from the primary reflection from the tissue/gas-fluid interface, and the second reverberated echo creates the far wall (Fig. 14-2). Because only one or two reverberated echoes may be

imaged because of a large interval, this type of reverberation artifact is much more difficult to recognize.

"Mirror-image" pseudomass

The "mirror-image" pseudomass type of artifact occurs adjacent to highly reflective acoustic interfaces, such as the diaphragm, the pleura, and the bowel because of reverberations that develop between the real mass and the reflective surface.[2] It is most frequently seen as a supradiaphragmatic projection of an infradiaphragmatic mass, and in this situation it is easily recognizable as artifact. The same situation may be created in the abdomen or pelvis adjacent to a highly reflective interface, usually the bowel wall. This artifact is more difficult to recognize because it can mimic an actual pathologic situation (Fig. 14-3). Mirror-image artifacts can also occur with pulsed and color Doppler imaging.

Comet-tail (ringdown) artifact

The comet-tail artifact appears as a line of intense nearly continuous echoes trailing behind a small reflector or behind the bands of a periodic reverberative artifact. It is speculated that this artifact arises from multiple short-path reverberations. The short path could arise within a cluster of microbubbles or within a lipid

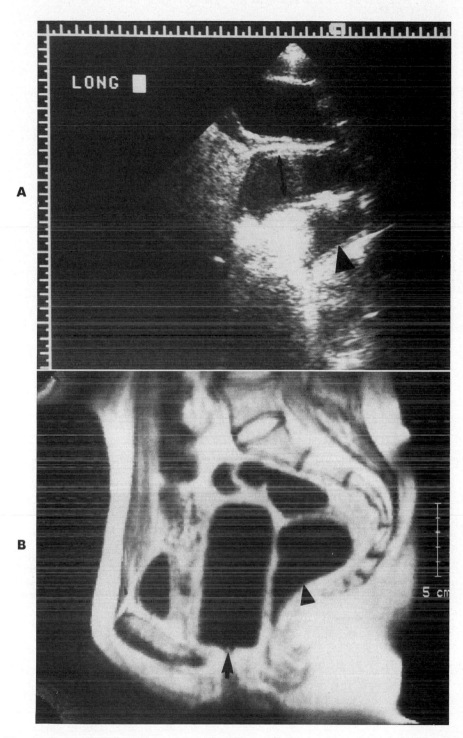

Fig. 14-2. A, Sagittal pelvis sonogram, midline view in a patient after vaginoplasty with a clinical question of pelvic abscess. Vaginal mold is identified posterior to the bladder, *doubled arrow.* A hypoechoic structure, *arrowhead,* posterior to the vaginal mold raised the question of an abscess. **B,** Magnetic resonance imaging scan 4 days later shows no fluid interposed between the vaginal mold, *arrow,* and rectum, *arrowhead.* The "abscess" was created by reverberation. (Courtesy Dr. Frederick Kelcz, Madison, Wis.; from Scanlan KA: *AJR* 156:1267-1272, 1991.)

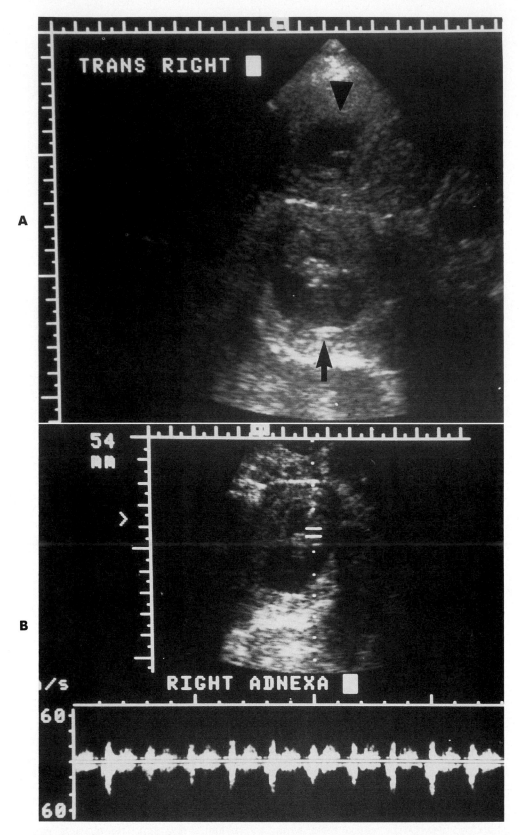

Fig. 14-3. Transabdominal pelvic ultrasonogram. **A,** An intrauterine gestation, *arrowhead, and* a duplicate gestational sac, *arrow,* complete with fetal pole are seen in an extrauterine location. The second gestation is likely "mirrored" from a highly reflective portion of sigmoid colon. The artifact disappeared on repeat scan. Water enema can be used in this situation if the colon is suspected as the "mirror." **B,** Artifactual image demonstrates an artifactual heartbeat with pulsed Doppler interrogation.

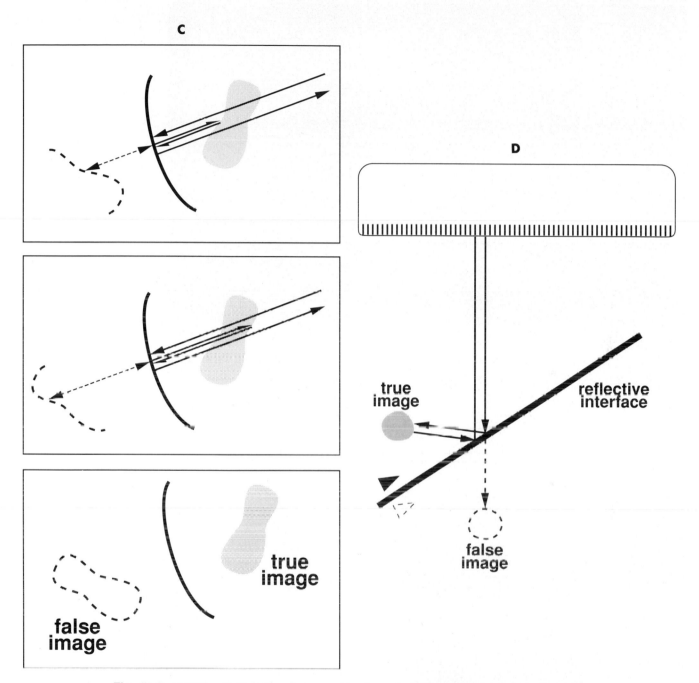

Fig. 14-3, cont'd. C, Drawing shows mechanism of mirror-image simulation of a mass. True mass is duplicated by additional round-trip reverberations that develop between points within mass and reflective interface. Additional distance traveled by reverberated sound registers spatially as a mirror image of mass appearing equidistant on opposite side of reflector. **D,** Drawing shows mechanism of mirror-image localization of a Doppler signal. If interrogating pulse first strikes a reflective interface such as pleura or gas-filled rectum and then interrogates a small moving reflector, returned frequency information will be spatially displaced, *dashed arrow,* by the distance of an additional round trip, *short arrows,* between specular reflector and small moving reflector. *Arrowheads* indicate direction of flow. (**B,** Courtesy Dr. Frederick Kelcz, Madison, Wis.; from Scanlan KA: *AJR* 156:1267-1272, 1991.)

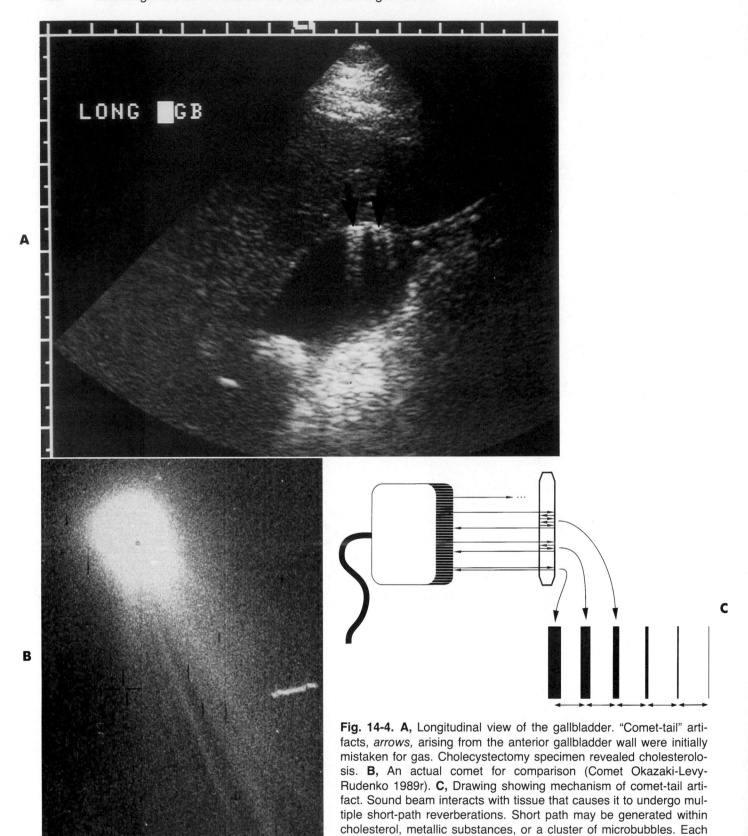

Fig. 14-4. **A,** Longitudinal view of the gallbladder. "Comet-tail" artifacts, *arrows,* arising from the anterior gallbladder wall were initially mistaken for gas. Cholecystectomy specimen revealed cholesterolosis. **B,** An actual comet for comparison (Comet Okazaki-Levy-Rudenko 1989r). **C,** Drawing showing mechanism of comet-tail artifact. Sound beam interacts with tissue that causes it to undergo multiple short-path reverberations. Short path may be generated within cholesterol, metallic substances, or a cluster of microbubbles. Each multiple of the short path is registered spatially as a bright line, resulting in a trail of closely spaced bright lines behind the source of the artifact. (**B,** Courtesy S. Larson and D. Levy; **A** and **C** from Scanlan KA: *AJR* 156:1267-1272, 1991.)

globule such as cholesterol (Fig. 14-4). The "comet tail" can also be identified behind substances that have a very large acoustic impedance mismatch with soft tissue, such as metal. Clinically, the comet tail is seen behind the gas collections, areas of cholesterolosis, and metallic clips, needles and IUDs.[3-5]

Speed-of-sound artifacts

Ultrasound equipment assigns spatial location based on round trip time, with the assumption of an average velocity of 1540 m/sec. Scanning through media with different speeds of sound will cause inaccurate depth assignment.[6,7] Such tissues include cartilage (>1540 m/sec), fluid (1480 m/sec), and fat (1459 m/sec). This artifact often also involves an element of refraction when media that have two different speeds of sound are traversed by the sound beam (Fig. 14-5).

Through-transmission artifacts

Tissue that lies deep to fluid-filled structures appears more echogenic than normal because the attenuation of sound is less in fluid than in soft tissue. This artifact can be encountered when one is scanning through ascites, large cystic masses, or a small fluid collection such as a hydrocele. Kidneys scanned through ascites may appear more echogenic than normal, leading to an erroneous diagnosis of medical-renal disease. The artifact can be particularly confusing when a nodular liver is scanned through ascites[8] (Fig. 14-6). Some refraction can also occur at the fluid/liver interface, further demarcating the protruding area. Scanning the "echogenic" area through a soft-tissue window will demonstrate the same echogenicity as the rest of the parenchyma.

Beam-width artifact

The ultrasound beam has a definite width that varies along the course of the beam depending on its focusing characteristics. With slice-width artifact one portion of the ultrasound beam may be interacting with a fluid-filled structure whereas another portion of the beam interacts with adjacent soft tissue. This will create spurious echoes registered within the cystic structure (Fig. 14-7). One can minimize the effect by using the narrowest sound beam available, focusing the beam at the site of interest, and scanning through the central portion of the cyst. Changing the patient's position relative to the sound beam will also reveal the echoes as spurious rather than gravity-dependent debris. This phenomenon will also cause masses of low echo contrast to be less apparent or missed entirely because of reduced contrast at the borders.

Side-lobe/grating-lobe artifacts

Several additional sound beams may be located outside the main axis of the ultrasound beam. They are usually of a much lower intensity than the main beam but create significant artifacts when they interact with highly reflective acoustic surfaces. Side lobes may cause specular or diffuse echoes within the image.[9] Specular artifacts occur adjacent to curved, highly reflective surfaces, such as the diaphragm, bladder, and gallbladder, whereas diffuse echoes tend to occur adjacent to bowel gas. The same phenomenon may cause the appearance of multiple needle paths during guided biopsy (Fig. 14-8). Because the off-axis portions of the beam are of lower intensity than that of the main beam, their potential for artifact generation is minimized at lower gain settings. If diffuse echoes are created in a cystic structure, their presence will be related to beam angle rather than gravity. A shift in acoustic window or changing patient position should reveal them as artifactual.

Focal zone banding

The ultrasound beam is of varying intensities along its course, and electronic focusing of the beam when it is transmitted can create bands of increased intensity[10] (Fig. 14-9). This may be particularly apparent in tissue of relatively low acoustic attenuation. The phenomenon can create bands of increased echogenicity in an organ that should be homogeneous. One can recognize the artifact by altering the level of focus within the area scanned.

Refraction

Refractive shadows occur when the sound beam is at an oblique angle of incidence to the boundary between two media, resulting in bending of the sound beam (Fig. 14-10). The amount of reflection and refraction that occurs depends on the angle at which the beam strikes the interface.[10] It also depends on whether the sound path is from a higher-velocity (soft tissue) to a lower-velocity medium (such as a cyst) or from a low-velocity medium to a higher-velocity medium, such as the path of a sound beam through ascites to the liver edge.

Refractive artifacts can mimic shadowing from calcified structures or simply can obscure evaluation of the tissue in the area of the artifact. Recognition of the physical cause of the artifact and altering the position of the transducer slightly can help to prevent misdiagnosis.

Attenuation

Partial attenuation of the sound beam by absorption and reflective mechanisms will cause a distal area of decreased echogenicity (Fig. 14-11). Clean acoustic shadowing behind gallstones aids in their recognition. However, when a fibroadipose area in the liver or spleen causes partial attenuation of the sound beam, an area of low echogenicity can occur in the usually uniform parenchyma. This finding may indicate an area of neoplastic involvement if the source of the artifact is not rec-

Text continued on p. 430.

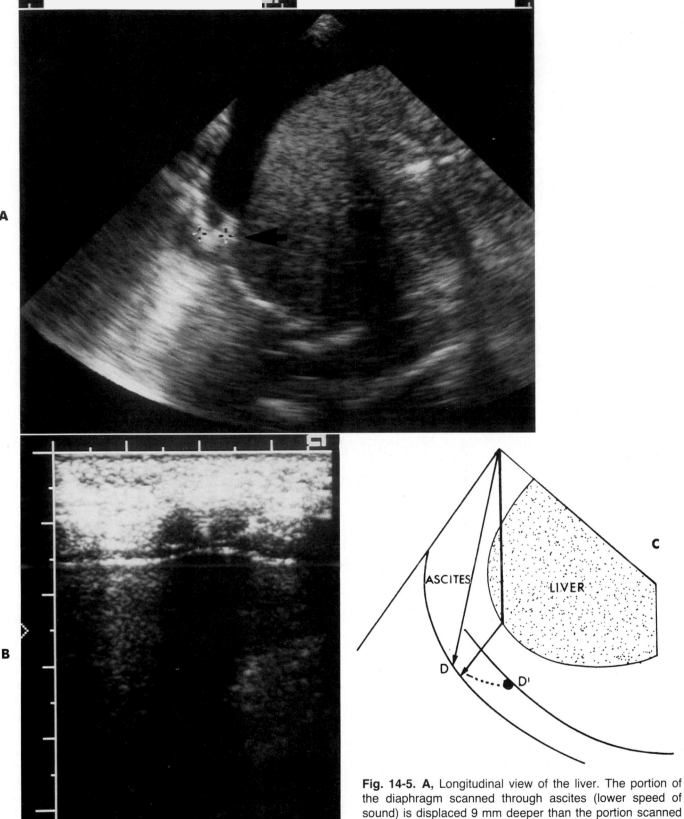

Fig. 14-5. A, Longitudinal view of the liver. The portion of the diaphragm scanned through ascites (lower speed of sound) is displaced 9 mm deeper than the portion scanned through liver, *arrow.* Refraction creates a short segment of double diaphragm. **B,** Longitudinal view of the liver. Because the speed of sound through cartilage is higher than 1540 m/sec, the subjacent liver capsule is artifactually placed closer to the transducer, creating a small pseudomass, *arrow.* **C,** Simplified illustration of origin of displaced and duplicated diaphragm. Sound beam is refracted by traveling through media that conduct sound at different speeds. **D** and **D¹** indicate two different spatial placements of a point on diaphragm caused by this phenomenon. (From Scanlan KA: *AJR* 156:1267-1272, 1991.)

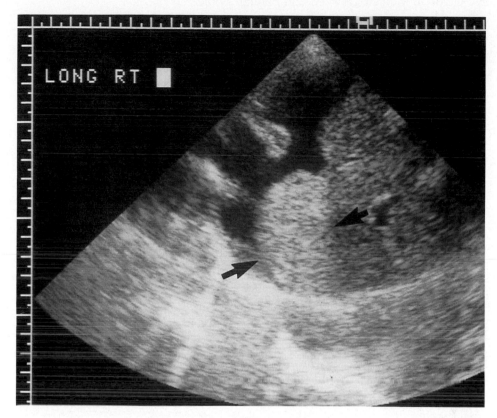

Fig. 14-6. Longitudinal view of the liver. A nodular projection at the liver dome appears to have higher echogenicity than the rest of the liver, creating a pseudomass, *arrows*. Scanning through ascites attenuates the beam much less than the liver does. (From Scanlan KA: *AJR* 156:1267-1272, 1991.)

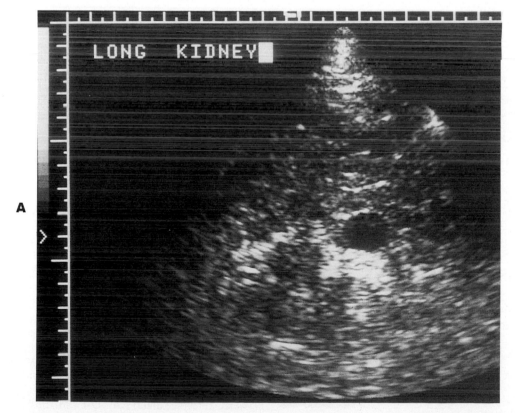

Fig. 14-7. A, Longitudinal view of a kidney. Cyst appears relatively echo-free with appropriate focusing.   *Continued.*

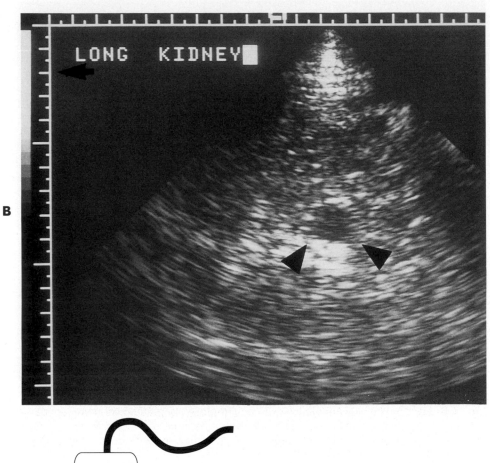

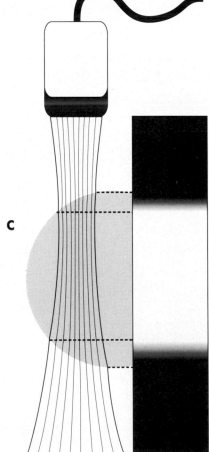

Fig. 14-7, cont'd. B, Poorly placed focal zone, *arrow,* creates internal echoes and irregular wall, *arrowheads.* **C,** Drawing shows that a wider portion of an ultrasound beam can interact partially with a cystic structure and partially with surrounding soft tissue, causing loss of definition of cyst walls. (From Scanlan KA: *AJR* 156:1267-1272, 1991.)

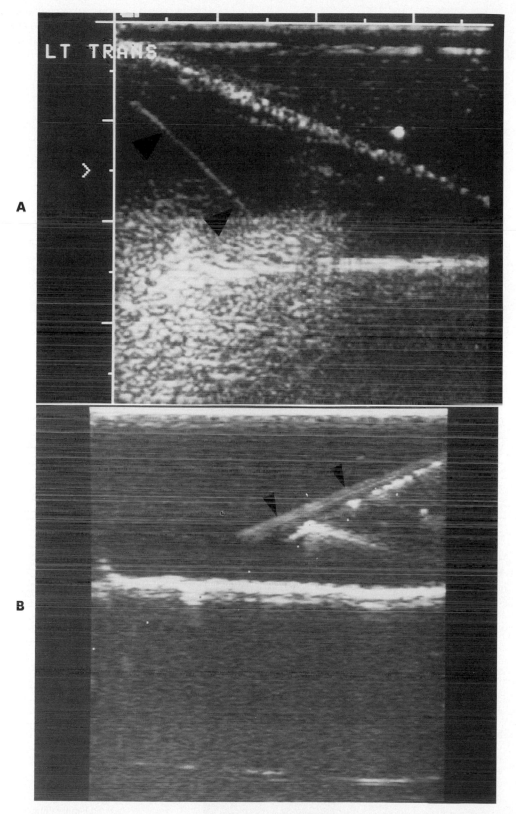

Fig. 14-8. A and **B,** Biopsy needle imaged with two different linear transducers shows side-lobe artifacts, *arrowheads,* created by off-axis grating lobes. *Continued.*

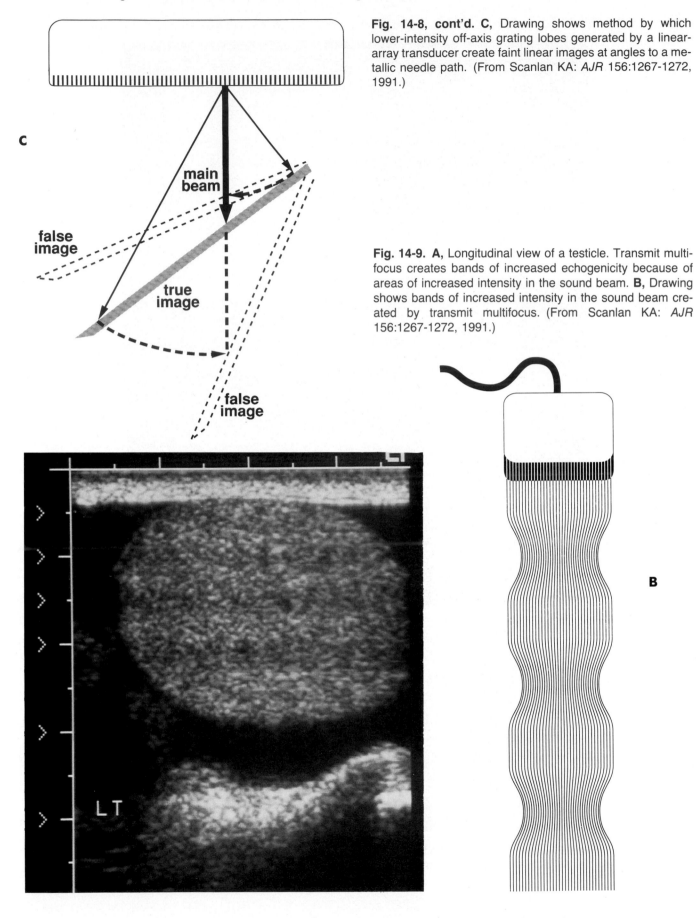

Fig. 14-8, cont'd. C, Drawing shows method by which lower-intensity off-axis grating lobes generated by a linear-array transducer create faint linear images at angles to a metallic needle path. (From Scanlan KA: *AJR* 156:1267-1272, 1991.)

Fig. 14-9. A, Longitudinal view of a testicle. Transmit multifocus creates bands of increased echogenicity because of areas of increased intensity in the sound beam. **B,** Drawing shows bands of increased intensity in the sound beam created by transmit multifocus. (From Scanlan KA: *AJR* 156:1267-1272, 1991.)

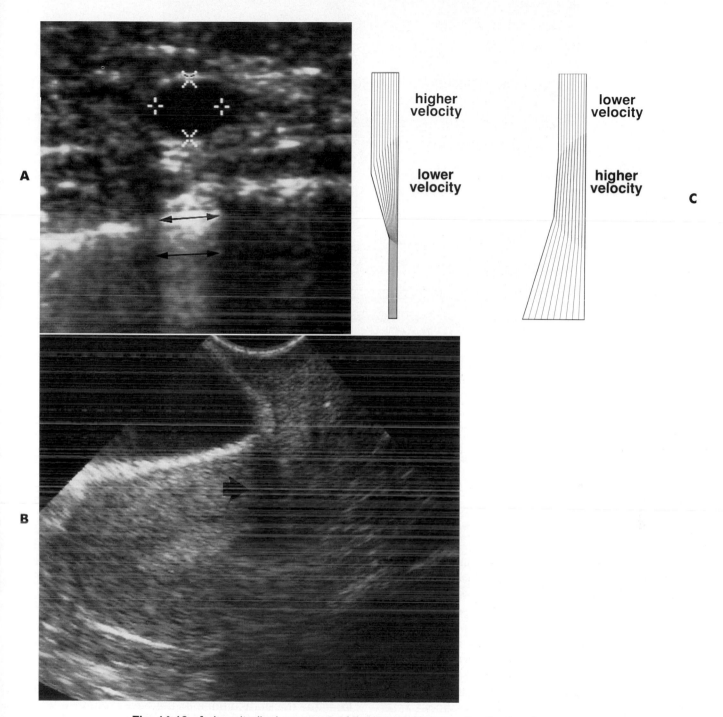

Fig. 14-10. A, Longitudinal sonogram of the breast. Narrow refractive bands, *arrows,* are seen at the margins of a simple cyst. **B,** Longitudinal transvaginal image of the uterus. Refractive band, *arrow,* from the bladder edge obscures the uterus. Scanning with an empty bladder minimizes this artifact. **C,** Simplified illustration shows how a relatively higher to lower velocity path will refract and narrow the sound beam, creating thin refractive artifacts at margin of lower-velocity cyst. A lower-to-higher velocity path in the same situation will cause spreading of the sound beam. (From Scanlan KA: *AJR* 156:1267-1272, 1991.)

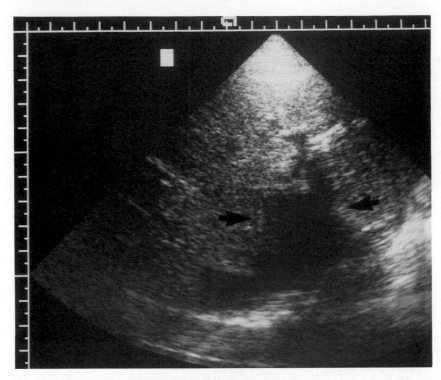

Fig. 14-11. Transverse view of the liver. Partial attenuation of the sound beam by portal structures creates an irregular hypoechoic area, *arrows,* which could be misconstrued as metastatic disease (From Scanlan KA: *AJR* 156:1267-1272, 1991.)

ognized. This phenomenon may occur behind fibroadipose areas, such as the porta hepatis, the falciform ligament, and the hilar area of the spleen. When this type of abnormality is suspected, scanning from multiple windows can resolve the issue.

Pulsed Range Gated Doppler Imaging

Simultaneous bidirectional flow artifact

This phenomenon of simultaneous bidirectional flow artifact produces the appearance of bidirectional simultaneous flow on both sides of the zero base line (Fig. 14-12). The artifact is most commonly produced when the Doppler signal is nearly perpendicular to the interrogated vessel and when the Doppler gain is relatively high.[11] The direction of blood flow relative to the transducer is assigned when the device analyzes small phase differences between the returning echo and the transmitted pulse. These small directional differences can be more difficult to assign when the vector component aligned with the axis of flow is reduced. One can correct this by decreasing gain and using a more favorable (closer to 60-degree) angle to the vessel. The bidirectional phenomenon may also be attributable in part to the presence of side-lobe/grating-lobe artifact. Off-axis portions of the Doppler signal may have access to phase and frequency information from the same vessel as the main beam, but these off-axis lobes "see" the information from a different direction.

Aliasing

Frequency aliasing occurs when the pulse-repetition rate is too low to adequately sample the Doppler frequency shift. This causes blood of highest velocity going in one direction to be displayed as low velocity in the opposite direction (Fig. 14-13). Increasing the pulse-repetition rate or switching to a lower frequency transducer may solve the problem. As a general rule, the minimum pulse-repetition rate must be two times the frequency of the Doppler frequency shift being measured.

Range-gate ambiguity

In this situation of a range-gate ambiguity the echoes from one transmitted burst do not have the time to dissipate before the next burst is sent. The overlap of signals from the bursts causes uncertainty about the depth of the reflector that produced them.[12] Although frequency aliasing sets a lower limit on the pulse-repetition frequency, range ambiguity sets an upper limit. At very high pulse repetition frequencies there is very limited range discrimination, with the most extreme example of this being continuous-wave Doppler imaging having no range discrimination.

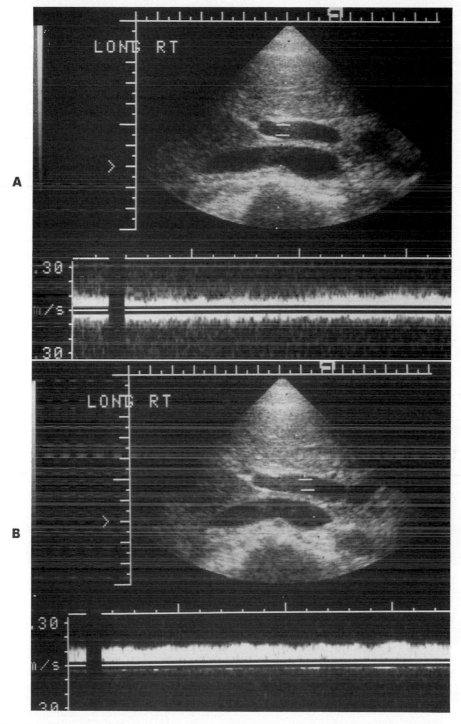

Fig. 14-12. A, Longitudinal view of the portal vein, pulsed Doppler image. Near perpendicular angle and relatively high gain create artifactual bidirectional flow. **B,** Slight improvement in angle and lowering the gain now demonstrates true direction.

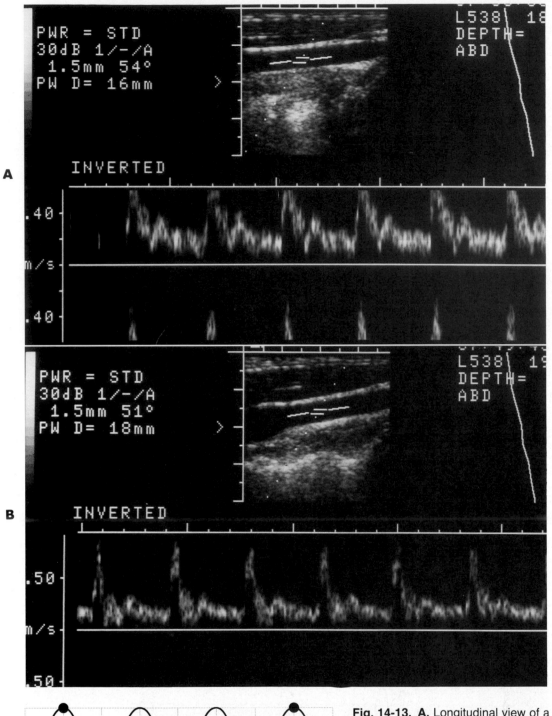

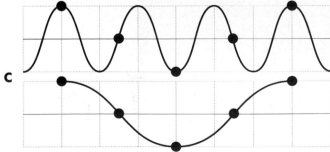

Fig. 14-13. A, Longitudinal view of a carotid artery. Aliasing is manifest as clipped peaks are displayed below the base line. **B,** Widening the velocity range increases the pulse-repetition frequency (PRF), and the entire spectral signal is properly displayed above base line. **C,** Drawing shows that inadequate sampling of the signal, *top,* will produce a resultant signal of lower frequency, *bottom.*

Most equipment should display the "phantom" range gates to make the sonographer aware of the problem (Fig. 14-14). Decreasing the pulse-repetition frequency (by decreasing the velocity scale) or decreasing the depth of the image may eliminate the phantom gate.

Gate placement

The cross-sectional velocity profile of each vessel is different. A small sample gate measures the velocity only in the portion of the vessel where it is placed. Slower velocities are most frequently encountered at the periphery of vessels with the highest velocity centrally.

In areas of nonlaminar flow it is possible to place a relatively small sample gate such that it registers authentic reversed velocity in an eddy of flow reversal, whereas the bulk of flow is in the opposite direction. This problem has been clarified recently by color flow

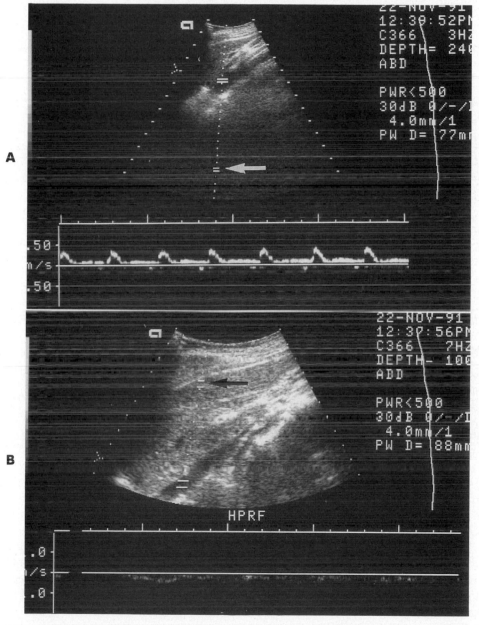

Fig. 14-14. A, Longitudinal view of the aorta. A second phantom gate, *arrow,* is displayed deep to the area of interest when a relatively superficial vessel is interrogated. This can be corrected by decreasing the depth of the image. **B,** Longitudinal view of inferior vena cava. A second superficial phantom range gate, *arrow,* is displayed when a deeper structure is interrogated. The PRF is too high for proper range discrimination. This can be corrected when the velocity range is decreased.   *Continued.*

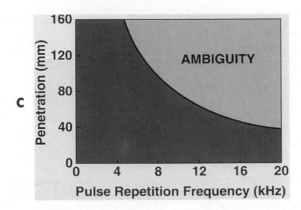

Fig. 14-14, con't. C, As the pulse-repetition frequency increases, the ability to localize the range gate without ambiguity is confined to more superficial tissues.

imaging, which can offer a more global picture of the velocity profile (Fig. 14-15).

Color Doppler Imaging

Color in nonvascular structures

Tissue or fluid motion for any reason can result in frequency shifts high enough to be registered in color where no blood flow is responsible for the signal. The problem most commonly occurs with tissue motion in the neck from speech, in areas adjacent to vascular turbulence, such as arteriovenous fistulas, and from bowel peristalsis. Color assignment can be noted in ureteral jets and with currents in peritoneal fluid (Fig. 14-16). The phenomenon is most pronounced in anechoic regions.[13-15]

Mirror-imaging artifact

Just as in gray-scale imaging, a mirror-image artifact may be created adjacent to a highly reflective acoustic interface (Fig. 14-17). This has been described at the lung apex where a duplicated image of the subclavian artery can be created.[16] If the artifactual image is sampled with a range gate, spectral Doppler signals identical to the real image will be obtained. Mirror-image artifacts should be suspected when duplicated structures are found adjacent to highly reflective acoustic interfaces such as the diaphragm, bowel, lung, and air-containing abscesses.

Velocity-range errors

Slower flow may not be assigned color when the range has been adjusted to a high setting (Fig. 14-18). An excessively high range setting will lower the dynamic range of the instrument and will filter out lower frequency shifts. This selection of technical factors may cause an erroneous diagnosis of vascular thrombosis when no color is assigned in a vessel, such as a portal vein with slow flow in chronic hepatic disease. The

range setting should be tailored to the expected velocity of flow in the interrogated vessel.

Aliasing

Aliasing in color Doppler imaging may occur just as in pulsed Doppler imaging when the pulse-repetition rate is too low for accurate sampling of the Doppler frequency shift. The highest velocities will be recorded as the slowest flow in the opposite direction. In vessels with laminar flow this will usually be evident in the center of the lumen, but if misinterpreted, the phenomenon may lead to an erroneous diagnosis of turbulence or reversed flow. One can correct aliasing by widening the velocity range to increase sampling frequency (Fig. 14-19).

ULTRASOUND VISUALIZATION OF MEDICAL DEVICES AND FOREIGN BODIES

Medical Devices (Iatrogenic Foreign Bodies)

Vascular catheters can often be visualized on ultrasound examinations, particularly if the examiner is aware of their existence and looks for them. They are identified as a two-walled echogenic structure within a vascular channel (Fig. 14-20). Ultrasound may be very useful in the assessment of the exact location of a catheter tip with respect to vascular anatomic landmarks, particularly in neonates where there is a need to limit the radiation dose and any interventional trauma to the patient.[17] Ureteral stents, biliary stents, chest tubes, as well as surgical drains can often be seen and have a similar appearance to each other and to vascular catheters (Figs. 14-21 to 14-24).

Occasionally a foreign body is visualized on a pelvic ultrasound examination. Usually, when one observes its location (vagina, cervix, or uterus) and speaks with the patient, the foreign body can be explained. A vaginal tampon is one of the most frequently encountered for-

Text continued on p. 443.

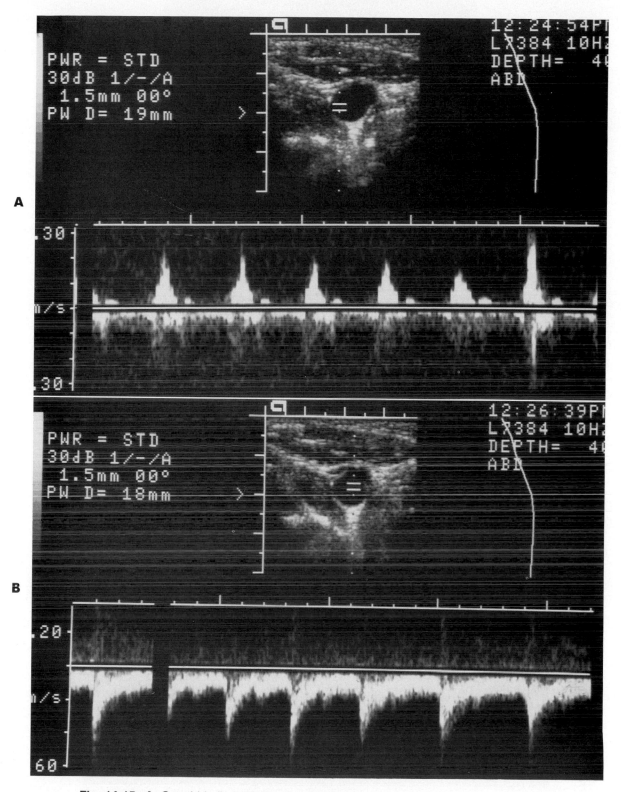

Fig. 14-15. A, Carotid bulb, transverse pulsed Doppler image. Interrogation of the lateral lumen shows flow toward the transducer and, **B,** of the medial lumen, flow away from the transducer.

Continued.

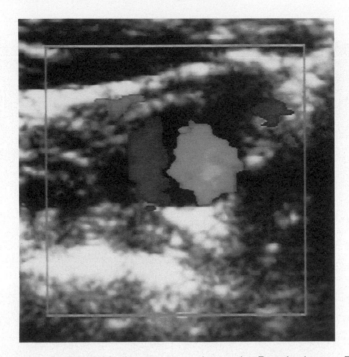

Fig. 14-15, cont'd. C, Carotid bulb transverse view, color Doppler image. Flow reversal in bulb is graphically demonstrated.

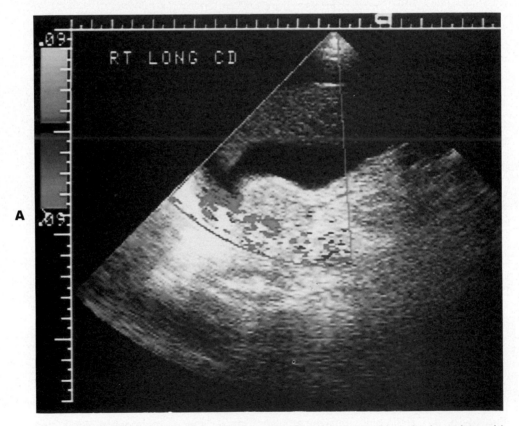

Fig. 14-16. A, Sagittal view of the spleen, color Doppler image. No color is registered in motionless ascites.

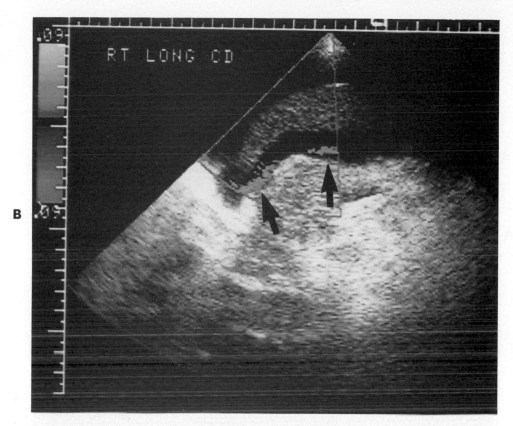

Fig. 14-16, cont'd.   B, Respirations cause rocking of the spleen on its pedicle resulting in fluid currents. The fluid motion is given color assignment, *arrows*. This artifact may be confused with varices.

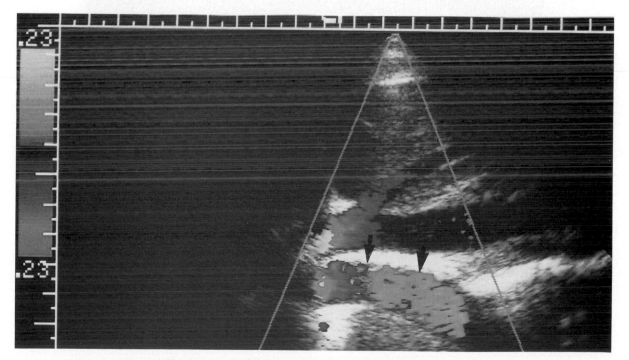

Fig. 14-17. Sagittal view of inferior vena cava, color Doppler image. A mirror image, *arrows,* of inferior vena cava is created, reflected from the diaphragmatic crus. Notice color change from red (light gray; toward) to blue (dark gray; away) near the central axis of the fluid.

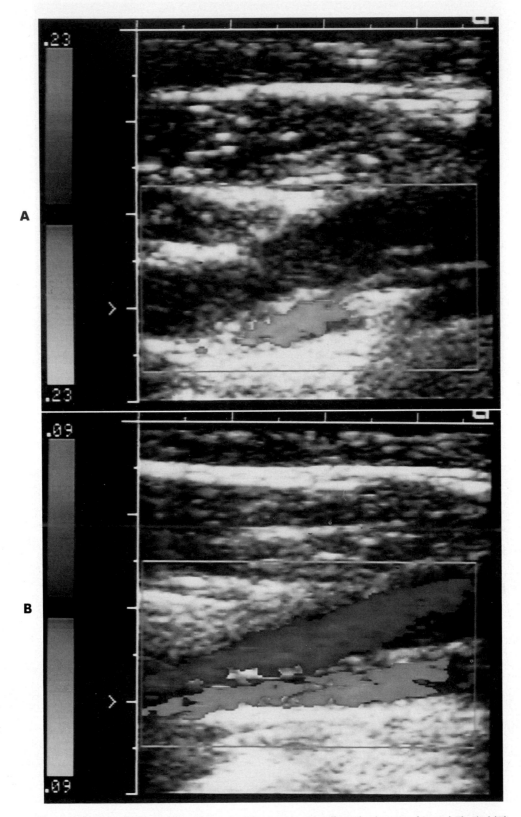

Fig. 14-18. Longitudinal view of the popliteal vein, color Doppler image. At a relatively high-velocity range setting, no color is displayed, suggestive of thrombosis. **B,** Adjusting the velocity range to the lowest setting correctly displays flow in the patent vein.

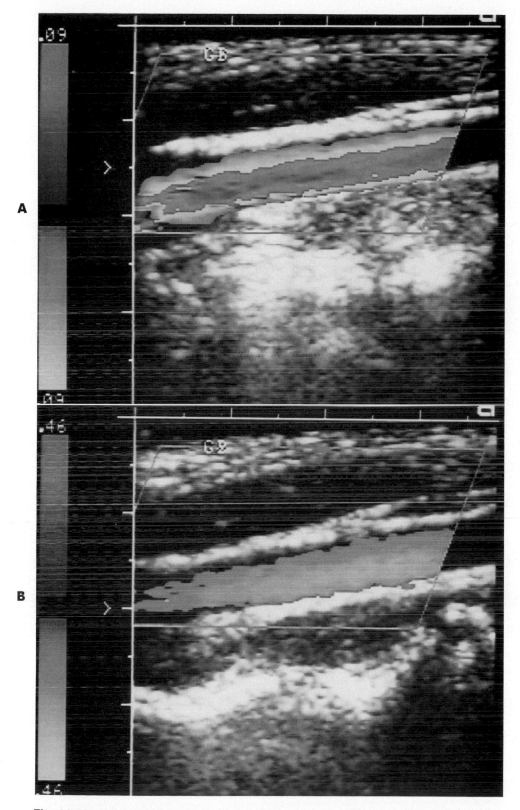

Fig. 14-19. A, Longitudinal view of the carotid artery, color Doppler image. Reversed flow (blue = dark gray) is registered in the central vessel with a low-velocity range (0.09). **B,** Aliasing is no longer displayed when velocity range is increased (0.46).

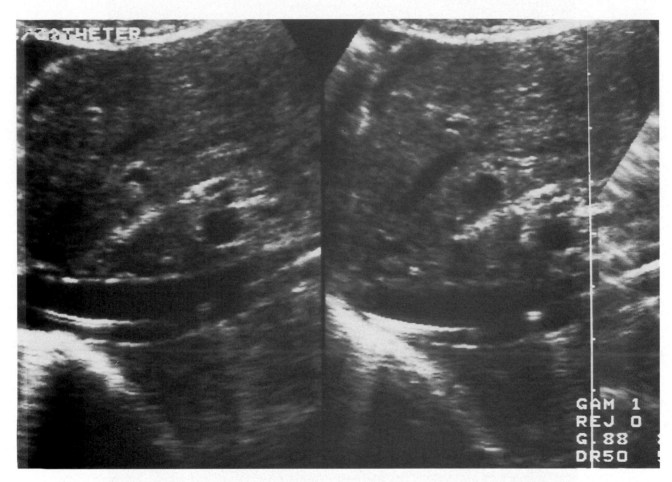

Fig. 14-20. Six-year-old child with acute myelogenous leukemia. Notice the Hickman catheter in the inferior vena cava.

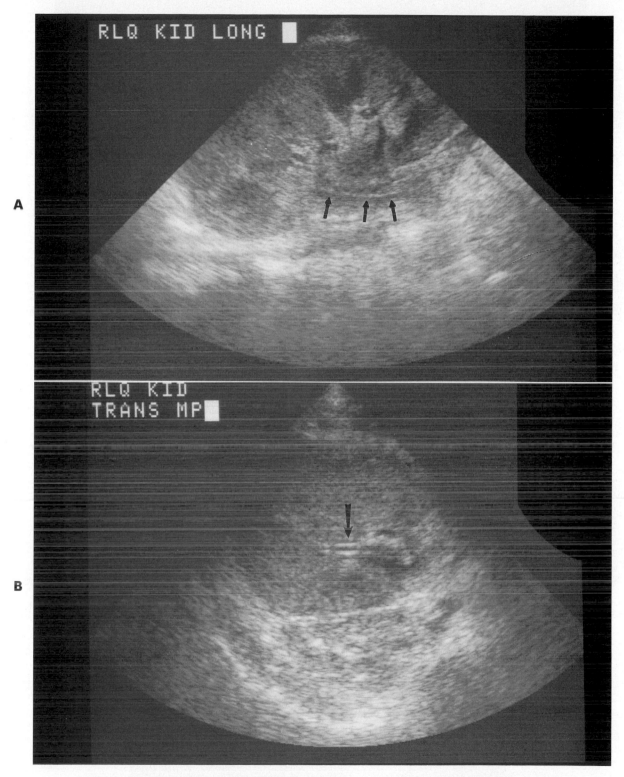

Fig. 14-21. A renal transplant kidney is located in the right iliac fossa. Longitudinal, **A,** and transverse, **B,** views show a ureteral stent, *arrows,* in place.

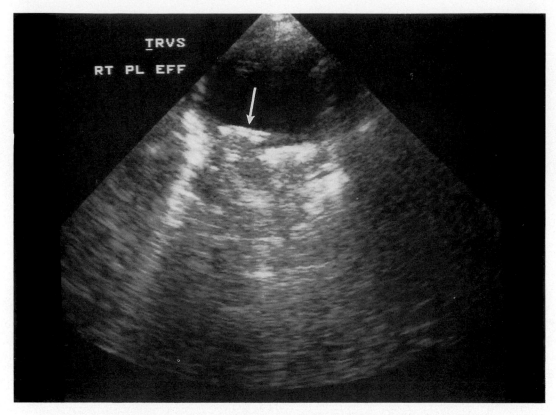

Fig. 14-22. A chest tube, *arrow,* is readily visualized within a large amount of right pleural effusion.

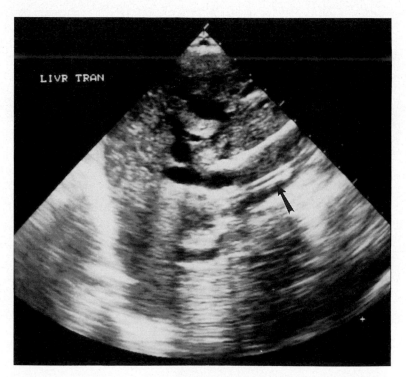

Fig. 14-23. Transverse view showing a biliary stent, *arrow,* in a greatly dilated tumor-filled common bile duct.

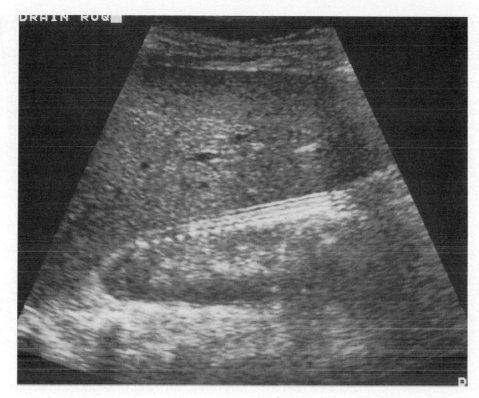

Fig. 14-24. Longitudinal view of the right kidney. A surgical drain is visible in Morrison's pouch.

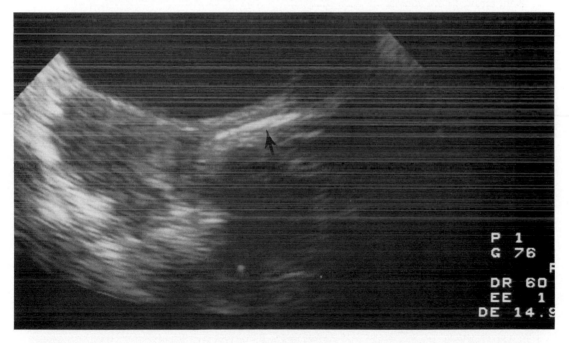

Fig. 14-25. A longitudinal transabdominal pelvic ultrasound scan shows an echogenic tampon, *arrow*, in the vagina.

eign body (Figs. 14-25 to 14-26). A somewhat rare foreign body encountered nowadays is a pessary (Fig. 14-27) (see also Chapter 8).

Cervical cerclages can sometimes be visualized in an obstetric patient as an echogenic suture (see below) on the lips of the cervix. Posterior shadowing is most prominent in the region of the surgical knot.[18] Cerclages are placed as therapy for cervical incompetence.

Intrauterine contraceptive devices (IUD) (see also Chapter 8) are readily visualized on pelvic sonography.

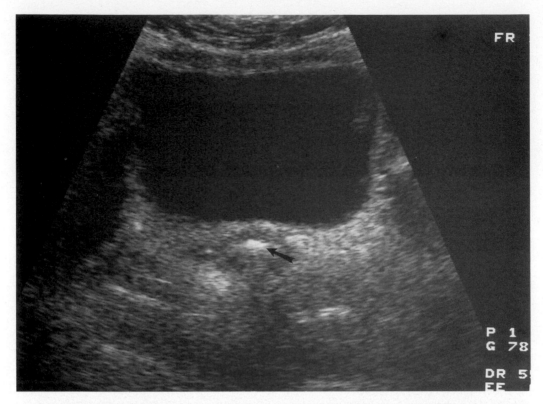

Fig. 14-26. A transverse transabdominal pelvic ultrasound scan shows an echogenic tampon, *arrow,* in the vagina.

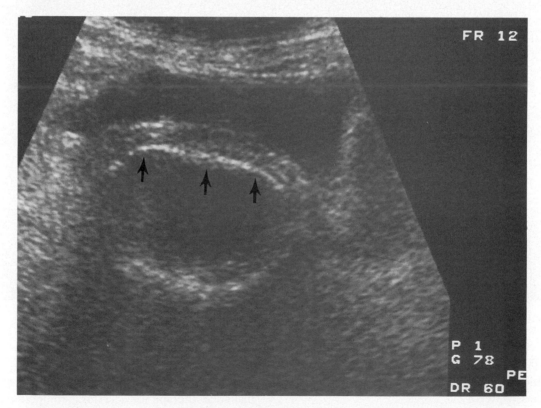

Fig. 14-27. A transverse transabdominal pelvic ultrasound scan shows a pessary, *arrows,* in the vagina of an elderly woman.

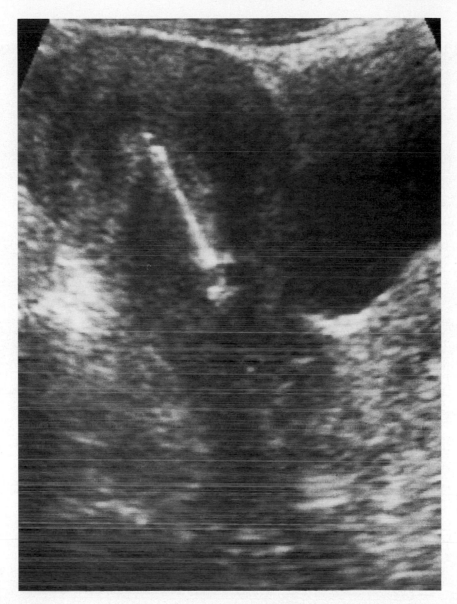

Fig. 14-28. Copper 7 intrauterine device in the endometrial cavity of a middle-aged woman.

They have a somewhat typical morphology and typical posterior acoustic shadowing.[19] It may even be possible to distinguish between various types, though this would be better accomplished by plain film radiography. Ultrasonography is an important tool in localizing an IUD to confirm its continued location in the endometrial canal, especially when the IUD string can no longer be found on physical exam (Figs. 14-28 and 14-29).

Accidental foreign bodies; surgical foreign bodies: sutures, staples, and clips

The acoustic impedances of standard foreign materials (glass particles, wood splinters, and bullet fragments) are different enough from soft tissues to make them readily visible on ultrasonography.[20-21] In fact, ultrasonography may be the most cost-effective method for localizing radiolucent foreign bodies (wood splinters or cactus thorns) in the upper and lower extremities (see also Chapter 3). Most foreign bodies present as a prominent echogenic focus, and they cannot be distinguished from each other.

Metallic objects, however, may produce a characteristic "comet-tail" artifact (see p. 418) (Fig. 14-30). Easily recognizable, the "comet-tail" artifact is a dense continuous echo distal to the foreign body, and it represents a type of reverberation artifact. Surgical sutures, clips, and staples, no matter where in the body, usually have this appearance (Figs. 14-31 and 14-32). Nonetheless, sutures, staple, and clips may be easily overlooked

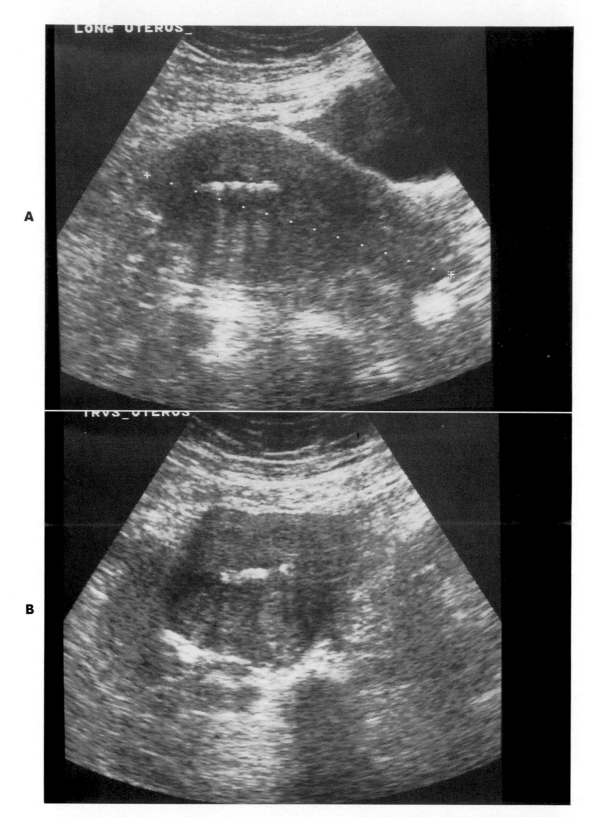

Fig. 14-29. Lippes loop intrauterine device in the uterine cavity of a middle-aged woman. Longitudinal, **A,** and transverse, **B,** views.

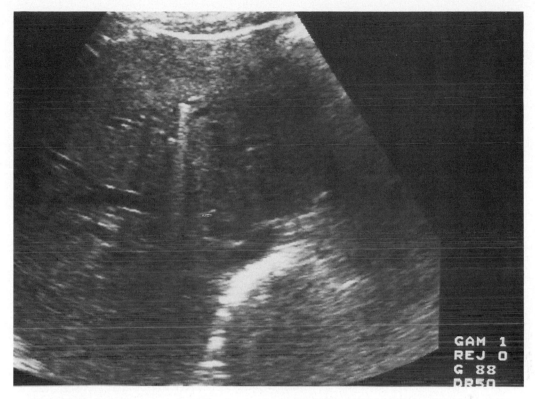

Fig. 14-30. Transverse view of the liver. A bullet fragment is imbedded in the liver of a gunshot-wound victim. Notice the typical "comet-tail" artifact.

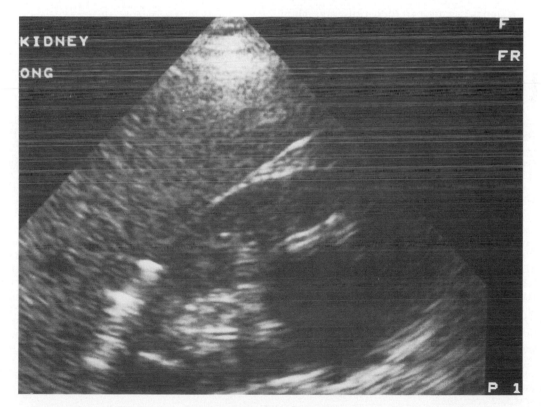

Fig. 14-31. Longitudinal view of the right kidney. Surgical clips are visible along the upper pole of the right kidney. The patient had a partial right adrenalectomy.

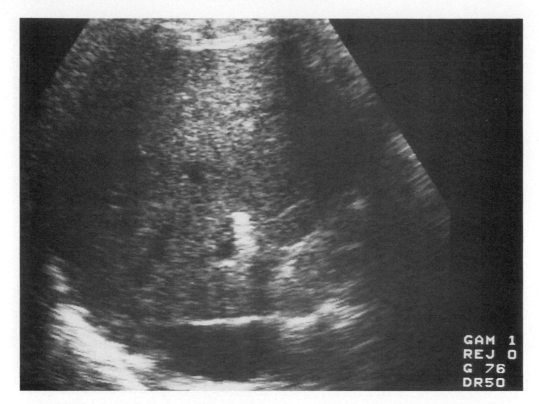

Fig. 14-32. Longitudinal view of the right lobe of the liver. Surgical clips are visible in a patient who had undergone a cholecystectomy.

at sonography if one is not alert to their presence. They may blend in with reverberations and shadowing from surrounding structures, such as the bowel and bone.

REFERENCES

1. Hykes D, Hedrick WR, Starchman DE: *Ultrasound physics and instrumentation,* New York, 1985, Churchill Livingstone.
2. Laing FC: Commonly encountered artifacts in clinical ultrasound, *Semin Ultrasound* 4(1):27-43, 1983.
3. Avruch L, Cooperberg PL: The ring-down artifact, *J Ultrasound Med* 4:21-28, 1985.
4. Shapiro RS, Winsberg F: Comet-tail artifact from cholesterol crystals: observations in the postlithotripsy gallbladder and an in vitro model, *Radiology* 177:153-156, 1990.
5. Cover KL, Slasky BS, Skolnick ML: Sonography of cholesterol in the biliary system, *J Ultrasound Med* 4:647-653, 1985.
6. Middleton WD, Melson GL: Diaphragmatic discontinuity associated with perihepatic ascites: a sonographic refractive artifact, *AJR* 151:709-711, 1988.
7. Bonhof JA, Linhart P: A pseudolesion of the liver caused by rib cartilage in B-mode ultrasonography, *J Ultrasound Med* 4:135-137, 1985.
8. Skwarok DJ, Goiney RC, Cooperberg PL: Hepatic pseudotumors in patients with ascites, *J Ultrasound Med* 5:5-8, 1986.
9. Laing FC, Kurtz AB: The importance of ultrasonic side-lobe artifacts, *Radiology* 145:763-768, 1982.
10. Kremkau FW, Taylor KJW: Artifacts in ultrasound imaging, *J Ultrasound Med* 5:227-237, 1986.
11. Parvey HR, Eisenberg RL, Giyanani V, Krebs CA: Duplex sonography of the portal venous system: pitfalls and limitations, *AJR* 152:765-770, 1989.
12. Gill RW, Kossoff MB, Kossoff G, Griffiths KA: New class of pulsed Doppler US ambiguity at short ranges, *Radiology* 173:272-275, 1989.
13. Pozniak MA, Zagzebski JA, Scanlan KA: Spectral and color Doppler artifacts, *RadioGraphics* 12:35-44, 1992.
14. Mitchell DG, Burns P, Needleman L: Color Doppler artifact in anechoic regions, *J Ultrasound Med* 9:255-260, 1990.
15. Middleton WD, Erickson S, Melson GL: Perivascular color artifact: pathologic significance and appearance on color Doppler US images, *Radiology* 171:647-652, 1989.
16. Reading CC, Charboneau JW, Allison JW, et al: Color and spectral Doppler mirror-image artifact of the subclavian artery, *Radiology* 174:41-42, 1990.
17. Oppenheimer D, Carroll B, Garth K, Parker B: Sonographic localization of neonatal umbilical catheters, *AJR* 138:1025-1032, 1982.
18. Parulekar SG, Kiwi R: Ultrasound evaluation of sutures following cervical cerclage for incompetent cervix uteri, *J Ultrasound Med* 1:223-228, 1982.
19. Callen P, Filly F, Munyer T: Intrauterine contraceptive devices: evaluation by sonography, *AJR* 135:797-800, 1980.
20. Fornage B, Schernberg F: Sonographic diagnosis of foreign bodies of the distal extremities, *AJR* 147:567-569, 1986.
21. Ziskin M, Thickman D, Goldenberg N, et al: The comet tail artifact, *J Ultrasound Med* 1:1, 1982.

15

Artifacts in Computed Tomography

· ·

Evan Charles Unger
Nicholas A. Awad

Artifacts are relatively common in computed tomography (CT). Their recognition and avoidance, where possible, helps prevent the making of diagnostic mistakes and improves the quality of the CT examination. This chapter discusses some of the common artifacts in CT and methods to minimize their effects.

RANDOM NOISE

Random noise is present in all CT images, at least to some extent. The CT information in the images is created by the photons registered by the detectors in the CT gantry.[1-3] Because of the CT reconstruction process, random noise becomes correlated in the final image and is presented as such[4] (Fig. 15-1). Although advances in technology have improved the efficiency of detection of photons by the CT detectors, there must still be abundant photons incident on the detectors to generate images with sufficient signal-to-noise ratios for acceptable image quality.

The number of photons received by the detector varies directly with the number of photons incident on the patient. Increasing the milliampere-seconds (mAs) will increase the number of photons received by the detectors and hence will improve image quality by increasing the signal-to-noise ratio; likewise, this will increase radiation dose to the patient. A smaller field of view and a smaller slice thickness will lead to images with a lower signal-to-noise ratio unless the number of milliampere-seconds is increased accordingly in the CT scanner. Image noise and image quality then are always a trade-off between patient radiation dose and tube cooling. The lowest number of milliampere-seconds possible that will still produce diagnostically acceptable CT images should be used.

LINEAR ARTIFACTS

Linear ("geometric") artifacts occur because, although the CT reconstruction algorithms assume an infinite number of views, in actual fact the number of views or sample points used to generate a working image is limited. Linear artifacts are seen at the edges of tissues with different densities, such as the dome of the liver and the lung bases. These linear artifacts present as streaks on the CT images at the margins of opposing structures with greatly different densities. Current-generation CT scanners have much less problem with these artifacts because the number of detectors (number of views) has increased relative to prior-generation CT scanners, and the reconstruction algorithms have also been improved.

BEAM-HARDENING ARTIFACT

A beam-hardening artifact (Fig. 15-2) occurs because the x-ray beam in CT scanners is not monochromatic. The x-ray beam is composed of multispectral energies of x-ray photons. The lower-energy photons are preferentially attenuated as they enter the patient. The preferential attenuation of lower-energy photons is even more severe as the x-ray beam passes through regions of very high density, such as bone or even more so in metal. Another manifestation of beam hardening is so-called cupping, which refers to an apparent decrease in

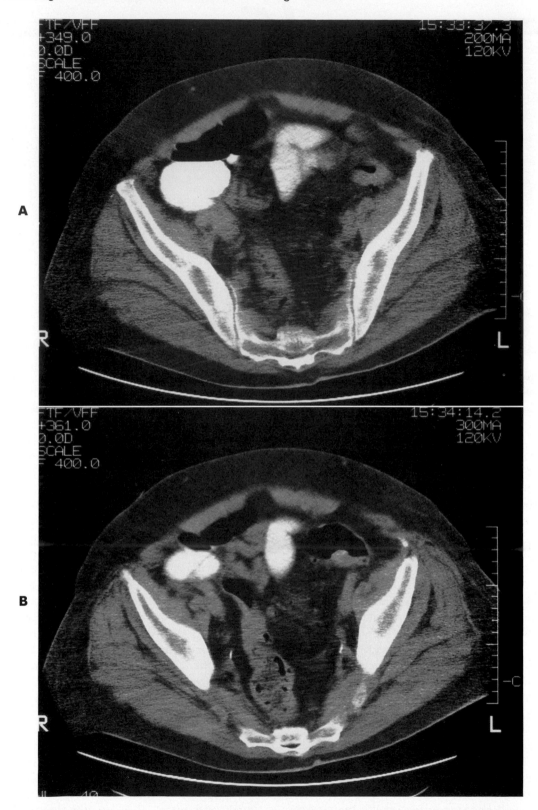

Fig. 15-1. Random noise. **A,** Computed tomographic (CT) scan of obese patient performed at 200 mA and 120 kVp is grainy. The image appears noisy, and there is also evidence of beam-hardening artifact. **B,** Image of same patient at a 10 mm lower position performed with 300 mA, also at 120 kVp. The image quality is improved because of higher signal-to-noise ratio. The increased milliamperes used in the CT acquisition resulted in a greater yield of x-ray photons striking the detectors.

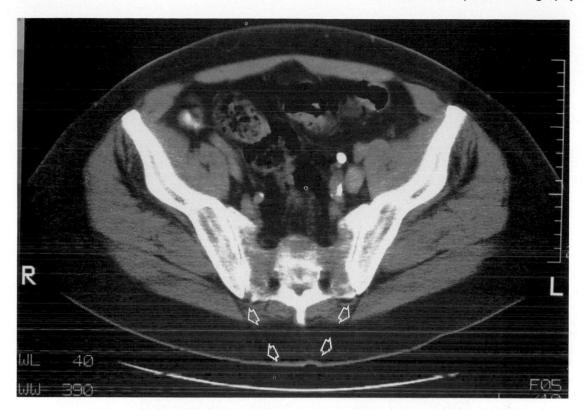

Fig. 15-2. Linear ("geometric") and beam-hardening artifacts. CT scan of obese patient shows linear low-density artifact emanating from the posterior iliac bones laterally, *arrows*. The artifact is produced by beam hardening with attenuation of the x-ray photons as they pass through the long axis of the iliac bone.

density of the scanned object in the center of the object as opposed to the periphery.[5] For example, a phantom of homogeneous high density, when scanned by CT, will show a characteristic decrease in density as measured by Hounsfield units in the center of the phantom compared to the periphery.[6]

Current-generation scanners contain algorithms to compensate for cupping. Compensation, however, is still incomplete and cupping may be present to some extent. Clinically, cupping is present in CT images of the brain where a measurement of brain density in the center of the brain may be artifactually lower than the true value secondary to cupping.

The other partial solution to cupping and beam-hardening artifact is to filter the x-ray beam highly to remove much of the spectrum of lower-energy photons, a solution already implemented by CT manufacturers. But even in current-generation CT scanners, the x-ray beam is not monochromatic but multispectral, and some degree of artifact remains because of beam hardening and cupping.

The dynamic range of the scanner corresponds to the range of different attenuation values or densities that a scanner will recognize in its reconstruction process. Current-generation scanners have extended dynamic range compared to older-generation CT scanners, and this has helped to decrease problems from the beam-hardening artifact. Despite increased dynamic range and improved reconstruction algorithms, the beam-hardening artifact is still problematic in regions of very high density, particularly in scans of patients with metal devices.[6-9]

The artifactual attenuation of an object is related to its electron density; the greater the electron density of the object, the greater will be its attenuation. Materials with lower x-ray attenuation coefficients have less artifact. Thus, in general, the artifact from plastic is the least, titanium is somewhat more, whereas stainless steel and cobalt-chromium alloy have the largest beam-hardening artifacts.

The degree of artifact from a metallic object is directly related to the path length of the photons through the metal object; that is, the longer the path length though the object, the greater the artifact will be and the greater the attenuation of the structure.[10,11] An example of minimal beam-hardening artifact caused by a metallic implanted device is shown in Fig. 15-3. In a patient in whom it is possible to select the type of implants, use of lower x-ray attenuation materials will help to minimize artifact and improve quality of follow-up CT

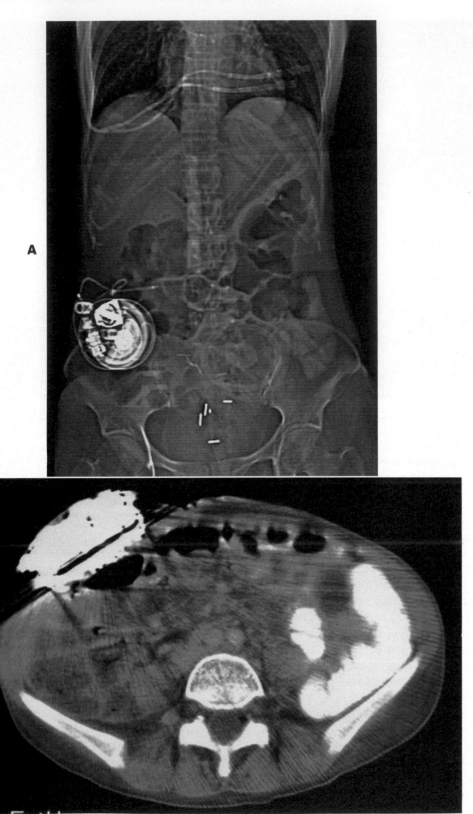

Fig. 15-3. Chemotherapy infusion pump. **A,** CT scan of abdomen and pelvis in a cancer patient shows a chemotherapy infusion pump with an intraperitoneal infusion catheter. **B,** CT image through the infusion pump shows slight image degradation because of beam-hardening artifact. One can improve image quality by increasing the milliampere-seconds.

examinations. Usually, however, we do not have the option of changing or preselecting the kind of material in an implanted device, and we are left with strategies of decreasing the artifact by modifying our CT technique.

In examinations of the head and neck, dental fillings are commonly a source of seriously degrading spray artifacts. The solution in this case is to perform the CT exam with two different degrees of angulation. The first set of images is acquired in the straight axial plane and then a second, limited set of images is acquired in a 15 to 20 degree–angled plane such that the area affected by artifact on the axial images is not obscured by artifact on the second set of angled images. Increasing the number of milliampere-seconds helps to decrease the artifact at a cost of increased radiation dose to the patient.

In other parts of the body where it is not possible to change the angulation of the gantry, another practical approach to decreasing the deleterious effects of the beam-hardening artifact is to use multiplanar reformatting.[7,8] This has been shown to be particularly useful in the assessment of pelvic fractures in patients with hip prostheses. The reformatted images are generally much less degraded by the beam-hardening artifact.[7,8] It also may be helpful to increase the number of milliampere-seconds when one is imaging patients with metal prostheses as shown in Fig. 15-4.

MOTION ARTIFACTS

Motion artifacts can have devastating effects on image quality and degrade studies to such an extent they are uninterpretable. More subtle degrees of motion degradation may not be readily appreciable and create sources of diagnostic error. Motion artifacts on CT scans are generally seen as streaks in the direction of the motion. These artifacts have been the primary impetus for the development of ultrafast CT scanners such as the Imatron (now Picker Fastrac, Picker International, Highland Heights, Ohio).

The most common source of motion artifact is patient motion (Fig. 15-5). The solutions to this are improved patient preparation, patient immobilization, and patient sedation when necessary. Selecting a faster scan speed, possibly at the cost of a decreased number of views, can be another solution to patient motion, albeit at the cost of some degradation in image quality when the number of views is decreased.

Motion artifact is usually seen as a streak or starburst

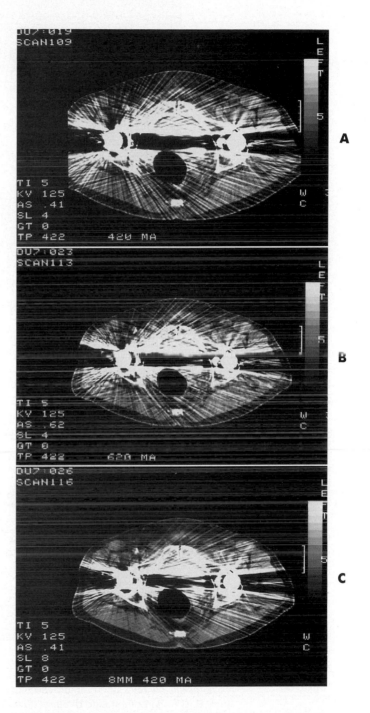

Fig. 15-4. Beam-hardening artifact. CT scans acquired over 5 seconds, each performed at different slice thicknesses and milliampere-second settings, show the dependence of beam-hardening artifact on slice thickness and milliampere-second setting. **A,** CT scan through hips in a patient with bilateral total hip prothesis. Image acquired with a 4 mm slice at 420 mA shows considerable degradation of image quality by beam-hardening artifact. **B,** Repeat scan at same level as in **A** at 620 mA shows slight decrease in artifact at higher milliampere setting. **C,** CT scan at same position as in **A.** It was acquired with an 8 mm slice thickness at 420 mA and shows improvement in image quality, that is, reduction in beam-hardening artifact compared to that in **A** and **B.**

Continued.

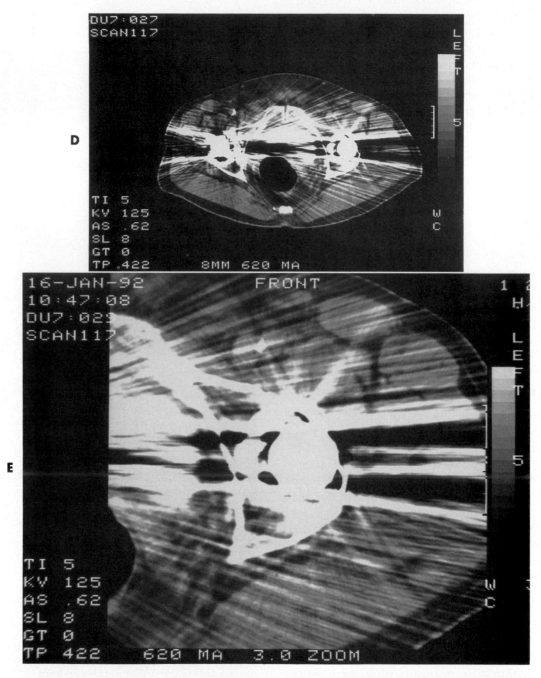

Fig. 15-4, cont'd.   D, Repeat scan at same plane as in **A** with an 8 mm slice thickness at 620 mA shows further improvement in image quality with reduction in artifact. The higher milliampere-second setting improved signal-to-noise and decreased beam-hardening artifact. **E,** CT scan of left side of hip acquired with 3 × Zoom, 8 mm slice thickness, and 620 mA shows essentially the same artifact as in **D.** Reduction in artifact could be obtained by multiplanar reformatting.

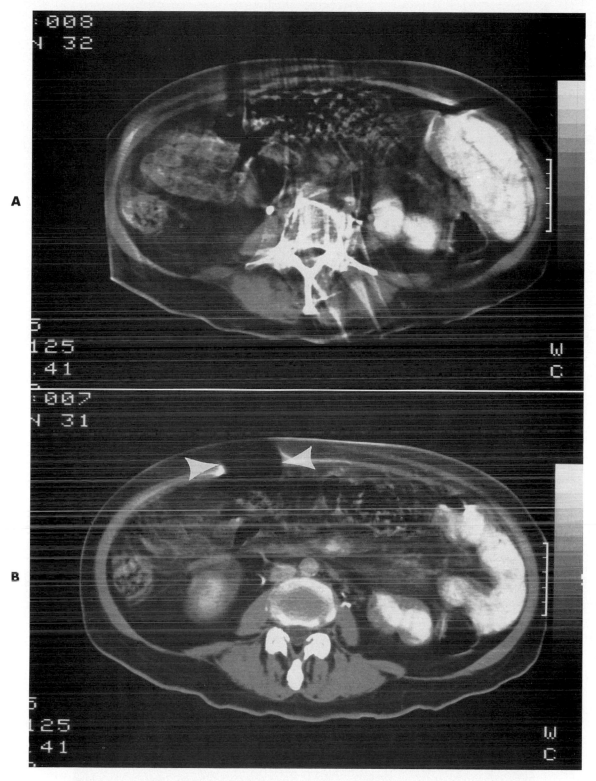

Fig. 15-5. Motion artifact. **A,** CT image of the lower abdomen in an uncooperative trauma patient is degraded by motion artifact. **B,** Image in same patient shows artifact in anterior abdomen, *arrowheads,* that is probably attributable to respiration and resultant movement of bowel.

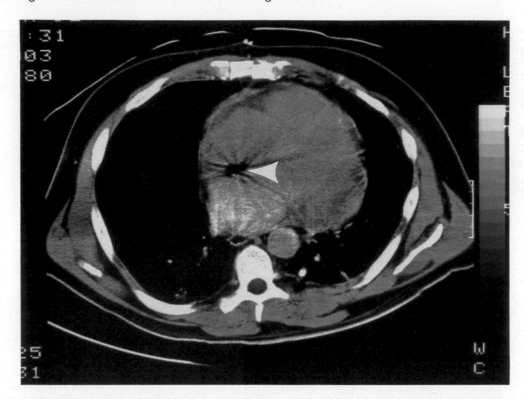

Fig. 15-6. Unusual artifact in a heart transplant patient. In heart transplantation the donor heart is sutured to the atria. This patient is approximately 1 week after operation and a small gas collection has presumably been left at the anastomotic site of the atria to the donor heart. The artifact, *arrowhead,* surrounding the small pocket of gas is probably caused by motion during the CT acquisition as well as possible CT dynamic range effects.

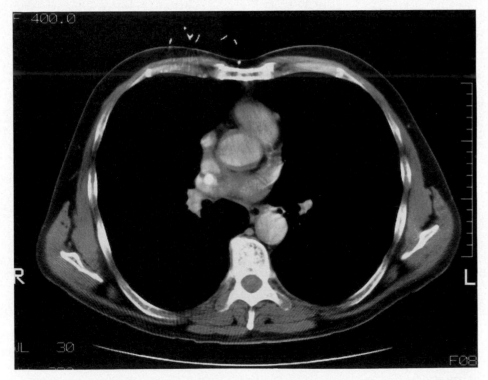

Fig. 15-7. Motion artifact in the ascending aorta might be misconstrued as an aortic dissection. This image was produced on a Toshiba TCT 900S scanner with a scan time of 1 second.

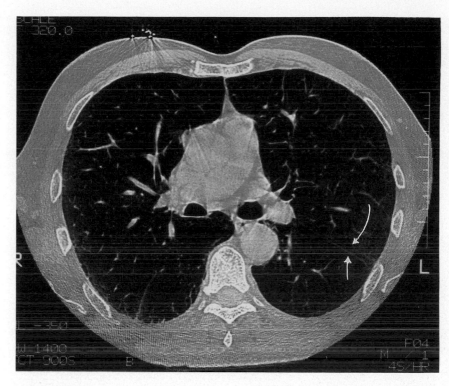

Fig. 15-8. Double-fissure sign. Notice the apparent double fissure, *arrows,* on the left. This is caused by transmitted cardiac motion during scanning.

in appearance and occurs where there are high or low density interfaces, for example, at the lung bases, or where there is gas in the bowel (Fig. 15-5). Motion artifact occurs when the CT image has acquired information from different views. This information does not add up correctly during the backprojection process, producing a streak or starburst superimposed on the image. Artifacts can occur even in the absence of movement. If there are regions in the object being imaged that have extremely high or extremely low attenuation values, nonlinearities in the reconstruction process may create motion artifacts.

Particularly troublesome artifacts result where there are moving structures containing very high or very low densities. Patient movement or organ motion combined with a focal interface of gas and tissue or gas and fluid may create very unusual artifacts (Fig. 15-6). Even with high-speed, fourth-generation scanners, motion artifacts may still create potential sources of diagnostic error.[12] In one study of CT scans of the thoracic aorta performed on a Siemens Somatom Plus scanner (1-second scan time), 10% of unenhanced and 18% of contrast-enhanced scans showed an artifact in the ascending aorta, which might be misconstrued to represent aortic dissection.[12] The artifact was seen as a linear low-density stripe through the ascending aorta and was visible on only one or two slices.

This same artifact was not visible on scans taken on a slower Siemens DRH scanner (4-second scan time) or a GE Highlight Quick Scanner (1.2-second scan time).[12] Apparently, the aortic motion occurred over a period of time coinciding with the scan time on the Somatom Plus scanner to produce the artifact. Differences in reconstruction algorithms may also account for the difference seen in artifacts between the different scanners despite relatively similar scan times (Fig. 15-7).

Cardiac motion has been reported to produce an artifact called the "double-fissure sign."[13] This is visible on high-resolution lung scans (such as 1.5 mm thick) as a double fissure in the lung (Fig. 15-8). Review of scans from 42 patients demonstrated that the double fissure occurred most frequently at the base of the left lung. However, in cases where the heart was central or to the right of midline, the artifact was noted on the right side.[13]

Slight respiratory motion has been attributed to cause motion artifacts that simulate bronchiectasis.[14] In one study of 475 chest scans taken on a Picker 1200SX scanner operating at scan times of 2.17 or 3.3 seconds, motion artifacts simulating bronchiectasis were seen in 20 patients. These artifacts were attributed to slight respiratory motion in 17 patients and to cardiac motion in 3 patients. The artifacts attributable to respiration were eliminated by better coordination of patient respiration and breath holding with the scanning. The artifacts attributable to cardiac motion were present on 2 or 5 mm

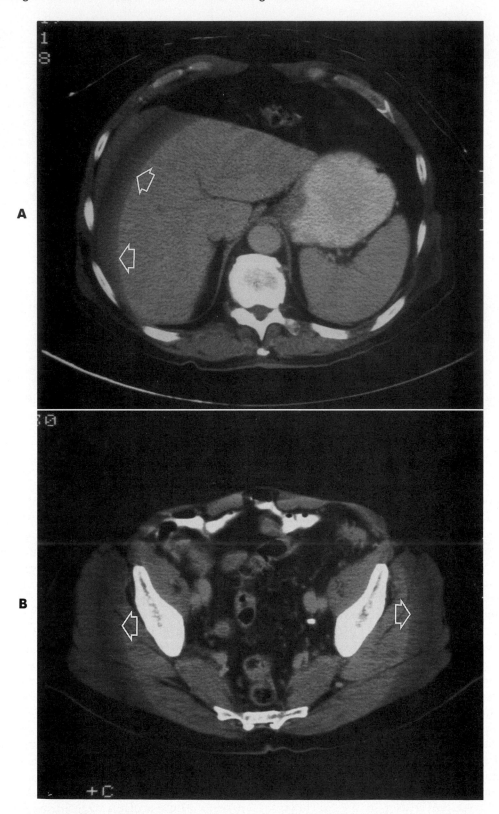

Fig. 15-9. Ring artifact. **A,** CT image through upper abdomen shows characteristic ring artifact, *arrows,* which might in some cases be misconstrued to represent ascites about the liver. **B,** CT scan in same patient acquired through the pelvis shows ring artifact bilaterally, *arrows,* through the buttocks. This is caused by a faulty detector that may be either miscalibrated or broken.

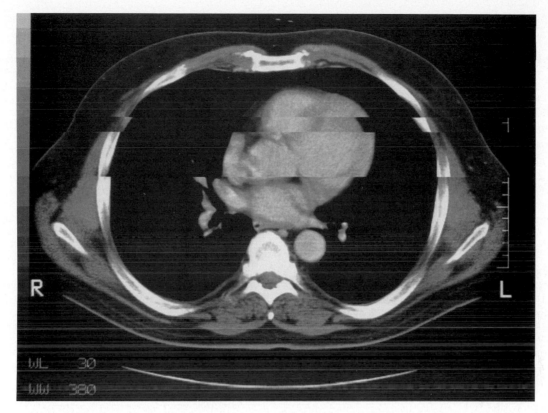

Fig. 15-10. Exuberant filming artifact. This artifact through the heart was produced by the technologist's filming too rapidly, such that the resulting image was produced from a composite of the previous and following images.

thick scans but disappeared on 10 mm thick scans.

Motion artifacts have also been noted on scans taken for CT pelvimetry.[15] These artifacts have appeared as abnormalities in fetal osseous anatomy visible on the scout images and have been attributed to fetal motion occurring during scan acquisition of the scout images. In the same study, the investigators also evaluated a phantom wherein they moved a bone along the long axis of the scanner and rotationally within the scanner. The type of artifact varied with the direction of the motion.

PARTIAL-VOLUME ARTIFACT

Partial-volume artifacts are very common for structures that are of smaller diameter than the slice thickness. Partial-volume averaging can obscure the true nature of a lesion and may cause some objects, such as the diaphragm at the lung base, to spuriously appear to have a higher CT density than is actually the case. Small cysts in the liver and kidney are particularly prone to suffer from this phenomenon.

RING ARTIFACT

The most common source of ring artifact is a faulty detector.[16] The detector may be either out of calibration or broken. The resulting ring artifacts present as crescent-shaped areas of low density, usually at the periphery of the image. Ring artifacts may superficially mimic a true diagnostic finding. It is easy, however, to recognize ring artifacts, because they appear on serial images and do not correspond to known anatomic structures (Fig. 15-9).

ROUND CT STATIC ARTIFACTS AND OTHER FILM-RELATED ARTIFACTS

Round CT film static artifacts are seen as spotlike or smudgelike low densities on film.[17] They are created by static electric discharges at points of contact between film and cassettes. These artifacts are usually produced during low-humidity midwinter conditions and present as low densities on CT films. They may be misconstrued to represent a true pathologic condition. Recognition of the potential for these artifacts to occur usually is enough to prevent a misdiagnosis. Review of the CT images on the viewing console should be sufficient to prove that the abnormality noted on the film is not a true finding and is an artifact that arose during the filming of the CT images. Sometimes, film-related artifacts can be quite bizarre, as shown in Fig. 15-10. This artifact was created by the technologist doing too rapid filming with a laser printer, thereby accidentally forming a composite picture with elements from two or more CT images.

CONCLUSIONS

There are many kinds of CT artifacts. They are a common problem, but they can be ameliorated or eliminated by understanding their causes and effects. This in turn leads to improved CT image quality and better patient diagnostic accuracy.

REFERENCES

1. Brooks RA: Comparative evaluation of CT scanner technology. In Medical Physics Monograph No. 6: *Medical physics of CT and ultrasound: tissue imaging and characterization,* American Institute of Physics, 335 E. 45 St., New York, NY 10017, pp 53-69, 1980.
2. Hendee WR: *The physical principals of computed tomography,* Boston, 1983, Little, Brown & Co.
3. Hounsfield, GN: Computerized transverse axial scanning (tomography): Part I. Description of system, *Br J Radiol* 46:1016-1022, 1973.
4. Hansen KM, Boyd DP: The characteristics of computed tomographic reconstruction noise and their effect on detectability, *IEEE Trans Nucl Sci* 25:160, 1978.
5. Curry TS, Dowdey JE, Murry RC: Computed tomography. In *Christensen's physics of diagnostic radiology,* Philadelphia, 1990, Lea & Febiger, p 319.
6. Moström U, Ytterbergh C: Artifacts in computed tomography of the posterior fossa: a comparative phantom study, *J Comput Assist Tomogr* 10(4):560-566, 1986.
7. Fishman EK, Magid D, Robertson DD, et al: Metallic hip implants: CT with multiplanar reconstruction, *Radiology* 160:675-681, 1986.
8. Robertson DD, Weiss PJ, Fishman EK, et al: Evaluation of CT techniques for reducing artifacts in the presence of metallic orthopedic implants, *J Comput Assist Tomogr* 12(2):236-241, 1988.
9. O'Donnell CJ, Yong K, Joplin GF: Assessment of computed tomographic artifact in the pituitary fossa following needle implantation of radioactive rods, *Clin Radiol* 40:154-157, 1989.
10. Kalender WA, Hebel R, Ebersberger J: Reduction of CT artifacts caused by metallic implants, *Radiology* 164(2):576-577, 1987.
11. Silverman PM, Spicer LD, McKinney R Jr, et al: Computed tomographic evaluation of surgical clip artifact: tissue phantom and experimental animal assessment, *Computerized Radiol* 10(1):37-40, 1986.
12. Burns MA, Molina PL, Gutierrez FR, et al: Motion artifact simulating aortic dissection on CT, *AJR* 157:465-467, 1991.
13. Mayo JR, Muller NL, Henkelman RM: The double-fissure sign: a motion artifact on thin-section CT scans, *Radiology* 165:580-581, 1987.
14. Tarver RD, Conces DJ, Godwin JD: Motion artifacts on CT simulate bronchiectasis, *AJR* 151:1117-1119, 1988.
15. Brody AS, Saks BJ, Field DR, et al: Artifacts seen during CT pelvimetry: implications for digital systems with scanning beams, *Radiology* 160:269-271, 1986.
16. Curry TS, Dowdey JE, Murry RC: Computed tomography. In *Christensen's physics of diagnostic radiology,* Philadelphia, 1990, Lea & Febiger, p 320.
17. Wilbur AC, Kriz RJ: Round CT film static artifacts: simulation of focal pathology, *J Comput Assist Tomogr* 13(4):730-731, 1989.

16

Artifacts in Magnetic Resonance Imaging

Evan Charles Unger
Ammar Darkazanli
Nicholas A. Awad

Artifacts in magnetic resonance imaging (MRI) are complex and fascinating. They are both partly under our control and partly beyond our control.[1,2] By understanding the genesis of MRI artifacts, we can minimize their deleterious effects on image quality and diagnostic information. To understand these artifacts it is necessary to have a basic understanding of magnetic resonance imaging. Accordingly, this chapter will first review the fundamentals of magnetic resonance (MR). It will explain how artifacts are related to the principles underlying MR and show how this information can be used to minimize these artifacts.

FUNDAMENTALS

MR images are made by the imposition of radiofrequency and gradient pulses upon a static main magnetic field.[3] It is important to ensure homogeneity of the main magnetic field. Typical specifications on a current-generation, superconducting, high–field strength magnet are in the order of a few parts per million (ppm). The stable, homogeneous magnetic field enables the resonant nuclei (such as water protons) to spin freely and reflect their intrinsic properties upon excitation. If the magnetic field is inhomogeneous, the spinning protons will be magnetically disturbed. Magnetic inhomogeneity will cause the spins to precess faster or slower than they are supposed to and to dephase more rapidly, resulting in signal misregistration and decrease in signal intensity.

The radiofrequency pulses that are applied to the object (such as the patient) within the magnetic field excite the spinning protons.[3] The excited protons act as a spinning magnet and induce a current signal in a receiver coil surrounding the imaging subject. The slice gradient as well as the radiofrequency pulses excite a thin slice of the object. The read gradient superimposed on the static magnetic field causes spins (along the frequency direction) to impart signals of unique frequency information. Repeating the experiment with changing phase-encoding gradients assigns unique phase information to spins along the phase-encoding direction.

To make an MR image, a device must collect the signals with the varying phase and frequency information and then process them into images.[3] In the process of receiving these signals with different phase and frequency signatures many possibilities for creating artifacts arise. As MR images are acquired, the phase and frequency information is projected onto the phase and frequency axes. By paying close attention to the pattern of the artifact on the axes, one can often determine the source of an artifact. The artifacts have various influences on image quality and can have severe diagnostic effects.[1,2] One can minimize some of these artifacts by changing MR parameters or by repeating the imaging sequence, allowing the physician to work around the artifact.

CHEMICAL SHIFT

Chemical-shift artifacts are some of the most common artifacts and are present on most MR images to some extent.[4-7] Examples of chemical-shift artifact are shown in Figs. 16-1 to 16-3. Chemical-shift artifacts are commonly seen at the interface of fat and soft tissue and can

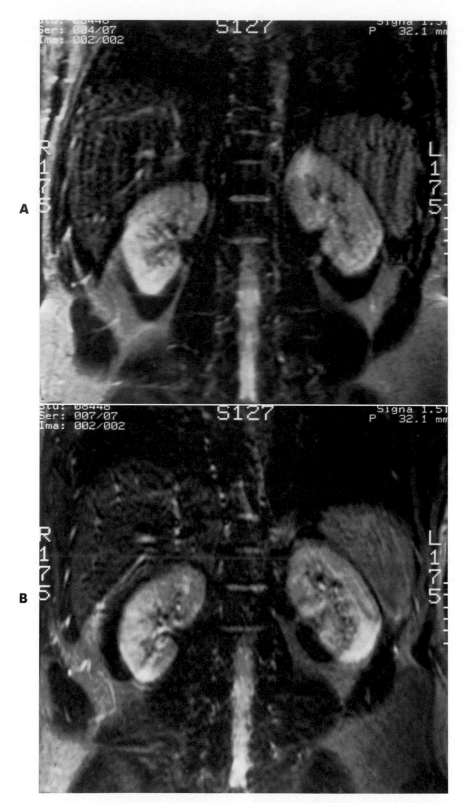

Fig. 16-1. Orientation of chemical shift artifact. **A,** T_2-weighted magnetic resonance image acquired at 1.5 tesla depicts chemical shift artifact at the interfaces of tissues containing varying concentrations of fat and water (in this case kidney and surrounding perirenal fat). The direction of the artifact is along the frequency-encoding axis and is most apparent as a band of low signal intensity inferior to the kidneys at the interface of each kidney with the perirenal fat. **B,** A second T_2-weighted image shows how switching the direction of the phase and frequency-encoding gradients cause the artifact to rotate by 90 degrees. Now the band of low signal intensity is best seen lateral to the right kidney and medial to the left kidney.

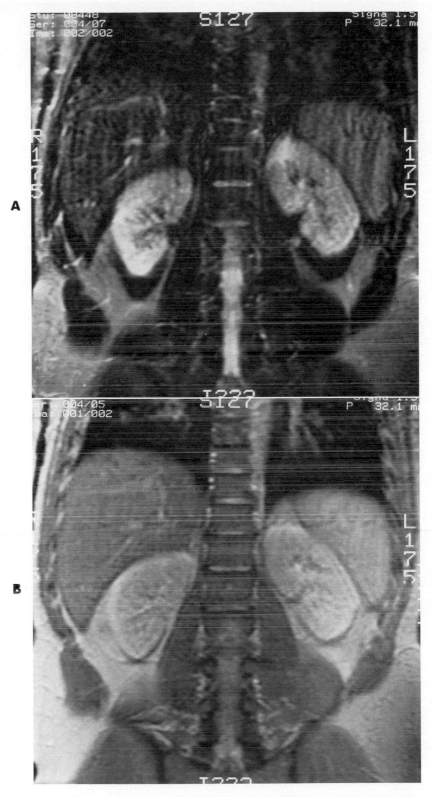

Fig. 16-2. Variation in chemical shift artifact with bandwidth. **A,** Chemical shift artifact at a low bandwidth of 4 kHz, on a spin-echo pulse sequence. The artifact is prominent on the narrow bandwidth image. **B,** Image from a wide bandwidth pulse sequence of 32 kHz (other imaging parameters held the same as in **A**) shows a reduction in chemical shift artifact.

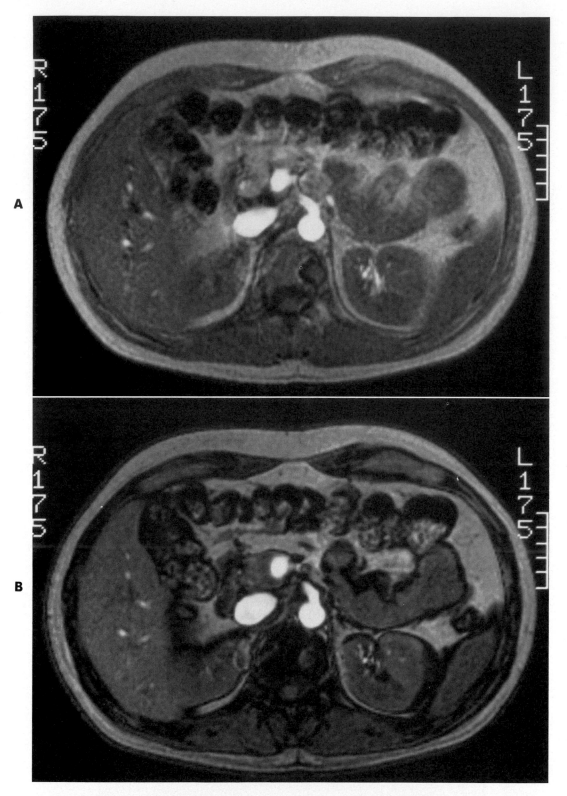

Fig. 16-3. Chemical shift artifact versus TE (echo time) on gradient-echo pulse sequences. **A,** Turbo Grass Gradient echo image from 1.5-tesla magnet at an echo time of 4.3 msec. Water and fat are in phase. **B,** Turbo Grass Gradient echo image using TE of 2.2 msec. Fat and water are out of phase and chemical shift artifact is shown at fat-water interface. Although **B** has increased chemical shift artifact relative to **A,** the shorter echo time image also has increased signal-to-noise ratio.

create diagnostic problems. In one report, chemical-shift artifact even led to a misdiagnosis of aortic dissection.[8] Chemical-shift artifacts arise because of the difference in resonant frequency between fat and water spins. Chemical shift is most pronounced when protons in free water are immediately adjacent to protons in fat. A difference of about 3.3 ppm has been measured between the precessional frequencies of fat and water. Parts per million is a method of normalizing frequency shifts; 3.3 ppm corresponds to a difference in precessional frequency of 3.3 hertz (Hz) per megahertz (MHz). A 1-tesla magnetic field causes spins to precess at about 42.6 MHz. This means there is a difference in precessional frequency of about 140 Hz per tesla. In other words, at 1.0 tesla the protons attached to a fatty molecule precess about 140 times per second slower than the protons in free water as they spin. The difference between fat and water frequencies is therefore field-strength dependent. For example, the difference between 0.1 tesla and 1.0 tesla precessional frequencies is that the latter is tenfold higher.

The frequency shift, however, is fixed at a given field strength and independent of the pulse sequence played. The effects of this frequency shift on image formation can, fortunately, be changed to lessen image degradation. The effect of the chemical shift on MR images can be illustrated with the following numerical example. Assume there is an image with a matrix of 256 × 256 on a 1.5-tesla scanner. Assume also a bandwidth of 25.6 kHz is used. This is actually the width of the image in hertz, and it implies a resolution of 100 Hz per pixel. The frequency shift is approximately 210 Hz between fat and water at this field strength. Therefore, if one chooses the resonant frequency to be that of water when prescanning, the fat signal will be misregistered by 2 pixels toward the direction of the lower frequency with respect to the actual signal (frequency shift − 210 Hz/100 Hz per pixel corresponds to a 2-pixel shift). If there is a field of view of 25 cm, there will be a shift of about 2 mm of the fat signal; this may disturb the diagnostic quality of the image. On the other hand, if the bandwidth is double to 51.2 kHz, the shift in signal will be less than 1 pixel (less than 1 mm for the same image). On the other hand, narrowing the bandwidth to about a 6.4 kHz will result in a shift of 8 pixels (almost 8 mm, which would probably be intolerable). However, wide bandwidth increases the power of the noise in the spectrum and therefore reduces the signal-to-noise ratio.

One can minimize chemical shift (see Fig. 16-2), then, by using wide-bandwidth pulse sequences, and it will be increased by using narrow-bandwidth pulse sequences. Were it a perfect world, one could use narrow-bandwidth pulse sequences more often to improve the signal-to-noise ratio, but chemical-shift artifact limits the use of narrow-bandwidth pulse sequences in parts of the body where there are high concentrations of both fat and water. In the brain, where there is little fat, narrow-bandwidth pulse sequences can be applied without as many problems with chemical-shift artifacts as in other parts of the body. Narrow-bandwidth pulse sequences are used routinely in the brain to increase the signal-to-noise ratio on the second-echo T_2-weighted images (T_2 is spin-spin, or transverse, relaxation time).

As shown in Fig. 16-1, chemical-shift artifact is usually projected onto the frequency-encoding axis and not onto the phase-encoding axis. One can switch this direction by changing the directions of the phase- and frequency-encoding axes. If need be, this may even be used for patient diagnosis. For example, a hematoma may appear bright, and so may a lipoma. By acquiring two sets of images, it is possible to see the direction of the chemical-shift artifact switch and to determine whether you are dealing with hemorrhage or fat. A lipoma will manifest a chemical-shift artifact along its margins in the direction of the frequency-encoding axis, whereas a hemorrhage will not (unless the hemorrhage is surrounded by fat). (Another way of differentiating between fat and hemorrhage is by using a fat saturation sequence or a short tau ('relaxation time') inversion recovery (STIR) pulse sequence with the appropriate inversion pulse, where the fat will appear dark and the subacute hemorrhage bright.)

The degree of chemical-shift artifact varies inversely with the bandwidth (Fig. 16-2). Narrow-bandwidth pulse sequences produce images with much more chemical-shift artifact than wide-bandwidth pulse sequences. On gradient-echo pulse sequences (Fig. 16-3), echo time (TE) as well as bandwidth affect the chemical shift. Like spin echo pulse sequences, narrow-bandwidth pulse sequences have more chemical-shift artifacts. Echo time, however, affects chemical shift in a cyclic way on gradient-echo images.

Fig. 16-4 shows the signal collected from a voxel (volume element) that contains 50% fat and 50% water. The fat was assumed to have a 20 msec T_2^* (free induction decay constant, dependent on both the physicochemical nature of tissue and any magnetic field inhomogeneities present) and the water to have a 60 msec T_2^*. The fat and water spins are cycling in and out of phase affecting chemical shift. The cycling time in which fat and water spins precess in and out of phase is field-strength dependent and is shorter at higher field strengths. At 1.5 tesla the first fat/water phase point is about 4.3 msec, and at 0.5 tesla the first fat/water phase point is about 13 msec. The cycling period is about 4.3 msec for 1.5 tesla magnets and 13 msec for 0.5 tesla scanners. Therefore in-phase images and out-of-phase images can be obtained when one chooses the appropriate echo time. Representative gradient-echo images depicting the relationship between chemical shift and

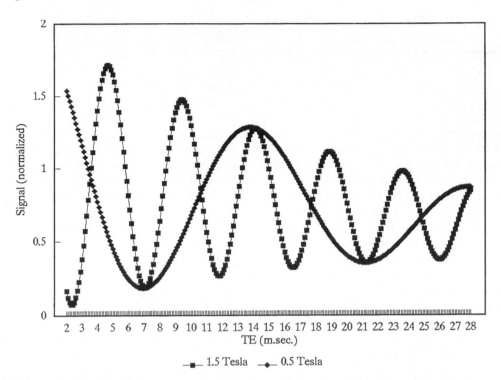

Fig. 16-4. Simulation of the signal intensity produced by a voxel (volume element) containing 50% water and 50% fat. Cycling is apparent in collected signal versus echo time. The period of cycling is field dependent and shorter at higher field strength.

echo times are shown in Fig. 16-3. As shown in these images, the chemical-shift artifact is minimum at in-phase points and greatest at fat/water out-of-phase points.

To minimize artifact from chemical shift, one must select the bandwidth carefully. From the above numerical example, it was noted that the chemical shift was 2 pixels (in case of the 25.6 kHz bandwidth). This implies the artifact will be more than 2 mm should there be a field of view of 25 cm. If the field of view is halved, the artifact will be spread over 1 mm. Thus smaller field of view images may be selected to minimize the area affected by chemical-shift artifact. However, small field-of-view imaging can introduce wraparound artifact (see p. 471).

On gradient-echo pulse sequences if chemical-shift artifact is a problem, an echo time at an in-phase point for fat and water spins may be selected. One can achieve this by either reducing the echo time to a shorter in-phase point or by increasing the echo time to a longer in-phase point. The latter is more practical, since the preceding solution demands higher gradient strength. The drawback to selecting a longer echo time to minimize chemical shift on gradient-echo pulse sequences is that the signal decays very quickly. Signal loss on gradient-echo pulse sequences decays exponentially with a time constant of T_2^* as opposed to the T_2 of tis-

sues on spin-echo images. Therefore longer echo times on gradient-echo images may cause unacceptable loss in the signal-to-noise ratio; a better way of minimizing chemical shift on gradient-echo images is generally to change the bandwidth rather than the echo time.

MAGNETIC SUSCEPTIBILITY ARTIFACT

Magnetic-susceptibility artifact is really a form of chemical-shift artifact wherein the artifacts may be attributable, not to the difference in the frequency precessions of fat and water, but to the magnetic susceptibilities of different materials, inhomogeneity in the static field, or the presence of magnetic materials.[4] Magnetic artifacts are projected along the frequency-encoding axis and may have "comet-tail" appearances depending on the shape of the magnetic inhomogeneity (Fig. 16-5). Metal is a common source of magnetic artifact and is seen as a signal void with bright and dark bands oriented along the frequency-encoding axis. Similar to chemical shift, superimposition of a magnetic field of tissues surrounding magnetic metal causes spins adjacent to the metal to give a signal at frequencies different from their assigned frequency. The signal produced from the tissues near the metal will be interpreted as a signal from other locations producing the same frequency, and therefore an increase in signal intensity is seen at the latter location.

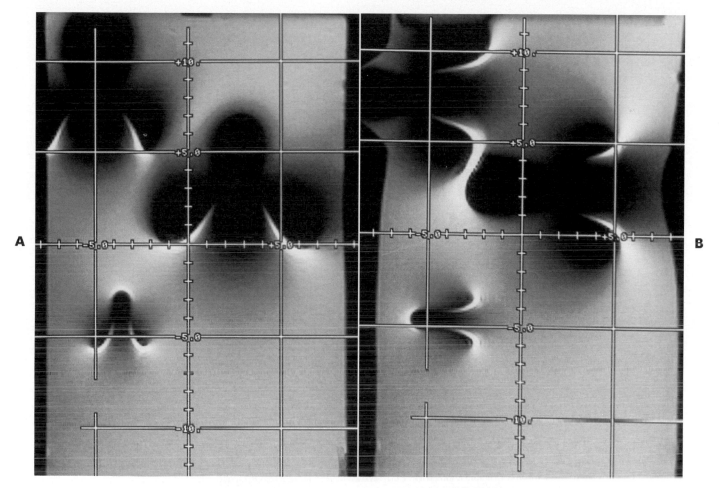

Fig. 16-5. Magnetic artifact. **A,** MR image from metal screw in gelatin phantom shows a comet-shaped or spear-shaped artifact composed of a central signal void circumscribed by bright and dark boundaries. The artifact is oriented in the direction of the frequency-encoding axis. **B,** MR image with identical technique as in **A** except that frequency- and phase-encoding directions have been switched. The direction of the magnetic artifact has switched by 90 degrees along the course of the new frequency-encoding axis.

A decrease in signal intensity is commonly seen at the center of magnetic artifacts and can be attributed to either spins that have gone wild and dephased completely or to the fact that there is no more signal at the actual location of the spins. Like chemical shift, magnetic artifact is much worse on narrow-bandwidth pulse sequences.

Magnetic artifacts caused by metal (Fig. 16-6) vary inversely with bandwidth and in spin-echo pulse sequences are independent of the echo time (TE). Gradient-echo pulse sequences (Fig. 16-6) are much more severely affected by magnetic artifact than spin-echo pulse sequences. On gradient-echo pulse sequences, a magnetic artifact increases with increasing TE and with decreasing bandwidth. Magnetic artifact may manifest itself as an extreme form of chemical shift and destroy the diagnostic quality of an image.

Different materials and different metals vary widely in their potential for creating magnetic artifacts[9,12] (see also Chapter 17). In large part, magnetic artifact is linearly related to the ferromagnetic nature of the magnetic material. One can test this by determining if a particular object will be deviated by a magnetic field.[9] The object (such as a metal pin) may be suspended from a string and placed in a magnetic field. The degree of torque, or movement, reflects the degree of ferromagnetism of the object. Objects with no demonstrable torque or effect from the magnetic field are generally not ferromagnetic and will usually not then produce large artifacts on MR images. Ferromagnetic objects generally create large artifacts.

Steel, iron, and stainless steel commonly produce magnetic artifacts on MR images.[10,11] Dental material containing stainless steel (such as caps, crowns, or pins)

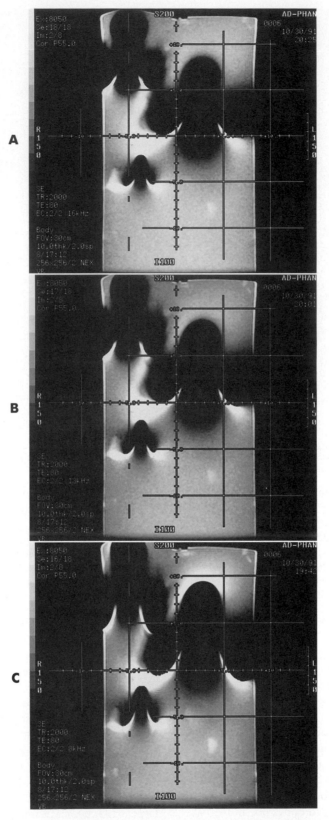

Fig. 16-6. Variation in size of magnetic artifact with bandwidth and TE (echo time) on spin-echo and gradient-echo pulse sequences. **A,** Image from spin-echo pulse sequence at wide bandwidth shows relatively small artifact. **B,** Medium bandwidth image, with other parameters being held constant, shows an increase in the size of the artifact relative to that in **A.** **C,** Narrow bandwidth image (other parameters held the same as in **B**) shows the largest size artifact.

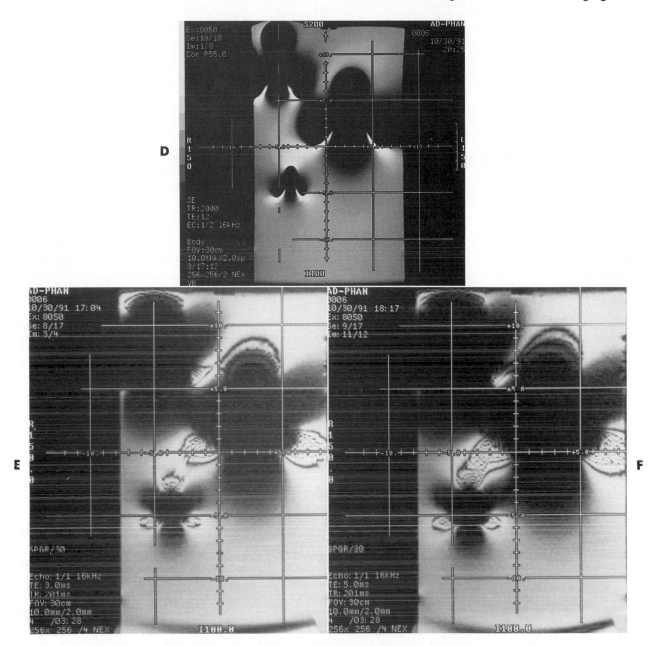

Fig. 16-6, cont'd. D, Short spin-echo time (TE = 12 msec) image shows the same size artifact as in **A** despite the short TE. On spin-echo images, the size of the magnetic field artifact varies inversely with the bandwidth and has no dependence on TE. **E,** Turbo Grass image (ultrashort TE) shows an artifact that is larger than the spin-echo images despite the extremely short TE of the gradient echo. **F,** Turbo Grass image with somewhat longer TE (5 msec) shows an increase in the size of the artifact relative to that in **E.** On gradient-echo images, both TE and bandwidth affect artifact size.

causes large artifacts. Materials such as amalgam, gold alloy, aluminum, microfilled resin, and polyvinyl acrylics do not generally cause artifacts.[10] Surgical clips, intravascular stents, filters, and coils generally cause magnetic artifacts if they are made of steel or stainless steel.[11] Alloys composed of tantalum or beta-3 titanium alloy (Ormco, Glendora, California), however, are not

ferromagnetic and cause either little or no appreciable artifacts on MRI.[9,11]

Bullets and metal ballistic fragments may also cause magnetic artifacts[12] (see also Chapter 19). The worst artifacts are generally caused by objects that contain steel. Lead bullets and casings with copper and nickel jackets may also cause noticeable artifacts because of metal impurities in the jacket casings. Lead bullets generally cause minimal artifacts unless they have jackets containing steel.[12]

Care should be taken when using MR to examine patients with ferromagnetic devices, clips, or metal fragments[13-15] (see Chapter 17). Magnetic torque may cause movement of metal objects such as ferromagnetic aneurysms clips within the patient's body.[15] Far more common than actual torque of metal in MRI is artifact production. A very small metal fragment, of which the patient might be unaware, may produce a large artifact on the MR images (Fig. 16-7).

Magnetic materials that are absolute contraindications to MRI include ferromagnetic intracranial aneurysm clips and shrapnel in vital locations. Many surgical clips are nonmagnetic. In a patient with brain aneu-

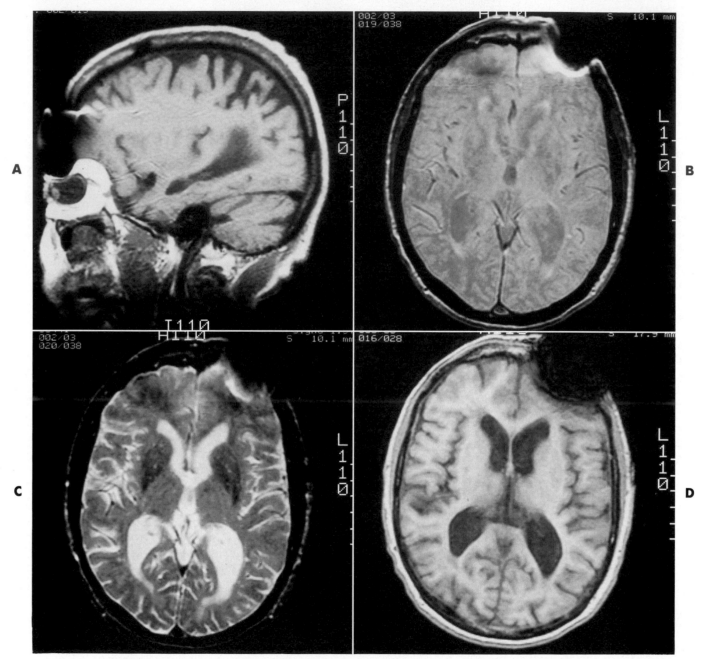

Fig. 16-7. MR images of a patients with a small metallic fragment in the scalp. **A,** Sagittal T₁-weighted (spin-lattice or longitudinal relaxation–weighted) image shows characteristic magnetic artifact with distortion of the superior portion of the orbit. **B,** Medium bandwidth proton-density spin-echo image shows distortion of the left frontal lobe. **C,** Narrow bandwidth T₂-weighted (spin-spin–weighted) image shows somewhat greater distortion of the frontal lobe. **D,** Gradient-echo Spoiled Grass MR image of the brain, with TE at 5 msec, shows greater degree of distortion than the spin-echo images despite the shorter TE.

rysm clips the radiologist should check to see what kind of clips the patient has and whether these clips are ferromagnetic before performing the MR examination. MR should not be performed in patients with brain ferromagnetic aneurysm clips or in patients whose type of clip is unknown.

Metal fragments in the eyes are another potential hazard. Metal workers may unknowingly have iron fillings in their eyes, and such fragments can injure the eye upon magnetic torque. In a patient with a history of possible metal fragments in the eyes anteroposterior and lateral skull x-ray films should be obtained. If these show a possible ferromagnetic metal fragment in the eyes, MR is generally contraindicated.

Metal is not the only substance to cause magnetic artifacts. Magnetic artifacts can commonly be seen on MR images as a result of the differing magnetic susceptibilities of adjacent structures. The sphenoid sinuses and petrous ridges are common sources of magnetic susceptibility artifact that may distort the anatomy of the temporal lobes. Similarly, gas and tissue interfaces or gas and liquid interfaces may be present as artifacts. These artifacts are seen to a greater extent on gradient-echo than on spin-echo pulse sequences.

Pulse sequences can be chosen carefully to minimize magnetic artifact. This is particularly important in MR imaging of patients with metal plates, screws, prostheses, and other devices as are commonly encountered in orthopedics. First, as wide a bandwidth as necessary should be used to minimize artifact. The axis of the phase and frequency encoding should be chosen carefully to minimize the detrimental effects of the artifact. The axes of the phase and frequency ending directions can be switched to change the direction of the magnetic artifact so that it does not project over crucial anatomy. Lastly, spin-echo rather than gradient-echo pulse sequences should be used to minimize artifact (see Fig. 16-6).

WRAPAROUND ARTIFACT

Wraparound (fold-in, foldover) artifact (Fig. 16-8) is actually a result of a phenomenon called "aliasing."[16] For the frequency-encoding direction, assume a signal is sampled at a fixed frequency. According to the Nyquist theorem, information for frequencies more than twice the sampling rate will not be sampled fast enough. This results in the information being folded over onto some other portion of the image. To overcome this problem, an electronic filter can be used to avoid aliasing in the frequency direction. A similar concept is also applicable in the phase-encoding direction. Aliasing also occurs in three-dimentional imaging when the slice information is encoded in the same way as the phase information. Aliasing results in information from slices outside the volume of interest folding into the field of view.

Two methods are used principally to minimize fold-in. First, pulse sequences with extended readout may be used. In extended readout pulse sequences, the data are oversampled along the phase-encoding axis, and then the spatial information outside the imaging field of view is thrown away.

This technique is very powerful, though it has two drawbacks. It cannot be done on some MRI machines because they are designed to collect two image averages to reduce ghosting. Two averages also reduce "DC" artifacts, which are lines passing through the center of the images. Manufacturers have recently developed method to reduce the necessity of collecting two averages, and this makes the technique of oversampling look rather attractive. The other drawback to oversampling is the need for very strong gradients. With oversampling, the machine must effectively image twice the field of view, which will cause the machine to encode twice as much.

The second principal method of minimizing fold-in is to use saturation pulses to suppress the signal from objects outside the imaging volume. The drawback to using saturation pulses is that the repetition time (TR) increases slightly, and the number of slices may be reduced on particular pulse sequences as well as producing an increased SAR (specific absorption rate in the patient), reflecting increased radio frequency power deposition. Transmit-receive as opposed to receive-only coils can also be used to minimize fold-in, since the use of a smaller and more localized coil results in selective excitation of spins in the imaging volume.

Fold-in may occur when the field of view or imaging volume is smaller than the size of the object being imaged (see Fig. 16-8). Saturation pulses decrease the degree of the fold-in artifact, but the artifact is still present. No-phasewrap techniques can eliminate the fold-in artifact.

GIBBS ARTIFACT

Gibbs artifact is another frequency artifact similar to chemical shift and magnetic artifact.[17-23] Gibbs artifact may present as a linear area of increased or decreased signal intensity in the cervical spinal cord.[17-19] Gibbs artifact is worse on coarse matrix MR images (such as 128×128). The artifact occurs because of truncation of information.[20,21] The echo cannot be sampled indefinitely; therefore the information must be truncated at some point in time.

Because edges between apposing tissues or fluids are formed of high-frequency information (which mainly results from collecting the information for a long time), Gibbs artifact is mostly seen at the edges of different tissues and fluids. Gibbs artifact can present as a linear high- or low-signal intensity in the cervical spinal cord and in severe cases may mimic a syrinx (Fig. 16-9). Us-

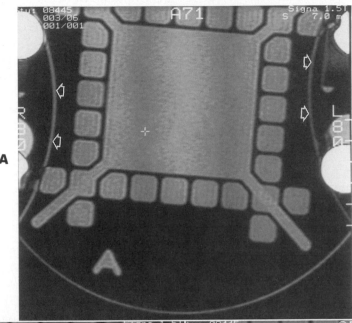

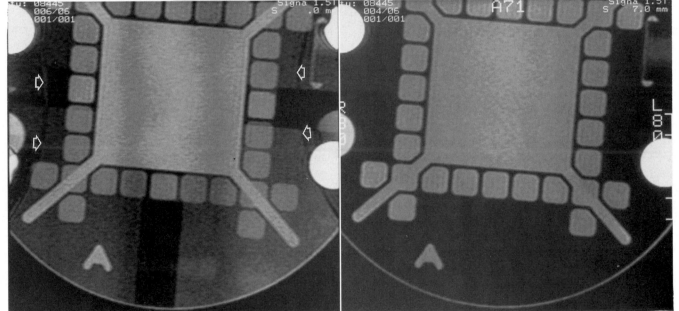

Fig. 16-8. Foldover (wraparound) artifact. **A,** MR image of the phantom shows foldover artifact, *arrows,* from edges of the phantom. **B,** MR image of same phantom as in **A** with saturation pulses (with other parameters being held constant). The artifacts, *arrows,* are diminished relative to those in **A.** The saturation pulses have somewhat decreased the signal from the edges of the phantom outside the field of view. Despite saturation pulses, however, the artifact is still noticeable, though to a much lesser extent. **C,** MR image of phantom with no-phase wrap (other parameters the same as in **A**). Foldover artifact is no longer visible.

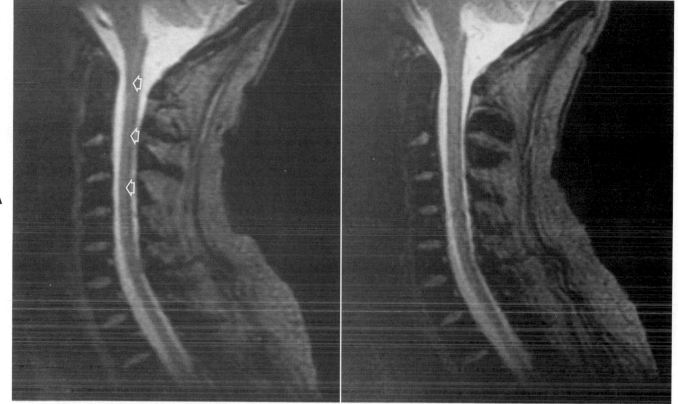

Fig. 16-9. Gibbs artifact. **A,** T_2-weighted sagittal image of the cervical spine shows Gibbs artifact within the central signal cord. This appears as a linear band of high signal intensity, *arrows,* which in more severe cases might be misconstrued to represent a syrinx. **B,** MR image of the cervical spine with identical parameters as in **A** except that a finer matrix (192 × 256) was used. The linear band of increase signal intensity shown in **A** is no longer visualized.

ing a finer matrix helps to ameliorate the artifact. In MR images of the abdomen acquired with a coarse matrix, ringing artifact can be seen as linear bands of low signal at the periphery of the liver. A finer matrix eliminates the artifact.

Several papers introduce and discuss postprocessing solutions to the Gibbs type of artifact.[20,22,23] However, the most convenient method of decreasing Gibbs artifact is to collect fine enough matrices during the minimum acquisition time to eliminate the artifact.[24] Currently, a 192 × 256 matrix seems to be optimum for minimizing image acquisition time while providing high-quality images with minimal Gibbs artifact.

MOTION ARTIFACT

Motion artifacts (Fig. 16-10) are projected along the phase-encoding direction and as such can be differentiated from frequency artifacts (such as chemical shift) that are projected along the frequency-encoding axis.[25] When moving spins, such as flowing blood, encounter a phase-encoding gradient, they impart a unique phase.

Spins that are moving will experience a phase shift, which may result in offset of the moving spins on the MR images. The speed of the flow and the magnitude and duration of the gradients determine the degree of offset of the signal from the moving spins. Motion artifacts can be caused by a variety of different movements. The most common kinds of motion artifact are caused by respiratory and cardiac motion, as well as vascular pulsation.

Motion artifact is a very significant problem. Manufacturers and independent researchers have devoted much effort to develop methods to overcome it.[26-33] Depending on the type of motion, various different pulse sequences can be used to decrease motion artifacts. Respiratory artifacts can be diminished by the use of respiration-compensated pulse sequences. As shown in Fig. 16-11, respiratory compensation improves the quality of abdominal and thoracic MR images. Respiratory compensation is accomplished when the phase acquisitions are ordered to correspond with respiration.

Pseudogating can be used to improve or eliminate pe-

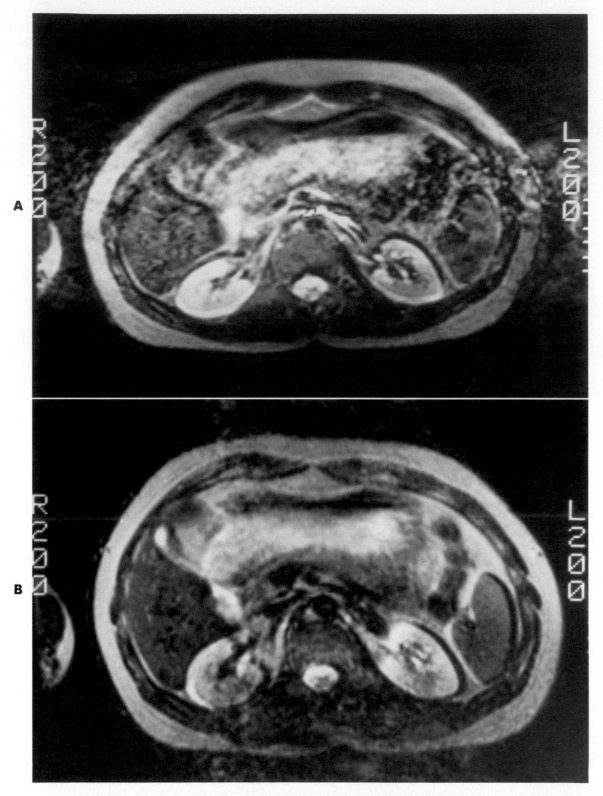

Fig. 16-10. Motion artifact on MR images. **A,** Transaxial image of the abdomen shows cardiac-motion artifacts projected along phase-encoding axis. **B,** Switching of phase and frequency gradients changes the direction of the motion artifacts. They are now projected in a different plane by 90 degrees.

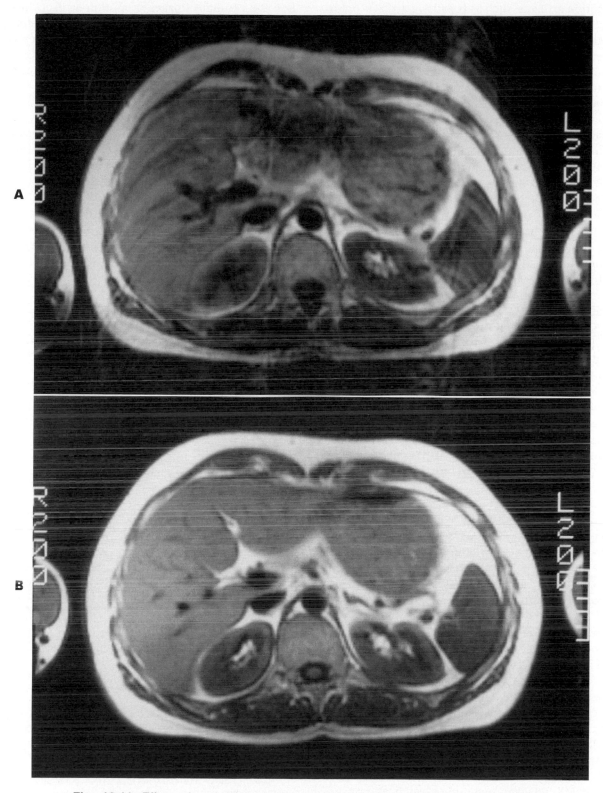

Fig. 16-11. Effect of respiratory compensation on motion artifact. **A,** Transaxial T_1-weighted spin-echo image of abdomen is severely degraded by respiratory-motion artifact. **B,** T_1-weighted spin-echo image obtained with identical parameters as those in **A** other than addition of respiratory compensation shows a considerable reduction in respiratory-motion artifact and a significant improvement in image quality.

riodic motion artifacts, such as breathing artifacts, without one having to do actual respiratory gating.[27] One accomplishes pseudogating by setting the product of the repetition time (TR) multiplied by the number of acquisitions to equal the time period for the periodic motion to be eliminated. For example, if the respiratory rate is one time each 4 seconds, a TR of 2 seconds with 2 acquisitions might be used for pseudogating.

Cardiac motion is also a common cause of artifacts on abdominal and thoracic MR images (see Fig. 16-10). The solution to cardiac motion artifact is to gate the acquisition of the MR images to the cardiac cycle. In so doing, motion artifact is greatly reduced.

Another way of suppressing artifacts from motion is to use radio frequency pulses to saturate the signal from tissues or fluids that are not of primary interest in the MR examination.[28] As an example, saturation pulses can be used to remove signals from anterior neck tissues (eliminating swallowing artifact) to improve visualization of anatomic detail in the cervical spine. Saturation pulses can be applied superiorly and inferiorly to an imaging volume to suppress artifact from vascular pulsation. Saturation pulses may often be used complimentarily with other motion-compensation techniques to improve image quality.

Depending on the pulse sequence used, blood vessels may appear dark or bright. Velocity-compensated pulse sequences can be used to make blood appear bright as well as to decrease artifact from vascular pulsation. Similar pulse sequences can be used for pulsatile cerebrospinal fluid.

Motion artifact is projected along the phase-encoding axis and can be minimized by use of an appropriate pulse sequence that includes first- or second-order flow-compensation gradients. Switching the phase and frequency axis can sometimes be used to project the motion artifact off the anatomic region of interest in the MR images. By selecting motion-compensation pulse sequences, one can minimize the artifacts.

In general, motion artifact is much worse on longer echo time images, since the spins are exposed longer to motion. When a spin moves during the application of a gradient, it retains a phase different from the localized phase assumed by the imaging software. Therefore, upon the application of the Fourier transform the spin will be displaced and be presented as an artifact projected along the phase-encoding axis. By holding the echo time short, one can obtain a diagnostic MR study even when gross patient motion is present.

Ultrafast MR imaging techniques, such as conventional ultrashort repetition time pulse sequences (such as FLASH or TURBO GRASS) or more advanced techniques (such as echo planar imaging) can also be used to decrease motion artifacts on MR. Fast single-slice techniques may be used to freeze physiologic motion and free the resultant images of motion artifact. In the abdomen, slices of one or two seconds of acquisition time are sufficient to nearly eliminate motion artifact from respiratory and bowel peristalsis. In the heart, image acquisition has to be much shorter, on the order of 100 msec or less.

CONCLUSIONS

MR artifacts occur during the process of obtaining MR images because of the presence of different tissue interfaces, the presence of artificial magnetic materials, or the presence of motion and aliasing. Close attention to the relationship of the artifact to adjacent structures on the MR images usually permits the determination of the type of artifact present. By manipulating the pulse sequences as described above, one can greatly reduce MRI artifacts and improve the clinical utility of the MR diagnostic examination.

REFERENCES

1. Hahn FJ, Chu W-K, Coleman PE, et al: Artifacts and diagnostic pitfalls on magnetic resonance imaging: a clinical review, *Imaging in Neuroradiology* 26(4):717-735, 1988.
2. Clark JA, Kelly WM: Common artifacts encountered in magnetic resonance imaging, *Imaging in Neuroradiology* 26(5):893-920, 1988.
3. Edelman RR, Kleefield R, Wentz KU, et al: Basic principles of magnetic resonance imaging. In Edelman RR, Hesselink JR, editors: Clinical magnetic resonance imaging, Philadelphia, 1990, Saunders.
4. Cox IJ, Bydder GM, Gadian DG, et al: The effect of magnetic susceptibility variations in NMR imaging and NMR spectroscopy *in vivo, J Magnetic Resonance* 70:163-168, 1986.
5. Farahani K, Sinha U, Sinha S, et al: Effect of field strength on susceptibility artifacts in magnetic resonance imaging, *Computer Med Imaging Graph* 14(6):409-413, 1990.
6. Twieg, DB, Katz J, Peshock RM: A general treatment of NMR imaging with chemical shifts and motion, *Magn Reson Med* 5:32-46, 1987.
7. Cho ZH, Nalcioglu O, Park HW, et al: Chemical-shift artifact correction scheme using echo-time encoding technique, *Magn Reson Med* 2:253-261, 1985.
8. Lotan CS, Cranney GB, Doyle M, et al: Fat-shift artifact simulating aortic dissection on MR images, *AJR* 152:385-386, 1989.
9. Teitelbaum GP, Raney M, Carvlin MJ, et al: Evaluation of ferromagnetism and magnetic resonance imaging artifacts of the Strecker tantalum vascular stent, *Cardiovasc Intervent Radiol* 12:125-127, 1989.
10. Hinshaw DB, Holshouser BA, Engstrom HI, et al: Dental material artifacts on MR images, *Radiology* 166:777-779, 1988.
11. Teitelbaum GP, Bradley WG, Klein BD: MR imaging artifacts, ferromagnetism, and magnetic torque of intravascular filters, stents, and coils, *Radiology* 166:657-664, 1988.
12. Teitelbaum GP, Yee CA, Van Horn DD, et al: Metallic ballistic fragments: MR imaging safety and artifacts, *Radiology* 175:855-859, 1990.
13. New PFJ, Rosen BR, Brady TJ, et al: Potential hazards and artifacts of ferromagnetic and non-ferromagnetic surgical and dental materials and devices in nuclear magnetic resonance imaging, *Radiology* 147:139-148, 1983.

14. Shellock FG, Crues JV: High-field-strength MR imaging and metallic biomedical implants: an ex vivo evaluation of deflection forces, *AJR* 151:389-392, 1988.

15. Dujovny M, Kossovsky N, Kossowsky R, et al: Aneurysm clip motion during magnetic resonance imaging: in vivo experimental study with metallurgical factor analysis, *Neurosurgery* 17:543-548, 1985.

16. Pusey E, Yoon C, Anselmo ML, et al: Aliasing artifacts in MR imaging, *Comput Med Imaging Graph* 12(4):219-224, 1988.

17. Levy LM, Chiro GD, Brooks RA, et al: Spinal cord artifacts from truncation errors during MR imaging, *Radiology* 166:479-483, 1988.

18. Bronskill MJ, McVeigh ER, Kucharczyk W, et al: Syrinx-like artifacts on MR images of the spinal cord, *Radiology* 166:485-488, 1988.

19. Yousem DV, Janick PA, Atlas SW: Pseudoatrophy of the cervical portion of the spinal cord on MR images: a manifestation of the truncation artifact? *AJR* 154:1069-1073, 1990.

20. Haacke EM: The effects of finite sampling in spin echo or field-echo magnetic resonance imaging. *Magn Reson Med* 4:407-421, 1987.

21. Wood ML, Hendelman RM: Truncation artifacts in magnetic resonance imaging, *Magn Reson Med* 2:517-526, 1985.

22. Constable RT, Henkelman RM: Data extrapolation for truncation artifact removal, *Magn Reson Med* 17:108-118, 1991.

23. Webb AG, Clarkson RB: Sensitivity enhancement and reduction of Gibbs artifact in T_2-weighted imaging using variable tip angle excitation, *Magn Reson Med* 21:308-312, 1991.

24. Bradley WG, Kortman KE, Crues JV: Central nervous system high resolution magnetic resonance imaging: effect of increasing spacial resolution on resolving power, *Radiology* 156:93-98, 1985.

25. Wedeen VJ, Wendt RE, Jerosch-Herold M: Motional phase artifacts in Fourier transform MRI, *Magn Reson Med* 11:114-120, 1989.

26. Dixon WT, Brummer ME, Malko JA: Acquisition order and motional artifact reduction in spin warp images, *Magn Reson Med* 6:74-83, 1988.

27. Haacke EM, Lenz GW, Nelson AD: Pseudo-gating: elimination of periodic motion artifacts in magnetic resonance imaging without gating, *Magn Reson Med* 4:162-174, 1987.

28. Edelman RR, Atkinson DJ, Silver MS, et al: FRODO pulse sequences: a new means of eliminating motion, flow, and wrap-around artifacts, *Radiology* 166:231-236, 1988.

29. Duerk JL, Pattany PM: Analysis of imaging axis significance in motion artifact suppression technique (MAST™): MRI of turbulent flow and motion, *Magn Reson Imaging* 7:251-263, 1989.

30. Silverman PM, Patt RH, Baum PA, et al: Ghost artifact on gradient-echo imaging: a potential pitfall in hepatic imaging, *AJR* 154:633-634, 1990.

31. Colletti PM, Raval JK, Benson RC, et al: The motion artifact suppression technique (MAST) in magnetic resonance imaging: clinical results, *Magn Reson Imaging* 6:293-299, 1988.

32. Haacke EM, Patrick JL: Reducing motion artifacts in two-dimensional Fourier transform imaging, *Magn Reson Imaging* 4:359-376, 1986.

33. Mitchell DG, Vinitski S, Burk DL, et al: Motion artifact reduction in MR imaging of the abdomen: gradient moment nulling versus respiratory-sorted phase encoding, *Radiology* 169:155-160, 1988.

17

Magnetic Resonance Imaging and Biomedical Implants, Materials, and Devices

Frank G. Shellock
Julie S. Curtis

Magnetic resonance (MR) imaging may be contraindicated for a patient with a ferromagnetic metallic implant, material, or device. This is primarily because of the risk associated with movement or dislodgment of the object as well as other possible hazards including the induction of electrical current, excessive heating, and the misinterpretation of an artifact produced by the presence of the object as an abnormality.[1-58] The potential for MR imaging to injure patients by inducing electric currents in conductive metallic materials or devices, such as gating leads, unused surface coils, halo vests, or improperly used physiologic monitors, is well known and has led to recommendations for patient protection during MR imaging.[15,49,54]

Internal heating associated with MR imaging of metallic implants, biomaterials, and devices has been extensively studied, and there does not appear to be any significant hazard related to the temperature changes measured thus far.[7,16,17] However, this is not necessarily true for monitoring equipment, surface coils, or other externally applied devices, which in some in-

stances can heat up enough to cause significant patient injury. The type and extent of various artifacts produced by metallic implants, materials, and devices have also been described (see also Chapter 16) and are typically well recognized on MR images.[9,10,13,18-21,38,40,46,52]

Numerous studies have involved assessment of the ferromagnetic qualities of various metallic implants, materials, or devices by measurement of deflection forces or movements associated with the static magnetic fields used for MR imaging.* In general, these investigations have demonstrated that MR imaging may be performed safely in patients with metallic implants, materials, or devices if the object is nonferromagnetic or if it is only minimally attracted by the static magnetic field in relation to its in vivo application (that is, the associated deflection force or attraction is insufficient to move or dislodge the implant or material in situ).* Prior knowledge of the relative degree of ferromagnetism that a specified type of metallic implant, material, or device possesses is essential for proper screening of patients before MR imaging.[15,44,45,54,60-65]

Table 17-1 lists data on over 260 different implants, materials, or devices that have been tested for ferromagnetism, whether the objects were deflected or attracted by static magnetic fields, and the highest static magnetic field strength (static magnetic field strengths ranged from 0.147 to 4.7 tesla) at which the objects were evaluated. It should be noted that, unless otherwise stated,

Text continued on p. 490.

The slightly modified material in this chapter is reprinted from Shellock FG, Curtis JS: MR imaging and biomedical implants, materials, and devices: an updated review, *Radiology* 180:541-550, 1991.

*References 1-14, 17, 21-30, 33, 35-43, 47, 51, 53, 55, 59.

Table 17-1 Metallic Implants, Materials, and Devices Tested for Movement/Deflection Forces During Exposure to Static Magnetic Fields

Metallic implant, material, or device	Movement/ deflection	Highest field strength (T)†	Reference
Aneurysm and Hemostatic Clips:			
Drake (DR 14, DR 24)	Yes	1.44	9, 29
Edward Weck,			
Research Triangle Park, NJ			
Drake (DR 16)	Yes	0.147	9, 29
Edward Weck			
Drake (301 SS)	Yes	1.5	11, 29
Edward Weck			
Downs multipositional (17-7PH)	Yes	1.44	9
Gastrointestinal anastomosis clip, Auto Suture SGIA (SS)	No	1.5	11
United States Surgical Corp.,			
Norwalk, CT			
Heifetz (17-7PH)	Yes	1.89	4, 42
Edward Weck			
Heifetz (Elgiloy)	No	1.89	4, 29, 42
Edward Weck			
Hemoclip, #10 (316L SS)	No	1.5	11
Edward Weck			
Hemoclip (tantalum)	No	1.5	11
Edward Weck			
Housepian	Yes	0.147	9
Kapp (405 SS)	Yes	1.89	4, 29
American V. Mueller			
Chicago, IL			
Kapp curved (404 SS)	Yes	1.44	9
American V. Mueller			
Ligaclip, #6 (316L SS)	No	1.5	11
Ethicon, Inc., Somerville, NJ			
Ligaclip (tantalum)	No	1.5	11
Ethicon			
Mayfield (301 SS)	Yes	1.5	11
Codman, Randolph, MA			
Mayfield (304 SS)	Yes	1.89	4
Codman			
McFadden (301 SS)	Yes	1.5	11, 29
Codman			
Olivecrona	No	1.44	9
Pivot (17-7PH)	Yes	1.89	4
Scoville (EN58J)	Yes	1.89	4, 29
Downs Surgical, Inc.,			
Decatur, GA (now in Keene, NH)			
Stevens (50-4190, silver alloy)	No	0.15	2
Sugita (Elgiloy)	No	1.89	4, 29
Downs Surgical			
Sundt-Kees (301 SS)	Yes	1.5	11, 29
Downs Surgical			

SS, Stainless steel. Material or materials used to construct the objecs are indicated if known. Manufacturer information is provided if known. Consult Appendix for full addresses.

*The asterisk denotes the metallic implants, materials, or devices that were considered to be safe for magnetic resonance imaging, despite being moved/deflected by the static magnetic fields. For example, certain heart valve prostheses were moved/deflected by the static magnetic fields, but the forces were considered to be less than that exerted on the prosthetic valves by the beating heart.

†"Highest field strength" refers to the highest intensity of the static magnetic field in tesla units (T) that was used for the evaluation of movement/deflection forces of the various implants, materials, and devices tested.

Continued.

Table 17-1 Metallic Implants, Materials, and Devices Tested for Movement/Deflection Forces During Exposure to Static Magnetic Fields—cont'd

Metallic implant, material, or device	Movement/ deflection	Highest field strength (T)†	Reference
Sundt-Kees Multi-Angle (17-7PH)	Yes	1.89	4, 29
Downs Surgical			
Surgiclip, Auto Suture M-9.5 (SS)	No	1.5	11
United States Surgical Corp.			
Vari-Angle (17-7PH)	Yes	1.89	4
Codman			
Vari-Angle McFadden (MP35N)	No	1.89	4, 29
Codman			
Vari-Angle Micro (17-7PM SS)	Yes	0.15	2, 29
Codman			
Vari-Angle Spring (17-7PM SS)	Yes	0.15	2, 29
Codman			
Yaşargil (316 SS)	No	1.89	4
Aesculap, South San Francisco, CA			
Yaşargil (Phynox)	No	1.89	4, 29
Aesculap			
Carotid Artery Vascular Clamps:			
Crutchfield (SS)	Yes*	1.5	22
Codman			
Kindt (SS)	Yes*	1.5	22
V. Mueller			
Poppen-Blaylock (SS)	Yes	1.5	22
Codman			
Salibi (SS)	Yes*	1.5	22
Codman			
Selverstone (SS)	Yes*	1.5	22
Codman			
Dental Devices and Materials:			
Brace band (SS)	Yes*	1.5	11
American Dental, Missoula, MT (now in Tualatin, OR)			
Brace wire (chrome alloy)	Yes*	1.5	11
Ormco Corp., San Marcos, CA (now in Glendora, CA)			
Castable alloy	Yes*	1.5	55
Cement-in keeper	Yes*	1.5	55
Dental amalgam	No	1.44	9
Keeper, preformed post	Yes*	1.5	55
Parkell Products, Inc., Farmingdale, NY			
GDP Direct Keeper, preformed post,	Yes*	1.5	55
Golden Dental Products, Inc.			
Magna-Dent, large indirect keeper,	Yes*	1.5	55
Dental Ventures of America, Anaheim, CA			
Palladium clad magnet	Yes	1.5	37
Parkell Products, Inc.			
Palladium/palladium keeper	Yes*	1.5	37
Parkell Products, Inc.			
Palladium/platinum casting alloy	Yes*	1.5	37
Parkell Products, Inc.			
Permanent crown (amalgam)	No	1.5	11
Ormco Corp., Glendora, CA			
Titanium clad magnet	Yes	1.5	37
Parkell Products, Inc.			

Table 17-1 Metallic Implants, Materials, and Devices Tested for Movement/Deflection Forces During Exposure to Static Magnetic Fields—cont'd

Metallic implant, material, or device	Movement/ deflection	Highest field strength (T)†	Reference
Stainless steel clad magnet	Yes	1.5	37
Parkell Products, Inc.			
Stainless steel keeper	Yes*	1.5	37
Parkell Products, Inc.			
Silver point	No	1.5	11
Union Broach Co., Inc.,			
New York, NY (now in Emigsville, PA)			
Heart Valve Prostheses:			
Beall	Yes*	2.35	12
Coratomic, Inc. (Biocontrol Technology, Inc.)			
Indiana, PA			
Bjork-Shiley (convexo/concave)	No	1.5	11
Shiley Inc.,			
Irvine, CA			
Bjork-Shiley (universal/spherical)	Yes*	1.5	11
Shiley Inc.			
Bjork-Shiley, Model MBC	Yes*	2.35	5
Shiley Inc.			
Bjork-Shiley,	Yes*	2.35	5
Model 25 MBRC 11030			
Shiley Inc.			
Carpentier-Edwards Model 2650	Yes*	2.35	5
American Edwards Laboratories,			
Santa Ana, CA			
Carpentier-Edwards (porcine)	Yes*	2.35	5
American Edwards Laboratories			
Hall-Kaster, Model A7700	Yes*	1.5	11
Medtronic, Minneapolis, MN			
Hancock I (porcine)	Yes*	1.5	11
Johnson & Johnson,			
Arlington, TX			
Hancock II (porcine)	Yes*	1.5	11
Johnson & Johnson			
Hancock extracorporeal, Model 242R	Yes*	2.35	5
Johnson & Johnson			
Hancock extracorporeal, Model M 4365-33	Yes*	2.35	5
Johnson & Johnson			
Hancock Vascor, Model 505	No	2.35	5
Johnson & Johnson			
Ionescu-Shiley, Universal ISM	Yes*	2.35	5
Lillehei-Kaster, Model 300S	Yes*	2.35	12
Medical Inc.,			
Inver Grove Heights, MN			
Lillehei-Kaster, Model 5009	Yes*	2.35	5
Medical Inc.			
Medtronic Hall	Yes*	2.35	5
Medtronic Inc., Minneapolis, MN			
Medtronic Hall, Model A7700-D-16	Yes*	2.35	5
Medtronic Inc.			
Omnicarbon, Model 3523T029	Yes*	2.35	5
Medical Inc.,			
Omniscience, Model 6522	Yes*	2.35	5
Medical Inc.			

Continued.

Table 17-1 Metallic Implants, Materials, and Devices Tested for Movement/Deflection Forces During Exposure to Static Magnetic Fields—cont'd

Metallic implant, material, or device	Movement/ deflection	Highest field strength (T)†	Reference
Smeloff-Cutter	Yes*	2.35	11
Cutter Biological,			
Berkeley, CA (now in Covina, CA)			
Starr-Edwards, Model 1260	Yes*	2.35	12
American Edwards Laboratories			
Starr-Edwards, Model 2320	Yes*	2.35	12
American Edwards Laboratories			
Starr-Edwards, Model 2400	No	1.5	11
American Edwards Laboratories			
Starr-Edwards, Model Pre 6000	Yes	2.35	12
American Edwards Laboratories			
Starr-Edwards, Model 6520	Yes*	2.35	5
American Edwards Laboratories			
St. Jude	No	1.5	11
St. Jude Medical, Inc.,			
St. Paul, MN			
St. Jude, Model A 101	Yes*	2.35	5
St. Jude Medical Inc.			
St. Jude, Model M 101	Yes*	2.35	5
St. Jude Medical Inc.			
Intravascular Coils, Filters, and Stents:			
Amplatz IVC filter	No	4.7	13
Cook, Inc., Bloomington, IN			
Cragg nitinol spiral filter	No	4.7	13
Gianturco embolization coil	Yes	1.5	13
Cook			
Gianturco bird nest IVC filter	Yes	1.5	13, 24
Cook			
Gianturco zig-zag stent	Yes	1.5	13
Cook			
Greenfield vena cava filter, stainless steel	Yes*	1.5	13, 40
Medi-tech, Watertown, MA			
Greenfield vena cava filter, titanium alloy	No	1.5	13
Ormco, Glendora, CA			
Gunther IVC filter	Yes	1.5	13
William Cook Europe A/S			
Bjaerverskov, Denmark			
Maas helical IVC filter	No	4.7	13
Medinvent, Lausanne,			
Switzerland (and Englewood, NJ)			
Maas helical endovascular stent	No	4.7	13
Medinvent			
Mobin-Uddin IVC/umbrella filter	No	4.7	13
American Edwards, Santa Ana, CA			
New retrievable IVC filter	Yes	1.5	13
Thomas Jefferson University,			
Philadelphia, PA			
Palmaz endovascular stent	Yes	1.5	13
Ethicon			
Strecker stent (tantalum)	No	1.5	25, 34
Medi-tech,			
Watertown, MA			

Table 17-1   Metallic Implants, Materials, and Devices Tested for Movement/Deflection Forces During Exposure to Static Magnetic Fields—cont'd

Metallic implant, material, or device	Movement/ deflection	Highest field strength (T)†	Reference
Ocular Implants:			
Fatio eyelid spring/wire	Yes	1.5	23
Intraocular lens implant, Binkhorst, iridocapsular lens, platinum-iridium loop	No	1.5	3
Intraocular lens implant, Binkhorst, iridocapsular lens, platinum-iridium loop	No	1.0	3
Intraocular lens implant, Binkhorst, iridocapsular lens, titanium loop	No	1.0	3
Intraocular lens implant	No	1.0	3
Worst, platinum clip lense			
Retinal tack (303SS)	No	1.5	27
Bascom Palmer Eye Institute			
Retinal tack (titanium alloy)	No	1.5	27, 41
Coopervision (= Alcon Surgical), Irvine, CA			
Retinal tack (303SS)	No	1.5	27
Duke (Beiersdorf, Inc., Norwalk, CT)			
Retinal tack (cobalt-nickel)	No	1.5	41
Grieshaber, Fallsington, PA (now in Langhorne, PA)			
Retinal tack, Norton staple (platinum-rhodium)	No	1.5	27
Retinal tack (aluminum tetraoxide)	No	1.5	27
Retinal tack (SS-martensitic)	Yes	1.5	27
Orthopedic Implants, Materials, and Devices:			
AML femoral component bipolar hip prothesis	No	1.5	11
Zimmer, Warsaw, IN			
Cervical wire, 20 gauge (316L SS)	No	0.3	35
Cortical bone screw, large (titanium, Ti-6AL-4V alloy)	No	1.5	59
Zimmer			
Cortical bone screw, small (titanium, Ti-6AL-4V alloy)	No	1.5	59
Zimmer			
Cotrel rods with hooks (316L SS)	No	0.3	35
DTT, device for transverse traction (316L SS)	No	0.3	35
Drummond wire (316L SS)	No	0.3	35
Endoscopic noncannulated interference screw (titanium)	No	1.5	59
Acufex Microsurgical, Inc.			
Norwood, MA (now Mansfield, MA)			
Fixation staple (cobalt-chromium alloy)	No	1.5	59
ASTM F 75			
Smith & Nephew Richards Medical,			
Memphis, TN			
Harrington compression rod with hooks and nuts (316L SS)	No	0.3	35
Harris hip prosthesis	No	1.5	11
Zimmer			
Jewett nail	No	1.5	11
Zimmer			
Large staple plate	No	1.5	59
Zimaloy			
Zimmer			
Kirschner intramedullary rod	No	1.5	11
Kirschner Medical Corp.			
Timonium, MD			
Perfix interence screw (17-4 stainless steel, AL 630-17 Cr)	Yes	1.5	59
Instrument Makar, Inc.			
Okemos, MI			
Stainless steel plate	No	1.5	11
Zimmer			

Continued.

Table 17-1   Metallic Implants, Materials, and Devices Tested for Movement/Deflection Forces During Exposure to Static Magnetic Fields—cont'd

Metallic implant, material, or device	Movement/ deflection	Highest field strength (T)†	Reference
Stainless steel screw	No	1.5	11
Zimmer			
Stainless steel mesh	No	1.5	11
Zimmer			
Stainless steel wire	No	1.5	11
Zimmer			
Zielke rod with screw, washer and nut (316L SS)	No	0.3	35
Otologic Implants:			
Austin Tytan Piston (titanium)	No	1.5	26
Treace Medical (new Xomed-Treace), Memphis, TN			
Berger "V" bobbin ventilation tube (titanium)	No	1.5	26
Smith & Nephew Richards, Inc.			
Memphis, TN			
Cochlear implant	Yes	0.6	8
3M Medical-Surgical Division, St. Paul, MN			
Cochlear implant	Yes	0.6	8
3M Medical-Surgical Division, St. Paul, MN			
Cochlear implant	Yes	1.5	53
Nucleus Mini 22-channel			
Cochlear Corporation,			
Engelwood, CO			
Cody tack	No	0.6	8
Ehmke hook stapes prosthesis (platinum)	No	1.5	26
Smith & Nephews Richards, Inc. Co.			
Fisch piston, (Teflon, stainless steel)	No	1.5	53
Smith & Nephew Richards, Inc.			
House single loop (ASTM-318-76 grade 2 stainless steel)	No	1.5	26
Storz Instrument Company			
St. Louis, MO			
House single loop (tantalum)	No	1.5	26
Storz			
House double loop (tantalum)	No	1.5	26
Storz			
House double loop (ASTM-318-76 grade 2 stainless steel)	No	1.5	26
Storz			
House-type wire loop stapes prosthesis (316L SS)	No	1.5	26, 53
Smith & Nephew Richards, Inc.			
House-type stainless steel piston and wire (ASTM-318-76 grade 2 stainless steel)	No	1.5	26
Xomed-Treace Inc.			
Jacksonville, FL			
House wire (tantalum)	No	0.5	36
Otomed			
House wire (stainless steel)	No	0.5	36
Otomed			
McGee piston stapes prosthesis (316L SS)	No	1.5	26, 53
Smith & Nephew Richards, Inc.			
McGee piston stapes prosthesis (platinum/316L SS)	No	1.5	26, 53
Smith & Nephew Richards, Inc.			
McGee piston stapes prosthesis (platinum/17Cr-4Ni SS)	Yes	1.5	53
(recalled by manufacturer)			
Smith & Nephew Richards, Inc.			

Table 17-1   Metallic Implants, Materials, and Devices Tested for Movement/Deflection Forces During Exposure to Static Magnetic Fields—cont'd

Metallic implant, material, or device	Movement/ deflection	Highest field strength (T)†	Reference
McGee Shepherd's Crook stapes prosthesis (316L SS) *Smith & Nephew Richards, Inc.*	No	1.5	26
Plasti-pore piston (316L SS/plasti-pore material) *Smith & Nephew Richards, Inc.*	No	1.5	26, 53
Platinum ribbon loop stapes prosthesis (platinum) *Smith & Nephew Richards, Inc.*	No	1.5	26
Reuter bobbin ventilation tube (316L SS) *Smith & Nephew Richards, Inc.*	No	1.5	26
Richards bucket handle stapes prosthesis (316L SS) *Smith & Nephew Richards, Inc.*	No	1.5	26, 53
Richards platinum Teflon piston 0.6 mm (Teflon, platinum) *Smith & Nephew Richards, Inc.*	No	1.5	53
Richards platinum Teflon piston 0.8 mm (Teflon, platinum) *Smith & Nephew Richards, Inc.*	No	1.5	53
Richards piston stapes prosthesis (platinum/fluoroplastic) *Smith & Nephew Richards, Inc.*	No	1.5	26
Richards Shephard's crook (platinum) *Smith & Nephew Richards, Inc.*	No	0.5	36
Richards Teflon piston (Teflon) *Smith & Nephew Richards, Inc.*	No	1.5	53
Robinson-Moon-Lippy offset stapes prosthesis (ASTM-318-76 grade 2 stainless steel) *Storz*	No	1.5	26
Robinson-Moon offset stapes prosthesis (ASTM-318-76 grade 2 stainless steel) *Storz*	No	1.5	26
Robinson incus replacement prosthesis (ASTM-318-76 grade 2 stainless steel) *Storz*	No	1.5	26
Robinson stapes prosthesis (ASTM-318-76 grade 2 stainless steel) *Storz*	No	1.5	26
Ronis piston stapes prosthesis (316L SS/fluoroplastic) *Smith & Nephew Richards, Inc.*	No	1.5	26
Schea cup piston stapes prosthesis (platinum/fluoroplastic) *Smith & Nephew Richards, Inc.*	No	1.5	26, 53
Schea malleus attachment piston (Teflon) *Smith & Nephew Richards, Inc.*	No	1.5	53
Schea stainless steel and Teflon wire prosthesis (Teflon, 316 L SS) *Smith & Nephew Richards, Inc.*	No	1.5	53
Scheer piston stapes prosthesis (316L SS/fluoroplastic) *Smith & Nephew Richards, Inc.*	No	1.5	26
Scheer piston (Teflon, 316L SS) *Smith & Nephew Richards, Inc.*	No	1.5	53
Schuknecht gelfoam and wire prosthesis, Armstrong style (316L SS) *Smith & Nephew Richards, Inc.*	No	1.5	6
Schuknecht piston stapes prosthesis (316L SS/fluoroplastic) *Smith & Nephew Richards, Inc.*	No	1.5	26
Schuknecht tef-wire incus attachment (ASTM-318-76 grade 2 stainless steel) *Storz*	No	1.5	26, 53
Schuknecht tef-wire malleus attachment (ASTM-318-76 grade 2 stainless steel) *Storz*	No	1.5	26, 53
Schuknecht Teflon wire piston 0.6 mm (Teflon, 316L SS) *Smith & Nephew Richards, Inc.*	No	1.5	53
Schuknecht Teflon wire piston 0.8 mm (Teflon, 316L SS) *Smith & Nephew Richards, Inc.*	No	1.5	53
Sheehy incus replacement (ASTM-318-76 grade 2 stainless steel) *Storz*	No	1.5	26

Continued.

Table 17-1   Metallic Implants, Materials, and Devices Tested for Movement/Deflection Forces During Exposure to Static Magnetic Fields—cont'd

Metallic implant, material, or device	Movement/ deflection	Highest field strength (T)†	Reference
Sheehy incus strut (316L SS) *Smith & Nephew Richards, Inc.*	No	1.5	53
Sheehy-type incus replacement strut (Teflon, 316L SS) *Smith & Nephew Richards, Inc.*	No	1.5	26
Silverstein malleus clip ventilation tube (Teflon, 316L SS) *Smith & Nephew Richards, Inc.*	No	1.5	53
Spoon bobbin ventilation tube (316L SS) *Smith & Nephew Richards, Inc.*	No	1.5	26
Tantalum wire loop stages prosthesis (tantalum) *Smith & Nephew Richards, Inc.*	No	1.5	26, 53
Tef-platinum piston (platinum) *Xomed-Treace Inc.*	No	1.5	26
Total ossicular replacement prosthesis (TORP) (316L SS) *Smith & Nephew Richards, Inc.*	No	1.5	53
Trapeze ribbon loop stapes prosthesis (platinum) *Smith & Nephew Richards, Inc.*	No	1.5	26
Williams microclip (316L SS) *Smith & Nephew Richards, Inc.*	No	1.5	26
Xomed stapes (ASTM-318-76 grade 2 stainless steel) *Xomed-Treace Inc.*	No	1.5	26
Pellets and Bullets:			
BB's *Daisy*	Yes	1.5	15
BB's *Crosman*	Yes	1.5	15
Bullet, .380 inch (copper, plastic, lead) *Glaser*	No	1.5	33
Bullet, .44 inch (Teflon, bronze) *North American Ordinance*	No	1.5	33
Bullet, 7.62 × 39 mm (copper, steel) *Norinco*	Yes	1.5	33
Bullet, .357 inch (copper, lead) *Cascade*	No	1.5	33
Bullet, .357 inch (lead) *Remington*	No	1.5	33
Bullet, .357 inch (aluminum, lead) *Winchester*	No	1.5	33
Bullet, 9 mm (copper, lead) *Remington*	No	1.5	33
Bullet, .380 inch (copper, nickel, lead) *Winchester*	Yes	1.5	33
Bullet, .357 inch (nylon, lead) *Smith & Wesson*	No	1.5	33
Bullet .45 inch (steel, lead) *Evansville Ordnance*	Yes	1.5	33
Bullet, .357 inch (steel, lead) *Fiocchi*	No	1.5	33
Bullet, .357 inch (copper, lead) *Hornady*	No	1.5	33
Bullet, 9 mm (copper, lead) *Norma*	Yes	1.5	33
Bullet, .357 inch (bronze, plastic) *Patton-Morgan*	No	1.5	33

Table 17-1 Metallic Implants, Materials, and Devices Tested for Movement/Deflection Forces During Exposure to Static Magnetic Fields—cont'd

Metallic implant, material, or device	Movement/ deflection	Highest field strength (T)†	Reference
Bullet, .357 inch (copper, lead)	No	1.5	33
Patton-Morgan			
Bullet, .45 inch (copper, lead)	No	1.5	33
Samson			
Shot, 12 gauge, size: 00 (copper, lead)	No	1.5	33
Federal			
Shot, 7½ (lead)	No	1.5	33
Shot, 4 (lead)	No	1.5	33
Shot, 00 buckshot (lead)	No	1.5	33
Penile Implants:			
Penile implant, AMS Malleable 600	No	1.5	10
American Medical Systems,			
Minnetonka, MN			
Penile implant, AMS 700 CX Inflatable	No	1.5	10
American Medical Systems			
Penile implant, Flexi-Flate	No	1.5	10
Medical Engineering Corp./Surgitek,			
Racine, WI			
Penile implant, Flexi-Rod (Standard)	No	1.5	10
Medical Engineering Corp./Surgitek			
Penile implant, Flex-Rod II (Firm)	No	1.5	10
Medical Engineering Corp./Surgitek			
Penile implant, Jonas	No	1.5	10
Dacomed Corporation,			
Minneapolis, MN			
Penile implant, Mentor Flexible	No	1.5	10
Mentor Corporation			
Stewartville, MN			
Penile implant, Mentor Inflatable	No	1.5	10
Mentor Corporation			
Penile implant, OmniPhase	Yes	1.5	10
Dacomed Corporation			
Vascular Access Ports:			
Button (polysulfone polymer, silicone)	No	1.5	21
Infusaid, Inc.,			
Norwood, MA			
Dome Port (titanium)	No	1.5	21
Davol Inc.			
Cranston, RI			
Dual MicroPort (polysulfone polymer, silicone)	No	1.5	21
Infusaid, Inc.,			
Dual MacroPort (polysulfone polymer, silicone)	No	1.5	21
Infusaid, Inc.			
Hickman Port (316L SS)	Yes*	1.5	21
Davol Inc.			
Hickman Port, Pediatric (titanium)	No	1.5	21
Davol Inc.			
Implantofix II (polysulfone)	No	1.5	21
Burron Medical, Inc.,			
Bethlehem, PA			
Infusaid, Model 400 (titanium)	No	1.5	21
Infusaid, Inc.			

Continued.

Table 17-1 Metallic Implants, Materials, and Devices Tested for Movement/Deflection Forces During Exposure to Static Magnetic Fields—cont'd

Metallic implant, material, or device	Movement/ deflection	Highest field strength (T)†	Reference
Infusaid, Model 600 (titanium)	No	1.5	21
Infusaid, Inc.			
Lifeport, Model 6013 (Delrin)	No	1.5	21
Strato Medical Corp.			
Beverly, MA			
Lifeport, Model 1013 (titanium)	No	1.5	21
Strato Medical Corp.			
MacroPort (polysulfone polymer, silicone)	No	1.5	21
Infusaid, Inc.			
MicroPort (polysulfone polymer, silicone)	No	1.5	21
Infusaid, Inc.			
MRI Port (Delrin plastic, silicone)	No	1.5	21
Davol Inc.			
Norport-AC (titanium)	No	1.5	21
Norfolk Medical Products Inc.			
Skokie, IL			
Norport-DL (316L SS)	No	1.5	21
Norfolk Medical Products Inc.			
Norport-LS (titanium)	No	1.5	21
Norfolk Medical Products Inc.			
Norport-LS (316L SS)	No	1.5	21
Norfolk Medical Products Inc.			
Norport-LS (polysulfone)	No	1.5	21
Norfolk Medical Products Inc.			
Norport-PT (titanium)	No	1.5	21
Norfolk Medical Products Inc.			
Norport-SP (polysulfone, silicone rubber, Dacron)	No	1.5	21
Norfolk Medical Products Inc.			
PeriPort (polysulfone, titanium)	No	1.5	21
Infusaid, Inc.			
Port-A-Cath, P.A.S. Port Portal (titanium)	No	1.5	21
Pharmacia Deltec Inc.			
St. Paul, MN			
Port-A-Cath, Titanium Dual Lumen Portal (titanium)	No	1.5	21
Pharmacia Deltec Inc.			
Port-A-Cath, Titanium Peritoneal Portal (titanium)	No	1.5	21
Pharmacia Deltec Inc.			
Port-A-Cath, Titanium Venous Low Profile Portal (titanium)	No	1.5	21
Pharmacia Deltec Inc.			
Port-A-Cath, Titanium Venous Portal (titanium)	No	1.5	21
Pharmacia Deltec Inc.			
Port-A-Cath, Venous Portal (316L SS)	No	1.5	21
Pharmacia Deltec Inc.			
Q-Port (316L SS)	Yes*	1.5	21
Quinton Instrument Co.,			
Seattle, WA			
S.E.A. (titanium)	No	1.5	21
Harbor Medical, Inc.,			
Boston, MA (now in St. Paul, MN)			
Snap-Lock (titanium, polysulfone polymer, silicone)	No	1.5	21
Infusaid, Inc.			

Table 17-1   Metallic Implants, Materials, and Devices Tested for Movement/Deflection Forces During Exposure to Static Magnetic Fields—cont'd

Metallic implant, material, or device	Movement/ deflection	Highest field strength (T)†	Reference
Synchromed, Model 8500-1 (titanium, thermoplastic, silicone) *Medtronic, Inc. Minneapolis, MN*	No	1.5	21
Vasport (titanium/fluoropolymer) *Gish Biomedical, Inc., Santa Ana, Ca*	No	1.5	21
Miscellaneous:			
Artificial urinary sphincter, AMS 800 *American Medical Systems Minnetonka, MN*	No	1.5	11
Cerebral ventricular shunt tube connector, Accu-Flow, straight *Codman, Randolph, MA*	No	1.5	11
Cerebral ventricular shunt tube connector, Accu-flow right angle *Codman*	No	1.5	11
Cerebral ventricular shunt tube connector, Accu-flow, T-connector *Codman*	No	1.5	11
Cerebral ventricular shunt tube connector (type unknown)	Yes	0.147	11
Contraceptive diaphragm, All Flex *Ortho Pharmaceutical, Raritan, NJ*	Yes*	1.5	11
Contraceptive diaphragm, Flat Spring *Ortho Pharmaceutical Corporation*	Yes*	1.5	11
Contraceptive diaphragm, Koroflex *Young Drug Products (now Carter-Wallace) Cranbury, NJ*	Yes*	1.5	11
Forceps (titanium)	No	1.44	10
Hakim valve and pump	No	1.44	10
Intrauterine contraceptive device (IUD), Copper T *G.D. Searle & Co. Skokie, IL*	No	1.5	7
Shunt valve, Holtertype *Holter-Hausner International (now Phoenix Bioengineering, Inc.) Bridgeport, PA*	Yes*	1.5	38
Shunt valve, Holter-Hausner type *Holter-Hausner International (now Phoenix Bioengineering, Inc.)*	No	1.5	38
Swan-Ganz thermodilution catheter *American Edwards Laboratories, Santa Ana, CA*	No‡	1.5	60
Tantalum powder	No	1.44	9
Tissue expander with magnetic port *McGhan Medical Corp., Santa Barbara, CA*	Yes	1.5	30
Vascular marker, O-ring washer (302 SS) *PIC Design, Middlebury, CT*	Yes*	1.5	58

‡Although there is no magnetic deflection associated with the triple-lumen thermodilution Swan-Ganz catheter, there has been a report of a catheter "melting" in a patient; therefore this would be considered a relative contraindication for MR imaging.

this information specifically pertains to the safety aspects of imaging a patient with respect to the ferromagnetic qualities of a metallic implant, material, or device (that is, its attraction to a magnetic field). Other issues related to electrical conductivity, artifact production, and so on are not discussed in this chapter.

Various factors influence the risk of performing MR imaging in a patient with a ferromagnetic implant, material, or device, including the strength of the static and gradient magnetic fields, the relative degree of ferromagnetism of the object, the mass of the object, the configuration of the object, the location and orientation of the object in situ, and the length of time the object has been in place.[*] These factors should be carefully considered before one subjects a patient with a ferromagnetic object to MR imaging, particularly if it is located in a potentially dangerous area of the body, as near a vital neural, vascular, of soft-tissue structure where movement or dislodgment could injure the patient.[*]

All biomedical implants, materials, and devices, particularly those made from unknown substances, should be evaluated by use of ex vivo techniques before one performs MR imaging in patients with them.[11] By following this procedure, the presence and amount of ferromagnetism may be determined so that a competent decision can be made concerning the potential associated risks.

ANEURYSM AND HEMOSTATIC CLIPS

Nineteen of the twenty-six aneurysm clips previously tested displayed ferromagnetic qualities and, therefore, are considered a contraindication for patients undergoing MR imaging.[4,9,11,29,32,38,42] Laboratory studies have demonstrated that there is a realistic hazard when subjecting ferromagnetic aneurysm clips to static magnetic fields insofar as these clips may be displaced and result in serious patient consequences.[4,38,42] Because of this, it is recommended that patients be examined only by MR imaging if the type of aneurysm clip is emphatically known to be nonferromagnetic. Four patients with nonferromagnetic or weakly ferromagnetic aneurysm clips have been scanned by MR imaging without incident.[29] None of the six hemostatic vascular clips evaluated were attracted by static magnetic fields used for MR imaging up to field strengths of 1.5 T.[11] These hemostatic clips are made from nonferromagnetic materials and therefore do not present a risk to patients during MR imaging.

CAROTID ARTERY VASCULAR CLAMPS

Each of the five carotid artery vascular clamps tested displayed magnetic deflection when in the presence of

a 1.5 T static magnetic field.[22] However, only the Poppen-Blaylock carotid artery vascular clamp was believed to be contraindicated for patients undergoing MRI because of the tremendous ferromagnetism of this particular device.[22] The others were believed to be safe because of the existence of only mild ferromagnetism.[22] Patients with metallic carotid artery vascular clamps have been imaged by MR systems with static magnetic fields ranging from 0.35 to 0.6 T without experiencing any discomfort or neurologic sequelae.[22]

DENTAL DEVICES AND MATERIALS

Of the 16 different dental devices and materials tested, 12 had measurable deflection forces, but only three of these represent a potential problem for patients during MR imaging because these are magnetically activated devices[9,11,37,55] (see p. 492).

HEART VALVE PROSTHESES

Twenty-nine different heart valve prostheses have been evaluated for magnetic deflection related to exposure to a 1.5 or 2.35 T static magnetic field.[5,11,12] Of these, four were nonferromagnetic and 25 had measurable deflection forces.[5,11,12] Because the magnetic deflection of these heart valves is minimal compared to the force exerted by the beating heart, MR imaging is not considered to be hazardous for patients with these valvular prostheses[5,11,12] (with the possible exception of performing MR imaging with a MR system greater than 0.35 T on a patient who has a Starr-Edwards Pre 600 valve when there is concern regarding the integrity of the annulus or presence of valvular dehiscence[12]).

INTRAVASCULAR COILS, FILTERS, AND STENTS

Fourteen different intravascular coils, filters, and stents have been assessed for ferromagnetic qualities.[13,25,28,31,40] Five of these are ferromagnetic. However, these devices typically become firmly incorporated into the vessel wall after approximately 6 weeks, and therefore it is unlikely that any of them would become dislodged by magnetic forces.[13,58] In fact, patients with most of the intravascular coils, filters, and stents listed in Table 17-1 have been imaged with 1.5 T MR scanners without incident.[13,24,25,31,40,58] Therefore it is considered to be safe to image patients with any of the intravascular coils, filters, and stents listed after a suitable time has elapsed to ensure stable positioning and retention of the device. MR imaging should not be performed if there is any possibility that an intravascular coil, filter, or stent is not held firmly in place.

OCULAR IMPLANTS

Of the 12 ocular implants tested, the Fatio eyelid spring[23] and the retinal tack made from martensitic

---

[*]References 9, 11, 15, 33, 44, 45, 49, 54, 62-64.

stainless steel (Western European)[27] were deflected by a 1.5 T static magnetic field. Both of these may be uncomfortable to (that is, the Fatio eyelid spring) or injure (that is, the Western European retinal tack) the patient during MR imaging. The case of a ferromagnetic object damaging the eye of a patient undergoing MR imaging has been previously described,[50] and such damage underscores the need for special diligence when one is subjecting a patient with any type of ferromagnetic material located near the eye to this imaging procedure.[49] (See also the discussion of magnetically activated implants and devices, p. 492.)

ORTHOPEDIC IMPLANTS, MATERIALS, AND DEVICES

Most of the various orthopedic materials and devices tested are made from nonferromagnetic materials and are safe for MR imaging.[11,35,59] Only the Perfix interference screw used for reconstruction of the anterior cruciate ligament displayed a substantial deflection force and caused extensive signal loss. This screw was the first orthopedic implant tested up to now that was substantially ferromagnetic and caused greater than the localized signal void typically observed with other metallic orthopedic implants. Images of the knee of one patient with two Perfix screws in place were not interpretable because of the image distortion caused by these implants.[59] Therefore alternative nonferromagnetic implants should be considered for reconstruction of the anterior cruciate ligament.

An additional concern of subjecting metallic orthopedic implants, which are typically large, to MR imaging is the potential heating that may develop as a result of exposure to the gradient or radiofrequency electromagnetic fields. However, studies have demonstrated that heating of these implants is relatively insignificant.[17]

OTOLOGIC IMPLANTS

The three cochlear implants tested are contraindicated for MR imaging because, in addition to being attracted by static magnetic fields, they are also electronically or magnetically activated.[8,53] Of the remaining otologic implants, only one of them displayed magnetic deflection during testing with a 1.5 T static magnetic field.[6,8,26,53] This implant, the McGee stapedectomy piston prosthesis, made from platinum and 17Cr-4Ni stainless steel (manufactured during mid-1987), has been recalled by the manufacturer.[53] In addition, patients who received this implant have been identified and issued cards warning them not to be examined by MR imaging.[53]

PELLETS AND BULLETS

Most of the pellets and bullets tested are composed of nonferromagnetic materials.[15,33] Ammunition that proved to be ferromagnetic tended to be manufactured in foreign countries or of the military variety.[33] Of note is that shrapnel typically contains steel and therefore presents a hazard for MR imaging.[33] Because pellets, bullets, and shrapnel may be contaminated with ferromagnetic materials, the risk versus benefits of performing MR imaging should be carefully considered as well as whether the pellet, bullet, or piece of shrapnel is located near a vital internal structure.[33-34]

Of further note is that, in an effort to reduce lead poisoning in the "puddling" type of ducks, there is a requirement by the federal government in many of the eastern United States to use steel shotgun pellets instead of lead.[34] This would present a potential hazard to patients undergoing MR imaging and cause severe artifacts.[34]

PENILE IMPLANTS

Only one of the nine penile implants, the Dacomed Omniphase, had a significant deflection force measured when exposed to a 1.5 T static magnetic field.[10] Although it is unlikely that this implant would severely injure a patient undergoing MR imaging because of the manner in which it is utilized, it would undoubtedly be uncomfortable for the patient and therefore scanning a patient with this implant is inadvisable.

VASCULAR ACCESS PORTS

Two of the 33 implantable vascular access ports tested had measurable deflection forces, but the forces were believed to be insignificant relative to the in vivo application of these implants.[21] Therefore it is safe to perform MR imaging in a patient who may have one of these implants. Future developments of this technology will include vascular access ports that are electronically activated, and these would obviously be contraindicated for MR imaging.

MISCELLANEOUS

Of the miscellaneous metallic implants, materials, and devices tested, the cerebral ventricular shunt tube connector (type unknown)[11] and tissue expander with magnetic port[30] have significant deflection forces, which may be hazardous to patients undergoing MR imaging. Another ferromagnetic implant, the O-ring washer vascular marker, displays only slight ferromagnetic qualities and therefore does not represent a risk to patients examined by MR imaging.[59] The contraceptive diaphragms were attracted strongly by the 1.5 T static magnetic field, but patients have been scanned with these devices and did not complain of any sensation related to the movement of these objects. Accordingly, the presence of a diaphragm is not believed to pose a hazard to a patient during MR imaging. There is, however, a remote possibility that the contraceptive properties of the diaphragm may be hindered if it is inadvertently moved during an MR imaging examination.

Although the triple-lumen thermodilution Swan-Ganz catheter is constructed of nonferromagnetic materials, the presence of this device may be injurious to the patient during MR imaging.[60] A report indicated that a portion of a thermodilution Swan-Ganz catheter that was outside the patient melted as a result of MR imaging.[60] It was postulated that the high-frequency electromagnetic fields generated by the MR imaging system caused eddy current heating of either the wires within the thermodilution catheter or the radiopaque material inside the catheter. This incident indicates that patients with triple-lumen thermodilution Swan-Ganz catheters or other similar devices could be injured during MR imaging.

MAGNETICALLY ACTIVATED IMPLANTS AND DEVICES

Certain ferromagnetic implants and devices, such as cochlear implants, tissue expanders, ocular prostheses, and dental implants are magnetically activated.[8,30,37,55,56,61] The majority of these are considered to be hazardous to patients undergoing MRI.[49,54,61] Besides dislodging these particular types of implants and devices, MR imaging may also alter or damage the operation of the magnetic component,[49,54,61] possibly requiring surgery for replacement. Furthermore, if the portion of the prosthesis that the magnet attracts is implanted in soft tissue (for example, with certain ocular prostheses, the magnet is contained in the prosthesis and a ferromagnetic "keeper"), it is inadvisable to perform MR imaging in a patient with this type of device because of potentially adverse effects associated with displacement of the "keeper."[61] MR imaging may be performed safely in patients with dental magnet appliances that are properly attached to supporting structures after the magnet-containing portion of the device is removed.[55]

SUMMARY AND CONCLUSIONS

According to the *Policies, Guidelines, and Recommendations for MR Imaging Safety and Patient Management* information issued by the Society for Magnetic Resonance Imaging Safety Committee,[49] patients with electronically, magnetically, or mechanically activated, or electrically conductive devices should be excluded from MR imaging unless the particular device has been previously shown (that is, usually by ex vivo testing procedures) to be unaffected by the electromagnetic fields used for clinical MR imaging and there is no possibility of injuring the patient. During the screening process for MR imaging, patients with these objects should be identified before examination by MR imaging or being exposed to the electromagnetic fields used for this imaging technique. In this chapter, the numerous implants and foreign bodies that are considered to be absolute or relative contraindications for MR imaging have been presented and discussed. It should be noted, however, that there are implants, materials, devices, or other foreign bodies that have yet to be evaluated for MR compatibility, which may be encountered in the clinical setting. Patients that have untested objects should not be allowed to undergo MR imaging.

ACKNOWLEDGMENT

We wish to acknowledge the editorial contributions of Mr. Wally Kappelman, Milwaukee, Wisconsin, and Stacy M. Myers at Cedars-Sinai Medical Center, Los Angeles, California.

REFERENCES

1. Applebaum EL, Valvassori GE: Effects of magnetic resonance imaging fields on stapedectomy prostheses, *Arch Otolaryngol* 111:820-821, 1985.
2. Barrafato D, Henkelman RM: Magnetic resonance imaging and surgical clips, *Can Surg* 27:509-512, 1984.
3. DeKeizer RJW, TeStrake L: Intraocular lens implants (pseudophakoi) and steelwire sutures: a contraindication for MRI? *Doc Ophthalmol* 61:281-284, 1986.
4. Dujovny M, Kossovsky N, Kossowsky R, et al: Aneurysm clip motion during magnetic resonance imaging: in vivo experimental study with metallurgical factor analysis, *Neurosurgery* 17:543-548, 1985.
5. Hassler M, Le Bas JF, Wolf JE, et al: Effects of magnetic fields used in MRI on 15 prosthetic heart valves, *J Radiol* 67:661-666, 1986.
6. Leon JA, Gabriele OF: Middle ear prosthesis: significance in magnetic resonance imaging, *Magn Reson Imaging* 5:405-406, 1987.
7. Mark AS, Hricak H: Intrauterine contraceptive devices: MR imaging, *Radiology* 162:311-314, 1987.
8. Mattucci KF, Setzen M, Hyman R, Chaturvedi G: The effect of nuclear magnetic resonance imaging on metallic middle ear prostheses, *Otolaryngnol Head Neck Surg* 94:441-443, 1986.
9. New PFJ, Rosen BR, Brady TJ, et al: Potential hazards and artifacts of ferromagnetic and nonferromagnetic surgical and dental materials and devices in nuclear magnetic resonance imaging, *Radiology* 147:139-148, 1983.
10. Shellock FG, Crues JV, Sacks SA: High-field magnetic resonance imaging of penile prostheses: in vitro evaluation of deflection forces and imaging artifacts. Abstract in *Book of abstracts*, Society of Magnetic Resonance in Medicine, vol 2, p 915, Berkeley, Calif., 1987.
11. Shellock FG, Crues JV: High-field-strength MR imaging and metallic biomedical implants: an ex vivo evaluation of deflection forces, *AJR* 151:389-392, 1988.
12. Soulen RL, Budinger TF, Higgins CB: Magnetic resonance imaging of prosthetic heart valves, *Radiology* 154:705-707, 1985.
13. Teitelbaum GP, Bradley WG, Klein BD: MR imaging artifacts, ferromagnetism, and magnetic torque of intravascular filters, stents, and coils, *Radiology* 166:657-664, 1988.
14. Zheutlin JD, Thompson JT, Shofner RS: The safety of magnetic resonance imaging with intraorbital metallic objects after retinal reattachment or trauma, *Am J Ophthalmol* 103:831, 1987 (letter).
15. Shellock FG: Biological effects and safety aspects of magnetic resonance imaging, *Magn Reson Q* 5:243-261, 1989.
16. Davis PL, Crooks L, Arakawa M, et al: Potential hazards in NMR imaging: heating effects of changing magnetic fields and RF fields on small metallic implants, *AJR* 137:857-860, 1981.

17. Shellock FG, Crues JV: High field MR imaging of metallic biomedical implants: an ex vivo evaluation of deflection forces, *AJR* 151:389-392, 1988.

18. Bellon EM, Haacke EM, Coleman PE, et al: MR artifacts: a review, *Magn Reson Imaging* 2:41-52, 1984.

19. Pusey E, Lufkin RB, Brown RKJ, et al: Magnetic resonance imaging artifacts: mechanism and clinical significance, *RadioGraphics* 6:891-911, 1986.

20. Yamanashi WS, Wheatley KK, Lester PD, Anderson DW: Technical artifacts in magnetic resonance imaging, *Physiol Chem Phys Med NMR* 16:237-250, 1984.

21. Shellock FG, Meeks T: Ex vivo evaluation of ferromagnetism and artifacts for implantable vascular access ports exposed to a 1.5 T MR scanner, *J Magn Reson Imaging* 1:243, 1991.

22. Teitelbaum GP, Lin MCW, Watanabe AT, et al: Ferromagnetism and MR imaging: safety of carotid vascular clamps, *AJNR* 11:267-272, 1990.

23. Shellock FG, Schatz C, Shelton C, Brown B: Ex vivo evaluation of ferromagnetism for metallic ocular and middle-ear prostheses exposed to a 1.5 T MR imager, *Radiology* 177(P):271, 1990.

24. Watanabe AT, Teitelbaum GP, Gomes AS, Roehm JOF: MR imaging of the bird's nest filter, *Radiology* 177:578-579, 1990.

25. Teitelbaum GP, Raney M, Carvlin MJ, et al: Evaluation of ferromagnetism and magnetic resonance imaging artifacts of the Strecker tantalum vascular stent, *Cardiovasc Intervent Radiol* 12:125-127, 1989.

26. Shellock FG, Schatz CJ: Metallic otologic implants: assessment of ferromagnetism at 1.5 T, *AJNR* 12:279-281, 1991.

27. Albert DW, Olson KR, Parel JM, et al: Magnetic resonance imaging and retinal tacks, *Arch Ophthalmol* 108:320-321, 1990.

28. Williamson MR, McCowan TC, Walker CW, Ferris EJ: Effect of a 1.5 tesla magnetic field on Greenfield filters in vitro and in dogs, *Angiology* 39:1022-1024, 1988.

29. Becker RL, Norfray JF, Teitelbaum GP, et al: MR imaging in patients with intracranial aneurysm clips, *AJNR* 9:885-889, 1988.

30. Liang MD, Narayanan K, Kanal E: Magnetic ports in tissue expanders—a caution for MRI, *Magn Reson Imaging* 7:541-542, 1989.

31. Teitelbaum GP, Ortega HV, Vinitski S, et al: Low-artifact intravascular devices: MR imaging evaluation, *Radiology* 168:713-719, 1988.

32. Gold JP, Pulsinelli W, Winchester P, et al: Safety of metallic surgical clips in patients undergoing high-field-strength magnetic resonance imaging, *Ann Thorac Surg* 48:643-645, 1989.

33. Teitelbaum GP, Yee CA, Van-Horn DD, et al: Metallic ballistic fragments: MR imaging safety and artifacts, *Radiology* 175:855-859, 1990.

34. Teitelbaum GP: Metallic ballistic fragments: MR imaging safety and artifacts, *Radiology* 177:883, 1990 (letter to the editor).

35. Lyons CJ, Betz RR, Mesgarzadeh M, et al: The effect of magnetic resonance imaging on metal spine implants, *Spine* 14:670-672, 1989.

36. White DW: Interaction between magnetic fields and metallic ossicular prostheses, *Am J Otolaryngol* 8:90-92, 1987.

37. Shellock FG: Ex vivo assessment of deflection forces and artifacts associated with high-field strength of "mini-magnet" dental prostheses, *Magn Reson Imaging* 7(suppl 1):38, 1989.

38. Go KG, Kamman RL, Mooyaart EL: Interaction of metallic neurosurgical implants with magnetic resonance imaging at 1.5 tesla as a cause of image distortion and of hazardous movement of the implant, *Clin Neurosurg* 91:109-115, 1989.

39. Matsumoto AH, Teitelbaum GP, Barth KH, et al: Tantalum vascular stents: in vivo evaluation with MR imaging, *Radiology* 170:753-755, 1989.

40. Liebman CE, Messersmith RN, Levin DN, Lu CT: MR imaging of inferior vena caval filter: safety and artifacts, *AJR* 150:1174-1176, 1988.

41. Joondeph BC, Peyman GA, Mafee MF, Joondeph HC: Magnetic resonance imaging and retinal tacks, *Arch Ophthalmol* 105:1479-1480, 1987.

42. Brown MA, Carden JA, Coleman RE, et al: Magnetic field effects on surgical ligation clips, *Magn Reson Imaging* 5:443-453, 1987.

43. Roberts CW, Haik BG, Cahill P: Magnetic resonance imaging of metal loop intraocular lenses, *Arch Ophthalmol* 108:320-321, 1990.

44. Shellock FG: MR imaging of metallic implants and materials: a compilation of the literature, *AJR* 151:811-814, 1988.

45. Shellock FG, Canal E, Talagala L: Safety considerations in magnetic resonance imaging, *Radiology* 176:593-606, 1990.

46. Fache JS, Price C, Hawbolt EB, Li DKB: MR imaging artifacts produced by dental materials, *AJNR* 8:837-840, 1987.

47. Laakman RW, Kaufman B, Han JS, et al: MR imaging in patients with metallic implants, *Radiology* 157:711-714, 1985.

48. Mechlin M, Thickman D, Kressel HY, et al: Magnetic resonance imaging of postoperative patients with metallic implants, *AJR* 143:1281-1284, 1984.

49. Shellock FG, Kanal E: SMRI Safety Committee: Policies, guidelines, and recommendations for MR imaging safety and patient management, *J Magn Reson Imaging* 1:97-101, 1991.

50. Kelly WM, Paglen PG, Pearson JA, et al: Ferromagnetism of intraocular foreign body causes unilateral blindness after MR study, *AJNR* 7:243-245, 1986.

51. Kuethe DO, Small KW, Blinder RA: Non-ferromagnetic retinal tacks are a tolerable risk in magnetic resonance imaging, *Invest Radiol* 26:1-7, 1991.

52. Lissac MI, Metrop D, Brugirard J, et al: Dental materials and magnetic resonance imaging, *Invest Radiol* 26:40-45, 1991.

53. Applebaum EL, Valvassori GE: Further studies on the effects of magnetic resonance imaging fields on middle ear implants, *Ann Otol Rhinol Laryngol* 99:801-804, 1990.

54. Kanal E, Shellock FG, Talagala L: Safety considerations in MR imaging, *Radiology* 176:593-606, 1990.

55. Gegauff, Laurell KA, Thavendrarajah A, Rosentiel SF: A potential MRI hazard: forces on dental magnet keepers, *J Oral Rehabil* 17:403-410, 1990.

56. Power W, Collum LMT: Magnetic resonance imaging and magnetic eye implants, *Lancet* 2:227, 1988.

57. Kanal E, Shellock FG, Sonnenblick D: MRI clinical site safety survey: phase I results and preliminary data, *Magn Reson Imaging* 7(suppl 1):106, 1988.

58. Personal communication with R.D. Becker, New Haven, Conn., 1989.

59. Shellock FG, Mink JH, Curtin S, Friedman MJ: MRI and orthopedic implants used for anterior cruciate ligament reconstruction: assessment of ferromagnetism and artifacts, *J Magn Reson Imaging* 2:225, 1992.

60. ECRI, Health Devices Alert: A new MRI complication? p 1, May 27, 1988, Emergency Care Research Institute, Plymouth Meeting, Penn.

61. Yuh WTC, Hanigan MT, Nerad JA, et al: Extrusion of eye socket magnetic implant after MR imaging: potential hazard to patient with eye prosthesis, *J Magn Reson Imaging* 1:711-713, 1991.

62. Shellock FG, Crues JV: Safety aspects of MRI in patients with metallic implants or foreign bodies: absolute and relative contraindications, *Appl Radiol*, pp 44-47, Nov 1992.

63. Shellock FG, Litwer C, Kanal E: MRI bioeffects, safety, and patient management: a review, *Reviews in Magnetic Resonance Imaging* 4:21-63, 1992.

64. Shellock FG: Biological effects and safety aspects of MRI. In Stark DD, Bradley WG, editors: *Magnetic resonance imaging*, ed 2, St. Louis, 1991, Mosby—Year Book.

65. Shellock FG, Kanal E: Safety considerations of cardiovascular MR studies. In *Cardiovascular applications of magnetic resonance imaging and spectroscopy*, New York, 1992, Futura Publishing.

18

Nuclear Medicine Imaging: Medical Devices and Artifacts

. . . .

Dennis D. Patton

Artifacts are so common in nuclear medicine that when there is an unusual finding, it is good judgment to think of an artifact first. Nuclear medicine imaging relies on the detection of photons. Unlike radiography, the photons originate within the body rather than outside of it. Therefore, the anterior view of the body may differ greatly from the posterior view. Artifacts caused by devices within the body generally appear in all views on radiographic images, but they may be evident on only one or no views on nuclear medicine studies.

The functional (physiologic) information in nuclear medicine images often makes them exquisitely sensitive for the detection of disease, such as a bone scan demonstrating the effects of bony metastases before there are any plain film radiographic changes, or a lung scan demonstrating the effects of a pulmonary embolus in the presence of a normal chest radiograph. As a result, physiologic alterations in body function may cause artifacts in nuclear medicine scintigrams, even though there are no morphologic (anatomic) changes in the patient.

Nuclear medicine studies suffer from poor anatomic detail in comparison with most other medical imaging techniques, though resolution has steadily improved over the years. Artifacts or devices that are easily identifiable on other imaging studies may be very difficult to identify on nuclear scintigrams. Those experienced in interpreting nuclear medicine images have learned that correlating them with other imaging studies is a good habit that saves more time than it costs.

Because nuclear medicine images are primarily functional and because artifacts caused by objects within the body usually cause more morphologic than physiologic change, these artifacts should not overly interfere with interpretation, if they are properly recognized. Most of the artifacts illustrated here are commonly seen in a busy nuclear medicine practice. A few of the images are "dated" but are included because they show a particular artifact well. This chapter stresses artifacts related to medical devices and foreign bodies. Many other nuclear medicine artifacts arise from the more technical aspects of nuclear medicine imaging (improper gamma camera settings, radiotracer quality control, drug effects, and so forth). Although a few examples will be shown, extensive discussion of artifacts of technique is beyond the scope of this chapter and is well covered elsewhere.[1-5]

ORTHOPEDIC APPLIANCES

Orthopedic devices may be particularly troublesome and may produce bizarre images because they cause reactive bone formation (hence a "positive" bone scan) and also block transmission of gamma rays originating deeper in the body (Figs. 18-1 to 18-7). Common devices are spine struts (Fig. 18-1), hip prostheses (Figs. 18-2 and 18-3), knee or femoral prostheses (Figs. 18-4 and 18-5), Harrington rods (Fig. 18-6), and skull plates (Fig. 18-7). Most of these artifacts have a characteristic appearance and are easy to recognize. They are also readily explained once the patient's history and radiographic studies are available.

Increased local osteoblastic activity may persist for months to years after bone surgery, especially during

Text continued on p. 501.

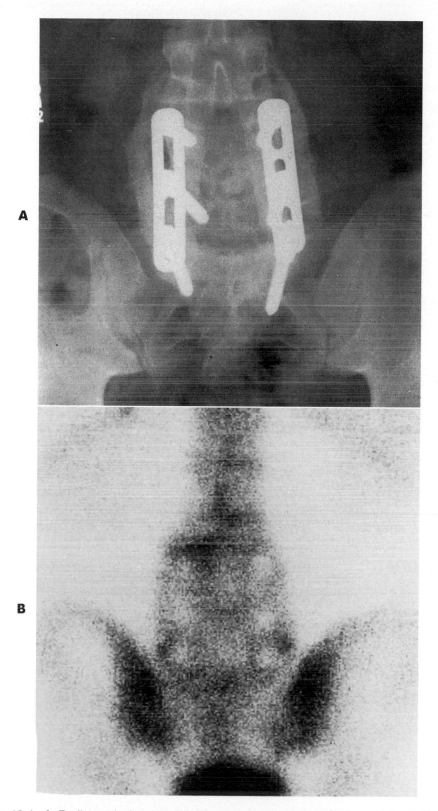

Fig. 18-1. A, Radiograph showing metal struts supporting spine after laminectomy. **B,** Bone scan showing attenuation of photons by the metal.

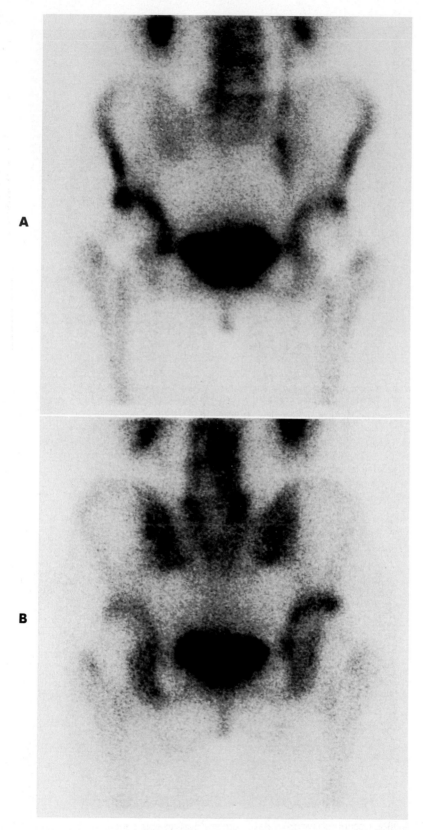

Fig. 18-2. Bone scan showing bilateral total hip prostheses. The artifacts are more readily seen in the anterior view, **A,** than in the posterior view, **B.**

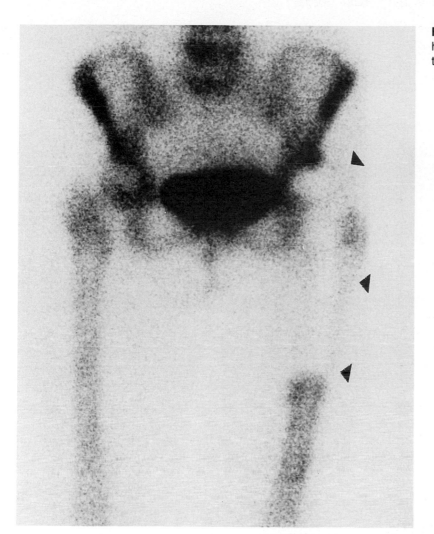

Fig. 18-3. Bone scan showing metal prosthetic hip, *arrowheads*, that was installed after resection of a fibrosarcoma.

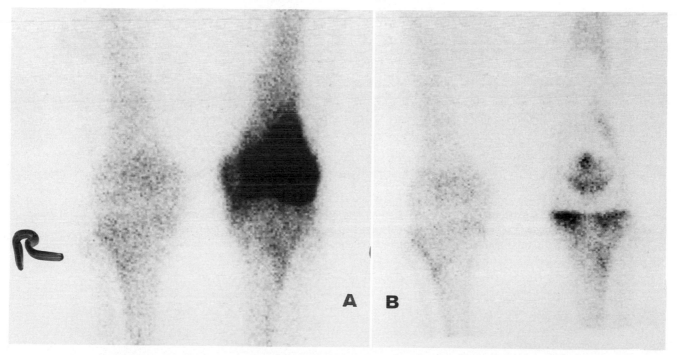

Fig. 18-4. A, Bone scan showing osteosarcoma in distal left femur. **B,** After removal, the distal femur and the knee were replaced by metal prostheses.

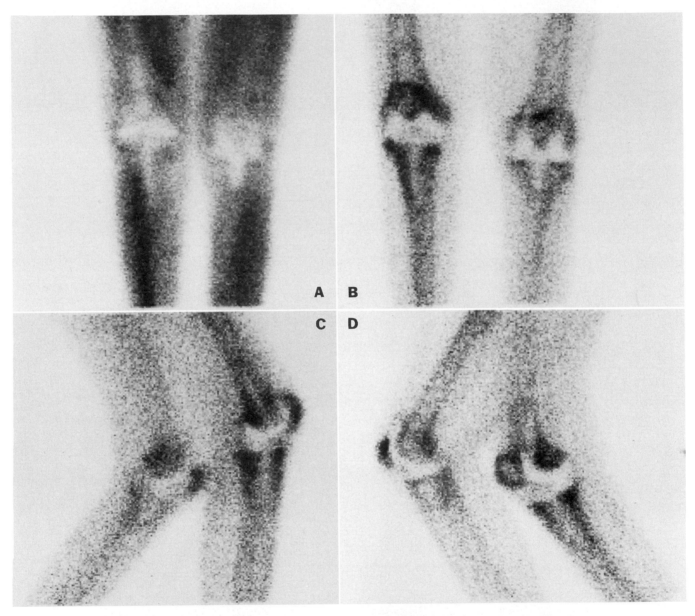

Fig. 18-5. Bone scan showing bilateral total knee replacements. **A,** Blood pool study. **B** to **D,** delayed views showing normal increased osteoblastic activity 6 months after surgery. A right lumbar sympathectomy has led to slightly increased blood pool activity on the right.

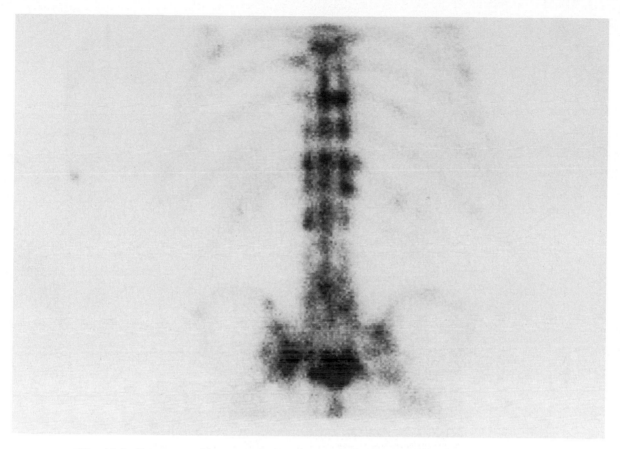

Fig. 18-6. Bone scan. Linear vertical lucent stripes represent bilateral Harrington rods.

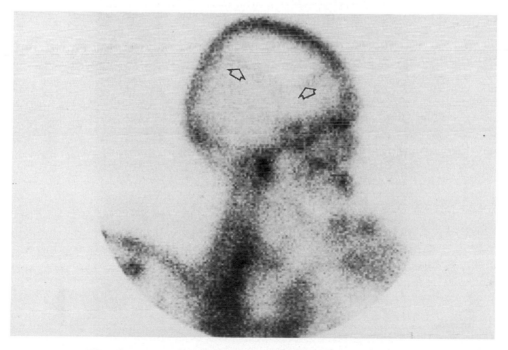

Fig. 18-7. Bone scan showing metallic skull plate, *arrowheads.*

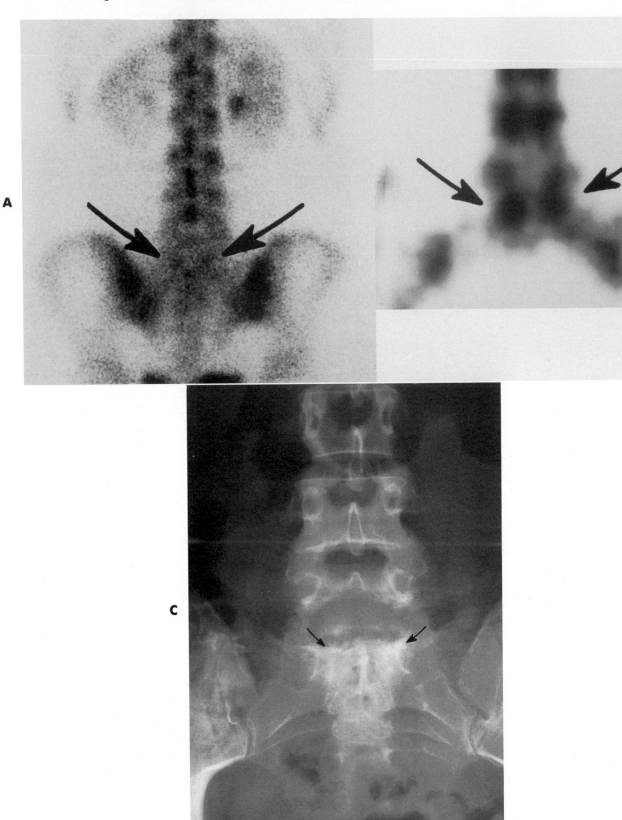

Fig. 18-8. Autologous bone dowels were placed on either side of L5-S1 for stabilization, *arrows.* There is good uptake of ^{99m}Tc-methylene diphosphonate in the grafts, seen better on the images using single-photon emission computerized tomography.

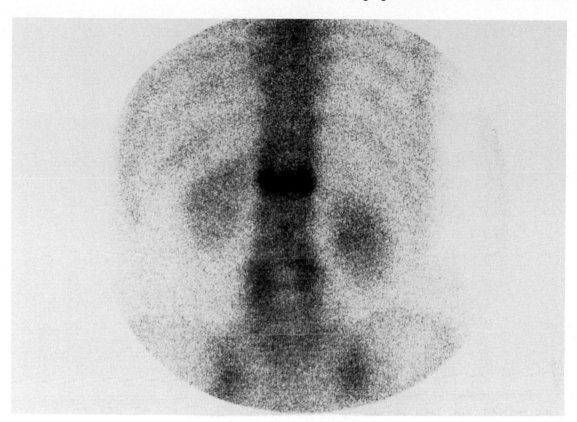

Fig. 18-9. After a standard laminectomy the posterior spinous processes in L4 and L5 are no longer present. There is active bone repair there, and in this case also an incidental compression fracture of L1.

the first 6 months, even in the absence of bone infection or other known pathologic conditions. This reflects normal bone repair and makes it difficult, for example, to distinguish loosening of a joint prosthesis or infection at the prosthesis site from a normal postoperative effect. White blood cells labeled with indium 111 or technetium 99m are helpful in detecting infection in the presence of postsurgical artifacts.[6]

Bone scans may be used to assess whether bone grafts are "taking." Fig. 18-8 illustrates a patient in whom autologous bone dowels had been inserted into the L5-S1 region for spine stabilization. The SPECT images in this case demonstrate good bone function. The localized absence of the posterior arch of the spine after a laminectomy produces a characteristic defect on nuclear medicine scans (Fig. 18-9).

BARIUM SULFATE

Barium sulfate used as a contrast agent in gastrointestinal radiographic studies may produce significant artifacts in nuclear medicine images because of its high coefficient of absorption for gamma rays. It may especially degrade bone scans (Fig. 18-10) and liver scans (Fig. 18-11). Barium remaining in the bowel can seri-

ously degrade or ruin CT, MRI, plain film radiography, and nuclear medicine studies; one should therefore complete these studies before barium examinations of the gastrointestinal tract. Abdominal ultrasound examinations may be significantly degraded by a recent barium enema, though surprisingly not by recent upper gastrointestinal series.[7,8] Iodinated contrast agents are used in concentrations thinner than those of barium mixtures and generally do not cause visible artifacts on nuclear medicine images, though they may profoundly affect thyroid function measurements.

THE BREAST AND BREAST PROSTHESES

The normal breast may cause confusing nuclear medicine artifacts by attenuating photons originating more deeply in the body, leading to lucent defects over the chest or upper abdomen in liver, bone, heart, and lung scans (Fig. 18-12). In patients with large breasts, it may be necessary to lift the breast away from the area being imaged. Pendulous breasts may cause confusing artifacts on lateral images when the patient lies supine. Small-angle Compton scatter can also cause a band of intensification, especially in large or fatty breasts.

Increased soft-tissue radionuclide uptake in the breast

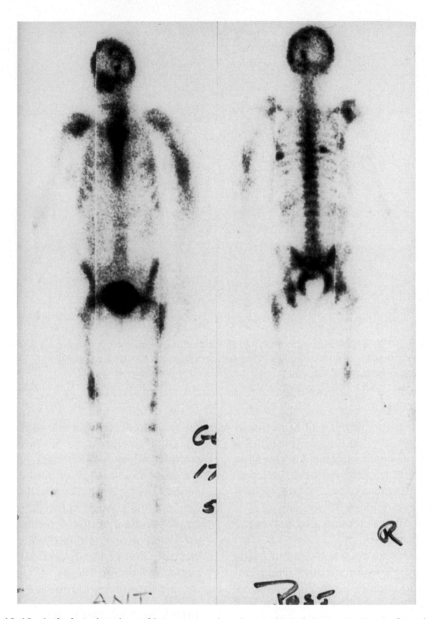

Fig. 18-10. *Left,* Anterior view of bone scan showing multiple bony metastases from breast cancer, and a full bladder. *Right,* Photons from the bladder are strongly attenuated by residual barium sulfate in the rectum from a recent radiologic study. These images also show the "zipper" artifact: vertical blank stripes running through the image caused by a small-field-of-view gamma camera that had to scan the patient three times to build up a full image of the body. The larger modern cameras do not suffer from this artifact.

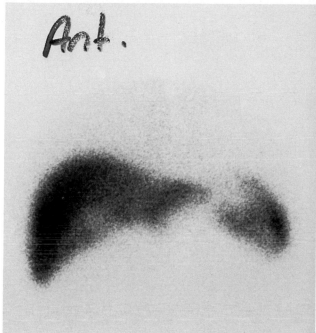

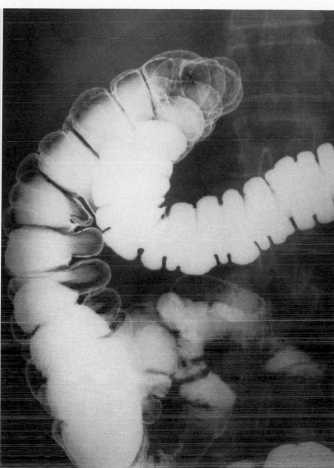

Fig. 18-11. A, Liver-spleen scan showing artifact caused by barium sulfate in the colon (central defect along inferior border of liver). **B,** The spleen is partly hidden by barium sulfate in the splenic flexure, or possibly by the stomach.

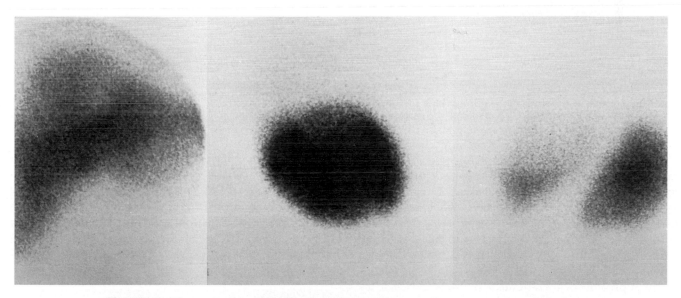

Fig. 18-12. The normal breast often produces a lucent artifact on liver scans. This montage of three different studies shows the artifact in anterior view *(left),* right lateral view *(center),* and left lateral view *(right;* liver is to the left, showing artifact, and spleen is to the right).

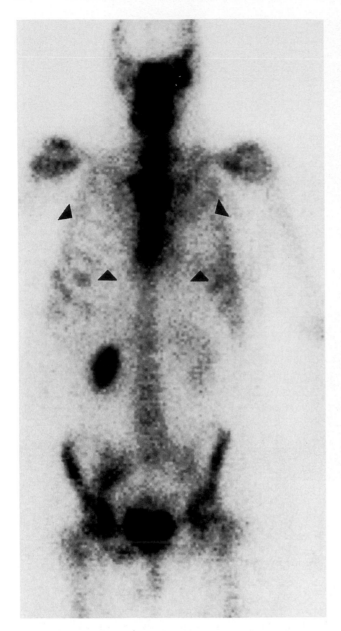

Fig. 18-13. Bone scan showing bilateral breast prostheses after bilateral mastectomy (*arrowheads* outline lucent areas). Patient has metastatic breast carcinoma.

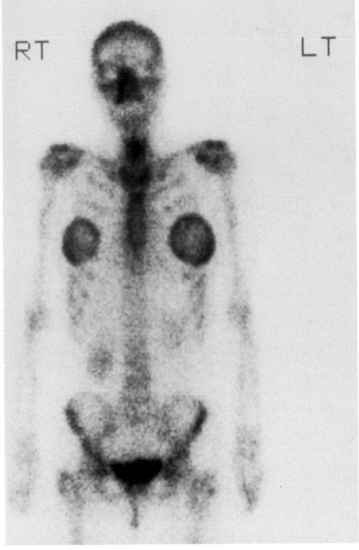

Fig. 18-14. Inflamed bilateral silicone breast prostheses. Inflammatory tissue often takes up the bone-seeking radiotracer, which is a form of phosphate and presumably follows calcium into necrotizing tissue.

may reflect inflammatory or even neoplastic disease, but in most cases it is a nonspecific finding of no particular significance. After mastectomy, there may appear to be increased tracer uptake in the ipsilateral ribs. This probably represents loss of attenuating tissue, but it also may reflect increased rib uptake caused by surgical manipulation.

Breast prostheses also attenuate photons and cause lucent defects similar to those in the normal breast (Fig. 18-13). Prostheses with associated complications, such as rupture, contracture, or chronic inflammation (see Chapter 7), may show up on radionuclide bone scans

as hot areas, probably reflecting inflammatory microcalcification (Fig. 18-14). This reflects the nonspecificity of present-day bone-seeking radiotracers, which can be taken up by inflammation, infection, tumor, and other foci of accelerated metabolic activity, as well as by osteoblasts.

PATIENTS WITH UNUSUAL OR ALTERED ANATOMY

Ectopic kidneys, severe kyphosis or scoliosis, situs inversus, and other anatomic variants may lead to bizarre images very difficult to interpret. Some patients cannot

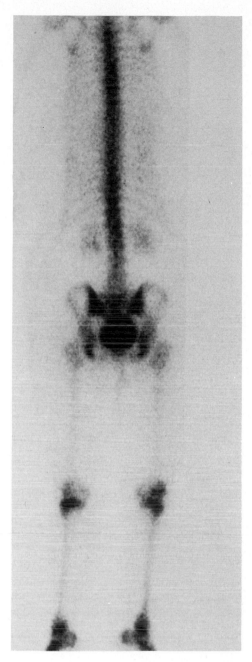

Fig. 18-15. Bone scan in an obese patient. The gamma camera normally passes beneath the supine patient from foot to head, building up a whole-body image. In this case, the imaging table sagged so much from the patient's weight that the camera caught it and traveled with it, repeating portions of the image until it slipped free.

tion?) and physical examination (scars, missing limbs, obesity, jaundice?) may save an hour of effort trying to understand and reconcile seeming discrepancies in anatomy.

Morbidly obese patients are often difficult to image adequately. Some patients are too large to fit into a CT or MRI scanner, or they cannot undergo imaging because their weight exceeds the maximum allowable load limit for the scanning table. For most gamma camera scanning tables, this load limit is about 300 pounds. Fig. 18-15 illustrates an artifact that resulted from trying to image a patient weighing 350 pounds on a table designed for 300 pounds.

Altered anatomy after bowel resection, bladder removal, lung resection or thoracoplasty, placement of indwelling catheters or shunts, or other significant surgical procedures may cause confusion and unusual patterns in tracer accumulation (Figs. 18-16 to 18-19). Again, examining the patient briefly can usually clear up the confusion.

Cerebrospinal fluid (CSF) shunts may be evaluated after injection of a small volume of radiotracer into the shunt reservoir (Figs. 18-20 to 18-22). If the volume of the reservoir is known, the flow of CSF in milliliters per minute can be calculated from the clearance rate. In CSF shunts it is helpful to distinguish between a shunt that is *patent* (not clogged or obstructed) and one that is *working* (carrying CSF as intended). When interpreting the images of a CSF shunt, it is important to know what the shunt looks like, where the ends are, and where the reservoir, if any, is located.

Radionuclide hepatobiliary studies are sensitive for detecting bile leaks that occur after biliary surgery (Fig. 18-23). This type of study can also be used to check T-tube bile flow after a cholecystectomy when the patient's postoperative recovery does not proceed normally.

Accumulation of tracer in a urine bag or an ostomy device is a very frequent artifact (see Figs. 18-17 to 18-19). Tracer may spill onto the skin, or into a body cavity, or into soft tissues. The nuclear medicine physician can often avoid misinterpreting these studies by examining the patient, obtaining information about prior surgery, and tailoring the examination to fit the specific clinical problem.

Vascular shunts produce artifacts when the blood is labeled with a radiotracer. The resulting images of blood flowing through the vascular shunt can show to what extent the shunt is working. Shunts may lead to secondary changes in function; for example, a Blalock-Taussig shunt anastomosing the left subclavian artery to the left pulmonary artery will lead to higher arterial pressure in the left lung than the right, with the result that in a perfusion lung scan the labeled particles will travel preferentially to the right lung. If the shunt is not working, however, perfusion will be symmetric.

Text continued on p. 510.

lie in certain standard positions, and others cannot lie still. The nuclear medicine physician who spends a few minutes with the patient is less likely to be led astray by abnormal or variant anatomy. A brief 5-minute history (any known abnormalities, prior surgery, radia-

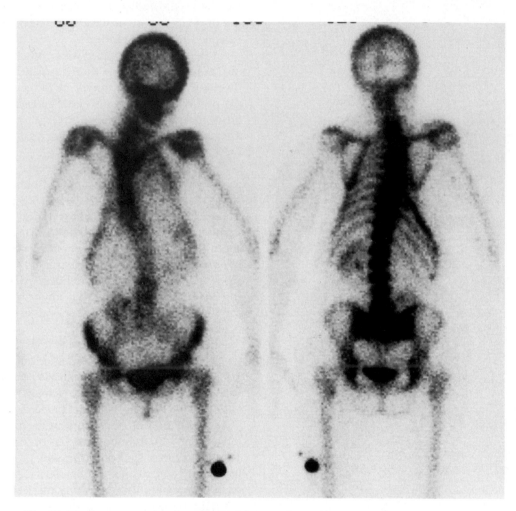

Fig. 18-16. Bone scan showing effect of thoracoplasty done 40 years previously for tuberculosis. Notice also right pelvic kidney. *Left,* Anterior view; *right,* posterior view.

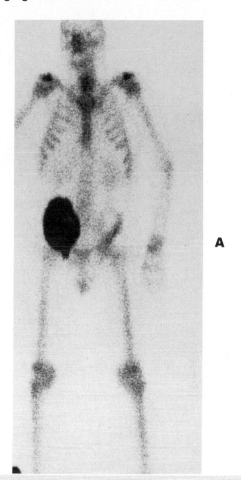

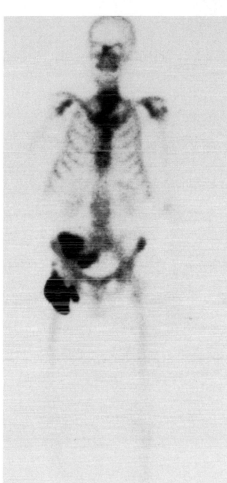

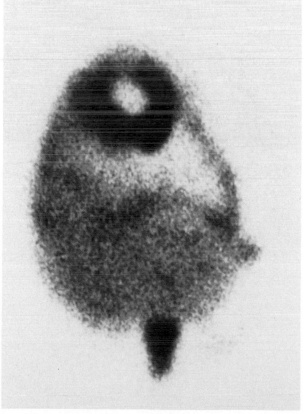

Fig. 18-17. Bone scan in a patient with an ileal loop and urine bag (patient with bladder resection for carcinoma). Notice absence of bladder activity.

Fig. 18-18. Bone scan in a patient with an ileostomy and urine bag. **A,** Bone scan. **B,** Detail scan of urine bag. Notice collection around stoma.

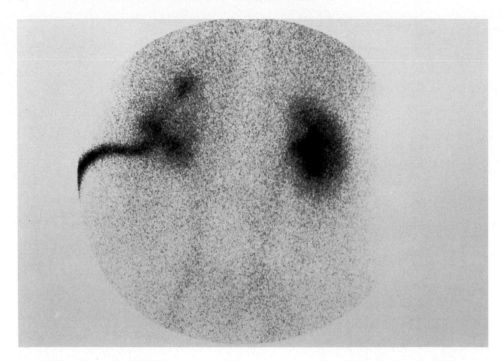

Fig. 18-19. Renal study (^{99m}Tc-glucoheptonate, posterior view) showing nephrostomy tube exiting from left kidney.

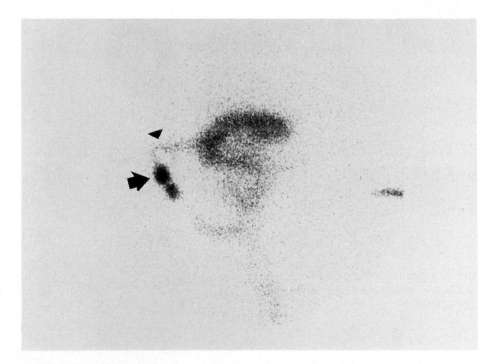

Fig. 18-20. Cerebrospinal fluid study in a 7-year-old child receiving intraventricular chemotherapy for *Coccidioides immitis* cerebritis (a coccidioidomycosis) by an intraventricular catheter, *arrowhead,* with reservoir, *arrow.* Tracer was injected into the reservoir to determine whether drugs so injected would reach the ventricles. The study shows that they would.

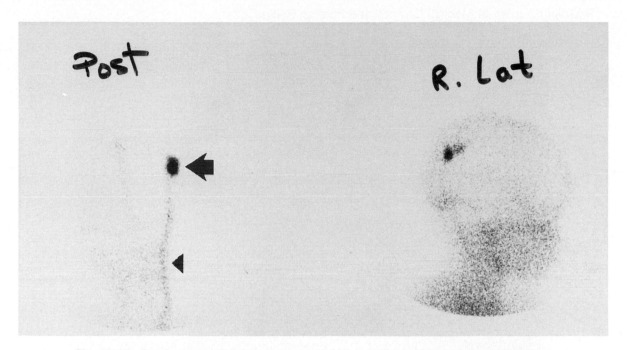

Fig. 18-21. Cerebrospinal fluid shunt in a child with pseudotumor cerebri. Tracer injected into the shunt reservoir, *arrow,* proceeds antegrade through the catheter, *arrowhead,* into the abdomen. If the volume of the shunt reservoir is known, the cerebrospinal fluid flow can be measured in milliliters per minute.

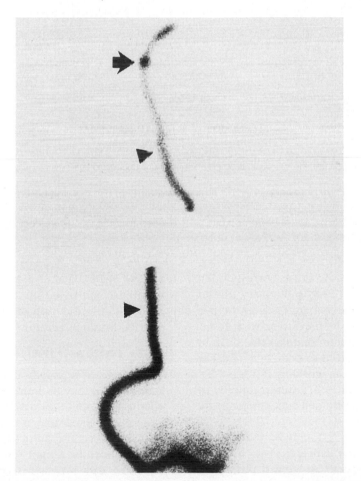

Fig. 18-22. Ventriculoperitoneal cerebrospinal fluid shunt in an elderly woman with communicating hydrocephalus and dementia. Tracer injected into the reservoir, *arrow,* proceeds antegrade through the shunt catheter, *arrowheads,* into the peritoneal cavity where it is absorbed.

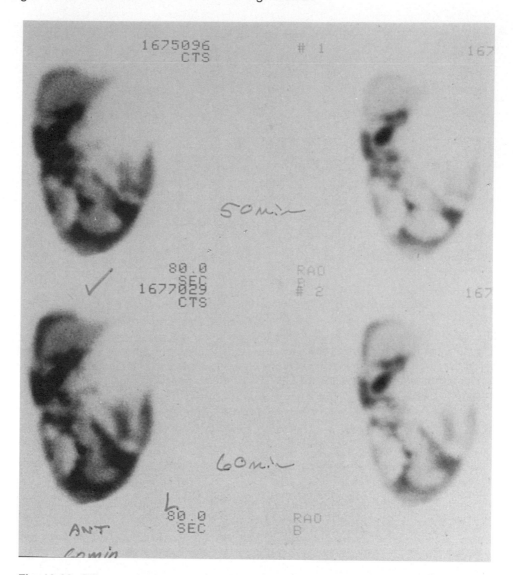

Fig. 18-23. Biliary study showing bile leak (notice labeled bile free in peritoneal cavity, outlining loops of bowel). After cholecystectomy there was leakage around the T-tube, which had been inserted into the common bile duct. Notice that the accumulation of tracer in the gallbladder fossa is not gallbladder but part of the bile leak.

Other types of vascular shunts cause corresponding secondary changes in the patient's pulmonary physiologic state. These indirect effects may show in the perfusion lung scan and can also be used to show whether the shunt is working. In addition, one can demonstrate whether a LeVeen shunt, inserted to drain peritoneal ascites into the subclavian vein, is working. If it is, ^{99m}Tc-macroaggregated albumin (or ^{99m}Tc-sulfur colloid) injected into the peritoneal cavity will accumulate in the lungs (or liver) (Fig. 18-24).

Sometimes, patient anatomy is totally normal, but the patient's physiology is altered. Nuclear medicine studies are very sensitive indicators of altered physiology and often pick up unexpected findings, such as old fractures (Fig. 18-25), drug-induced nephrotoxicity (Fig. 18-26), or the effects of a radiation port (Figs. 18-27 and

18-28). Ischemia after exposure to severe cold can lead to intense soft-tissue uptake of bone-seeking radiotracers,[9] and thyroid uptake of radioiodine is easily depressed by small amounts of exogenous iodine.

INJECTION ARTIFACTS

Radiotracer is usually injected into an arm vein, but sometimes it may be more feasible to use an indwelling venous catheter (Figs. 18-29 to 18-31). On very rare occasions, the tracer may mistakenly be injected into a peripheral artery instead of a vein (Fig. 18-32). Limb ischemia induced by a tight tourniquet before radioisotope injection can increase tracer uptake.[10] When some tracer is extravasated on injection, it may wind up in local lymph nodes[11] (Fig. 18-33).

Text continued on p. 515.

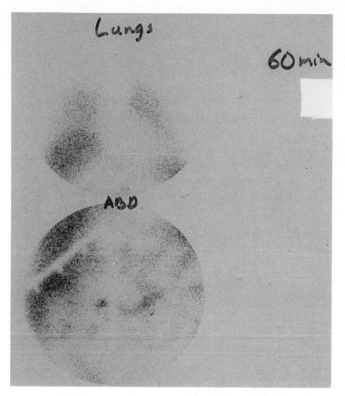

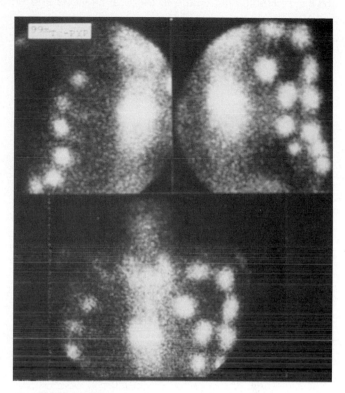

Fig. 18-24. LeVeen shunt study. ^{99m}Tc-macroaggregated albumin (MAA) particles were instilled into the peritoneal cavity. In the lower image *(ABD)* one can see the tracer free in the ascitic fluid, outlining the liver and loops of bowel. A marker outlines the costal margin. In the upper image *(Lungs)* one can see faint accumulation of tracer in the lungs, indicating that the MAA has entered the bloodstream and therefore that the shunt is working. Occasionally, the shunt itself can be seen.

Fig. 18-25. Bone scan showing multiple rib fractures in a patient who received cardiac resuscitation. The procedure was evidently successful.

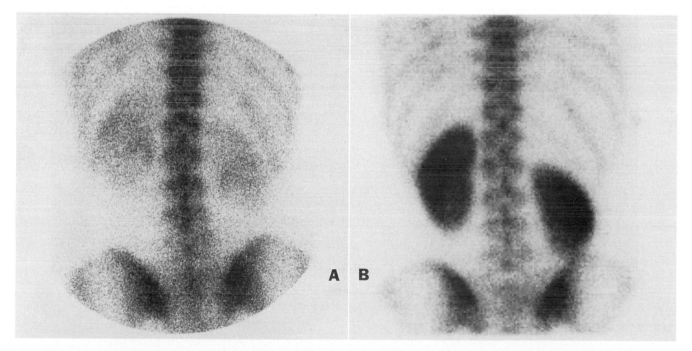

Fig. 18-26. A, Bone scan showing normal kidneys. **B,** Same patient after treatment of non-Hodgkin's lymphoma and *Coccidioides immitis* pneumonia with amphotericin B. The nephrotoxicity of several chemotherapeutic agents can be seen as abnormally increased uptake of the bone-seeking radiotracer by renal parenchyma.

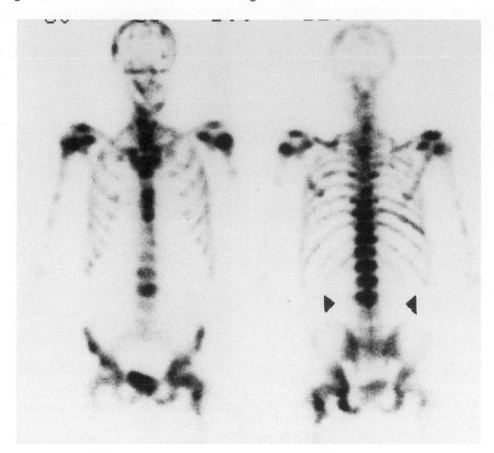

Fig. 18-27. Bone scan showing radiation port, *arrowheads,* which included entire pelvis and L4-5 in a 65-year-old man with widespread metastases from prostate cancer. *Left,* Anterior view; *right,* posterior view.

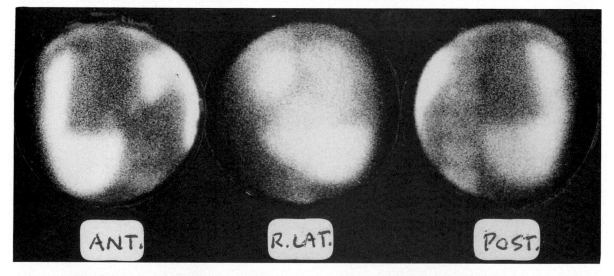

Fig. 18-28. Liver scan *(activity in white against black background)* showing radiation port. Straight lines and right angles almost always represent some sort of artifact.

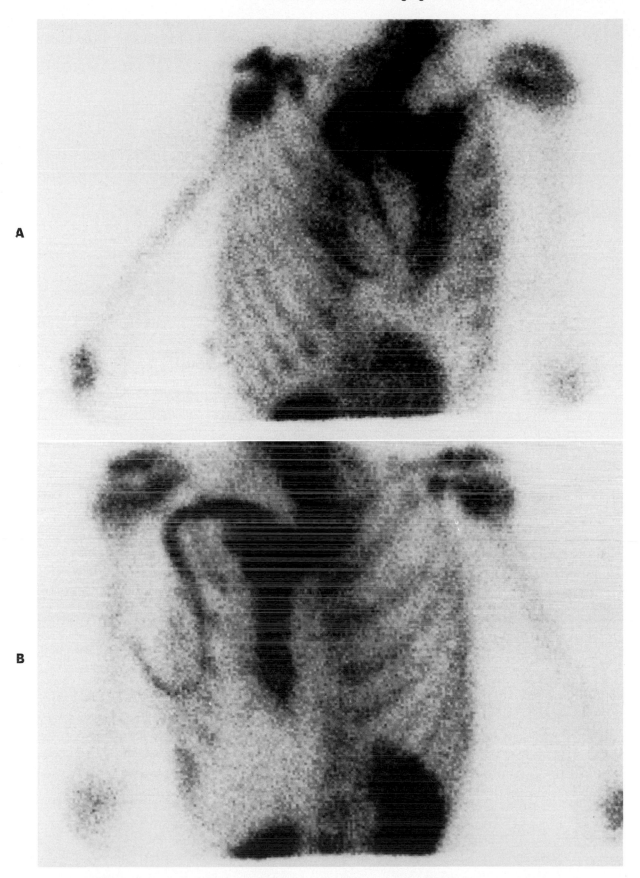

Fig. 18-29. Oblique views of the chest from a bone scan showing injection of radiotracer through a Hickman catheter placed in the sternum.

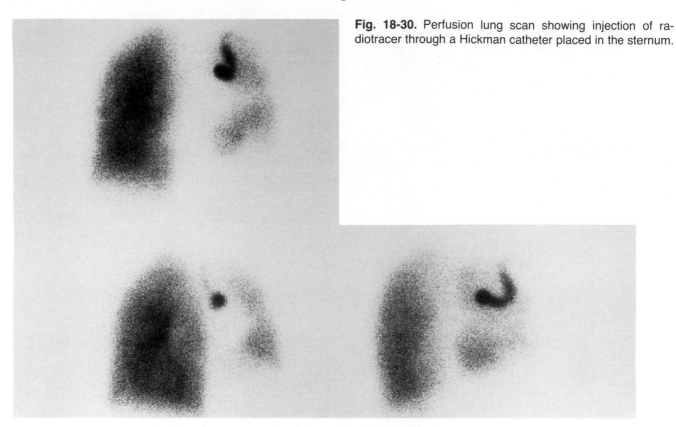

Fig. 18-30. Perfusion lung scan showing injection of radiotracer through a Hickman catheter placed in the sternum.

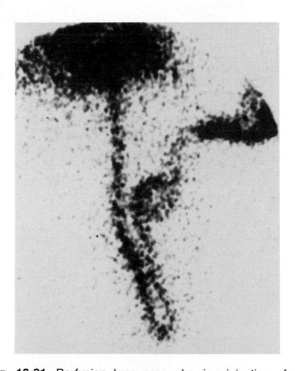

Fig. 18-31. Perfusion lung scan showing injection of radiotracer through an indwelling Broviac catheter placed in the inferior vena cava. The loop shows the slack in the catheter.

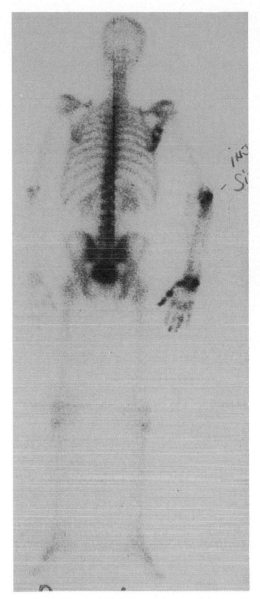

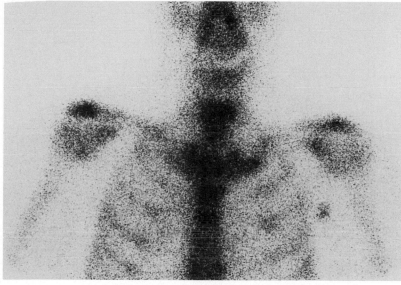

Fig. 18-33. Bone scan (anterior view) showing tracer accumulation in lymph node in left axilla after partial extravasation during injection. In some projections, the lymph node can mimic a lesion in the ribs or scapula.

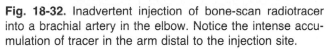

Fig. 18-32. Inadvertent injection of bone-scan radiotracer into a brachial artery in the elbow. Notice the intense accumulation of tracer in the arm distal to the injection site.

For chemotherapy of malignancies involving the liver, a catheter may be placed in the hepatic artery; its reservoir can appear on liver scans. Images of the liver made after infusion of ^{99m}Tc-macroaggregated albumin can even be used to predict the distribution of infused chemotherapy and to make sure there is no arteriovenous shunting through the tumor (Fig. 18-34).

In perfusion lung scans, the macroaggregated albumin (MAA) may mix with the patient's blood during injection, especially if needle placement is uncertain, and there is prolonged contact between the MAA and the patient's blood. This can lead to the formation of small clots ("hot clots"), which appear large in the images be-

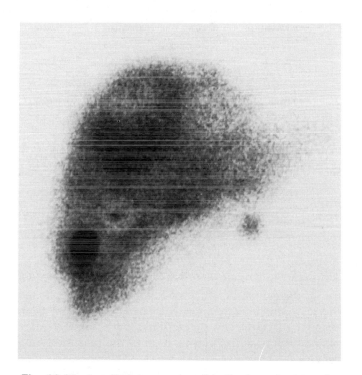

Fig. 18-34. A catheter was placed in the hepatic artery for chemotherapy infusion, and a test dose of ^{99m}Tc-macroaggregated albumin was injected into the reservoir, *dark spot*. There is good distribution throughout the liver, which is riddled with metastases. The absence of lung activity shows that there is no intrahepatic shunting.

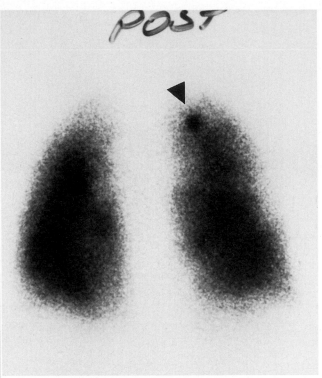

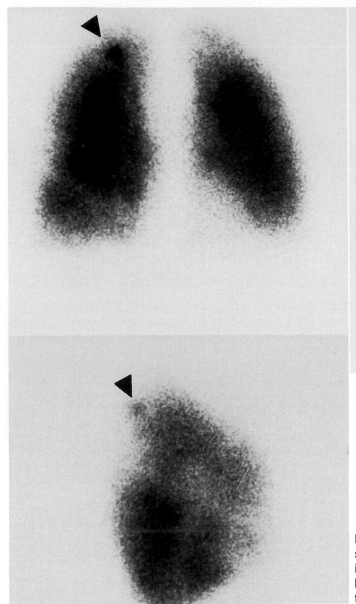

Fig. 18-35. "Hot clot," *arrowhead.* This intense focus is a small clot that formed when macroaggregated albumin being injected for a perfusion lung scan mixed with the patient's blood. The "hot clot" looks large but is actually small enough to have passed through the bore of the injection needle.

cause of their intense activity (Fig. 18-35), but obviously they must be small enough to pass through the bore of the injection needle. They have never been known to cause any deleterious effects, though they may interfere with interpretation of the perfusion lung scan.

PATIENT MOTION

To keep the radiation dose to the patient as small as possible, the amount of radiotracer given is kept as low as feasible. As a result, it often takes a long time to complete a study. The long times are necessary for the accumulation of enough photons to produce good images. Imaging times range from a few minutes to as long as an hour. For many patients, it is difficult to hold still for

this long, especially for those in pain, or those who are confused or sedated. Motion artifacts therefore are common.

In planar imaging, patient motion appears as blurring or duplication, sometimes with bizarre effects such as floating hands or doubled heads (Fig. 18-36). In SPECT imaging, patient motion often leads to streaking artifacts of the type seen also in CT and MRI studies (see Chapters 15 and 16). SPECT studies that include the kidneys or bladder often suffer from reconstruction artifacts caused by activity that changes during acquisition, leading to inconsistent data sets.

URINE CONTAMINATION

Roughly half of the radionuclide dose administered for a bone scan is excreted through the kidneys. The

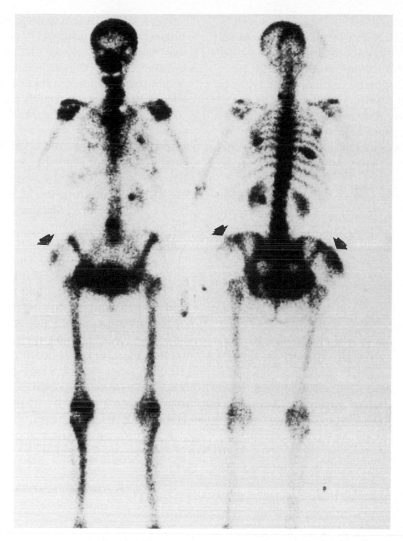

Fig. 18-36. Bone scan (older technique) showing accumulation of bone-seeking radiotracer in the buttocks, *arrows*. Chronic inflammatory reaction to iron injections. The patient moved her head during acquisition, creating another artifact.

body also excretes several other radiotracers through the urine. Patients are usually instructed to empty their bladders immediately before imaging. Urine carries with it a surprising potential for contamination leading to imaging artifacts. Many radiotracers are concentrated by the kidneys, so that even small droplets of urine can produce intense artifacts. After someone voids, there is always a drop or two of urine remaining on their undergarments. In patients with some degree of incontinence this effect may be pronounced. For example, an artifact mimicking osteitis pubis was traced to a tampon.[12]

Careless aiming during urination may lead to marked contamination (Fig. 18-37). Patients who do not wash their hands after voiding can leave "imageable" contamination anywhere on their body. We have even seen it in a patient's hair overlying the skull on a bone scan. It

mimicked skull metastases, but multiple projections showed that the activity was external to the skull, giving away the artifact. One should consider urine contamination whenever abnormal activity appears in the form of spots or streaks and especially in images of infants (Fig. 18-38).

MISCELLANEOUS ARTIFACTS

Bone scans seem to carry more than their share of artifacts, partly because they have high-detail images and partly because they view the entire body, which allows artifacts more of a chance to appear. Patients often wear jewelry or items of clothing with metal or other dense materials in them. These objects should be removed before imaging because they may cause artifacts. Such items include belt buckles (Fig. 18-39), earrings (Fig. 18-40), pendants, necklaces, bracelets, watches, large rings, and corsets. Metallic objects in patient's pockets or about their body also should be removed. These include keys, coins, and weapons!

Eyeglasses should be removed because some types of glass contain lead. Dentures usually can be left in place; they have a characteristic pattern and are easily recognized. They should be removed if the facial bones are to be examined. Glass eyes and facial or dental prostheses cause characteristic artifacts and are usually recognized without problem.

In patients with thyroid cancer undergoing imaging

surveys, labeled saliva may cause artifacts difficult to distinguish from metastases.[13] Likewise, labeled secretions may wind up in pocket handkerchiefs, causing false-positive images (the "radioactive handkerchief sign").[14] When images indicate metastases, the initial response should be a rigorous search for artifacts.

Pacemakers cause characteristic artifacts and are easy to identify by their shape and sharp margins. On pyrophosphate images of the heart for acute myocardial infarction, skin burns attributable to defibrillation paddles may mimic myocardial damage on planar views but are easy to separate from the heart on SPECT studies (Fig. 18-41). An artifact in thallium myocardial images caused by mitral valve annulus calcification has even been described.[15] The artifact mimicked a myocardial scar in the posterolateral and inferoposterior walls.

On whole-body images (for example, for bone scans, gallium-67 scans) the patient may eat between injection and imaging, and the unlabeled food in the stomach may appear as a lucent left upper quadrant defect ("lunch sign," Fig. 18-42).[16] This is distinguished from the breast by its appearance on both anterior and posterior views. Healing surgical scars may accumulate bone-seeking tracers and mimic metastases, ureters, and ribs. Indwelling venous catheters may also sometimes mimic a bone lesion (Fig. 18-43).

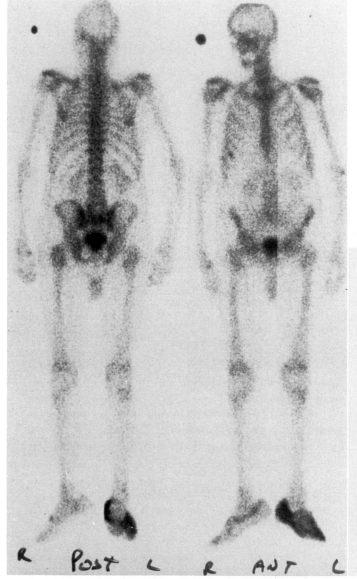

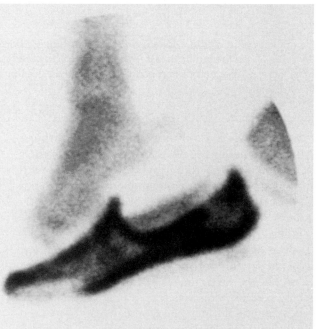

Fig. 18-37. Bone scan, **A,** and detail scan, **B,** showing urine contamination in a slipper. The bone-seeking tracer, a form of phosphate, is efficiently excreted by the kidneys, and urine contamination is a common artifact.

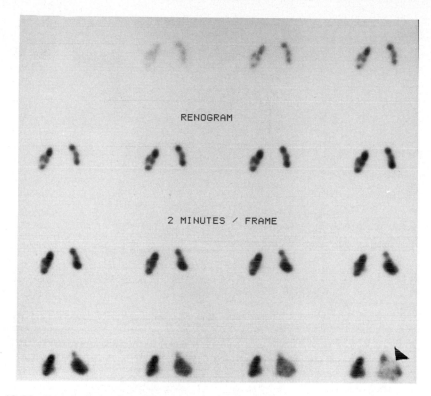

Fig. 18-38. Renal study showing urine contamination in an infant with a nephrostomy in the right collecting system. Labeled urine collects in the diaper, *arrowheads*.

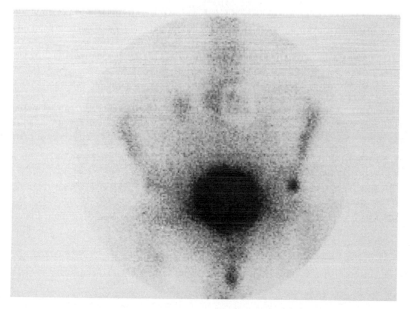

Fig. 18-39. Belt buckle. Western-style belts with their massive metal shields may cause large artifacts on anterior views.

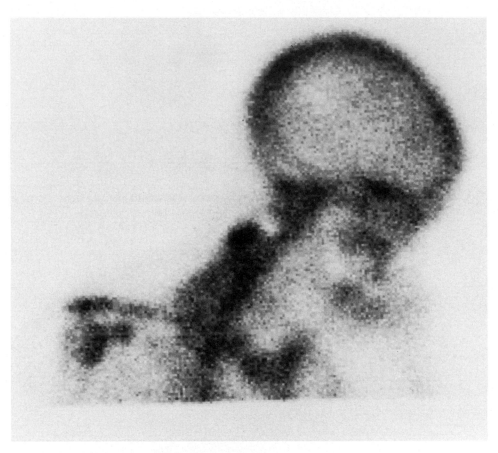

Fig. 18-40. Metal earring projected over upper cervical spine. All vertebrae are present, though there are degenerative changes posteriorly.

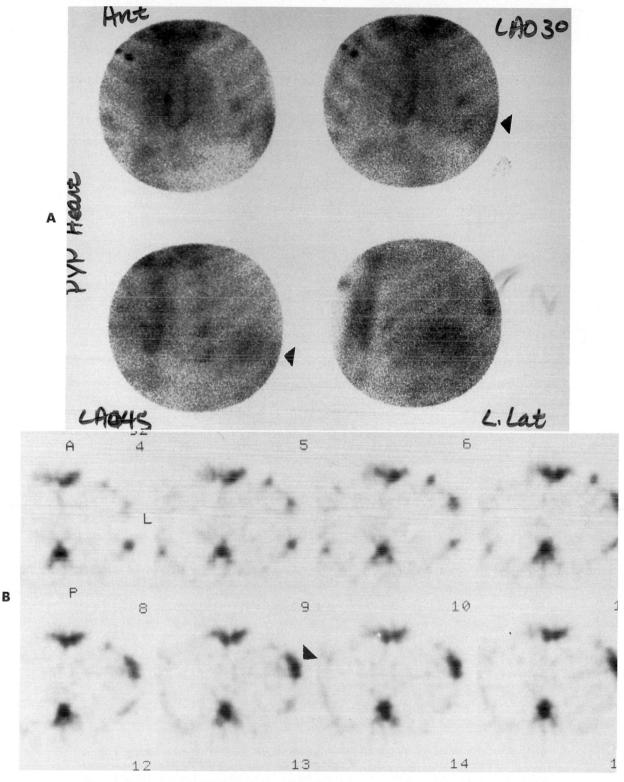

Fig. 18-41. A, Planar pyrophosphate cardiac study in a patient with a history of cardiac arrest, showing abnormal uptake in a location too far lateral to be heart, *arrowheads*. **B,** SPECT study shows location on chest wall, *arrowhead*. The uptake represents surface burns from an electrical defibrillating paddle.

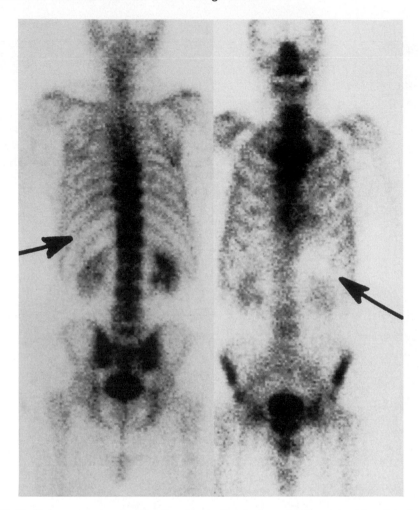

Fig. 18-42. Bone scan showing the "lunch sign," a photopenic stomach with unlabeled food eaten after injection of radioisotope.

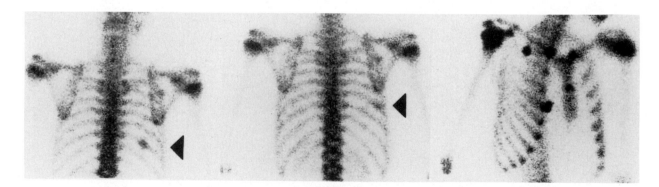

Fig. 18-43. Bone scan showing an indwelling venous access catheter mimicking a rib lesion. *Left,* Posterior view indicates possible metastasis in the right ninth rib, *arrowhead. Center,* After repositioning of the catheter, the "lesion" is more lateral and in the eighth rib, *arrowhead. Right,* Right anterior oblique (RAO) view showing catheter and reservoir.

CONCLUSION

This has been a brief review of some of the artifacts found in nuclear medicine images. A literature search under "artifacts" (or "artefacts") and "radioisotope imaging" will convince the reader that artifacts truly abound in this field. As imaging equipment becomes more complex, new types of artifacts will surely appear.

REFERENCES

1. Ryo UY, Bekerman C, Pinsky SM: *Atlas of nuclear medicine artifacts,* ed 2, St. Louis, 1990, Mosby–Year Book.
2. Fogelman I, editor: *Bone scanning in clinical practice,* London, 1987, Springer-Verlag.
3. DePuey EG, García EV: Optimal specificity of thallium-201 SPECT through recognition of imaging artifacts, *J Nucl Med* 30:441-449, 1989.
4. Tsui BM, Gullberg GT, Edgerton ER, et al: Correction of nonuniform attenuation in cardiac SPECT imaging, *J Nucl Med* 30:497-507, 1989.
5. Gillen GJ, Gilmore B, Elliott AT: An investigation of the magnitude and causes of count loss artifacts in SPECT imaging, *J Nucl Med* 32:1771-1776, 1991.
6. Schauwecker DS: Osteomyelitis: diagnosis with In-111-labeled leukocytes, *Radiology* 171:141-146, 1989.
7. Friedman DL, Hunter TB, Elam EA, Hunt KR, Fajardo LL: Sonographic image degradation after barium emema, *Invest Radiol* 28:295-296, 1993.
8. Elam EA, Hunter TB, Hunt KR, Fajardo LL: Barium interference with the abdominal ultrasound examination: myth versus reality, *AJR* 153:993-994, 1989.
9. Shih WJ, Riley C, Magoun S, Ryo UY: Intense bone imaging agent uptake in the soft tissues of the lower legs and feet relating to ischemia and cold exposure, *Eur J Nucl Med* 14:419-421, 1988.
10. Lecklitner ML, Douglas KP: Increased extremity uptake on three-phase bone scans caused by peripherally induced ischemia prior to injection, *J Nucl Med* 28:108-111, 1987.
11. Chatterton BE, Vannitamby M, Cook DJ: Lymph node visualization: an unusual artifact in the ^{99m}Tc-pyrophosphate bone scan, *Eur J Nucl Med* 5:187-188, 1980.
12. Murray IPC, Bass S: A false-positive artifact in the investigation of osteitis pubis, *Clin Nucl Med* 16:597-598, 1991.
13. Park HM, Tarver RD, Schauwecker DS, Burt R: Spurious thyroid cancer metastasis: saliva contamination artifact in high dose iodine-131 metastases survey, *J Nucl Med* 27:634-636, 1986.
14. Pochis WT, Krasnow AZ, Isitman AT, et al: The radioactive handkerchief sign: a contamination artifact in I-131 images for metastatic thyroid carcinoma, *Clin Nucl Med* 15:491-494, 1990.
15. Wagoner LE, Movahed A, Reeves WC: Myocardial imaging artifacts caused by mitral valve annulus calcification, *Clin Nucl Med* 16:94-97, 1991.
16. Croft BY, Teates CD: "Lunch syndrome," a bone-scanning artifact: case report, *Clin Nucl Med* 3:137-138, 1978.

19

Bullets, Pellets, and Wound Ballistics

Jeremy J. Hollerman
Martin L. Fackler

PRINCIPLES OF WOUND BALLISTICS

Violence involving firearms is a significant problem in the United States. In 1988, handgun deaths in various countries were as follows: Great Britain 7, Sweden 19, Switzerland 53, Israel 25, Austria 13, Canada 8, and the United States 8915. By 1990, the United States figure was more than 17,000.[1] Fifty percent of all murders in the United States occur with handguns, and there are 60 million handguns in the country. Only 26 million of them are legally owned; 100,000 handguns are stolen annually. There are approximately 22 homicides per 100,000 persons. This means, on the average, every day in the United States, there are 59 murders. For every death, more than three people are injured. Multiple gunshot wounds account for 30% of all gunshot cases; 10 years ago it was only 5%.[1]

To properly diagnose and treat victims of gunshot injuries, it is necessary to understand the principles of wound ballistics. It is very important to realize that it is not possible to predict the severity of a wound merely by knowing the type of bullet involved and whether the bullet had a "high velocity" or a "low velocity." The medical literature is, unfortunately, full of erroneous articles in this regard. Bullet velocity is certainly an important factor in determining the extent of injury, but other bullet and tissue characteristics are at least as important as velocity.[2-5] Bullet mass, bullet construction, bullet shape and center of mass, wounded body-part thickness (Fig. 19-1), tissue type (such as femur versus lung), tissue elasticity, tissue density, tissue specific

Fig. 19-1. **A°,** Five examples of wound profiles. This technique was developed at the Letterman Army Institute of Research to measure the amount, type, and location of tissue disruption produced by a given projectile.[6] The entire missile path is captured in one or more blocks of 10% ballistic (ordnance) gelatin at 4° Celsius. The gelatin reproduces the penetration depth, projectile deformation, fragmentation pattern, site of yaw, and size and site of the temporary cavity produced by the missile in living swine muscle. Measurements are taken from cut sections of the blocks after mapping of the fragmentation pattern with two x-ray views at 90 degrees (see **B°**). These data are then reproduced on a wound-profile diagram, as shown here. A centimeter (cm) scale is included. The centimeter scale on the x-axis is the same as the centimeter scale on the y-axis, not shown.

This figure is a comparison of the wound profiles of; A, .22 long rifle bullet; B, .38 special lead round nose bullet; C, .45 automatic full metal case (full metal jacket) bullet; D, M16 full metal case bullet; and E, 7.62 NATO full metal case bullet. In each wound profile diagram the temporary cavity maximum size is outlined and the permanent cavity (permanent wound channel) is shaded.

The vertical lines drawn at 12 cm (the diameter of an average human thigh) and at 25 cm (the diameter of an average human abdomen) facilitate comparison. The disruption in the first 12 cm varies little among the bullets compared, despite a fourfold difference in striking velocity and a 24-fold difference in striking kinetic energy.[7] These bullets have very different amounts of wounding potential but may produce soft tissue wounds of thin body parts, which are very similar. At 25 cm there is a pronounced difference in the wounds produced by the different bullets. (From Fackler ML: *Ann Emerg Med* 15[12]:1451, 1986.)

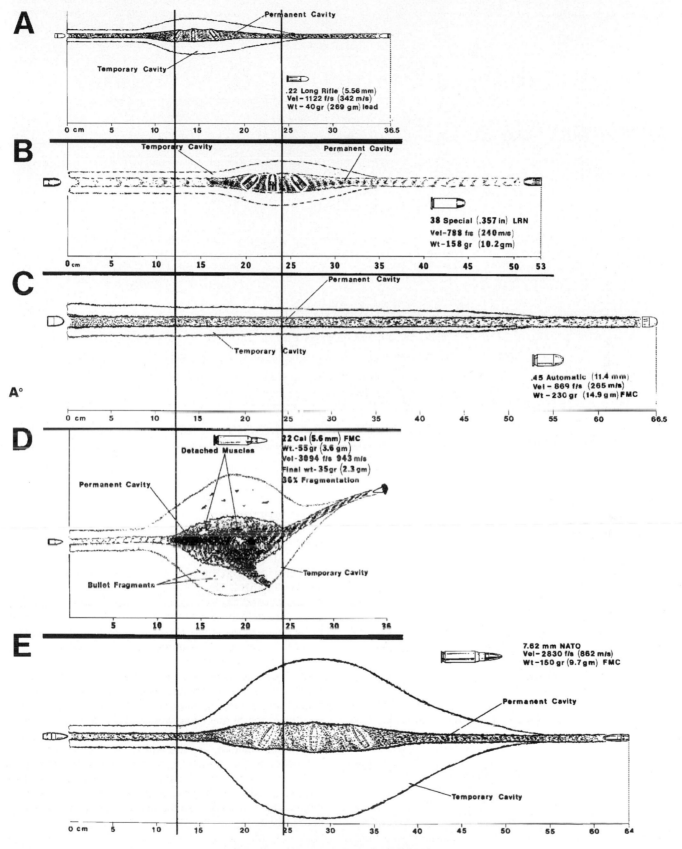

Fig. 19-1. For legend see opposite page.

Continued.

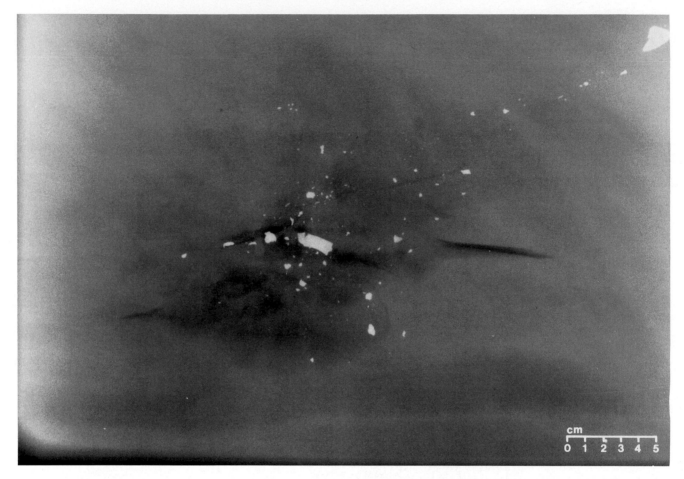

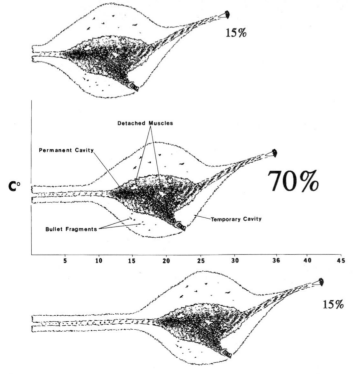

Fig. 19-1, cont'd. B°, A radiograph of a block of 10% gelatin used in wound-profile research.[6] A number of such shots would be averaged for the final composite diagram. This is a shot from the M16A1 rifle firing a full metal jacket M193 bullet at a range of 10 ft. Note the characteristic tapelike fragment in the center of the permanent cavity (seen in Fig. 19-24, *A*). After the bullet breaks at the cannelure, the copper bullet jacket on the back part of the bullet unwinds forming this fragment. The bullet tip is flattened (see Fig. 19-24, *A*) and pointed backwards, at the upper right of the figure. Notice the air in the permanent cavity and radial gelatin splits in the center of the figure. Cross sections of the gelatin block show the maximum size of the temporary cavity by the diameter of the radial splits.

C°, Figure demonstrating that there is a normal statistical distribution of wound characteristics produced by a number of shots of the same ammunition. The magnitude of the standard deviation of any given wound characteristic will be determined by bullet type, shape, and construction, the uniformity of manufacture, and the age of the ammunition. The final wound-profile diagram represents an average of many shots. In the distribution illustrated here, 15% of these M16 bullets yawed to 90 degrees and fragmented several centimeters earlier or later than the average performance shown in the center.

gravity, and tissue internal cohesiveness are all also extremely important in determining the nature of the wound produced. In addition, the amount of kinetic energy "deposited" or "retained" in a victim wounded by a projectile is not a reliable predictor of wound severity.[6-10]

There have been many papers printed that suggest harmful and unnecessary treatment for gunshot wounds based on common misconceptions about wound ballistics.[3,11] An example of such a misconception is the recommendation for mandatory surgical excision of the tissue surrounding an extremity wound tract, whenever the extremity wound is caused by a "high-velocity" bullet. This is based on the belief that these tissues will become necrotic. Clinical experience and research show this to be false.[2,12]

Mechanisms of Wounding

Missiles passing through tissue wound by only two mechanisms. These are *crush* and *stretch*. Tissue *crush* refers to the crushing of tissues struck by the projectile with the resultant formation of a permanent cavity. Tissue *stretch* refers to radial stretching of tissues along the projectile path with the formation of a temporary cavity (Fig. 19-2). The sonic pressure wave preceding the missile as it passes through tissue does not damage tissue.[13]

Both missile and tissue characteristics determine the nature of the wound. Missile characteristics are partly inherent in the nature of the bullet (mass, shape, construction) and are partly conferred by the weapon involved as it imparts a longitudinal and rotational velocity to the bullet. Tissue characteristics (elasticity, density, anatomic relationships) also strongly affect the nature of the wound. Moreover, the severity of a bullet wound is influenced by the bullet's orientation during its flight through tissue and by whether the bullet fragments[8] or deforms. For example, if a radiograph shows a cluster of small bullet fragments present at a site, this is a strong indicator of significant tissue damage at that site.[8]

Bullet yaw

Bullet yaw is an important concept and is defined as the angle between the long axis of the bullet and its flight path. If the bullet is traveling with its pointed end forward and its long axis parallel to the longitudinal axis of flight (0 degrees of yaw), it crushes a tube of tissue no greater than its approximate diameter. If the bullet yaws to 90 degrees, the entire long axis of the bullet strikes tissue. The amount of tissue crushed at 90 degrees of yaw may be three times greater than at 0 degrees of yaw. If the bullet strikes an intermediate target before striking the patient, the bullet may yaw, deform, or decelerate. Its wounding properties will be altered,

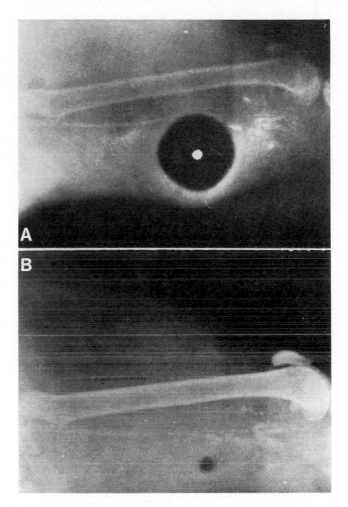

Fig. 19-2. High-speed roentgenograms of the thigh of a cat during and after the passage of a ¹⁄₃₂-inch steel sphere whose impact velocity was 3200 feet/second. The sciatic nerve of the cat's thigh has been made radiopaque with iodobenzene. The images are obtained with the beam parallel to the path of the missile. **A,** Microsecond roentgenogram showing anterior displacement of the sciatic nerve by the temporary cavity. The tissues surrounding the tract of the projectile are undergoing local blunt trauma and tissue stretch because of temporary cavity formation. **B,** Roentgenogram made immediately after the shot. The permanent cavity (wound channel) is considerably smaller than the temporary cavity. The sciatic nerve is in its usual anatomic position. (Courtesy General Leonard D. Heaton, Col. James B. Coates, Jr., and Major James C. Beyer, MC; reprinted from *Wound Ballistics,* Office of the Surgeon General, Department of the Army, 1962, p 209.)

sometimes increasing wound severity, sometimes decreasing it.

Soft point or hollow point bullets

Civilian weapons often use hollow point or soft point bullets. Hollow point bullets have a hole in the jacket at the bullet tip, and soft point bullets have some of the

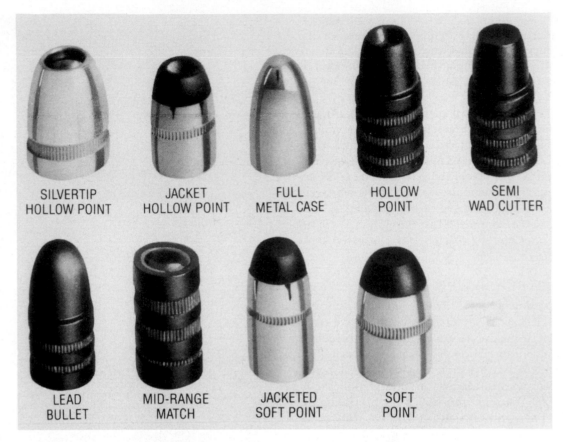

SILVERTIP HOLLOW POINT   JACKET HOLLOW POINT   FULL METAL CASE   HOLLOW POINT   SEMI WAD CUTTER

LEAD BULLET   MID-RANGE MATCH   JACKETED SOFT POINT   SOFT POINT

Fig. 19-3. A variety of standard bullet types are shown. (Courtesy Winchester Division, Olin Corporation, East Alton, Ill.)

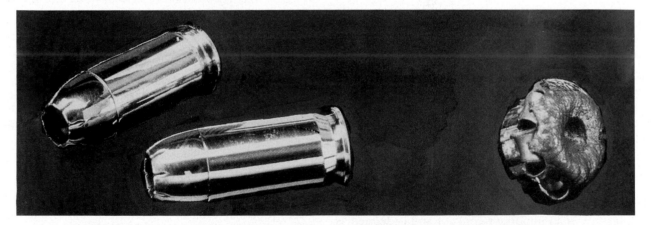

Fig. 19-4. When a hollow-point or soft-point semijacketed bullet strikes a thick body part with sufficient velocity, it will usually flatten on impact. This flattening increases bullet diameter resulting in a mushroom-shaped projectile, causing more tissue to be crushed. A larger hole in tissue (the permanent bullet tract) is made than would be made by the original unexpanded bullet.

All projectiles penetrate more deeply as projectile velocity is increased, only up to the point where velocity becomes high enough to deform the projectile; penetration decreases greatly from that point on. The greater the bullet-diameter expansion from mushrooming, the less the depth of penetration.[14] (Courtesy Winchester Division, Olin Corporation, East Alton, Ill.)

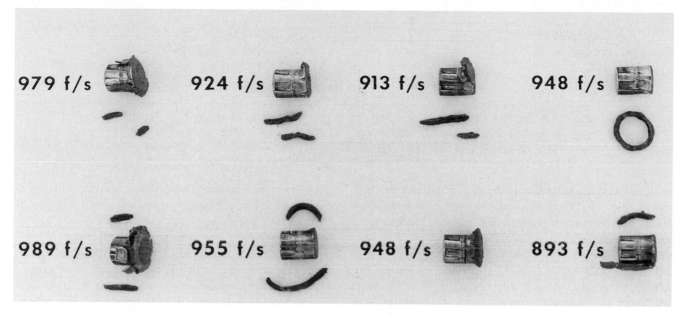

Fig. 19-5. Eight shots from a handgun into 10% ballistic gelatin at muzzle velocity (range 4 feet), using Winchester Western .38 Special+P 125 grain jacketed hollow point ammunition. This ammunition is supposed to mushroom reliably, but as can be seen from its performance, it is highly variable from shot to shot, and some of the bullets did not expand at all. This is typical of much civilian handgun ammunition.

lead core of the bullet exposed at the bullet tip (Fig. 19-3). Soft point and hollow point bullets are designed to deform into a mushroom shape if they strike soft tissue with sufficient velocity (Fig. 19-4). This greatly increased surface increases the amount of tissue crushed. If the mushroomed diameter is 2.5 times greater than the initial diameter of the bullet, the area of tissue crushed by the bullet is 6.25 times greater than the amount that would have been crushed by the undeformed bullet. For most big-game hunting, such bullets are mandated by law.

Although soft point and hollow point bullets from center-fire rifle rounds usually expand into a mushroom shape in tissue, even the magnum versions of some soft point and hollow point handgun bullets from various manufacturers sometimes fail to expand.[15] This is often because of insufficient striking velocity, an excessively thick or unbending bullet jacket, or construction variability in manufacture. This lack of expansion is most likely with short-barreled handguns and those of less potent calibers (such as .25 and .32) because of slower bullet velocity. Overall, about one third of soft point and hollow point handgun bullets fail to expand in human soft tissue [16] (Fig. 19-5).

Bullet jacket

Under the terms of the convention of the Hague of 1899, the jacket of a military bullet must completely cover the bullet tip.[17] This is called a full metal jacket

(or full metal case) bullet. Unjacketed lead bullets cannot be driven faster than about 2000 ft/sec (610 m/sec) without some of the lead stripping off in the barrel. This is avoided if a jacket made of a harder metal, such as copper or a copper alloy, is used to surround the lead.

If a bullet is jacketed, the bullet jacket usually cannot be distinguished from the lead core on standard radiographs because the entire bullet is of metallic density. Occasionally, as the bullet deforms or fragments, the bullet jacket separates from the bullet and is visible on a radiograph.

The shorter the barrel length, the shorter is the time available for bullet acceleration by the expanding gases created by burning gunpowder. Therefore, when identical rounds are fired, the gun with the shorter barrel produces a lower-velocity bullet. Its velocity may be too low to induce mushrooming after impact.

Bullets of the hollow point or soft point variety are also more likely to fragment in tissue than a full metal jacket bullet, adding to tissue disruption. Because of bullet mushrooming and fragmenting, the hollow point and soft point bullets used in civilian rifles and large handguns are often more damaging to tissue than military bullets fired from rounds otherwise configured identically.[4,8,18]

Bullet penetration depth

Penetration depth is inversely proportional to bullet expansion. Inadequate expansion (mushrooming) may

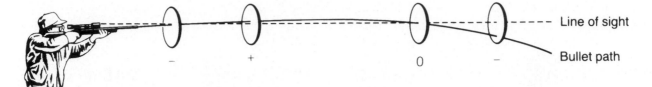

Fig. 19-6. Once a bullet leaves the barrel of a gun, it starts to drop slowly because of gravity. To hit a distant target, a bullet must travel in a trajectory. Although the line of sight remains a straight line to the target, the muzzle must be elevated slightly to launch the bullet in an arched path. (Courtesy Winchester Division, Olin Corporation, East Alton, Ill.)

result in overpenetration and the wounding of bystanders (see Fig. 19-5). Overexpansion can result in inadequate penetration depth for the bullet to reach and disrupt vital structures. Usually 12 to 20 inches of bullet penetration depth (approximately 30 to 50 cm) is required to reliably reach and disrupt vital structures in humans. Projectiles of any sort penetrate more deeply as velocity increases, only up to the point where velocity increases enough to deform the projectile; penetration depth decreases greatly from that point on.

Bullet sterilization

Bullets are not sterilized by the heat of firing. They can carry bacteria from the body surface deep into the wound. They can also spread bacteria from perforated organs (such as the colon) along their entire tissue path.

Bullet stabilization

Fired from an appropriate and well-designed weapon, a bullet flies in air with its nose pointed forward; it yaws only 1 to 3 degrees. Yaw occurs around the bullet's center of mass. In pointed rifle bullets, the center of mass is behind the midpoint of the bullet's long axis. Although the bullet's most naturally stable in-flight orientation would be with its heaviest part (its base) forward, for aerodynamically efficient flight it must fly point forward. It travels in an arched path called a "trajectory" (Fig. 19-6).

During flight, a bullet is stabilized against yaw by the spin imparted to it by the spiral grooves (rifling) in the gun barrel. Although the bullet's spin is adequate to stabilize it gyroscopically against yaw in its flight through air, it is not adequate to stabilize it in a point-forward position in tissue because of the higher density of tissue relative to air.[19]

The temporary cavity

If it does not deform in tissue, a pointed bullet eventually yaws to a base-forward position (180 degrees of yaw). Expanding bullets lose the physical stimulus to yaw because, after "mushrooming," their heaviest part is forward. As a bullet passes through 90 degrees of yaw, it is crushing its maximal amount of tissue (unless it fragments, which will crush more). It is slowed down rapidly, as its wounding potential is used up moving tissue radially away from its path. This force creates the temporary cavity.

Temporary cavitation is a splash in tissue: a bullet yawing to near 90 degrees causes a much larger "splash" than one with little yaw. This is entirely analogous to the minimal splash a diver makes with a "good" dive compared to the large splash produced by a bellyflopper. In tissue, this splash, the temporary cavity, produces localized blunt trauma.[2,8]

The maximal temporary cavity occurs several milliseconds after the bullet has passed through the tissue.[4] Because forces follow paths of least resistance, temporary cavitation can be asymmetric as it spreads out in tissue planes. The temporary cavity caused by common handgun bullets is generally too small to be a significant wounding factor in all but the most sensitive tissues (brain and liver).[2]

Center-fire rifle bullets and large handgun bullets (such as .44 magnum) often induce a large temporary cavity 10 to 25 cm in diameter (4 to 10 inches) in tissue. This can be a significant wounding factor, depending on the characteristics of the tissue in which it forms.

In general, the wounding effect of temporary cavitation has been greatly exaggerated in the literature,[2,11] particularly with regard to extremity wounds. Injuries of vessels, bones, nerves, and organs "remote," or "distant," from the projectile path but within the area displaced by the temporary cavity are commonly mentioned (as in reference 20), but in fact are extremely rare. A review of 1400 rifle wounds from Vietnam (the Wound Data and Munitions Effectiveness Team study) found no cases of bones being broken or major vessels being torn that were not penetrated by the bullet, bullet fragments, or secondary missiles.[21] In only two cases, an organ that was not hit (but was within a few centimeters of the projectile path) suffered some disruption.

Near-water-density, less-elastic tissue (such as brain, liver, or spleen), fluid-filled organs (including the heart, bladder, or fluid-filled intestine), and dense tissue (such as bone) may be damaged severely when a large temporary cavity contacts them or forms within them. More elastic tissue (such as skeletal muscle) and lower-density elastic tissue (such as lung) are less affected by the formation of a temporary cavity.[22,23] Because of these tissue differences, transmitted blunt trauma from temporary cavitation caused by a bullet traveling 800 to 950 m/sec can cause a more severe pulmonary contusion when the bullet traverses the chest wall musculature than the pulmonary contusion it would have caused if passing through the lung.[22]

Splenosis

After any type of trauma that fragments the spleen, there is the potential for the long-term complication of thoracic or abdominal splenosis. Abdominal splenosis can lead to abdominal pain, small bowel obstruction, or hematologic abnormality. Thoracic splenosis may present as a noncalcified coin lesion or a pleura-based mass anywhere in the thorax, including the apices.[24] Splenosis may be diagnosed by a nuclear medicine liver-spleen scan.

Bullet Caliber

Bullet caliber is defined as bullet diameter in decimals of an inch or in millimeters. It is only one indicator of missile wounding potential and not a very good one (Fig. 19-7). Caliber doesn't disclose bullet mass or bullet length; caliber specifies only bullet diameter. The bullet's composition and construction (and therefore tendency to yaw, fragment, or deform) do not relate to caliber.

Bullet caliber also doesn't disclose how much powder is in the cartridge case. The cartridge case may have a considerably larger diameter than the bullet and may be of any length. The amount of powder in the cartridge case is strongly correlated with bullet velocity.

A gun with a shorter barrel will generally produce a bullet of lower velocity than a weapon with a longer barrel would when its round is being fired. With shorter barrel length, the expanding gases of the burning gunpowder have less time to accelerate the bullet before they are discharged into the atmosphere. When identical rounds are fired by a rifle and a handgun, bullet velocity is often significantly different because of different barrel lengths. A .22 long rifle round fired in a rifle will produce a bullet with up to 300 ft/sec more velocity than the same round fired in a handgun. However, it is always important to remember that missile velocity is only one factor in determining the extent of wounding.[4,10,25]

Unfortunately, commonly used weapon and bullet designations are often numerically incorrect (Table 19-1). Rounds are named for the cartridge case used, not the bullet. One would expect the numerical part of the name to correspond to bullet diameter; often it does

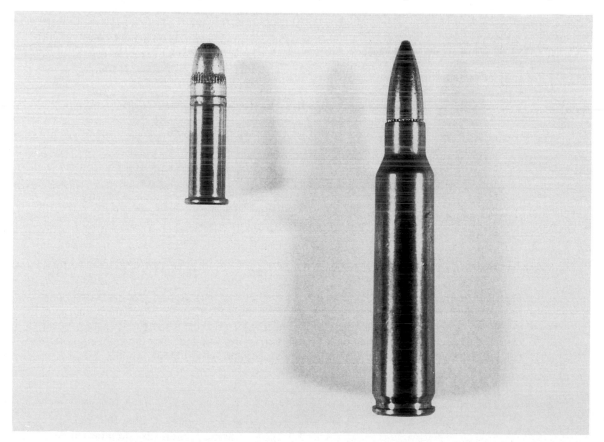

Fig. 19-7. A shows a .22 long rifle round, *left,* and an M16 round, *right.*
Continued.

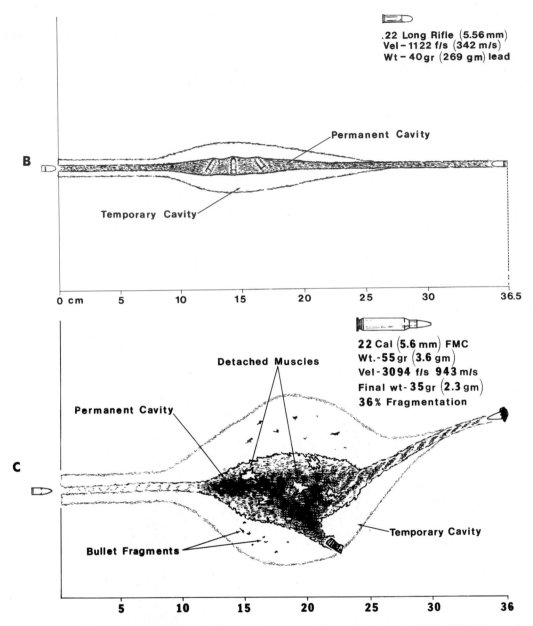

.22 Long Rifle (5.56 mm)
Vel – 1122 f/s (342 m/s)
Wt – 40 gr (269 gm) lead

Permanent Cavity

B

Temporary Cavity

0 cm   5   10   15   20   25   30   36.5

22 Cal (5.6 mm) FMC
Wt.-55 gr (3.6 gm)
Vel-3094 f/s 943 m/s
Final wt-35 gr (2.3 gm)
36% Fragmentation

Detached Muscles

Permanent Cavity

C

Temporary Cavity

Bullet Fragments

5   10   15   20   25   30   36

Fig. 19-7. cont'd. The wound profiles of the same .22 long rifle, **B,** and .224 cal M193 round of the M16A1 rifle, **C,** are illustrated. (Full metal case [FMC] is a synonym of full metal jacket [FMJ], the type of bullet used in the military.) This figure shows that caliber (bullet diameter in decimals of an inch or in millimeters) is only one indicator of wounding potential and not a very good one. (From Hollerman JJ et al: *AJR* 155:686, 1990.)

Table 19-1   Cartridge Case Name and Actual Bullet Diameter Used

Cartridge Cases of Common Interest	Actual Bullet Diameter (inch)
32 Auto (ACP) [Automatic Colt Pistol]	.312
380 Auto (ACP)	.355
38 Super	.355 or .357
38 Special	.357
357 Magnum	.357
44 Special	.4295
44 Magnum	.4295
444 Marlin	.4295

Others Cartridge Cases of Interest	Actual Bullet Diameter (inch)
22 Hornet	.223 and .224
218 Bee	.224
219 Donaldson Wasp	.224
219 Zipper	.224
221 Remington Fireball	.224
222 Remington	.224
222 Remington Magnum	.224
223 Remington	.224
224 Weatherby Magnum	.224
225 Winchester	.224
22-250 Remington	.224
220 Swift	.224
243 Winchester	.243
244 Remington/ 6 mm Remington	.243
240 Weatherby Magnum	.243
256 Winchester Magnum	.257
250/3000 Savage	.257
257 Roberts	.257
25/06 Remington	.257
257 Weatherby Magnum	.257

Table 19-1—cont'd   Cartridge Case Name and Actual Bullet Diameter Used

30-06	.308
30-30 Winchester	.308
30 M1 Carbine	.308
7.62 × 39 mm (AK-47 rifle)	.308
30/40 Krag	.308
7.5 × 55 mm Swiss (Schmidt-Rubin)	.308
300 Savage	.308
7.62 mm Russian	.308
308 Winchester	.308
7.62 mm NATO	.308
30-06 Springfield	.308
300 H & H Magnum	.308
30-338	.308
300 Winchester Magnum	.308
308 Norma Magnum	.308
300 Weatherby Magnum	.308
303 British	.311
7.65 mm Mauser	.311
7.7 mm Japanese	.311

From *Sierra Rifle Reloading Manual* and *Sierra Handgun Reloading Manual* (both ed 3, 1989), Sierra Bullets, L.P., 10532 South Painter Avenue, Santa Fe Springs, CA 90670.

Often, both the numerical designation associated with the bullet and the cartridge case do not reflect exact measurements. As an example, the 44 Remington Magnum Pistol cartridge is .456-inch diameter at its distal end and uses a bullet with a .43-inch diameter.[1] Both the 38 special and the 357 magnum use bullets that have the same diameter, .357 inch (9.07 mm). These bullets often have exactly the same weight. When trying to determine the bullet type from a radiograph, in addition to correcting for magnification or deformation, one must look up actual bullet diameter, rather than relying on the bullet name for its size.

not. For example, the 44 Remington Magnum uses a bullet with a .429-inch diameter.[26] Both the .38 special and the .357 magnum use bullets that have the same diameter (.357 inch) and weight. The longer cartridge case of the magnum can hold more powder, giving the bullet higher velocity and greater wounding potential.

Wounding Potential and Wound Therapy

Often it is not possible to determine missile type from radiographs, particularly when the bullet has passed out of the body leaving a few small metallic fragments or none at all (Fig. 19-8). Does this matter to patients? Not if they have a good doctor. The history of what type of weapon caused the wound is more often wrong than right and, even if correct, does not determine the therapy needed.

Many factors determine wound severity. Some "high-velocity" wounds are minor, and some "low-velocity" wounds are devastating. A simple stab wound of a vital structure, the heart, spinal cord, or aorta, has proper-

ties similar to a small handgun bullet wound and is frequently lethal (Figs. 19-9 and 19-10). An AK-47 military "assault" rifle wound of an extremity often is like an ice-pick stab wound and may have little effect if it traverses only muscle.

For proper treatment of gunshot wounds, it is essential that treatment be based on the physical examination of the patient and the results of radiologic studies, not on the history of what weapon inflicted the wound. It is the condition of the patient that determines the treatment needed.

When an undeformed bullet is visualized on a radiograph, it is usually not possible to state accurately whether it is fully jacketed (Fig. 19-11). It may not have become deformed because it entered the patient with insufficient velocity, because it did not strike a structure causing it to deform, or because it is a full metal jacket bullet. On standard radiographs, the bullet jacket cannot be differentiated from the bullet core unless it has separated from the bullet.

Text continued on p. 539.

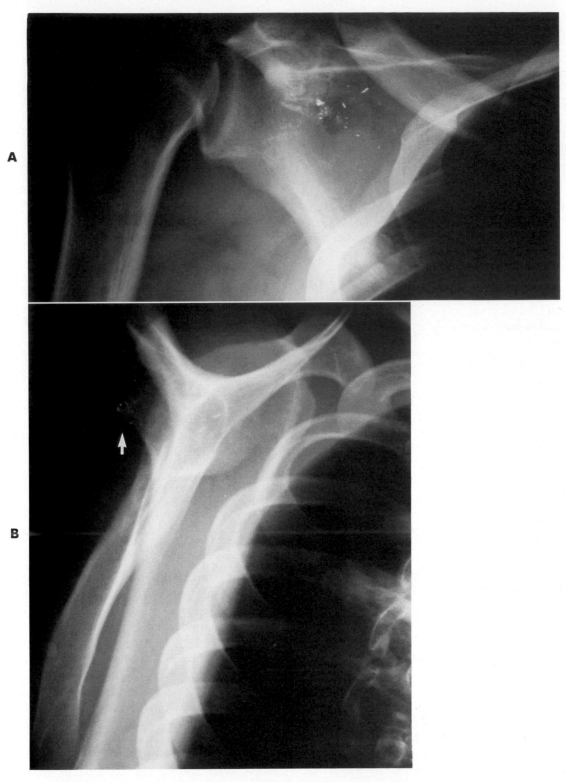

Fig. 19-8. It is not possible to adequately assess from these radiographs (**A,** frontal view; **B,** lateral scapular view) the type of weapon causing this bullet wound of the shoulder. The bullet entered from the anterior body surface and exited posteriorly leaving small lead fragments in the posterior soft tissues (**B,** *arrow*). Because of the location of the wound tract, the possibility of arterial or brachial plexus injury should be suspected.[27] The direction of fire, from anterior to posterior, is disclosed by the posteriorly located bullet fragments, sheared off after bullet deformation when passing through the scapula.

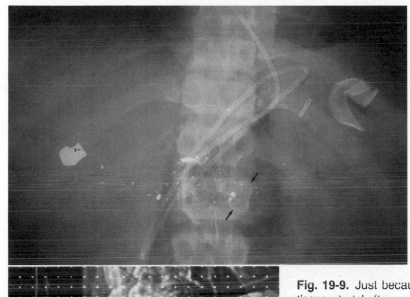

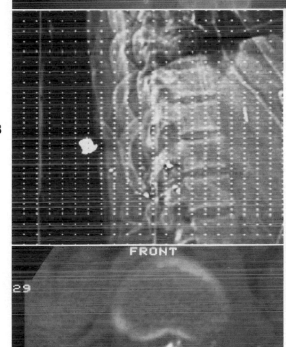

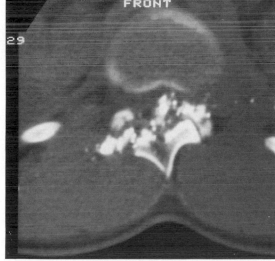

Fig. 19-9. Just because a handgun bullet does not induce much tissue stretch (temporary cavitation), it cannot be concluded that the wound will be minor. This patient was shot in the abdomen. The bullet tract was from the left anterolaterally to the right flank posteriorly. The bullet passed directly through the spinal canal, producing paraplegia. **A,** Anteroposterior view of the thoracolumbar junction. Notice the absence of visualization of the superior portion of the cortex of the left pedicle of L1, *arrows,* with adjacent bullet fragments, consistent with fracture by the bullet. A trail of fragments extends to the right, with a moderately deformed, "mushroomed" bullet projecting over the right upper quadrant. Its anteroposterior location cannot be determined without a lateral view. **B,** Lateral digital scout radiograph obtained on the CT scanner without moving the patient. It shows that the deformed bullet is in the posterior soft tissues of the right flank. Because of this position, the bullet was very close to the x-ray cassette used to film the anteroposterior (AP) view, **A.** Therefore, even though portable technique was used for the AP view, with its relatively short focus-film distance (FFD), the degree of magnification of the bullet is minimal. The diameter of the bullet measures 1 cm (0.39 inch) in the AP view. The bullet may be either a .38 caliber bullet (actual diameter .357 inch; see Table 19-1), or a 9 mm bullet (actual diameter .355 inch), slightly magnified. Bullet fragments project over the spinal canal in both the AP and lateral views, consistent with the possibility of cord injury. **C,** CT scan at the level of the T12-L1 disk.

Continued.

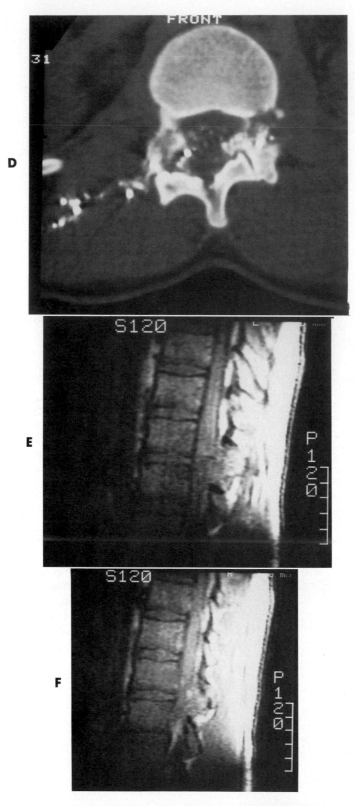

Fig. 19-9, cont'd. D, CT scan at the level of the L1 pedicles. This demonstrates the comminuted fractures resulting from bullet passage through the spinal canal and cord. Small metallic bullet fragments, bone fragments (which act as secondary missiles), and foci of hemorrhage are seen. The fracture of the left pedicle of L1, visible in the AP plain film, **A,** is confirmed in **D. E** and **F,** T_1-weighted magnetic resonance images of the same patient (T_1 is spin-lattice, or longitudinal, relaxation time). They show disruption of the spinal cord and dural sac at T12-L1.

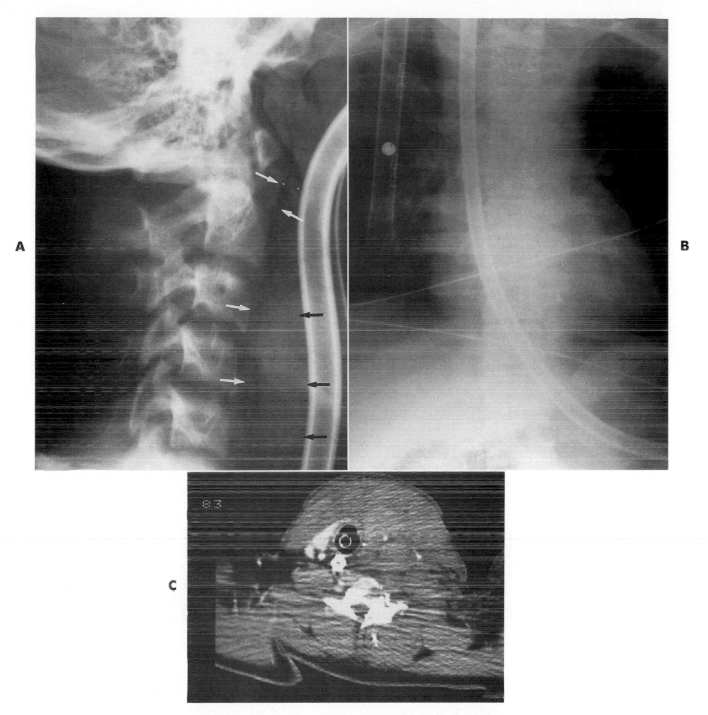

Fig. 19-10. This figure illustrates a fatal outcome from a small-caliber handgun wound with properties similar to a stab wound. In this case the vital structures hit were the left lobe of the thyroid gland and the left vertebral artery. Although these don't sound vital, the hematoma resulting from their bleeding displaced the trachea to the right, compressing it sufficiently to cause lethal anoxic brain damage. **A,** Lateral cervical spine film showing prevertebral soft tissue swelling caused by neck hematoma, *black arrows,* anteriorly displacing the Ewald large-caliber nasogastric tube. Prevertebral linear gas densities, *white arrows,* may have spread from the bullet wound tract itself, but esophageal injury must be ruled out. The bullet wound tract is lower in the neck, at the level of C6-7, obscured by overlying shoulders. **B,** Detail from the patient's portable chest radiograph, showing several signs of mediastinal hematoma. The Ewald tube is deviated to the right by the mass effect of the hematoma. The contours of the main pulmonary artery and aortopulmonic window are lost because of the hematoma. Left paraspinal and left prevascular soft tissues are widened and dense because of the hematoma. This hematoma had spread into the mediastinum from the bleeding in the lower area of the neck. There were no injuries in the chest. **C,** Avulsion of the left lobe of the thyroid gland.

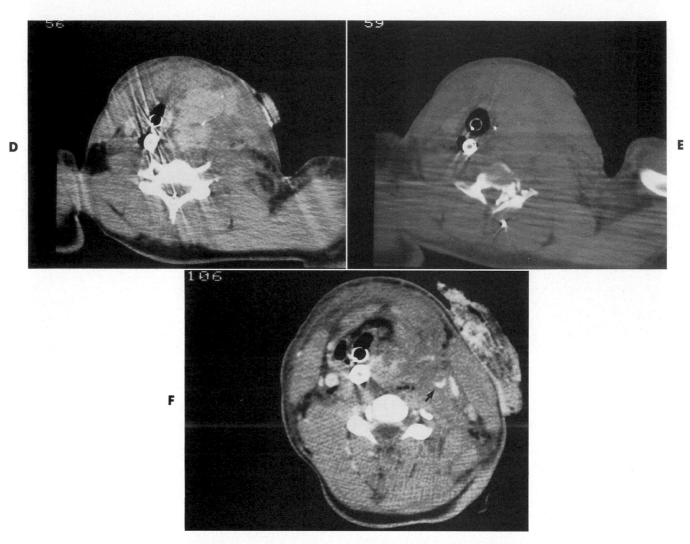

Fig. 19-10, cont'd. The thyroid gland and airway are greatly displaced to the right by the mass effect of the hematoma in the left neck, better shown in **D. E,** Bullet tract through the left foramen transversarium and left lamina of C6. There was no injury to the spinal cord. **F,** Thrombus partially occluding the left common carotid artery, *black arrow.* An angiogram showed no flow in either internal carotid artery because of brain death. There was no injury to the vessel itself. The brain swelling from anoxic injury caused by tracheal compression by the neck hematoma caused intracranial pressure to rise above arterial pressure, eliminating cerebral perfusion.

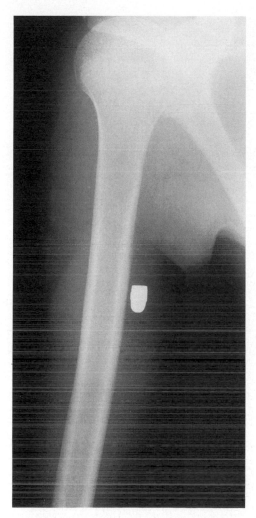

Fig. 19-11. Radiograph shows a small-caliber handgun bullet that lacked sufficient velocity to exit child's upper arm. No hard object (such as bone) stopped the bullet, and it did not traverse any other body part before the arm. The bullet had little wounding potential when it entered the patient. In extremity wounds, when a radiograph reveals an undeformed bullet lying in the soft tissues and no fracture is present, tissue disruption is usually minor; however, even a missile such as this can produce a serious wound if it divides a major vessel or nerve, similar to a stab wound. (From Hollerman JJ et al: *AJR* 155:695, 1990.)

Recent controlled animal experiments using military rifle bullets[12] have clearly disproved the assertion that all tissue exposed to temporary cavitation is destroyed. These studies also show that not only does the 14 cm diameter temporary cavity produced by the AK-74 assault rifle not destroy a great amount of muscle, but also the sizable stellate exit wound it causes in the uncomplicated thigh wound ensures excellent wound drainage.[12,23] This assists healing. A history that the wound

was caused by a "high-velocity bullet" does *not* mandate radical excision of the wound path.[2,10,11,23]

The characteristics of the wounded tissue, the thickness of the body part, the point in the path of the bullet at which yaw or fragmentation occurs, and other factors strongly influence the wound produced (see Fig. 19-1, *A*). Every moving bullet has a maximum wounding potential determined by its mass and velocity. Bullets of equal wounding potential may produce wounds of very different severity, depending on their shape, internal and external construction, and which tissues they traverse (Fig. 19-12).

In the first 12 cm of a soft-tissue wound path (the average thickness of an adult human thigh), there is often little or no difference between the wounding effect of low- and high-velocity bullets when the high-velocity bullet is of the military full metal jacket type[2,7] (see Fig. 19-1, *A*). This is particularly true of the relatively heavier military rifle bullets such as those fired by the AK-47 and NATO 7.62 mm (USA version) rifles.[2] A wound of an extremity caused by an AK-47 bullet that does not hit bone is often similar to a handgun bullet wound.

Civilian soft or hollow point bullets fired from a rifle deform soon after entering tissue and produce a much more severe extremity wound. If a "high-velocity," heavy bullet does not become deformed or fragmented or hit a bone, it may leave an extremity with much of its wounding potential unspent. These same bullets are often lethal in chest or abdominal wounds because the trunk is thicker than an extremity and allows the bullet a sufficiently long path through tissue to yaw. Maximal temporary cavitation induced by the AK-47 bullet usually occurs at a tissue depth around 28 cm, much greater than the diameter of a human extremity[30,31] (Fig. 19-13).

Radiologic Assessment of Missile Type

On a radiograph, assessment of missile caliber can be difficult because of magnification (Figs. 19-9 and 19-14) and missile deformation (Figs. 19-9 and 19-14). Sometimes even deformed bullets can be accurately characterized radiologically for intact bullet caliber and weight.[32] When determining bullet type from measurements, it is important to remember that bullet nomenclature is inexact and frequently illogical (see Table 19-1). Often, both the numerical designation of the bullet and that of the cartridge case do not reflect exact measurements. In addition to correcting for magnification or deformation, one must look up the actual bullet diameter, rather than relying on the bullet name for its size.

If an undeformed bullet is seen on two views at 90 degrees and its degree of magnification is known, it is possible to determine the approximate caliber of the

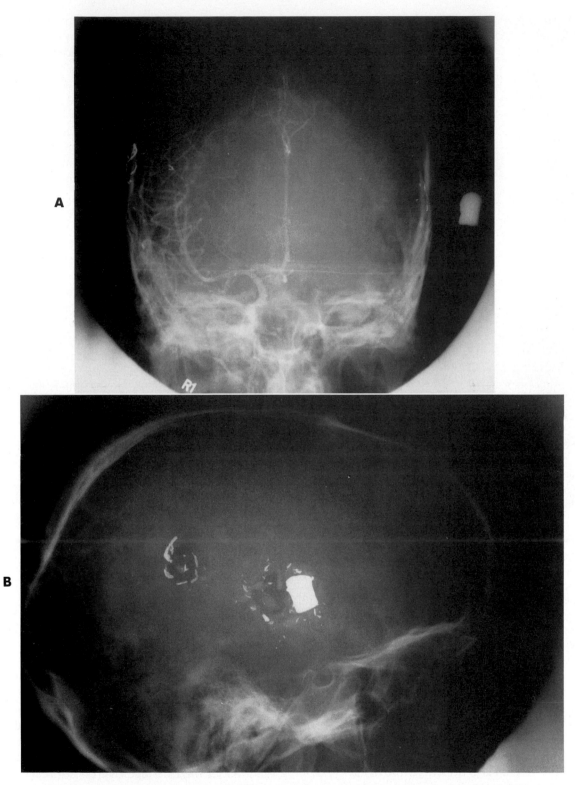

Fig. 19-12. Frontal, **A,** and lateral, **B,** views of the skull in a self-inflicted gunshot wound to the head with the bullet crossing the midline and coming to rest beneath the scalp on the side of exit. The elastic properties of the scalp (and skin in general) are such that it is not uncommon for bullets nearly out of velocity to be arrested immediately beneath the skin, as seen here. The large distance between the major bullet fragment on the side of exit and the calvarium is attributable to a hematoma that formed in the subcutaneous tissues. Self-inflicted gunshot wounds are more frequently lethal than gunshot wounds sustained during an assault.[28,29]

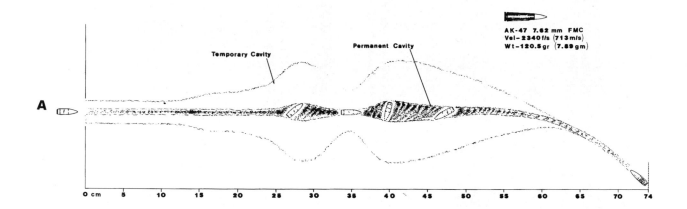

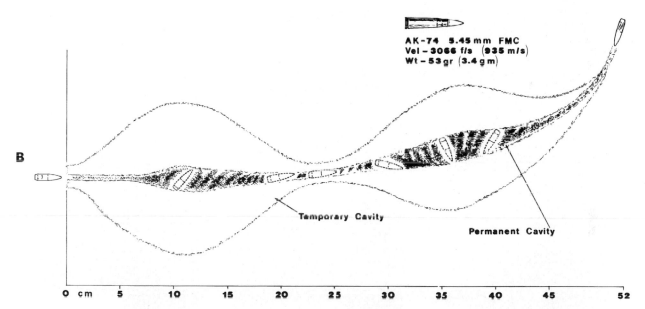

Fig. 19-13. The wound profiles of the AK-47, **A**, and AK-74, **B**, bullets in ballistic gelatin. The AK-47 has been the standard military rifle of the Soviet Block but is being replaced with the AK-74. The AK-74 bullet is quite similar in size and weight to the M16 bullet, but unlike the M16 bullet it doesn't fragment when at 90 degrees of yaw. Notice that the maximum temporary cavity of the AK-47 bullet during the first cycle of bullet yaw is at approximately 29 cm deep in tissue (the second cycle of bullet yaw is at a depth too great for the thickness of a human and doesn't count for human wounding). The AK-74 bullet, which is lighter, has internal construction to cause early yaw.[30] It causes its maximum temporary cavity at an 11 cm tissue depth. Extremity wounds from AK-74 bullets, in which a large bone is not hit, should be more severe than those from AK-47 bullets.[30,31] Trunk wounds at long range should be less severe because of the smaller wounding potential of the AK-74 compared to the AK-47. (From Hollerman JJ et al: *AJR* 155:689, 1990.)

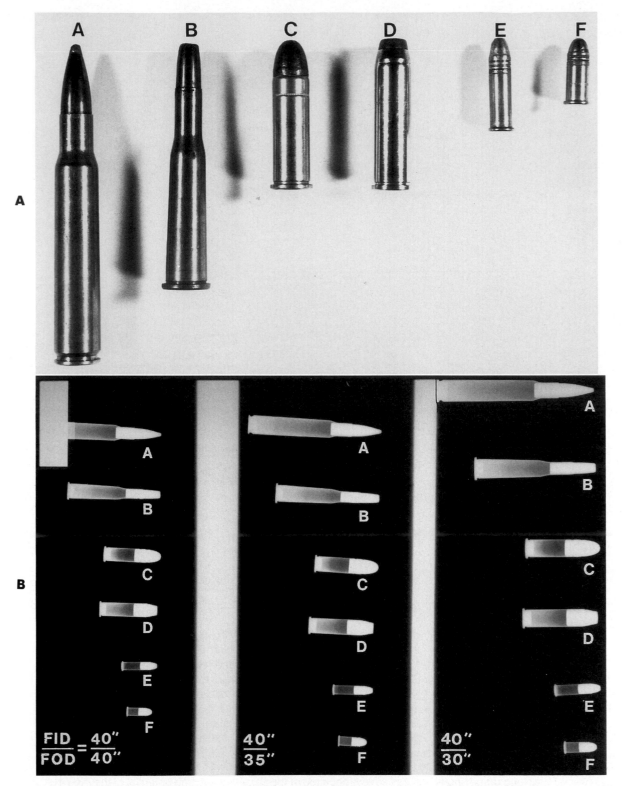

Fig. 19-14. Photograph, **A,** and radiograph, **B,** of same six rounds *(A-F)* at three different distances from the x-ray film. *A* is .30-06 (the version of this round with a full metal jacket bullet was the military round of the United States in World Wars I and II); *B,*.25-35; *C,* .38 special; *D,*.357 magnum; *E,* .22 long rifle; and *F,*.22 short. Percent magnification equals focus-image distance (FID) (also known as focus-film distance) divided by focus-object distance (FOD) times 100. In **B,** *left column,* FID is 40 inches (101.6 cm), and FOD is also 40 inches (101.6 cm) (no magnification). *In center column,* FID and FOD are 40 inches (101.6 cm) and 35 inches (88.9 cm) respectively (14% diameter magnification). *In right column,* FID and FOD are 40 inches (101.6 cm) and 30 inches (76.2 cm) respectively (33% diameter magnification). The visual impression is of a much greater magnification, probably because of visual perception of area rather than diameter. (Courtesy Dr. Bradford Allan and Larry Algiers, R.T. [R], Minneapolis; from Hollerman JJ et al: *AJR* 155:692, 1990.)

bullet. The focus-object distance (FOD) and focus-image distance (FID) (also known as the focus-film distance, FFD) must be known. This requires knowing the position of the bullet in the patient's body and its location relative to the film.[5,33] Percent magnification equals FID divided by FOD times 100:

$$\text{Mag \%} = \frac{\text{FID}}{\text{FOD}} \times 100.$$

It is usually possible to distinguish an undeformed .22 from a .25 and a .38 from a .44, but it is not possible to distinguish a .357 from a 9 mm (.355 inch) because they are too similar in diameter (see Fig. 19-9, *B*).

Radiolucent material, including plastic and paper, is present in some missile wounds, particularly those inflicted by shotguns at ranges under 15 feet (see the discussion of shotgun [pellet] wounds, p. 566). The surgical wound exploration must also include a search for this nonradiopaque material, which is often fragmented.

Radiolucent rubber or plastic bullets also exist[34-39] and can cause severe injury. They are rarely seen in the United States. The 40 mm plastic baton round or the 15 cm long rubber baton round usually do not penetrate the skin because of their ballistic properties including large size. Some other riot-control bullets are metal with a plastic coating,[40] and therefore are partly radiopaque.

Many radiographs show only fragments of the bullet and do not allow determination of the type of weapon and projectile causing the wound (see Fig. 19-8). However, certain bullets become fragmented in a characteristic pattern (such as the M16 military bullet or the .357 magnum 125-grain Remington semijacketed hollow point). Sometimes the pattern of fragments can be used to identify the bullet (see the discussion of characteristic fragments, p. 554). It should be noted that deformation of large lead shotgun pellets (such as 00 buckshot) after contact with bone can cause these to be confused with deformed bullet fragments.[41]

Gas between muscle bundles or within tissue planes often indicates that temporary-cavitation blunt trauma has occurred at that site (Fig. 19-15). However, other causes of gas in tissue planes exist, including direct spread of air from the projectile path (see Fig. 19-10, *A*), spread of gas from injury to the esophagus, stomach, or intestine, or spread of gas introduced iatrogenically during procedures such as chest tube insertion (Fig. 19-16).

Gas in tissue planes resulting from temporary cavitation can be useful in the radiologic assessment of missile type. Full metal jacket bullets typically penetrate at least 10 cm before the bullet yaws. With this type of bullet, only after significant yaw does a large temporary cavity form. In contrast, civilian soft point or hollow point bullets that expand into a mushroom shape do so

within the first 10 cm of penetration. They cause their cavitation and associated soft-tissue gas collections at this more superficial depth. Soft-tissue radiographs can be used for assessment of the depth of the bullet tract at which temporary cavitation occurred. Military rifle bullets (full metal jacket bullets) are more variable (the standard deviation is greater) than civilian soft point or hollow point bullets in the tissue depth at which temporary cavitation will occur (see Fig. 19-1, *C*).

Missile Path and Missile Location

Bullet localization requires two views at 90 degrees, or a tomographic image. Computed tomography of the head and body is often useful for analysis of a bullet path[5,42] (Figs. 19-17, 19-18, 19-29, and 19-30). When one is assessing a bullet wound with CT, it is important to realize that what appears to represent blood clots or bone fragments may not in fact be these materials. Semiradiopaque foreign bodies carried into the wound, such as stones, wood, plastic, and clothing, may have the same CT density as these biologic materials. Intracranial wood fragments can even resemble air at some display settings.[43]

In trunk wounds, an analysis of the bullet path is mandatory to determine whether a laparotomy is needed. Radiographs, CT, clinical examination, and peritoneal lavage are all useful.[42] If peritoneal penetration by a bullet is suspected, laparotomy is indicated.[44,45] The morbidity and mortality of an exploratory laparotomy is low compared with that of a missed intestinal injury. Any bullet wound below the nipple line should raise the question of whether the diaphragm or abdomen has been penetrated (Fig. 19-19).

Abdominal CT is more accurate if performed before peritoneal lavage because at this point there is no introduced free air but one has the ability to assess the volume of hemoperitoneum without additional introduced fluid and there is preservation of "sentinel clot" signs.[42,46,47]

Because of the skin's toughness and elastic properties, a bullet that might have the capacity to penetrate 4 or 5 inches farther into tissue is often arrested subcutaneously at the end of the wound path (see Fig. 19-12); it is held in by a trampoline-like action of the skin. This "holding-in" action of the skin is fortunate; it reduces the danger to other persons from a perforating bullet leaving one individual and going on to strike another.

Whenever a gunshot wound traverses the midline of the neck or the width of the mediastinum, perforation of the esophagus should be suspected (see Fig. 19-10). Esophageal evaluation must not be overlooked after angiographic evaluation of the neck or chest.

CT is particularly useful when only a body wall or retroperitoneal path is suspected because nonoperative therapy is often appropriate. CT has largely replaced ex-

Text continued on p. 548.

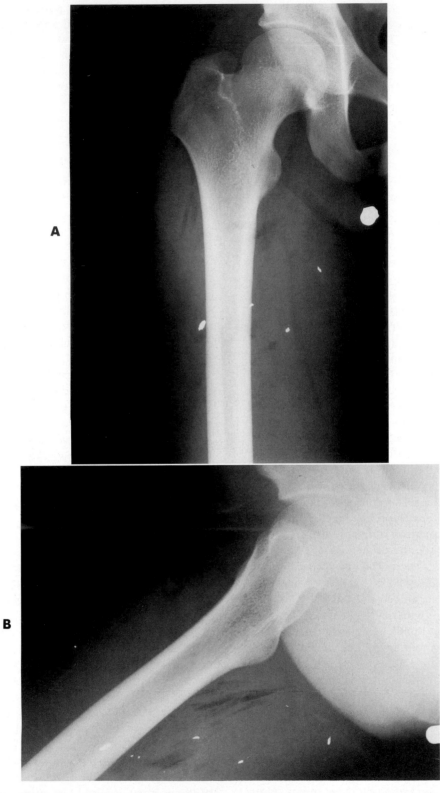

Fig. 19-15. Gas between muscle bundles or within tissue planes often indicates that temporary-cavitation blunt trauma has occurred at that site. **A,** A deformed partially fragmented bullet has traversed the thigh and groin. **B,** Linear and oval gas densities in the posterior soft tissues of the thigh along the bullet tract are shown to advantage on the frog-leg lateral view.

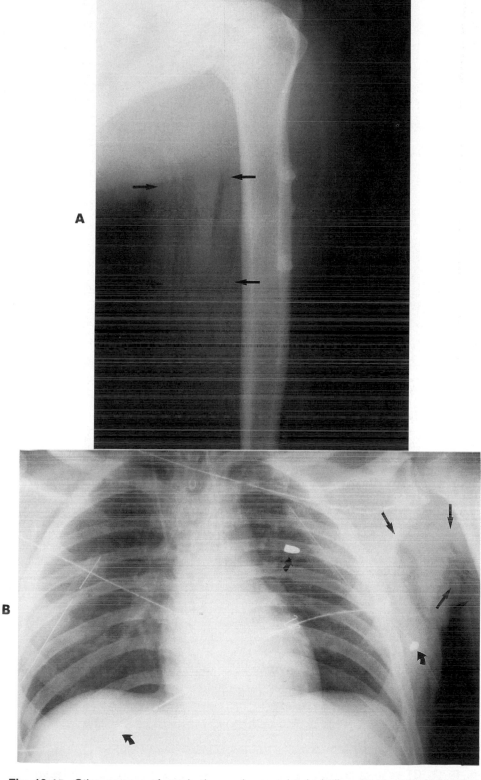

Fig. 19-16. Other causes of gas in tissue planes exist, including direct spread of air from the projectile path, spread of gas from injury to the esophagus, stomach, or intestine, or spread of gas introduced iatrogenically during procedures such as chest tube insertion. **A,** Gas, *arrows,* between muscle planes in the left upper arm after a gunshot wound that traversed the arm. In this case, the gas is from the left chest tube insertion site dissecting into the axilla and the upper arm, **B,** *straight black arrows.* Two bullets in the patient's chest and one in the right upper quadrant of the abdomen, *curved arrows,* are evident.

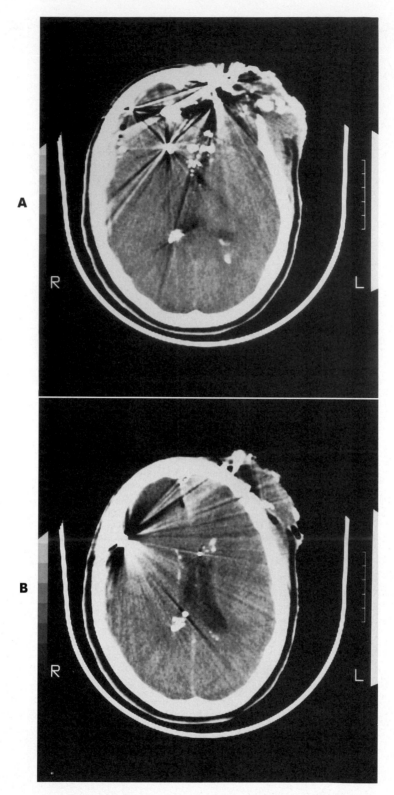

Fig. 19-17. CT scan of the head after a gunshot wound. **A,** Left frontal soft-tissue and bone damage and metallic star artifacts from dense bullet fragments. Some oval densities in the midline near the genu of the corpus callosum and others in the posterior portion of the right lateral ventricle may not be clot, bone, or bullet fragments. Semiradiopaque foreign bodies carried into the wound such as stones, wood, plastic, and clothing may have the same CT density as biologic structures. **B,** Notice also the right subdural hematoma and the anterior interhemispheric subdural hematoma.

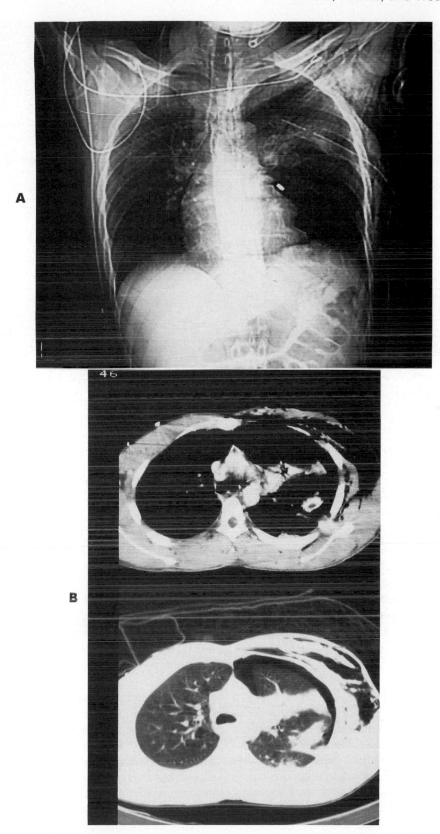

Fig. 19-18. Because of the position of the small-caliber handgun bullet in the left side of the chest on posteroanterior and lateral radiographs, CT scanning was done to determine whether the left pulmonary artery had been injured. **A,** Posteroanterior view. **B,** Path of the bullet through the left lung. The bullet tract is well marked by the hemorrhage it caused. The bullet went immediately adjacent to the left pulmonary artery, but no active bleeding was seen at the time of the dynamic CT scan. Left pneumothorax and left posterior pulmonary contusion associated with chest tube placement are also visible.

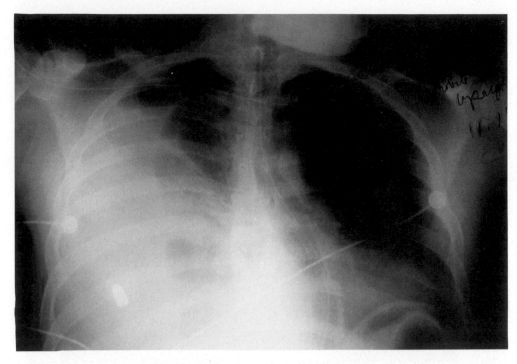

Fig. 19-19. Any bullet that penetrates the trunk below the nipple line may have passed through the abdomen. If it did pass through the abdomen, a laparotomy is required. Here a small-caliber handgun bullet has entered the left upper quadrant of the abdomen coming to rest in the right side of the chest. Notice the free air beneath the left hemidiaphragm, suggestive of a hollow viscus injury. A tension right hemopneumothorax is present, shifting the mediastinum to the left. There is displacement to the left of the nasogastric tube in the lower thorax. This patient has wounds of both the chest and abdomen, different from a wound that externally might be thought to be only a chest wound. Appropriate treatment of this patient includes exploratory laparotomy.

cretory urography as the preferred means of evaluating the urinary tract after penetrating trauma.

The CT digital scout radiograph may be used for missile localization (Figs. 19-9, 19-20, *B,* and 19-30). It usually can be taken in anteroposterior and lateral projections without moving the patient. The ability to manipulate the display window and level allows visualization of bullets seen through dense structures, such as the shoulders, pelvis, or spine.

Bullet embolization

It must always be determined if a bullet's current location can be accounted for by its traveling over a path from the entrance wound to the present location because the bullet may have reached its present location by embolization (see Fig. 3-57). Arterial and venous embolization of bullets and shotgun pellets, as well as bullet movement within the subarachnoid space in the head and spine are possible.

It is generally accepted that a missile freely floating within the left atrium or ventricle of the heart should be removed to prevent embolization.[59-61] Missiles floating in the right atrium or ventricle, except those that

embolized to the heart after first traversing an intestinal viscus, may be observed in anticipation of their embolization to the pulmonary artery, from which they can be removed.[61]

Missiles completely embedded in cardiac chamber walls are relatively safe.[60,61] Partially embedded missiles should be removed if seen soon after injury, but if they are seen late, studies to determine whether the missile is completely encapsulated by fibrous tissue should be done. If completely encapsulated, the patient may be followed rather than operated on.[61] In the rest of the body, symptomatic missiles, especially those manifesting with sepsis, or missiles located next to a major artery, should be removed.[61] In one case, a shotgun pellet was probably dislodged from the heart during cardiopulmonary resuscitation, and embolized to the intracranial circulation, with a fatal result.[62]

Missile size does not seem to be especially important because all sizes can produce morbidity after embolization. Two-dimensional echocardiography is useful in determining whether a missile is embedded in a chamber wall.[60] CT (particularly high-speed CT) and MR imaging for nonmagnetic missiles also have a role. On chest

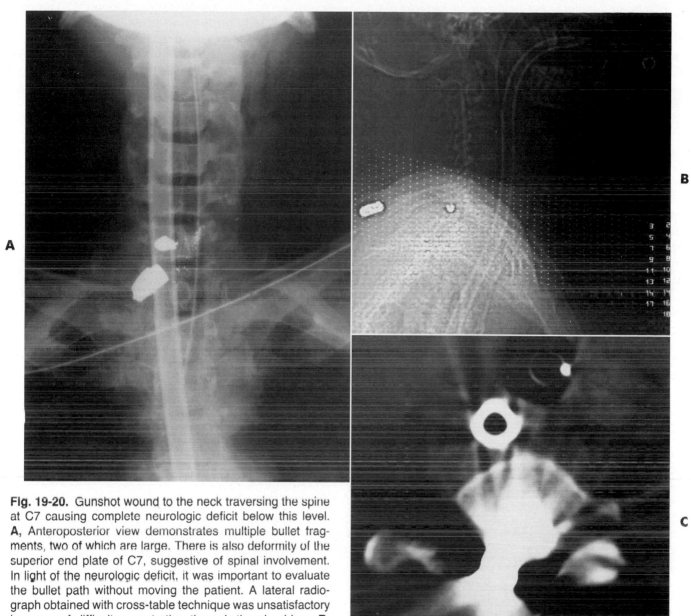

Fig. 19-20. Gunshot wound to the neck traversing the spine at C7 causing complete neurologic deficit below this level. **A,** Anteroposterior view demonstrates multiple bullet fragments, two of which are large. There is also deformity of the superior end plate of C7, suggestive of spinal involvement. In light of the neurologic deficit, it was important to evaluate the bullet path without moving the patient. A lateral radiograph obtained with cross-table technique was unsatisfactory because of difficulty penetrating through the shoulders. **B,** Lateral digital CT scout radiograph shows the location of the major fragments in the lateral projection. **C,** CT image at C7. CT was useful to determine the extent of the fracture and the location of the bullet fragments in the spinal canal. Typical CT star artifact from a large dense metallic bullet fragment causes difficulty with visualization. If one is sure that no steel or other magnetic material is in the bullet (see text), magnetic resonance imaging may be very useful. It is controversial whether to operate on patients with gunshot wounds of the spine.[48-58]

radiographs, blurring of the margins of a pericardiac missile or fragment is grounds for suspecting that the missile is in or next to the heart.[33,59]

Whenever a bullet is not found on radiographs of the body part predicted to contain it based on the entrance wound, the bullet's location is not known, and there is no exit wound, additional radiographs or fluoroscopy to find the bullet are mandatory. Immediately before surgery for removal of a missile, repeat radiographic confirmation of the exact location of the missile is usually indicated.

Most bullets follow fairly straight paths through the body. However, even in the absence of embolization, bullets, particularly handgun bullets, do not always follow a straight path. They may ricochet off body structures, especially bone, or may follow fascial or tissue planes. Bullets traveling less than 900 ft/sec (274 m/sec) are the ones most likely to be deflected by anatomic structures or to follow tissue planes.

Interventional radiologic techniques are useful in bullet removal, including the removal of intravascular and intrarenal bullets.[63-66] Significant deformation of an intravascular bullet is a relative contraindication to retrieval using a transarterial catheter because of potential damage to the intima.[67,68] Arthroscopy sometimes can be used for removing bullets from joints, especially the knee.[69]

Lead Fragments and Lead Poisoning

Lead fragments in soft tissue usually become encapsulated with fibrous tissue and do not cause problems. Lead intoxication has been reported from soft-tissue wounds, particularly those containing many lead pellets.[70] However, usually the lead must be intra-articular, bursal, or in a disk space for lead poisoning to occur.[71-74]

Lead fragments left in the brain usually follow a benign course unless they are copper plated (as are many civilian .22 caliber bullets).[75] Copper-plated lead pellets produced a sterile abscess or granuloma in the brain of cats surgically implanted with missiles of this type.[75] This was often associated with downward migration of the missile, resorption of copper from the surface of the missile, progressive neurologic deficit, and often death. These findings were absent in cats whose brains were implanted with uncoated lead pellets. The reaction of the brain to other metals has also been studied.[76]

Intra-articular fragments should be removed to avoid the destructive synovitis lead may cause.[73,77-79] Lead is relatively soluble in synovial fluid.[71-73,80,81] Fragments within a joint space may be distributed by joint mechanics such that they create an arthrogram-like effect on radiographs, delineating cartilage surfaces and joint capsule recesses (Fig. 19-21, A and B). Significant damage to the articular cartilage visible at surgery may be present as a result of lead synovitis, even when radiographs remain normal except for bullet fragments.[73] If large fragments are present in the joint, they can cause severe mechanical trauma during motion.[78,81] This motion may lead to further lead fragmentation.

A bullet completely or nearly completely embedded in a bone is less of a risk both for lead poisoning and mechanical traumatic arthropathy (see Fig. 19-21, C and D). A clinical decision must be made as to whether removal is necessary.

Whether lead poisoning occurs depends largely on the surface area of the retained lead particles and their location in the body.[71,72,83,84] In several cases, a fibrotic mass containing gray fluid with a high lead content has been observed adjacent to the site of a large bullet fragment or fragments.[71,72,74] Sometimes the onset of clinical lead poisoning can be quite rapid,[83,84] but usually it takes years.

Death from lead poisoning caused by bullets or lead fragments occurs because the diagnosis is not considered. Presenting symptoms may be bizarre, leading the physician to consider them psychogenic in origin. A patient who has retained lead, particularly near a joint, should be made aware of the possibility of late lead poisoning, especially if the lead migrates or erodes to a position where it has contact with synovial fluid. The patient should be reassured that if this does happen, the lead fragment can then be easily removed. It poses no acute threat to life and lead toxicity can be diagnosed by measurement of the patient's blood lead level.

Magnetic Resonance Imaging of Missile Wounds

(See also Chapters 15 to 17.)

MR imaging can be useful in the evaluation of gunshot wounds, particularly when star artifact from a dense metallic bullet fragment limits the usefulness of CT.[49] Damage to the brain or spinal cord is often well shown (see Fig. 19-9, E and F). Vascular abnormalities, including arteriovenous fistula[85] (Fig. 19-22) or aneurysm,[86] sometimes are revealed. Missiles composed of ferromagnetic or paramagnetic materials may produce MR artifacts disproportionate to the missile's size. This can sometimes obscure important information.

Small, nonmagnetic metallic foreign bodies (such as surgical clips and wires) are generally not a problem. Large-volume, nonmagnetic conducting materials inside or outside the body may generate eddy-current artifacts that obscure image detail. For nonferrous missiles, image artifacts are usually less severe on MR than on CT.

One potential problem in performing MR imaging studies on patients with missile wounds comes from the fact that a missile or bullet fragment may be significantly torqued or moved inside the body during the exam because of the large magnetic forces it is subjected to dur-

Fig. 19-21. A and **B,** Radiographs of the knee after a bullet traversed the patella. Bullet fragmentation within the joint space has created an arthrogram effect, which has been referred to as a plumbogram.[81,82] The articular cartilage of the tibiofemoral joint is outlined by fragments, best seen in the lateral compartment. A large fragment has become partially embedded in the anterior articular surface of the lateral femoral condyle.

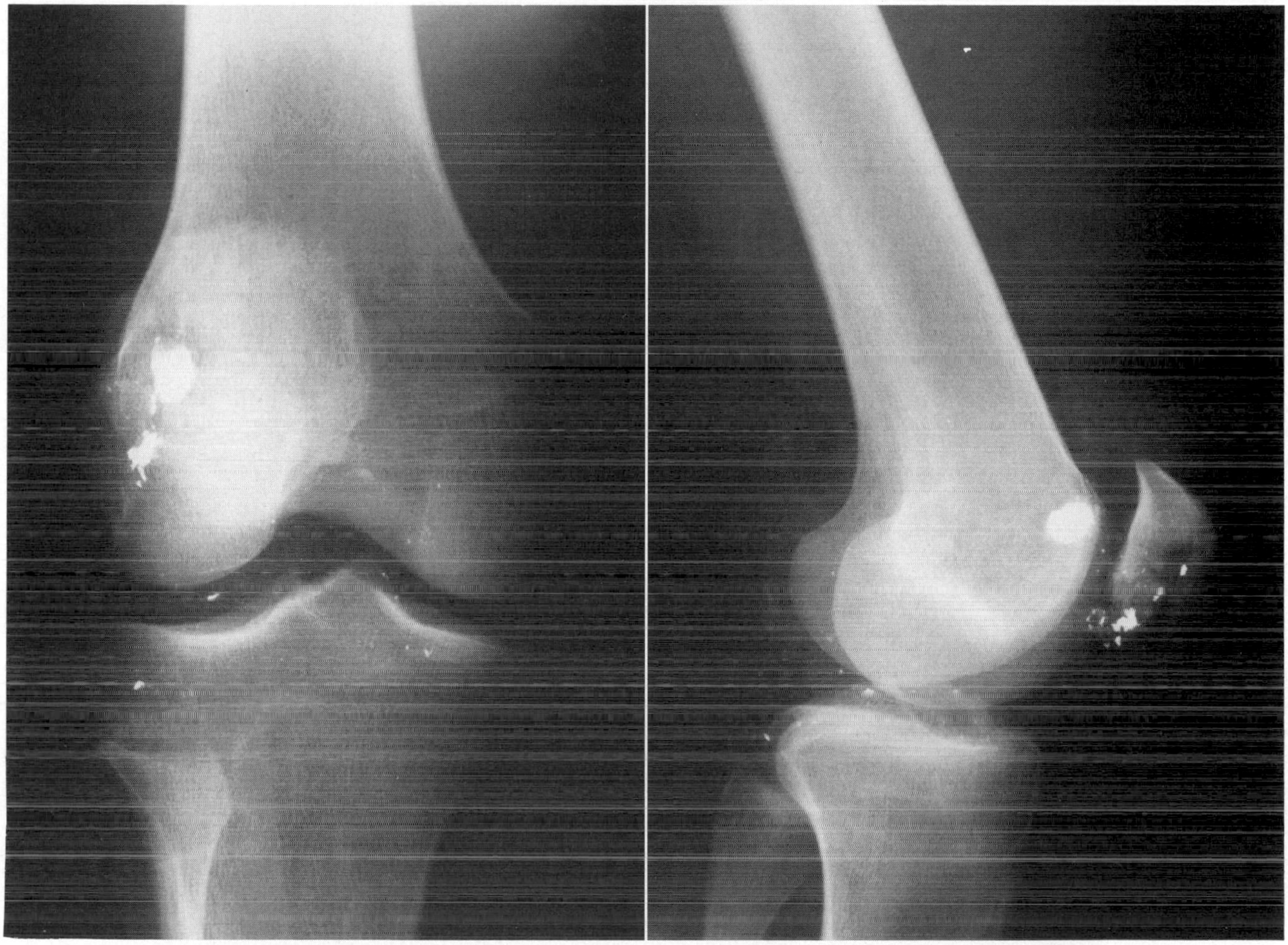

Continued.

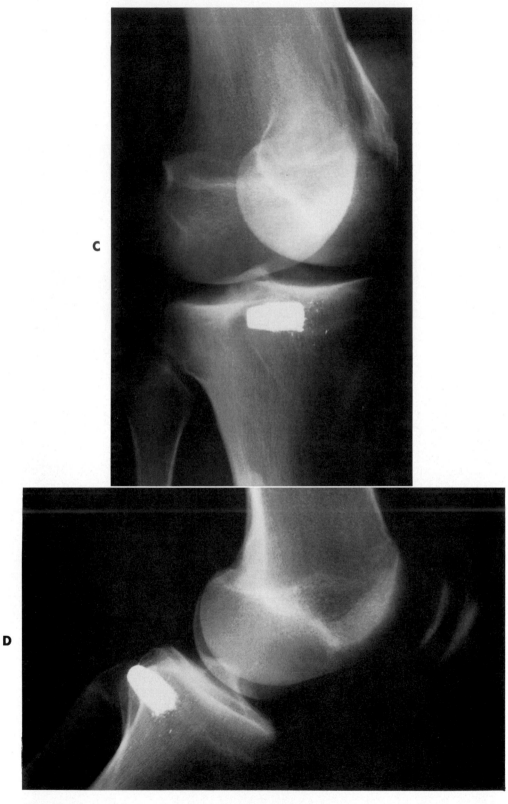

Fig. 19-21, cont'd. C and **D,** This medium-sized handgun bullet has embedded itself in the proximal area of the tibia. No fracture comminution or bullet fragmentation is present. (**A** and **B** from Hollerman JJ et al: *AJR* 155:695, 1990.)

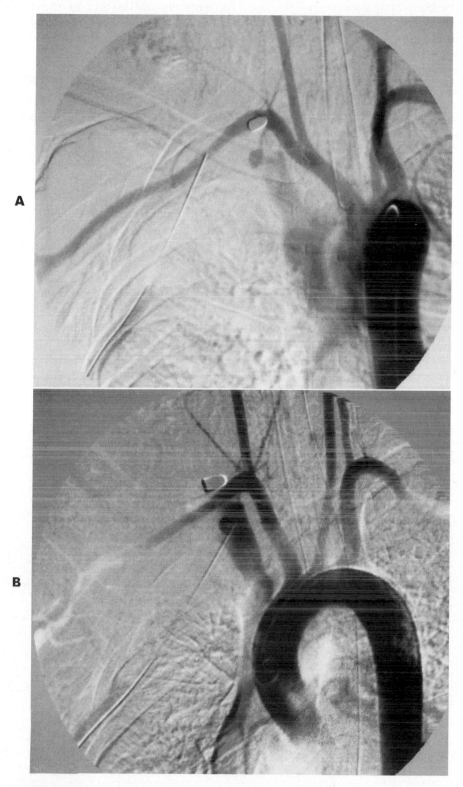

Fig. 19-22. After a handgun bullet wound of the thorax, digital subtraction angiography reveals an unsuspected arteriovenous fistula from the right internal mammary artery to the right brachiocephalic vein.

ing MR imaging. Any time a patient with a missile or bullet lodged inside the body is to undergo an MR examination, the question must be asked, Will it potentially harm this patient if this missile is moved from its present position? If the missile is in the brain or spinal cord, the answer may be yes. If it is in skeletal muscle of the thigh, the danger is much less.[87,88]

In the United States, the most common missile that can be affected by a large magnet is steel shot, required by law for hunting waterfowl.[5] Steel shot should be considered a possibility if a radiograph shows shot that is undeformed, remaining round in shape. Steel shot is harder than lead shot and does not deform, even if it strikes bone. Moreover, there are more pellets in a 1-ounce load of steel shot than in a 1-ounce load of lead shot (see Fig. 19-37).

Other missiles potentially containing metal subject to the effects of strong magnetic fields include some AK-47 ammunition, particularly that from China, which often is sold in the United States. These bullets contain a steel penetrator surrounded by a steel bullet jacket. AK-74 ammunition also has a steel penetrator within the bullet. Most armor-piercing ammunition contains steel and is ferromagnetic (Fig. 19-23). The M855/SS109 M16A2 bullet contains a steel penetrator as well (Fig. 19-24, *B*).

This bullet is designed for use in the M16A2 rifle, which is replacing the M16A1 as the standard-issue United States military rifle. The AK-47 round is unlikely to stay in the body of the wounded person unless it hits a large bone.

CHARACTERISTIC FRAGMENTS

A physician or health care worker asked to assist in a firearms case should be aware that an experienced firearms examiner at the local police criminalistics laboratory is a valuable source of technical expertise on bullets. Also, the International Wound Ballistics Association (RR 4, Box 264, Hawthorne, FL 32640; telephone [904] 481-5661) is available to assist in firearms cases.

When military full metal jacket bullets break and fragment, they do so as a result of yawing to 90 degrees. The resulting stresses cause flattening of the sides of the bullet as if it had been squeezed in a vise (Fig. 19-24, *A*).

Full metal jacket bullets do not mushroom at the bullet tip as soft point or hollow point bullets do. Although the M193 military bullet of the M16 rifle fragments in soft-tissue wounds with a characteristic pattern depending on range[30] (Figure 19-24, *A*), most other full metal jacket military bullets, such as those fired from the AK-

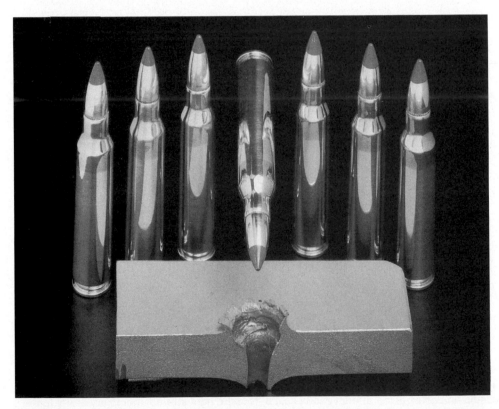

Fig. 19-23. Armor-piercing ammunition often contains steel and is ferromagnetic. If the bullet is located in proximity to a vital structure, magnetic resonance imaging may be contraindicated.[87] (Courtesy Winchester Division, Olin Corporation, East Alton, Ill.)

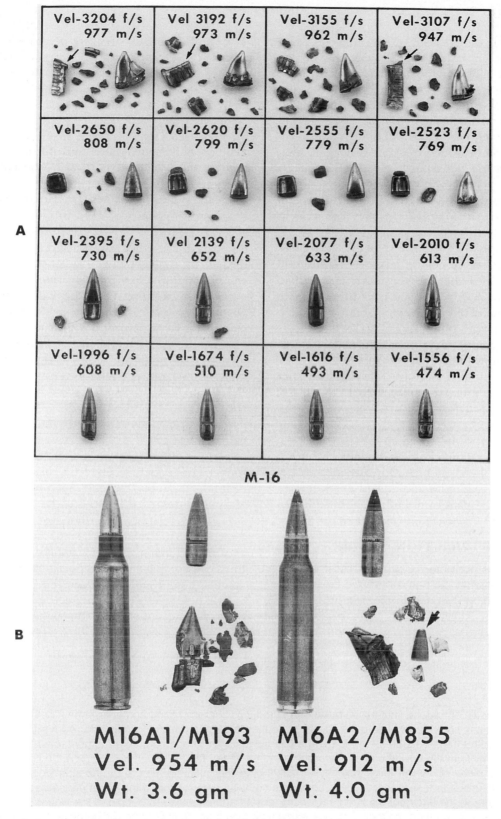

Fig. 19-24. A, Bullet velocity is directly related to range. This series of "step-down" shots illustrates the fragmentation and deformation pattern of the M193 bullet of the M16A1 rifle at different velocities. **B,** The M16A1 rifle/M193 bullet combination is being replaced by the U.S. military with the M16A2 rifle/M855 bullet combination. The M855 bullet was originally developed in an attempt to produce a more "humane" military bullet.[89] It was touted as a full metal jacket bullet that would not fragment in tissue. It does fragment, however, to a very similar extent as the M193 bullet. These shots were into ballistic gelatin at a 10-foot range. The small trapezoidal steel penetrator, *black arrow,* housed inside the full metal jacket of the intact M855 bullet will be identifiable after the bullet breaks and fragments, if the penetrator remains in the body. It is steel and ferromagnetic. If it is in or near a vital structure, magnetic resonance imaging might be contraindicated.

47, the AK-74, and the NATO 7.62 mm rifle (USA version) do not fragment unless they strike a large bone.

The absence of bullet fragments can sometimes assist in determining where the shots came from. Consider, for example, the case of an individual accidentally killed by an M16 bullet on a military training course. The bullet passed completely through the abdomen of the soldier, creating a 25 cm wound tract and leaving no fragments. The bullet was not recovered. Only two groups of other trainees were on the course at the same time, one 60 meters from the deceased and one 200 meters from the deceased. The M16 bullet makes fragments in a characteristic pattern depending on range (Fig. 19-24, A). Range correlates with striking velocity. Shots done with M16 bullets at up to 120 meters consistently showed considerable bullet breaking and fragmentation, and those shots at 200 meters and over showed some flattening of the bullet but no breaking or fragmentation. Because there were no bullet fragments in the soldier and because the wound tract through the abdomen was long enough to allow bullet fragmentation if it were going to occur, it could be determined that the fatal shot originated from the group at 200 meters.

Some other bullets fragmenting in a characteristic pattern include the .45 cal Federal Hydrashok bullet (Fig. 19-25), the Remington .357 Magnum JSP (partially jacketed soft point) and Remington .44 Magnum JSP handgun bullets (Fig. 19-26), and the Hornady STX hollow point bullet (Fig. 19-27). In addition to characteristic bullet fragments, the pattern of bullet deformation can be used in forensic investigation (Fig. 19-28).

ASSESSMENT OF DIRECTION OF FIRE

When projectiles perforate bone, they cause inward beveling of the entrance hole and outward beveling at the exit.[90] This is demonstrated in the proximal femur, the skull, and the proximal humerus (Figs. 19-29 to 19-31). The two-surface structure of a pane of glass causes a similar beveling pattern when penetrated by a missile such as a BB. Bone fragments can become secondary missiles and are propelled along the bullet tract, or radially out from it, creating a distal spray of bone fragments adjacent to the surface of the bone from which the bullet left (see Figs. 19-8, 19-29, and 19-31).

When bullets penetrate thin portions of the skull, such as the squamous portion of the temporal bone, characteristic beveling may not be evident. In those cases and others, characteristic fracture patterns of the skull can sometimes be used to differentiate entrance and exit holes.[90,94-97] Skull fractures propagate across the calvarium much faster than the bullet travels through the brain. Fractures radiating from the entrance wound extend across the calvarium unimpeded; however, those radiating from the exit wound will stop when they meet a previously made fracture from the entrance hole (they will not propagate across a previous fracture). This technique of analysis is most often used to determine the order of shots when there are multiple calvarium penetrations or perforations.[96,97]

GUNSHOT FRACTURES

Handgun wounds of the extremities yield characteristic fracture patterns. Some are discussed above in the "direction of fire" section. Other frequently seen gunshot fractures include divot fractures of cortical bone, drill hole fractures, butterfly fractures, and double butterfly fractures.[5,98,99]

Fractures related to gunshot wounds vary greatly in their severity. However, at some hospitals, outpatient treatment is being used successfully for extremity fractures caused by handguns if no significant neurologic or vascular compromise has occurred.[100]

Drill hole fractures are characterized by a cylindrical core of bone removed by the bullet, with a diameter

Text continued on p. 563.

Fig. 19-25. The .45 caliber Federal Hydrashok bullet often produces characteristic fragments when it deforms. It has a post in the center of this hollow point bullet. The bullet jacket of copper forms the rim of the bullet tip. As the bullet deforms into a mushroom shape, jacket fragments break off, forming a characteristically shaped pointed fragment, often five sided. **A,** Six of these jacket fragments form the full circumference of the distal portion of the bullet jacket shown on the right. The linear score marks placed in the distal portion of the copper bullet jacket near the bullet tip, visible on the side view of the bullet at the upper left, cause the jacket to tear at reproducible points during bullet deformation. If the bullet penetrates through a shooting victim and is no longer in the body but these characteristic jacket fragments are left behind in the wound tract, the bullet type can be identified. Because they are copper, they are less dense than lead fragments on radiographs. Sometimes, a fragment of lead is attached to the copper jacket fragment, increasing radiographic density. They may separate, and no lead is attached to the copper jacket fragment. In addition to the characteristic jacket fragments, the Hydrashok may sometimes be identified as a deformed bullet with a post projecting from its center. **B,** Results of 28 shots with .45 caliber Federal Hydrashok bullets from 10 feet into ballistic gelatin. This bullet is touted as deforming in a very consistent fashion. Notice, however, that there is considerable shot-to-shot variation in the pattern of deformation and fragmentation, even when shot into the very consistent medium of ballistic gelatin. This is very common with handgun ammunition (see also Fig. 19-5).

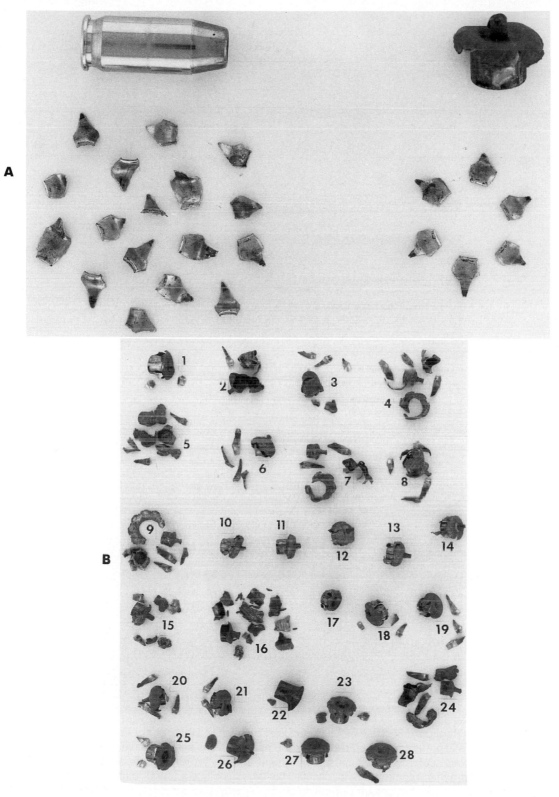

Fig. 19-25. For legend see opposite page.

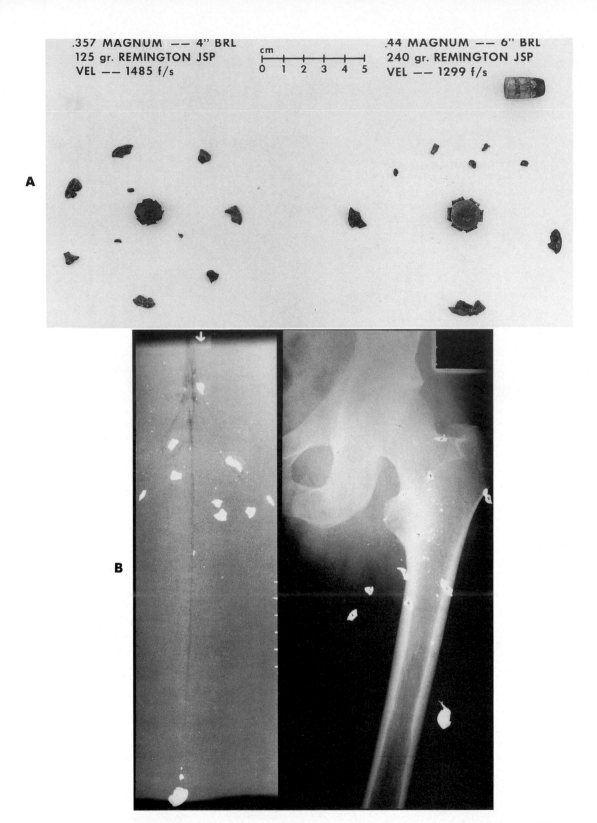

Fig. 19-26. Remington .357 Magnum JSP (partially jacketed soft point) and Remington .44 Magnum JSP handgun bullets often fragment in a characteristic pattern. **A,** The distal end of the bullet jacket is scalloped (see side view of intact round in the upper right corner). As the bullet deforms into a mushroom shape and the jacket folds backward, bilobed "B-shaped" lead fragments are broken off. Not every fragment has this shape, but when some are found, they very strongly indicate this ammunition. This jacket edge construction is unique to Remington. **B,** Side-by-side photograph of a shot into ballistic gelatin *(on left)* and a shot into a patient *(on right)* with Remington .357 Magnum JSP ammunition. There are bilobed fragments in both. The fragment just inferolateral to the greater trochanter is particularly characteristic. This appearance could be simulated by two small adjacent fragments, and so some caution is warranted. Sometimes other projections or fluoroscopy should be done to confirm that one is viewing a bilobed characteristic fragment and not two adjacent oval fragments.

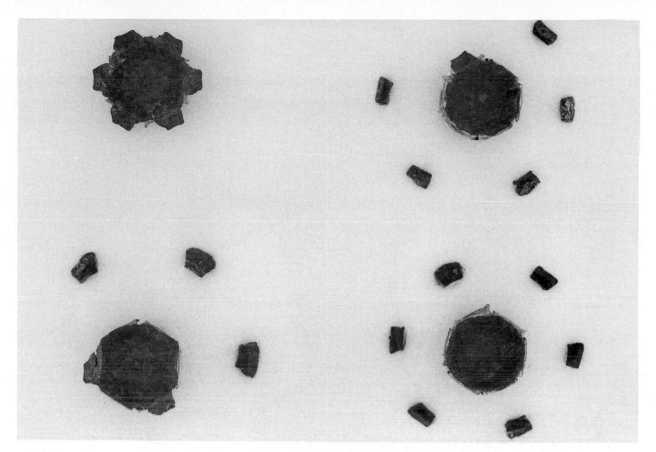

Fig. 19-27. Characteristic trapezoidal fragments of the Hornady .45 and .38 caliber STX hollow point bullet. The trapezoidal fragments are larger and weigh more if they are from the larger caliber STX bullet. During bullet deformation in tissue, each leaf of this bullet jacket bends back, taking a characteristically shaped fragment of lead with it. The fragment of bullet lead may separate from the adjacent bullet jacket fragment or stay attached.

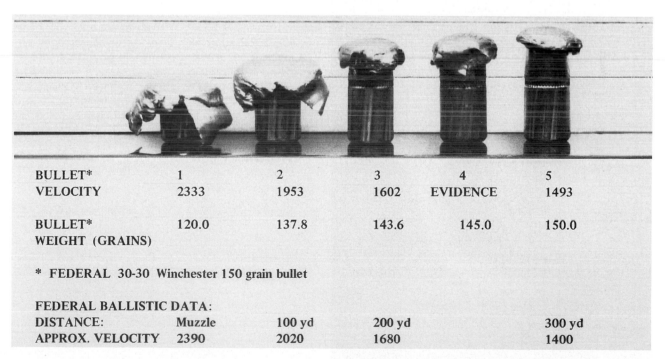

BULLET*	1	2	3	4	5
VELOCITY	2333	1953	1602	EVIDENCE	1493
BULLET* WEIGHT (GRAINS)	120.0	137.8	143.6	145.0	150.0

* FEDERAL 30-30 Winchester 150 grain bullet

FEDERAL BALLISTIC DATA:

DISTANCE:	Muzzle	100 yd	200 yd		300 yd
APPROX. VELOCITY	2390	2020	1680		1400

Fig. 19-28. In this case a person with many enemies was fatally shot while hunting on the first day of deer season. The bullet passed through the victim's abdomen, through the full thickness of the liver, and out the posterior flank, being caught in the patient's backpack, which it partially penetrated. Was this an accident or an assassination? It was determined that the bullet was a Federal 30-30 Winchester 150 grain bullet. The 30-30 is not accurate at long range, and in the opinion of the investigators, if fired from a distance of greater than 100 yards, it was consistent with an accident and not a professional murder. "Step-down" shots at different bullet velocities were done as illustrated. It was found that the deformed bullet recovered from the backpack of the victim had length and diameter between that of the test bullets at simulated ranges of 200 and 300 yards. The shooting was ruled accidental, and the investigation closed.

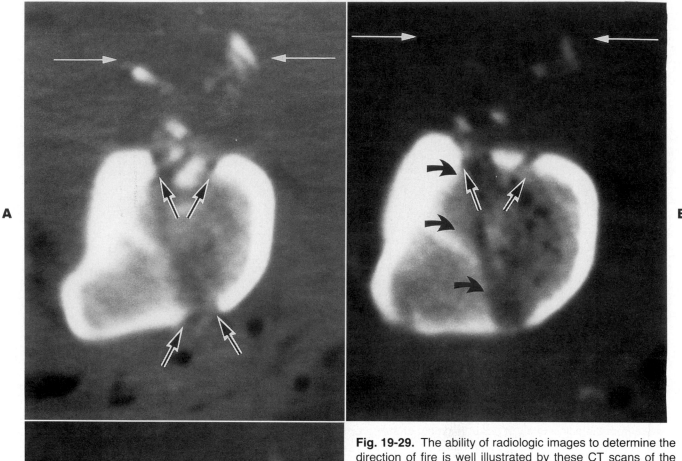

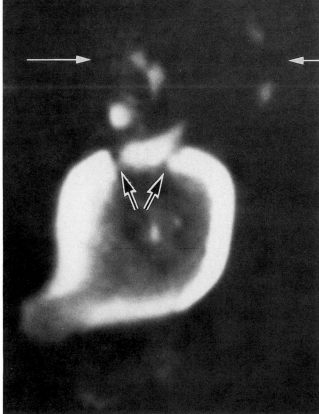

Fig. 19-29. The ability of radiologic images to determine the direction of fire is well illustrated by these CT scans of the proximal femur of a patient shot from the back. They show inward beveling of bone at the bullet entrance and outward beveling at the bullet exit (*black and white straight arrows* in **A** to **C**). There is also a permanent wound channel in the femur (a drill-hole fracture, *curved black arrows* in **B**) and outwardly driven bone fragments in the soft tissues of the thigh anterior to the bullet exit from the femur (*white arrows* in **A** to **C**). Some oval foci of soft-tissue gas are also visible posterior to the femur on scan **A**.

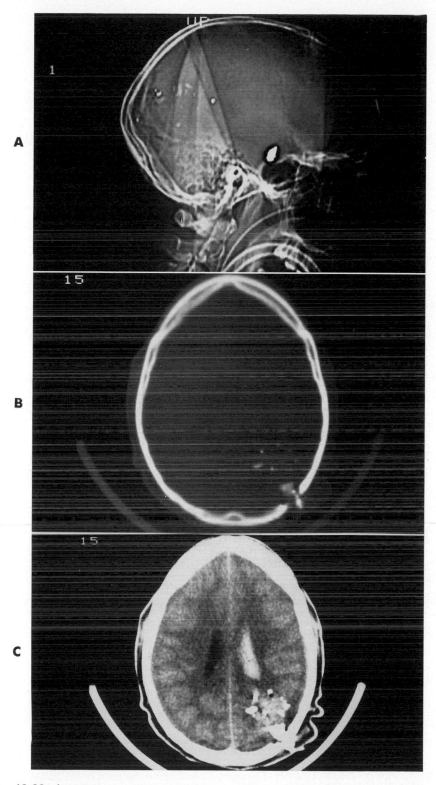

Fig. 19-30. A recent execution-style murder victim is shown here. A small-caliber handgun was held to the victim's left occiput. The lateral scout radiograph, **A,** obtained before CT scanning of the head, shows inwardly driven bone fragments posteriorly and the small-caliber undeformed bullet. Notice the inward beveling at the bullet entrance wound, displayed at bone-window settings in **B.**   *Continued.*

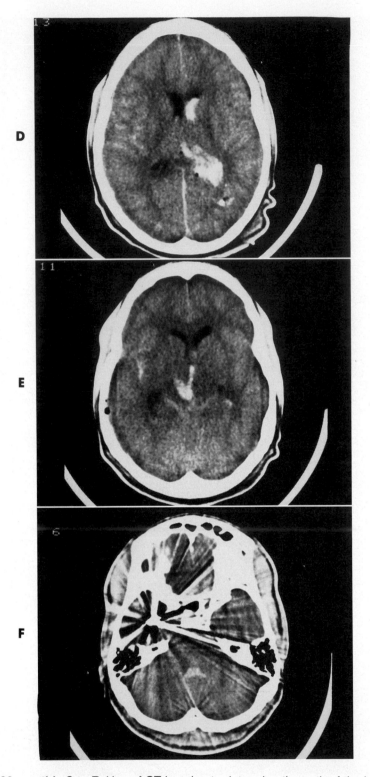

Fig. 19-30, cont'd. C to **F,** Use of CT imaging to determine the path of the bullet through the brain. This bullet entered in the left occiput, with skull fragments becoming secondary missiles injuring the left parieto-occipital area of the brain. It passed through the atrium of the left lateral ventricle, the third ventricle, and the right thalamus and came to rest in the right middle cranial fossa within the right temporal lobe. Bullets crossing the midline either sagittally or coronally are usually lethal.[28,29,91-93]

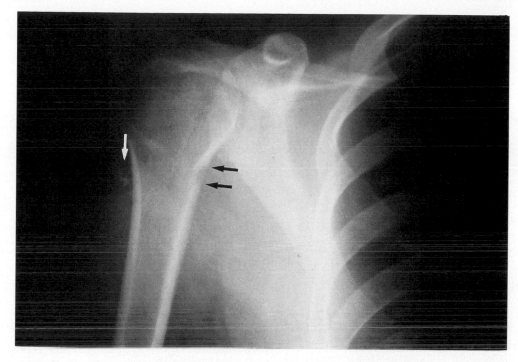

Fig. 19-31. A gunshot wound to the proximal right humerus, from medial to lateral. The humeral entrance wound with inward beveling, *black arrows,* and the outwardly driven bone fragments, *white arrow,* adjacent to the humeral exit wound are marked.

approximating the bullet diameter on the entrance side and usually a larger defect on the exit side[98] (Figs. 19-29 and 19-32). Nondisplaced fracture lines sometimes radiate from these defects (Fig. 19-32). These usually heal well.

Divot fractures are the removal of a divotlike portion of bone, always involving the cortex and occasionally some adjacent medullary bone. A longitudinal fracture line or lines may extend along the bone from the point of the divot fracture.

Spiral fractures may extend proximally or distally to the site of the bullet impact on bone (Fig. 19-33). This type of gunshot fracture is especially common in bones under torsional stress at the time of impact. Torsional stress can result from twisting of an extremity, can be attributable to the normal shape of some bones, or can result from normal biomechanical forces acting on a bone placed under a load.[99] Torsion is always present, for example, in the femur.

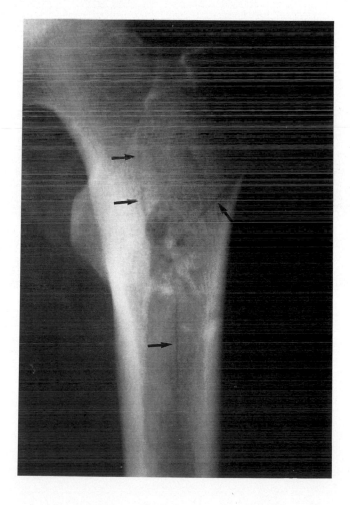

Fig. 19-32. Handgun wounds of the extremities yield characteristic fracture patterns. One is the drill-hole fracture (seen here and also in Fig. 19-29) caused by bullet passage through the bone. Drill-hole fractures are characterized by a cylindrical core of bone removed by the bullet, with a diameter approximating the bullet diameter on the entrance side and usually a larger defect on the exit side. Nondisplaced fracture lines often radiate from these defects, *black arrows.*

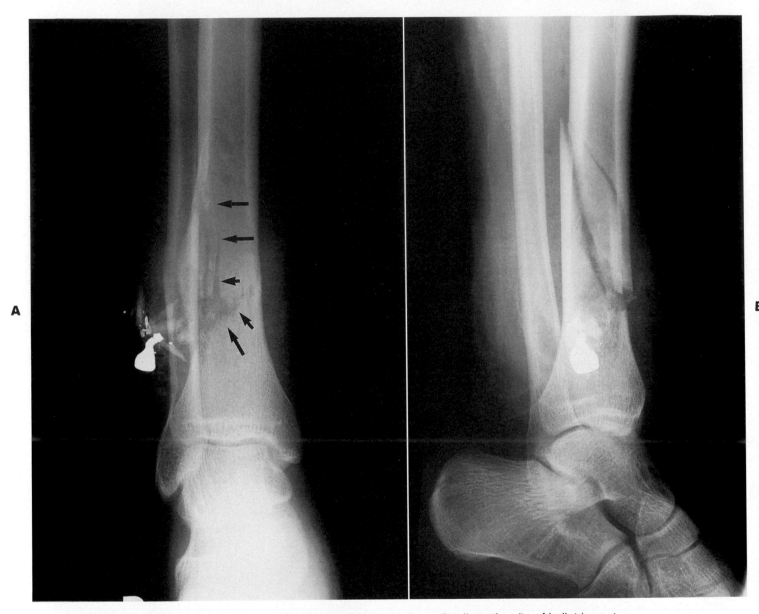

Fig. 19-33. Spiral fractures can extend proximally or distally to the site of bullet impact on the bone. This type of gunshot fracture is especially common in bones under load and torsional stress at the time of bullet impact. Here, a handgun bullet has impacted on the tibia creating linear and spiral fractures, *arrows*, extending cephalad from the point of impact.

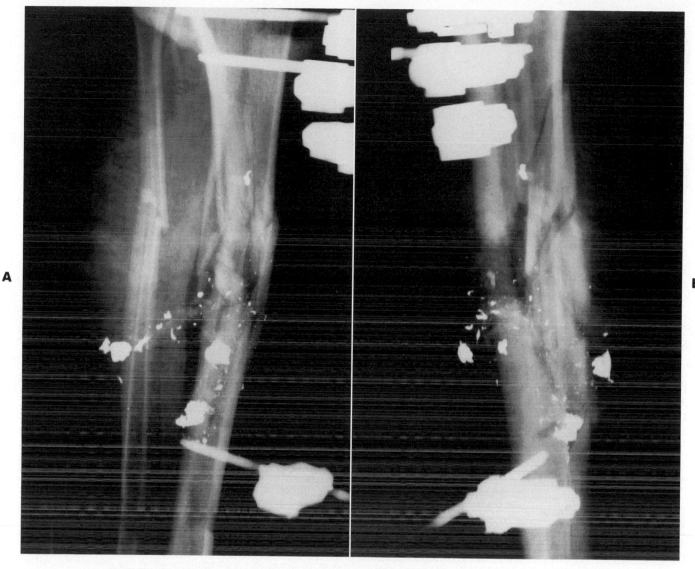

Fig. 19-34. Frontal, **A,** and lateral, **B,** views show comminuted tibial and fibular fractures. Such fractures may be created by rifle and large handgun bullets striking bone. Bone fragments become secondary missiles, crushing tissue. The bullet fragmentation resulting from striking bone also increases wound severity. The greater the extent of fracture comminution, the greater the extent of the associated soft-tissue damage. When a large bone is struck, it is likely that the bullet will expend its wounding potential in the patient and will not exit. Many handgun bullets are unable to significantly fragment large bones.

Especially interesting are the spiral fractures, which can occur at variable distances proximally or distally to the fracture occurring at the site of the bullet passage. Sometimes there is a considerable length of normal intervening bone, particularly in the femur. These remote fractures probably occur because the bone was under load or stress at the time of impact.[99,101] This type of fracture has occasionally been attributed to the fall that some patients report after being wounded. This is rarely the mechanism of the injury.[99]

Gunshot fractures from rifles and large handguns may produce a greater extent of comminution (Fig. 19-34). The magnitude of bone fragmentation depends on the amount of pressure generated within the bone.[99] These comminuted fractures often have further complications because of the soft-tissue damage, including macrovascular and microvascular injury, these bullets cause.[5,102] Wound infections are also more common in this group.

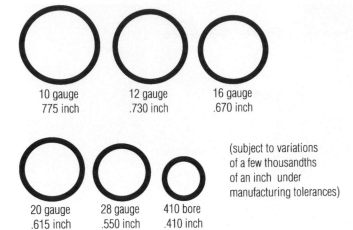

Fig. 19-35. Some common standard shotgun-bore diameters. (Courtesy Winchester Division, Olin Corporation, East Alton, Ill.)

SHOTGUN (PELLET) WOUNDS

Shotguns are smooth-bore weapons (without rifling grooves in the barrel). The gauge or bore size of a shotgun is named by the weight (in fractions of a pound) of the round lead ball of maximum size that will fit in the barrel. A 12-gauge shotgun will accept a lead ball weighing $\frac{1}{12}$ lb. (Fig. 19-35). There are two common exceptions to this rule, the 9 mm shotgun and the .410 shotgun, both named for caliber.

Compared with the pointed rifle bullet, the spherical pellet slows rapidly in its flight through air or tissue. When it hits tissue, the entire wounding potential of the shot pellet at its resulting entrance velocity is likely to be delivered to the target, usually with no exit wound.

At long range (greater than 100 meters), air resistance slows smaller spherical pellets so much that little wounding potential remains. On the other hand, at close range (less than 3 meters), shotgun pellets remain tightly clustered. Shot-pellet size makes little difference because the entire load of the pellets functions as a unit, with a velocity virtually equal to muzzle velocity (Fig. 19-36). It makes no difference whether the shell contained 2981 pellets of number 12 birdshot with a total weight of 1¼ ounces or 11 pellets of 00 buckshot with a total weight of 1¼ ounces (Fig. 19-37).

At longer ranges, the pellets spread out. The size and mass of each pellet determines the proportion of the wounding potential of the load that each pellet will carry. The shot charge radiates from the gun muzzle in a cone-shaped distribution with the pellets nearly evenly distributed at the base of the cone. The choke of a shotgun refers to the degree of constriction at the end of the barrel. Choke is used to reduce the spread of the shot pattern, causing a greater number of shot to

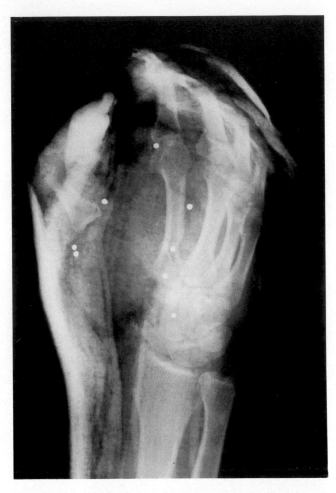

Fig. 19-36. A close-range shotgun wound has completely avulsed the thenar eminence of the hand, the first metacarpal, and the distal portion of the navicular. The shot pellets were tightly clustered together and functioned as a unit, punching out a large oval soft-tissue defect. The thenar eminence is too thin a structure to allow the "billiard-ball effect" (see text) to occur during the passage of the load.

strike a given target at a distance. Choke functions like the nozzle of a garden hose, constricting the flow pattern and increasing range. Improved, modified, and full choke distributions are shown in Fig. 19-38.

Shotgun wounds at ranges less than 5 meters consist of multiple parallel wound channels[2] (Fig. 19-39). This pattern grossly disrupts the blood supply to tissue between the wound channels. The most severe civilian firearm wounds typically seen are those inflicted by a shotgun from close range.[103-107] Preoperative angiography of most close-range shotgun extremity wounds is recommended.[105,107-112] Major neural injury after shotgun wounding may be more important than fracture or major vascular injury in determining the final outcome.[113]

During surgical exploration of a close-range shotgun wound, it is important to search for wadding, plastic

						Buckshot Sizes
#4	#3	#1	0	00	000	Shot Number
.24	.25	.30	.32	.33	.36	Diameter in Inches
338	299	173	143	130	100	Pellets/Lb.,Lead

													Shot Sizes
9	8	7½	6	5	4	3	2	1	BB	BBB	T	F	Shot Number
.08	.09	.095	.11	.12	.13	.14	.15	.16	.18	.19	.20	.22	Diameter in Inches
585	410	350	225	170	135	—	87	—	50	—	—	—	Pellets/Oz.,Lead
—	—	—	316	243	191	153	125	103	72	61	53	39	Steel

Fig. 19-37. This illustration shows various shot-pellet sizes, their nomenclature designation (shot number), their diameter in inches, and the number of lead or steel pellets per unit weight. (Courtesy Winchester Division, Olin Corporation, East Alton, Ill.)

shot cup, plastic flake buffers (packed with the shot charge to decrease shot deformation from the charge being squeezed together by the initial acceleration in the barrel), and surface materials carried into the wound (such as clothing, glass, or wood). Many of these are radiolucent.[5,114] At close or intermediate range (up to 7 meters), the wadding or wad column, or shot cup, or both, are often in the wound.[106,107,113,114] The wadding may be cardboard, felt, fiber, plastic, cork, or cattle hair and is usually radiolucent.[106,110,114] Most shotgun rounds have more than one wad.

The radiographic diagnosis of long-range versus close-range shotgun injury based on the pattern of pellet spread is sometimes problematic. When the shotgun pellets are tightly clustered, close-range injury is suspected. When they are widely spread out, long-range injury is usually suspected. However, in close-range injuries, the "billiard-ball" effect may cause considerable pellet spread.[33] On radiographs, particularly in trunk wounds, this effect can simulate the pellet spread of a longer-range injury.[33] As the shotgun pellets enter tissue in a mass (at short range, that is, a few meters), the leading pellets are rapidly slowed and then struck by the pellets behind them, causing pellet spread because

Shotshell Pattern

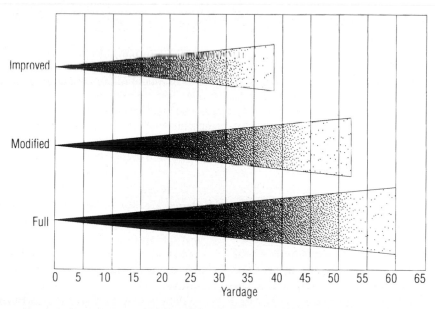

Fig. 19-38. Shotshell pattern. The spatial distribution of a load of shotgun pellets at various ranges with different types of choke boring of the shotgun barrel. (Courtesy Winchester Division, Olin Corporation, East Alton, Ill.)

Fig. 19-39. Frontal, **A,** and lateral, **B,** views of a shotgun wound to the knee. A shotgun fired from close range (less than 3 meters) causes the most severe firearm wounds typically seen in civilian practice. At this range, the heavy weight of the shot charge functions as a unit. There is rapid deceleration in tissue, often with no exit wound. The multiple parallel wound channels formed by the pellets cause severe local vascular disruption, inhibiting healing and increasing the probability of complications. In the case illustrated here, there are extensive fractures of the distal area of the femur and proximal area of the tibia. The knee-joint surface is grossly disrupted, and there was severe injury of the neurovascular structures of the popliteal space.

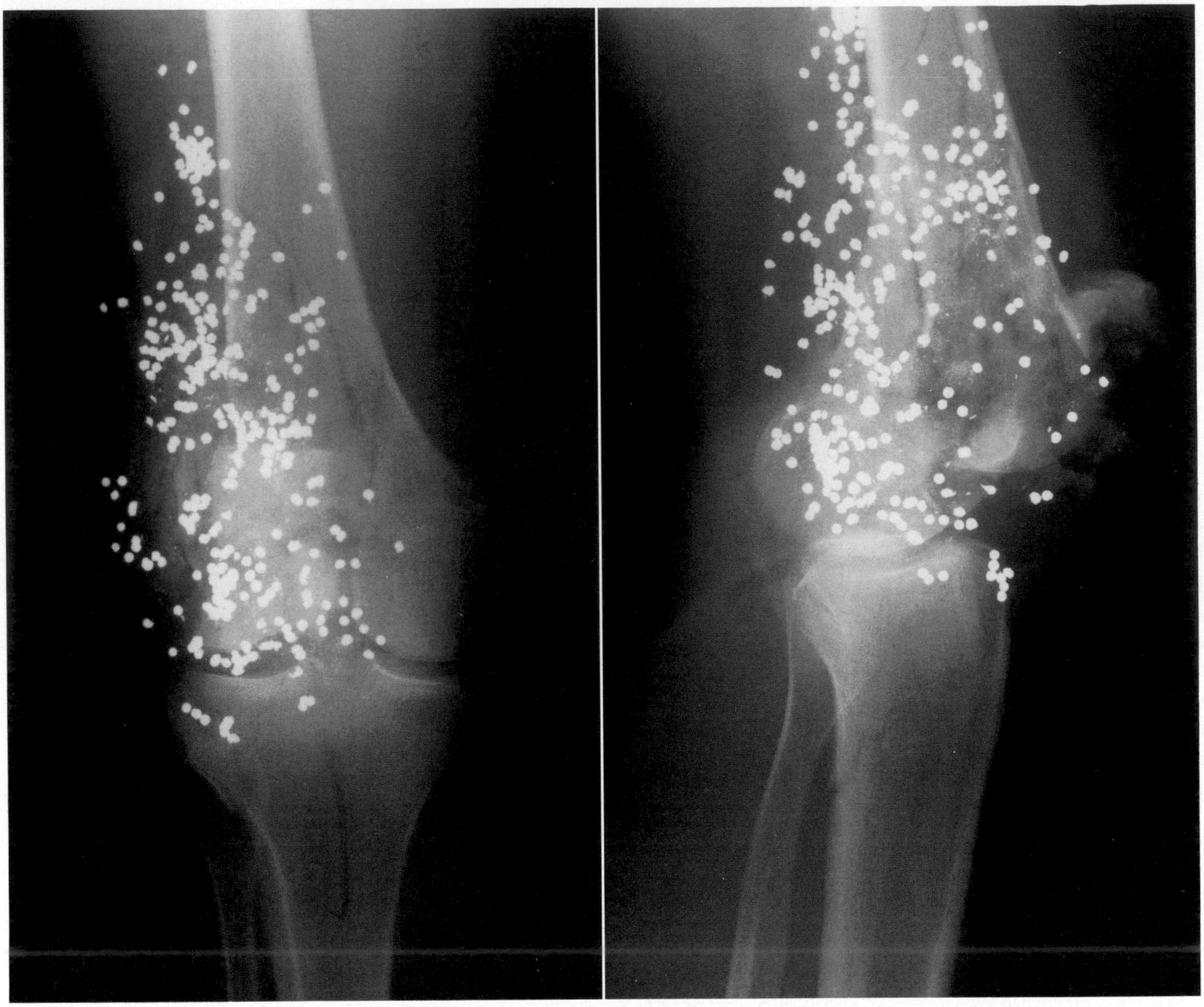

of a ricochet effect. This is much like a billiard ball striking a cluster of others, causing them to spread out at various angles. This effect can produce a wide pellet-distribution pattern that radiographically simulates the pellet spread from a much longer distance of fire. The billiard-ball pitfall can sometimes be avoided if the spread of the entrance wounds on the skin is correlated with the radiologic findings.

At close range, the pellets at the front of the clustered mass of the load enter tissue, are slowed, and then are struck by the pellets behind them. This collision deforms both the leading and trailing pellets from their normal spherical shape (if one assumes they are lead, not steel) (Fig. 19-40). This deformation increases their surface area and decreases their chance of leaving the body.

Pellets may be flattened to twice their initial diameter, resulting in a considerable decrease in their depth of tissue penetration. This effect is most noticeable with shots fired from as close as skin contact to as far away

#4 BUCKSHOT

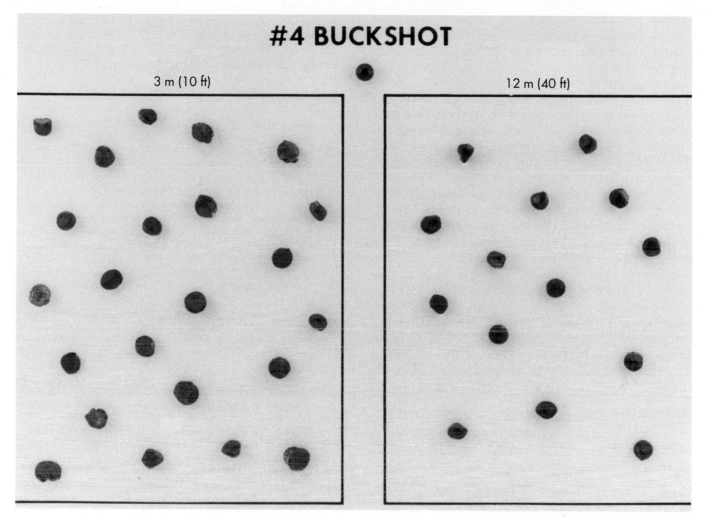

3 m (10 ft)   12 m (40 ft)

Fig. 19-40. Number 4 buckshot recovered from 10% ballistic gelatin. At 40 feet, all the buckshot pellets hit separately and do not deform by contact with each other. At 10 feet, there is far more pellet deformation because of the "billiard-ball effect." Most of the pellets at 10 feet are severely deformed. Two seen at the lower right corner of the group have fused together by impact. At ranges of 10 ft or less, this commonly occurs. This same effect occurs with body armor.

as 5 or 6 feet, but it still occurs somewhat at 10 feet. One might believe that at close range, higher pellet velocity would increase the chance of pellets leaving the body, but the increased pellet diameter caused by deformation from collision with other pellets decreases penetration depth, substantially compensating for the effect of the higher pellet velocity at close range. The entire wounding potential of the load is often imparted to the tissues with no exit wound even at close range.

Also, at close range, shotgun pellets often become fused together with other pellets (see Fig. 19-40). This probably occurs by impact. The pellets in the front of the load are slowed as they contact the body. The pellets behind run into them and sometimes fuse with them.

Recent BB guns and airguns that fire small pellets have considerably higher muzzle velocity than older guns of this type.[115,116] Penetrating injuries from these weapons are sometimes fatal.[116-118] These weapons should not be considered toys. Occasionally, body penetration of a pellet or BB fired from a pneumatic rifle will be unsuspected by both the victim and the doctor (see Fig. 3-51). Both may think that only a skin wound is present. Even brain penetration can have this presentation, with no neurologic deficit.[115] Radiographs of the injured part should always be obtained after a missile injury with a visible skin wound but no visible missile.

The Glaser Safety Slug consists of hundreds of pellets of number 12 birdshot in a copper cup with a nonradiopaque fiberglass-Teflon cap.[119] It may cause severe superficial wounds because of its relatively high velocity and because of the spherical pellets of the load (already in a prefragmented form).[119] Because of this, it sometimes does not penetrate to a lethal depth. It travels through air with the properties of a bullet, since the pellets are enclosed by the cup and cap. However, it behaves like pellet ammunition when it enters the body, usually without leaving. This type of ammunition should be considered if a radiograph is encountered with shotgun pellets and a metallic cup (often fragmented) in the wound.

The shot cup of shotgun ammunition is almost never radiopaque, whereas the cup of the Glasser Safety Slug is metallic and visible. This shot cup should be removed for examination by a firearms examiner because it may allow a positive weapon identification attributable to rifling marks. The surgeon should also be aware that wound exploration must include a search for the nonradiopaque cap material (often fragmented), which is expected to be in the wound.[119] This is a similar clinical problem to the nonradiopaque parts of shotgun ammunition, particularly the wads.[114] Other handgun rounds loaded with pellets are also available in various calibers.[120]

CONCLUSIONS

Bullet velocity is only one factor in wounding, and in some wounds may be a minor factor. If a bullet expands to such an extent that it uses up its wounding potential by crushing superficial tissues and causing temporary cavitation stretch, it may not reach the depth of vital structures.[3-5] A heavier, slower bullet may penetrate more deeply, reaching vital structures. Missile mass and velocity establish an upper limit of *possible* tissue damage, the bullet's *wounding potential*. The amount of the *wounding potential* actually used in disrupting tissue depends on bullet construction and the physical properties of the tissue it penetrates.

Gunshot wound treatment should be based on the physical examination of the patient and the results of radiologic studies, not on the history of what weapon inflicted the wound. One must "treat the wound not the weapon."[10] The history reported to the physician of what type of weapon inflicted the wound and at what range is usually wrong and, even if accurate, is usually irrelevant in determining treatment. Weapon type does not determine wound severity. Wound severity is determined by what anatomic structures are injured. Missiles with great wounding potential can produce very minor wounds. It is the condition of the patient that determines the treatment needed.

ACKNOWLEDGMENTS

We gratefully acknowledge the assistance of Toni Williams for aid in literature retrieval, Bradford Allan and Larry Algiers for the use of the radiograph in Fig. 19-14, Irwin Weisman for review of magnetic resonance metallic artifacts, and Kim Vojacek of the Minnesota Medical Research Foundation art department for assistance with photographs.

REFERENCES

1. Allison EJ Jr: Violence in America: a shameful epidemic, *ACEP News* 11(3):4, 1992 (American College of Emergency Physicians).
2. Bowen TE, Bellamy RF: *Emergency war surgery: second United States revision of the emergency war surgery NATO handbook,* ed 2, Washington, DC, 1988, United States Department of Defense, United States Government Printing Office.
3. Hollerman JJ, Fackler ML: Wound ballistics. In Tintinalli JE, Krome RL, Ruiz E, editors: *Emergency medicine: a comprehensive study guide (American College of Emergency Physicians),* ed 3, New York, 1992, McGraw-Hill, pp 1019-1025.
4. Hollerman JJ, Fackler ML, Coldwell DM, et al: Gunshot wounds: 1. Bullets, ballistics and mechanisms of injury, *AJR* 155:685, 1990.
5. Hollerman JJ, Fackler ML, Coldwell DM, et al: Gunshot wounds: 2. Radiology, *AJR* 155:691, 1990.
6. Fackler ML, Bellamy RF, Malinowski JA: The wound profile: illustration of the missile-tissue interaction, *J Trauma* 28(suppl 1):S21, 1988.
7. Fackler ML: Ballistic injury, *Ann Emerg Med* 15(12):1451, 1986.
8. Fackler ML, Surinchak JS, Malinowski JA, et al: Bullet fragmentation: a major cause of tissue disruption, *J Trauma* 24(1):35, 1984.
9. Knudsen PJT: Author's comment, *Z Rechtsmed* 103:69, 1989.
10. Lindsey D: The idolatry of velocity, or lies, damn lies, and ballistics, *J Trauma* 20(12):1068, 1980 (editorial).
11. Fackler ML: Wound ballistics: a review of common misconceptions, *JAMA* 259(18):2730, 1988.
12. Fackler ML, Breteau JPL, Courbil LJ, et al: Open wound drainage versus wound excision in treating the modern assault rifle wound, *Surgery* 105(5):576, 1989.
13. Harvey EN, Korr IM, Oster G, et al: Secondary damage in wounding due to pressure changes accompanying the passage of high velocity missiles, *Surgery* 21:218, 1947.
14. Wolberg EJ: Performance of the Winchester 9mm 147 grain subsonic jacketed hollow point bullet in human tissue and tissue simulant, *J International Wound Ballistics Assoc* 1(1):10, 1991.
15. Fackler ML: Handgun bullet performance, *International Defense Rev* 21(5):555, 1988.
16. Fackler ML: The ideal police bullet, *Internal Security & Counterintelligence* (Suppl to *International Defense Rev*) November: 45, 1990.
17. Fackler ML, Dougherty PJ: Theodor Kocher and the scientific foundation of wound ballistics, *Surg Gynecol Obstet* 172:153, 1991.
18. DeMuth WE Jr: Bullet velocity and design as determinants of wounding capability: an experimental study, *J Trauma* 6(2):222, 1966.
19. Fackler ML: Physics of missile injuries. In McSwain NE Jr, Kerstein MD, editors: *Evaluation and management of trauma,* Norwalk, CT, 1987, Appleton-Century-Crofts, pp 25-41.
20. Owen-Smith MS: Mechanism of injury. In *High velocity missile wounds,* London, 1981, Edward Arnold, pp 22-32.
21. Fackler ML, Peters CE: Letter to the editor, *J Trauma* 29(10):1455, 1989.
22. Daniel RA Jr: Bullet wounds of the lungs, *Surgery* 15:774, 1944.
23. Hampton OP Jr: The indications for debridement of gun shot (bullet) wounds of the extremities in civilian practice, *J Trauma* 1:368, 1961.

24. Roucos S, Tabet G, Jebara VA, et al: Thoracic splenosis: case report and literature review, *J Thorac Cardiovasc Surg* 99(2):361, 1990.

25. Wang ZG, Feng JX, Liu YQ: Pathomorphological observations of gunshot wounds, *Acta Chir Scand Suppl* 508:185, 1982.

26. *Hornady handbook of cartridge reloading: rifle-pistol,* ed 3, Grand Island, Nebraska 68801, 1980, Hornady Manufacturing Company.

27. Benzel EC, Prejean CA, Hadden TA: Pulsatile dysesthesia and an axillary artery pseudoaneurysm associated with a penetrating axillary artery injury, *Surg Neurol* 31:400, 1989.

28. Nagib MG, Rockswold GL, Sherman RS, et al: Civilian gunshot wounds to the brain: prognosis and management, *Neurosurgery* 18(5):533, 1986.

29. Selden BS, Goodman JM, Cordell W, et al: Outcome of self-inflicted gunshot wounds of the brain, *Ann Emerg Med* 17(3):247, 1988.

30. Fackler ML: Wounding patterns of military rifle bullets, *International Defense Rev* 22(1):59, 1989.

31. Fackler ML, Surinchak JS, Malinowski JA, et al: Wounding potential of the Russian AK-74 assault rifle, *J Trauma* 24(3):263, 1984.

32. Bixler RP, Ahrens CR, Rossi RP, et al: Bullet identification with radiography, *Radiology* 178:563, 1991.

33. Messmer JM, Fierro MF: Radiologic forensic investigation of fatal gunshot wounds, *RadioGraphics* 6(3):457, 1986.

34. Cohen MA: Plastic bullet injuries of the face and jaws, *S Afr Med J* 68(12):849, 1985.

35. Millar R, Rutherford WH, Johnston S, et al: Injuries caused by rubber bullets: a report on 90 patients, *Br J Surg* 62:480, 1975.

36. Phillips JG: Plastic bullet injury: a case report, *Br J Oral Surg* 14:199, 1977.

37. Redgrave AP: Plastic bullets in riot control, *Lancet* 1:1224, 1983.

38. Rocke L: Injuries caused by plastic bullets compared with those caused by rubber bullets, *Lancet* 1:919, 1983.

39. Roy D: Gunshot and bomb blast injuries: a review of experience in Belfast, *J R Soc Med* 75:542, 1982.

40. Balouris CA: Rubber and plastic bullet eye injuries in Palestine, *Lancet* 335(8686):415, 1990.

41. Froede RC, Pitt MJ, Bridgemon RR: Shotgun diagnosis: "It ought to be something else," *J Forensic Sci* 27(2):428, 1982.

42. Hollerman JJ: Computed tomography. In Tintinalli JE, Krome RL, Ruiz E, editors: *Emergency medicine: a comprehensive study guide (American College of Emergency Physicians),* ed 3, New York, 1992, McGraw-Hill, pp 1126-1136.

43. Jooma R, Bradshaw JR, Coakham HB: Computed tomography in penetrating cranial injury by a wooden foreign body, *Surg Neurol* 21(3):236, 1984.

44. Feliciano DV, Burch JM, Spjut-Patrinely V, et al: Abdominal gunshot wounds: an urban trauma center's experience with 300 consecutive patients, *Ann Surg* 208(3):362, 1988.

45. Moore EE, Moore JB, VanDuzer-Moore S, et al: Mandatory laparotomy for gunshot wounds penetrating the abdomen, *Am J Surg* 140:847, 1980.

46. Kelly J, Raptopoulos V, Davidoff A, et al: On the value of non-contrast-enhanced CT in blunt abdominal trauma, *AJR* 152(1):41, 1989.

47. Orwig D, Federle MP: Localized clotted blood as evidence of visceral trauma on CT: the sentinel clot sign, *AJR* 153(4):747, 1989.

48. Benzel EC, Hadden TA, Coleman JE: Civilian gunshot wounds to the spinal cord and cauda equina, *Neurosurgery* 20(2):281, 1987.

49. Ebraheim NA, Savolaine ER, Jackson WT, et al: Magnetic resonance imaging in the evaluation of a gunshot wound to the cervical spine, *J Orthop Trauma* 3(1):19, 1989.

50. Engel A, Rosenberger A: Injuries of the spine, *Acta Radiol Suppl (Stockh)* 367:49, 1986.

51. Jones FD, Woosley RE: Delayed myelopathy secondary to retained intraspinal metallic fragment, *J Neurosurg* 55:979, 1981.

52. Kaiser MC, Capesius P: Gunshot wounds to the spine as evaluated by CT-scanning: two illustrative case reports, *Comput Radiol* 9(2):121, 1985.

53. Plumley TF, Kilcoyne RF, Mack LA: Computed tomography in evaluation of gunshot wounds of the spine, *J Comput Assist Tomogr* 7(2):310, 1983.

54. Romanick CR, Smith TK, Kopaniky DR, et al: Infection about the spine associated with low-velocity-missile injury to the abdomen, *J Bone Joint Surg [Am]* 67-A(8):1195, 1985.

55. Simpson RK, Venger BH, Narayan RK: Treatment of acute penetrating injuries of the spine: a retrospective analysis, *J Trauma* 29(1):42, 1989.

56. Six E, Alexander E Jr, Kelly DL Jr, et al: Gunshot wounds to the spinal cord, *South Med J* 72(6):699, 1979.

57. Venger BH, Simpson RK, Narayan RK: Neurosurgical intervention in penetrating spinal trauma with associated visceral injury, *J Neurosurg* 70(4):514, 1989.

58. Waters RL: Gunshot wounds to the spine: the effects of bullet fragments in the spinal canal, *J Am Paraplegia Soc* 7(2):30, 1984.

59. Fragomeni LSM, Azambuja PC: Bullets retained within the heart: diagnosis and management in three cases, *Thorax* 42(12):980, 1987.

60. Robison RJ, Brown JW, Caldwell R, et al: Management of asymptomatic intracardiac missiles using echocardiography, *J Trauma* 28(9):1402, 1988.

61. Symbas PN, Picone AL, Hatcher CR Jr, et al: Cardiac missiles: a review of the literature and personal experience, *Ann Surg* 211(5):639, 1990.

62. Kase CS, White RL, Vinson TL, et al: Shotgun pellet embolus to the middle cerebral artery, *Neurology* 31:458, 1981.

63. Sclafani SJA, Mitchell WG: Retrograde venous bullet embolism, *J Trauma* 21(8):656, 1981.

64. Thomas R, Suarez G: Percutaneous removal of intrarenal bullet, *J Urol* 140:806, 1988.

65. Uflacker R, Lima S, Melichar AC: Intravascular foreign bodies: percutaneous retrieval, *Radiology* 160:731, 1986.

66. Wallace KL, Slovis CM: Hepatic vein bullet embolus as a complication of left thoracic gunshot injury, *Ann Emerg Med* 16:102, 1987.

67. Ben-Menachem Y: Angiography in diagnosis of vascular trauma. In Taveras JM, Ferrucci JT, editors: *Radiology: diagnosis, imaging, intervention,* ed 2, Philadelphia, 1988, Lippincott, pp 1 14.

68. Shannon JJ Jr, Vo NM, Stanton PE Jr, et al: Peripheral arterial missile embolization: a case report and 22-year literature review, *J Vasc Surg* 5(5):773, 1987.

69. White RR: Arthroscopic bullet retrieval, *J Trauma* 27(4):455, 1987.

70. Alho A, Husebo AAO, Viste A, et al: Lead poisoning after a shotgun femoral fracture, *Ann Chir Gynaecol* 71:130, 1982.

71. Grogan DP, Bucholz RW: Acute lead intoxication from a bullet in an intervertebral disc space, *J Bone Joint Surg [Am]* 63-A(7):1180, 1981.

72. Linden MA, Manton WI, Stewart RM, et al: Lead poisoning from retained bullets: pathogenesis, diagnosis, and management, *Ann Surg* 195(3):305, 1982.

73. Sclafani SJA, Vuletin JC, Twersky J: Lead arthropathy: arthritis caused by retained intra-articular bullets, *Radiology* 156:299, 1985.

74. Staniforth P, Watt I: Extradural plumboma: a rare cause of acquired spinal stenosis, *Br J Radiol* 55:772, 1982.

75. Sights WP, Bye RJ: The fate of retained intracerebral shotgun pellets: an experimental study, *J Neurosurg* 33:646, 1970.

76. McFadden JT: Tissue reactions to standard neurosurgical metallic implants, *J Neurosurg* 36:598, 1972.

77. Barros D'Sa AA: A decade of missile-induced vascular trauma, *Ann R Coll Surg Engl* 64(1):37, 1982.

78. Dean L, Dvonch V: Gun shot wound to the knee, *Orthopedics* 11(6):963, 1988.

79. Hughes JL, VanderGriend RV, Bennett TL: Gunshot fractures, *Unfallchirurg* 89:515, 1986.

80. Senturia HR: The roentgen findings in increased lead absorption due to retained projectiles, *AJR* 47(3):381, 1942.

81. Weston WJ: The vanishing lead arthrogram: plumbography, *Australas Radiol* 24(1):80, 1980.

82. Weston WJ: The lead arthrogram: plumbography, *Skeletal Radiol* 2:169, 1978.

83. Ovartlarnporn B, Prakaitip D: Lead intoxication due to retained bullet in right hip: a case report, *J Med Assoc Thai* 68(11):612, 1985.

84. Selbst S, Henretig F, Fee M, et al: Lead poisoning in a child with a gunshot wound, *Pediatrics* 77(3):413, 1986.

85. Conces DJ Jr, Kreipke DL, Tarver RD: MR of superior mesenteric artery–renal vein fistula, *Comput Radiol* 10(6):279, 1986.

86. Hanigan WC, Wright RM, Berkman WA, et al: MR imaging of a false carotid aneurysm, *Stroke* 17(6):1317, 1986.

87. Smith AS, Hurst GC, Duerk JL, et al: MR of ballistic materials: imaging artifacts and potential hazards, *AJNR* 12(3):567, 1991.

88. Teitelbaum GP, Yee CA, Van Horn DD, et al: Metallic ballistic fragments: MR imaging safety and artifacts, *Radiology* 175(3):855, 1990.

89. deVeth C: Development of the new second NATO calibre: the 5.56 with the SS109 projectile, *Acta Chir Scand Suppl* 508:129, 1982.

90. Dei Poli G, Baima Bollone PL: An interpretation of the discrepancy between the entry and exit holes made by bullets in the skull, *Panminerva Med* 20:181, 1978.

91. Clark WC, Muhlbauer MS, Watridge CB, et al: Analysis of 76 civilian craniocerebral gunshot wounds, *J Neurosurg* 65:9, 1986.

92. Kaufman HH, Makela ME, Lee KF, et al: Gunshot wounds to the head: a perspective, *Neurosurgery* 18(6):689, 1986.

93. Suddaby L, Weir B, Forsyth C: The management of .22 caliber gunshot wounds of the brain: a review of 49 cases, *Can J Neurol Sci* 14:268, 1987.

94. Dixon DS: Keyhole lesions in gunshot wounds of the skull and direction of fire, *J Forensic Sci* 27(3):555, 1982.

95. Dixon DS: Exit keyhole lesion and direction of fire in a gunshot wound of the skull, *J Forensic Sci* 29(1):336, 1984.

96. Dixon DS: Pattern of intersecting fractures and direction of fire, *J Forensic Sci* 29(2):651, 1984.

97. Smith OC, Berryman HE, Lahren CH: Cranial fracture patterns and estimate of direction from low velocity gunshot wounds, *J Forensic Sci* 32(5):1416, 1987.

98. Rose SC, Fujisaki CK, Moore EE: Incomplete fractures associated with penetrating trauma: etiology, appearance, and natural history, *J Trauma* 28(1):106, 1988.

99. Smith HW, Wheatley KK Jr: Biomechanics of femur fractures secondary to gunshot wounds, *J Trauma* 24(11):970, 1984.

100. Woloszyn JT, Uitvlugt GM, Castle ME: Management of civilian gunshot fractures of the extremities, *Clin Orthop* 226:247, 1988.

101. Ryan JR, Hensel RT, Salciccioli GG, et al: Fractures of the femur secondary to low-velocity gunshot wounds, *J Trauma* 21(2):160, 1981.

102. Leffers D, Chandler RW: Tibial fractures associated with civilian gunshot injuries, *J Trauma* 25(11):1059, 1985.

103. Brandner MD, Bunkis J: Shotgun blast injuries to the groin: reconstruction using the rectus abdominis flap, *Ann Plast Surg* 18(6):541, 1987.

104. Hooper TL, Scott NA: Self-inflicted shotgun wounds of the abdomen, *Injury* 16:330, 1985.

105. Meyer JP, Lim LT, Schuler JJ, et al: Peripheral vascular trauma from close-range shotgun injuries, *Arch Surg* 120:1126, 1985.

106. Shepard GH: High-energy, low-velocity close-range shotgun wounds, *J Trauma* 20(12):1065, 1980.

107. Wilson J: Shotgun ballistics and shotgun injuries, *West J Med* 129(2):149, 1978.

108. Flint LM, Cryer HM, Howard DA, et al: Approaches to the management of shotgun injuries, *J Trauma* 24(5):415, 1984.

109. Frykberg ER, Crump JM, Vines FS, et al: A reassessment of the role of arteriography in penetrating proximity extremity trauma: a prospective study, *J Trauma* 29(8):1041, 1989.

110. Mandal AK, Boitano MA: Principles and management of penetrating vascular injuries secondary to shotgun wounds, *Am Surg* 44(3):165, 1978.

111. Mandal AK, Boitano MA, Lundy IJ, et al: Shotgun wounds of the abdomen: revisited, *Am Surg* 45(1):5, 1979.

112. Roberts RM, String ST: Arterial injuries in extremity shotgun wounds: requisite factors for successful management, *Surgery* 96(5):902, 1984.

113. Deitch EA, Grimes WR: Experience with 112 shotgun wounds of the extremities, *J Trauma* 24(7):600, 1984.

114. Beverly MC, Pring DJ, Coombs RRH: Radiolucent plastic in gunshot wounds, *Injury* 16:461, 1985.

115. Lucas RM, Mitterer D: Pneumatic firearm injuries: trivial trauma or perilous pitfalls?, *J Emerg Med* 8(4):433, 1990.

116. Miner ME, Cabrera JA, Ford E, et al: Intracranial penetration due to BB air rifle injuries, *Neurosurgery* 19(6):952, 1986.

117. Jacobs NA, Morgan LH: On the management of retained airgun pellets: a survey of 11 orbital cases, *Br J Ophthalmol* 72:97, 1988.

118. Reddick EJ, Carter PL, Bickerstaff L: Air gun injuries in children, *Ann Emerg Med* 14(11):1108, 1985.

119. Jones AM, Reyna M Jr, Sperry K, et al: Suicidal contact gunshot wounds to the head with .38 special Glaser safety slug ammunition, *J Forensic Sci* 32(6):1604, 1987.

120. Leffers B, Jeanty D: Handgun pellet ammunition ("snake shot") wounds: report of three cases, *J Forensic Sci* 27(2):433, 1982.

20

How This Book Was Illustrated

· ·

Linda J. Goodwill
Tim B. Hunter

This book contains hundreds of illustrations of medical devices and radiologic studies. Biomedical Communications at the University of Arizona Health Sciences Center provided the superb drawings by Fred Anderson (The BioMechanical Man and Woman, The Foreign Body Woman, and the figures in Chapter 10), the wonderful computer-generated figures by Stacey K. Lane in the Gallery of Medical Devices, p. 1, and 10% of the photographs in the book. Individual chapter authors and manufacturers each generously furnished 5% of the illustrations. Approximately 80% of all the figures in the book represent devices or radiographs photographed by Linda Goodwill under the supervision of the chapter authors and the book editors.

Neither of us are professional photographers but undertook the task of doing most of the book's illustrations ourselves in order to save money. The publisher did provide a generous grant for the figures and illustrations, but this had to be spent very conservatively to prevent our running out of funds. By doing the illustrations ourselves, we estimate we reduced our expenses by a factor of two to four over that required by using professional audiovisual services. Mr. Richard McBain of Scot Photo, Tucson, Arizona, provided us with technical expertise throughout the project. Scot Photo performed all film processing and print development.

This short chapter is a brief description of our techniques and equipment. This is furnished to give useful background information for others attempting similar photographic challenges. The required equipment is not expensive (Table 20-1), and the procedures, once learned and standardized, are simple. However, there are a several pitfalls one has to take care to avoid.

Table 20-1 Equipment

1. Camera—35 mm Nikon F	$350-$400
2. Lens—Sigma Macro 50 mm f/2.8	$179.00
3. Film—Kodak EKTAR 25 Ultra Sharp Color Print	$ 4.80/roll
NOTE: Film should be stored in a refrigerator for optimum color balance and life but should not be frozen.	
4. Tripod—SLIK Insta-Lok Lightweight	$ 64.95
5. Lightstands—PHOTOFLEX	
a. Two heavyweight 11'	$ 67.96
b. Two lightweight 8'	$ 39.96
6. Light disks—PHOTOFLEX—two 52" white/white	$ 71.96
7. Lamps—photoflood—two	$ 95.96
8. Bulbs—BCA 250w Daylight Photoflood	$ 4.10 each
NOTE: The life-span for one bulb is approximately 1 hour per bulb. Be sure to have several on hand when doing long-term photography.	
9. Strong arms—two	$ 23.64
10. Cable Release—20 inches	$ 5.56
11. Copy Stand—Testrite No. C5-3 (Testrite Instrument Co., Inc., Newark, NJ 07105)	$108.50
12. X-ray view box for photographing radiographs	
13. Background material	
a. Gray Foam Board	
b. Gray Backdrop Paper (39 cm × 59 m)	$ 49.00
14. Miscellaneous	
a. White card reflectors covered with crumpled foil	
b. Small hand mirror	
c. Molding clay	
d. Supports (drinking straw cut into small pieces)	

The selection of the devices and radiographs to be photographed was the sole responsibility of each author. They were chosen to provide the reader with a quick and easy reference guide for identification of important, common everyday devices. Moreover, devices that have a unique appearance or are especially important and difficult to recognize on radiographs were also chosen.

CAMERA AND FILM

A 20-year-old Nikon F camera with a new Sigma Macro 50 mm f/2.8 lens was used for the photography. The camera's built-in light meter proved to be accurate and was followed for most exposures. Typical exposures were 1 second at f/16 for medical devices and 1 to 2 seconds for radiographs using Kodak Ektar 25 Ultra Sharp Color Print Film. This particular film was chosen because of its compatibility with the light source used (Photo-BCA 250-watt bulbs), and it has extremely fine grain, wide latitude, and ready availability at almost all cameras stores and many supermarkets. It is a standard C-41 print film and can be developed at any "one-hour" processor found in a shopping mall. Its negatives are easily processed to produce high-contrast black-and-white prints, and they can also be converted into gorgeous color slides.

LG photographed all medical devices and radiographs in a homemade studio. The films were processed in standard fashion and color proof sheets were made for the negatives. These were periodically examined by LG, TBH, or the chapter authors for technique and desired devices. Then, 7 by 5−inch black and white glossy prints were made for the illustrations to be included in the book.

PHOTOGRAPHIC TECHNIQUES

Controlling Shadows

Harsh shadows and dark hidden areas are a significant obstacle to overcome when one is photographing still-life objects. It is necessary to use reflectors to fill in shadows. This is less expensive and often more effective than adding more lights. Hand mirrors were tried at first. They effectively throw back most of the reflected light, but their effect is often very obvious. Crumpled cooking foil pasted to a rigid card gives slightly weaker, softer reflections. Plain white cards give an even softer fill-in and are particularly helpful when a device itself has reflective surfaces.

There is so much choice when working with reflectors that it is better to optimize technique with your main light sources before moving on to add reflected light to the scene. A basic principle to strive for is to choose and employ reflectors in such a manner that anyone viewing the final photograph is not aware they were used.

The most difficult objects to photograph are usually highly polished. Polished, bright metal surfaces reflect images of the lights, camera, and everything in the studio as effectively as a mirror (Fig. 20-1). Rounded surfaces often act like convex or concave mirrors as well. Without special care the photograph will show a distracting collection of highlights and irrelevant reflections. We avoided these problems in many cases by using one of the following tricks:

1. Constructing a "light tent" around the device by making a cone out of tracing paper and leaving a hole just large enough for the lens to poke through.

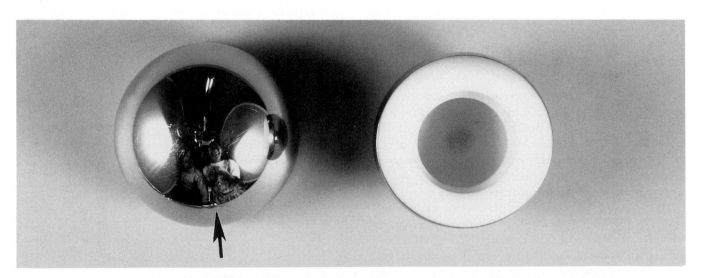

Fig. 20-1. Hip prosthesis with polished reflective surface. Notice the reflection of the photographer, *arrow,* and the glare from the femoral head component on the left.

2. Spraying the device surface with a dulling spray.
3. Putting the device in the freezer for a half hour before photographing it.

Lighting

Inevitably, there is nearly always less light available than desirable. This reduces your flexibility in most cases, and you must optimize a combination of lens speed, lens depth of focus, film speed, and shutter speed. Most of the time there will be some compromise, such as reducing the zoom magnification in order to achieve a better depth of focus and more light.

Kodak Ektar 25 Ultra Sharp Color Film is very slow. Its use requires a rigid tripod or copy stand, shutter release cable, and a strong light source. However, if these are available, the long exposures are not troublesome. Once the techniques have become established, it is possible to produce satisfactory photographs nearly 100% of the time.

Two photoflood lights were used with BCA Daylight Photoflood bulbs. The bulb type has to be carefully matched to the film used, or contrast and color may suffer greatly. Photoflood bulbs are fragile and expensive. They last only about 1 hour and therefore must be used very carefully. They also become too hot to touch and give off much heat. Moreover, they may produce a glaring point-source lighting effect and are best used in combination with large light disks to spread out the light into an even, nonglare distribution.

Image Sharpness and Depth of Focus

Most lenses are designed to operate within a narrow range of focusing distances. When they are adapted for other uses, such as performing close-up photography with a standard outdoor 35 mm camera lens, they generally give poor results with a very unsharp focus. Macro lenses are a must for close-up photography. At high magnifications and short f-ratios (f/1.5, f/2, and so on) the depth of focus is extremely shallow. It is often not possible to keep the entire object in sharp focus. To maximize the depth of field, it is best to use small lens apertures and large f-ratios (f/11, f/22, and so on) (Fig. 20-2). This in turn requires increasing the light source or lengthening the exposure.

THE STUDIO

Studios usually have to conform to available space. The minimum requirements of space and shape are determined by the type of work that will be done in the studio. The principal items of studio equipment are the lighting and the background (see Table 20-1). A specialized technique of some importance is even lighting of the background drop. The best method is to use two photoflood lamps placed directly behind light disks (each arranged vertically on either side) and to aim each light beam at the opposite edge of the background. This results in even illumination.

Backgrounds vary from seamless paper rolls for photographing large objects (Fig. 20-3) to using copy stands

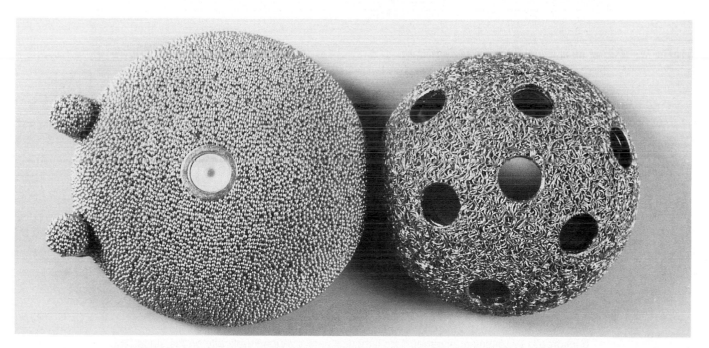

Fig. 20-2. Close-up photograph of the complex surface of two types of porous-coated acetabular components of hip prostheses. The fine detail in the image was obtained by using careful focusing, large f-ratio (f/22), long exposure (4 seconds), and an increased lighting level.

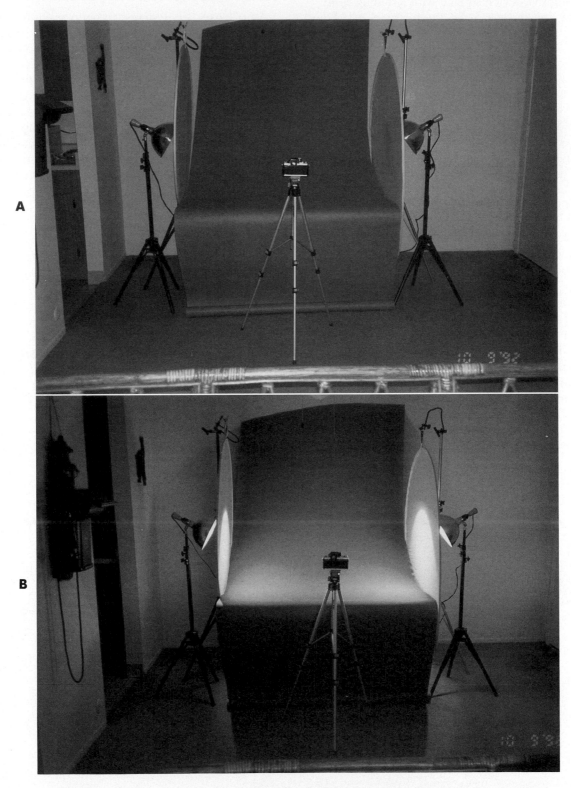

Fig. 20-3. Studio and background setup for photographing large objects. Notice that the backdrop is seamless gray paper. Two light disks are arranged vertically on the sides. The camera is supported with a tripod. **A,** Room lights on and flood lights off. **B,** Room lights off and flood lights on.

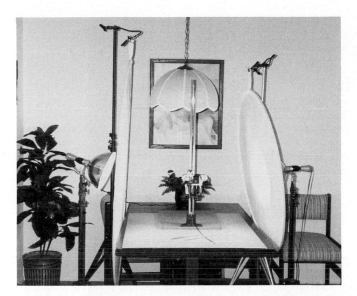

Fig. 20-4. Studio and background setup for photographing small objects. Notice that the copystand is arranged on top of a gray foam board.

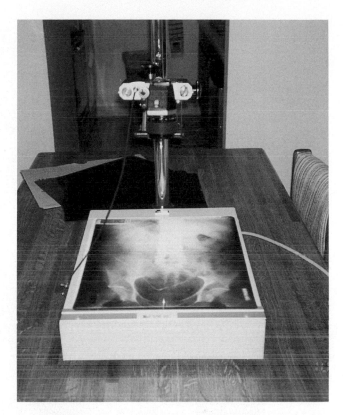

Fig. 20-5. Studio setup for photographing radiographs. There is a copystand with a light box.

covered with gray foam boards for small objects (Fig. 20-4).

In addition to lighting and backgrounds, studios also require a range of other tools, such as white cards, reflectors, small hand mirrors, molding clay, and supports. The basic setup for photographing radiographic images consists of a light box and a copy stand (Fig. 20-5). To prevent excess light entering the picture from around the margins of the radiograph, black borders made out of heavy paper or blackened x-ray film should be placed around the radiograph. Best results are obtained from photographing the original films if they are available. We found that photographing copy films produced much poorer results with uneven illumination and harsh contrasts.

A studio works best if it is left permanently set up. LG initially tried to photograph the medical devices in the University Medical Center (UMC) Central Services. This proved to be impractical because the studio had to be constantly set up and taken down depending on the work flow in the Central Services area. It became more efficient to set up the studio in her apartment and transport devices and radiographs for photography back and forth from UMC.

The fewer the distractions and the more ample the working space, the more efficient the operation will become. Photography at home in the company of your pet is fun and exciting as long as your pet is not in the same room (Fig. 20-6).

RECORD KEEPING

Meticulous records are mandatory when you are photographing large numbers of radiographs and devices.

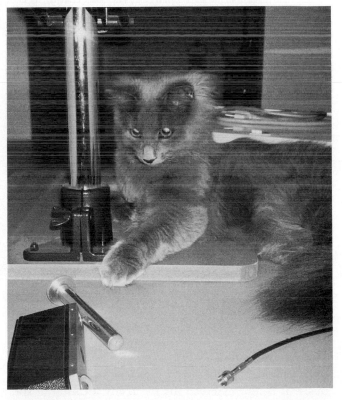

Fig. 20-6. When a studio is setup at home, pets can become a problem.

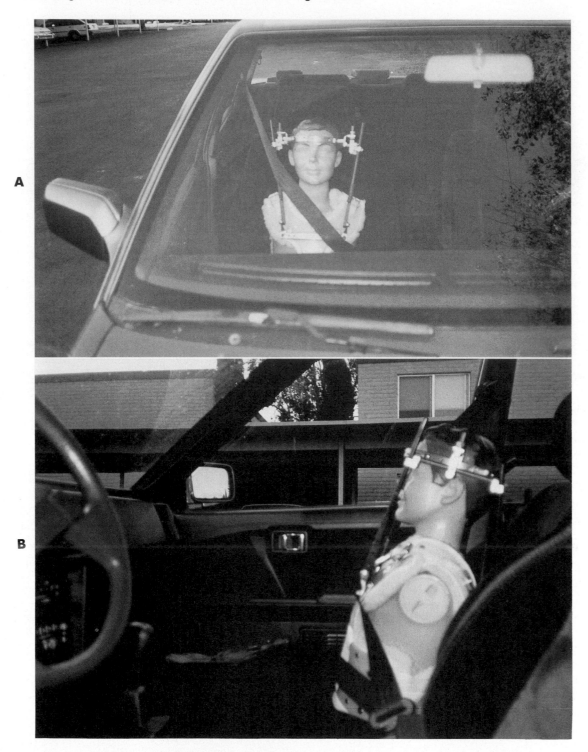

Fig. 20-7. The dummy model with the "halo brace" was transported with great care.

This is essential for the later duplication of a complex photographic task performed weeks or months previously. It is also essential for the ready location of specific photographs or for the identification of objects contained on a specific print or negative.

These are some suggestions:
1. Purchase large three-ring binders and photograph pages to hold proof sheets, glossy prints, and the original negatives respectively. Also keep one or more binders listing each roll of film taken, noting

which negative corresponds to which object or radiograph.

2. Have two proof sheets printed for each roll of film. These are invaluable for gaining a rapid assessment of image quality. When photographing many subjects at one time, it is quite helpful to photograph all the same objects per roll of film. For example, rolls 1 to 4 might contain radiographs; rolls 5 to 7 might feature devices.

3. Label every print on the back with the roll number and negative number. For example, roll 1, #26 might be a photograph of an intramedullary rod fixation device. Correlate the roll number and negative number with the corresponding proof sheet. Keep all package inserts. They often contain valuable information not easily found elsewhere.

4. Maintain identification lists of the devices or radiographs photographed correlated with their respective film roll and negative numbers.

TRANSPORTING ITEMS

At times, it may be necessary to borrow an expensive item or device and transport it to your studio. It is wise to obtain from the institution, manufacturer, or individual lending you the item a written statement granting you permission to borrow it and to use photographs of it for publication. The condition of the item, its approximate worth, and the procedure for reimbursing the owner in case of damage should be delineated. If a device is too large to fit into a protective container, one must exercise great care in ensuring its adequate protection during transportation (Fig. 20-7).

PROCESSING PRINTS

It is difficult to make adequate black-and-white prints of radiographs. The extreme density differences between light and dark areas on a radiograph are hard to reproduce on a print. Most photo labs use computerized processors programmed for negatives of everyday scenes. The technicians processing the prints for our radiographs and medical devices were not familiar with what our images represented and did not initially appreciate what we needed to illustrate. Therefore a significant percentage of our initial prints suffered from poor contrast, necessitating frequent reprints (Fig. 20-8).

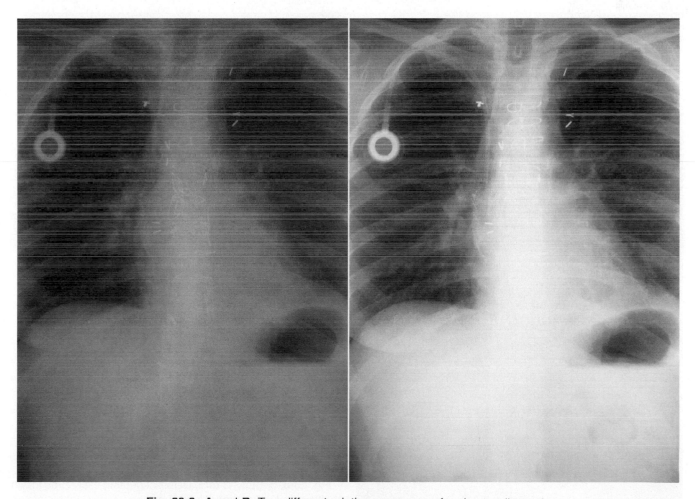

Fig. 20-8. A and **B,** Two different printing exposures of a chest radiograph.

Continued.

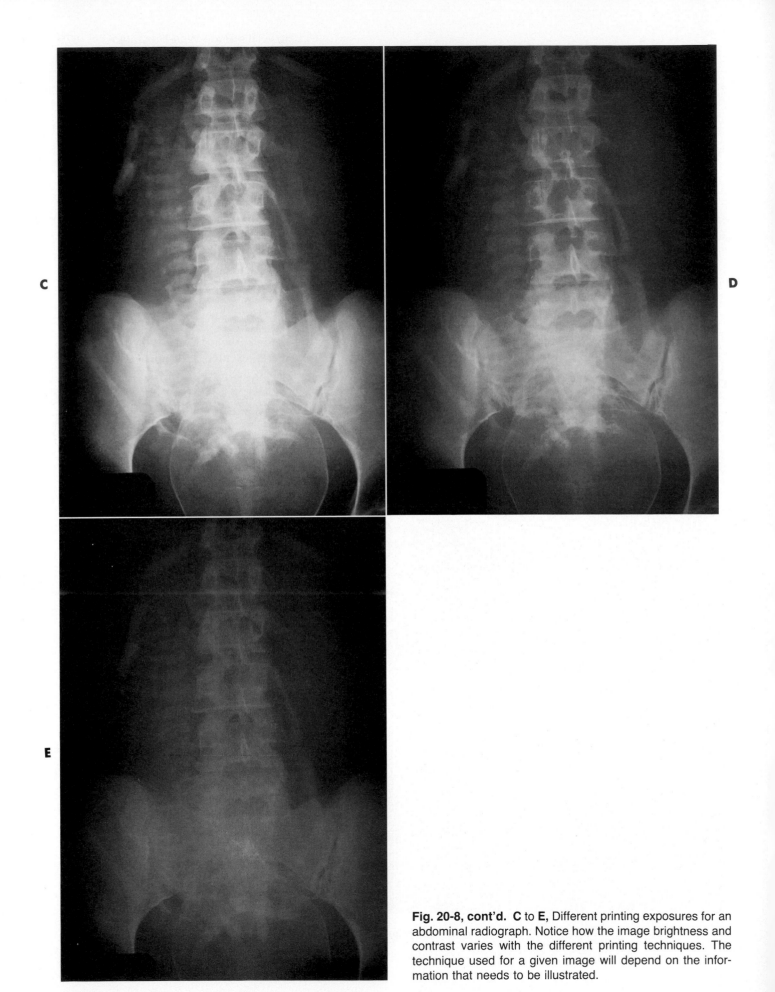

Fig. 20-8, cont'd. C to E, Different printing exposures for an abdominal radiograph. Notice how the image brightness and contrast varies with the different printing techniques. The technique used for a given image will depend on the information that needs to be illustrated.

This problem was not solved until we took the time to show some original radiographs and medical devices to the photo-processing personnel. LG also learned how to run one of the computerized processors and sometimes worked directly with the personnel as prints were being made.

These are some suggestions:

1. Whenever possible, make an appointment with the photo lab for you to be present when your prints are being processed. This will allow you to monitor the prints as they come out of the processor and enable you to adjust them on line to meet your specifications.
2. If you are unable to be at the lab, it is very helpful for the processor technicians to have the actual radiographs there for reference.
   a. Mark the area of interest with a wax pen.
   b. Arrange the radiographs in the order they were photographed.
   c. Make a list of any special instructions.
   d. For difficult cases, request several prints of each negative be made with settings considerably lighter and darker than normal.

REFERENCES

1. Freeman M: *The 35 mm handbook,* London, 1980, Quarto Publishing; reprinted 1991 by Courage Books, Philadelphia.
2. Kerr N: *Technique of photographic lighting,* New York, 1982, AMPHOTO.

Glossary

· ·

Tim B. Hunter
David H. Levy

The following words, abbreviations, and eponyms were chosen for inclusion in this glossary because they represent either an important device or material discussed in this book, or common medical device terminology used in everyday practice but not defined in standard medical reference texts or dictionaries (see bibliography, p. 591). The definitions are our own. We believe they conform to general usage, but their meanings may vary somewhat depending on locale or specialty. For example, the abbreviation CT means "computed (or computerized) tomography" to a radiologist, but it may signify "cardiothoracic" or "carotid tracing" to a surgeon.

Many terms now in general medical usage originally were strictly applied to a device introduced by a particular inventor or manufacturer. Over time, these terms have acquired a generic meaning having come to represent a class of devices, with their original restricted meaning being lost. Examples of this phenomenon include Jackson-Pratt drain, Hickman catheter, and Dobbhoff tube. Many of these terms could not be found in the standard medical dictionaries, or even in leading specialty textbooks. Moreover, package inserts supplied with many devices often cite references detailing the use and complications of the device, but frequently these references do not describe the device's origin, even when it carries an individual's name. The definitions (and spellings) for such terms were usually derived from our own experience, from discussions with the chapter authors and other medical colleagues, or from one of the excellent terminology texts available (see bibliography).

~ Symbol for 'about' or 'approximately'.

AAPM American Association of Physicists in Medicine.

AAWR American Association for Women Radiologists.

Abbott-Rawson tube A double-channeled tube for aspiration of fluid from or injection of fluid into the stomach.

ABF Aortobifemoral bypass graft or surgery.

ABR American Board of Radiology.

Acorn-tip (acorn-tipped) catheter Common term for any drainage catheter with a bulbous end having the appearance of an acorn. A typical example is a Malecot catheter. Also, a term used for a catheter employed in cystourethrography or retrograde pyelography.

ACR American College of Radiology.

ACUTENS Acupuncture/transcutaneous nerve stimulation.

ADA American Dental Association, American Diabetic Association, American Dietetic Association, or Americans with Disabilities Act.

ADR Adverse drug reaction.

AFB Aortofemoral bypass graft or surgery.

AHRA American Healthcare Radiology Administrators.

AICD Automatic implantable cardioverter defibrillator.

AIUM American Institute of Ultrasound in Medicine.

ALARA As low as reasonably achievable.

Aliasing *See* Wraparound artifact.

Allograft A tissue graft between donor and recipient of the same species but of disparate genotypes.

Alumina Aluminum oxide, which occurs in bauxite, rubies, and sapphires.

AMA American Medical Association.

Amalgam An alloy of two or more metals, one of which is mercury.

Amplatz filter A type of inferior vena cava (IVC) filter.

AMS 800 A type of artificial urinary sphincter.

AMS Hydroflex A type of penile prosthesis.

AMS 600 A type of penile prosthesis.

Angiocath A type of intravenous catheter.

ANSI American National Standards Institute, a nongovernmental, voluntary federation of trade associations, professional societies, and individuals. ANSI organizes and publishes national standards.

Anterior cervical plates A system of plates and screws placed anteriorly in the spine for fixation of unstable spine fractures and dislocations or to stabilize the spine after surgery.

Antibiotic beads Any beadlike material impregnated with antibiotics for use in treating bone and joint infections. The beads, typically composed of poly(methyl methacrylate), are packed into the area of infection. The antibiotics help treat the infection, and the bead packing material provides mechanical support in an area of missing or weakened bone.

AOBR American Osteopathic Board of Radiology.

ARRS American Roentgen Ray Society.

ARRT American Registry of Radiologic Technologists.

Arthroplasty A generic term for any joint surgery that is designed to restore joint function. In many cases, a prosthetic device is used to totally or partially replace the native joint.

ASAP As soon as possible.

ASTRO American Society for Therapeutic Radiology and Oncology.

Augmentation mammoplasty implant A general term for a breast implant.

AUR Association of University Radiologists.

AUS Artificial urinary sphincter.

Austin-Moore Eponym for a type of hip prosthesis.

Autograft A graft in which material is transferred from one part of a person's body to another part.

Automatic implantable cardioverter defibrillator (AICD) This device consists of two shocking electrodes, two sensing electrodes, and a generator implanted into the abdominal wall. It is being increasingly used for the long-term treatment of ventricular arrhythmias and is easily recognized on chest films.

AVR Aortic valve replacement.

BI, BII Abbreviations for Billroth I and Billroth II gastric surgeries respectively.

Beall valve A type of prosthetic heart valve.

Beam width artifact An artifact that may be created by the varying width of an ultrasound beam along its course.

Beam-hardening artifact A type of computed tomographic (CT) artifact that occurs because the x-ray beam in CT scanners is not monochromatic and gets progressively "harder" (of shorter wavelength) as it passes through tissue.

Bee cell A type of pessary.

BICAP Bipolar electrocoagulation therapy.

Bilbao-Dotter tube An intestinal tube placed into the duodenum or jejunum for performing various gastrointestinal radiologic studies, such as hypotonic duodenography or enteroclysis (high enema). It is placed with the aid of a stiffening guide wire.

Billroth Christian Albert Theodor (1829-1894) was a famous Austrian surgeon who introduced the most commonly used operations for gastric resection, the Billroth I and Billroth II (see illustration under surgical procedures).

Biomaterial A material that is brought into contact with living tissue for the purpose of treating medical and dental conditions.

Biopty Gun A type of biopsy gun using a spring-loaded mechanism for rapidly taking tissue samples with a cutting needle. It is popular for obtaining histologic core biopsy samples from the liver, kidneys, breast, and masses in the abdomen and pelvis.

Bipolar electrocoagulation therapy (BICAP) A form of endoscopic palliation therapy for esophageal neoplasms.

Bjork-Shiley valve A type of prosthetic heart valve.

Blade plate A type of orthopedic fixation plate with a sharp-angled extension at the end of the plate that is placed into the metaphysis for fracture fixation.

BNL Breast needle localization.

Body packers *See* Mules.

Bohlman technique A type of posterior cervical spine fixation using interspinous wiring with bone grafting to stabilize the spine.

Bone cement A biomaterial used to secure a firm fixation of joint prostheses, such as hip and knee joints. It is primarily made of poly(methyl methacrylate) powder and monomer methyl methacrylate liquid.

Bovine graft (valve) A biologic body part derived from a cow.

Brachytherapy A type of radiation therapy in which the source of the ionizing radiation is applied directly to or is only a short distance away from the body area being treated.

BRH Bureau of Radiological Health.

Broviac catheter A type of central venous catheter. Broviac is a trademark of C.R. Bard, Inc. (Tewksbury, Mass.). Dr. J.W. Broviac and associates in 1973 described the use of a silicone rubber atrial catheter for parenteral alimentation. The term "Broviac" is used by some generically to refer to any indwelling central venous catheter.

Buck's traction (extension) A skin traction system in which a fractured leg is extended and held in traction by weights with the bed raised at the foot to enable the body to act as a counterweight.

Buttress plate An orthopedic fixation plate used for bony alignment rather than compression. Typically, buttress plates are used in metaphyseal regions, such as the distal radius or the proximal tibia, whereas neutralization plates are used in the shafts of long bones.

Butyl cyanoacrylate An embolic material used to treat arteriovenous malformations, vascular fistulas, and so forth.

Bx Biopsy.

c̄ Abbreviation of Latin *cum*, meaning 'with', such as "51-year-old patient c̄ history of heavy smoking."

CABG Coronary artery bypass graft procedure.

CAD Computer-aided design or computer-aided diagnosis.

CAI Computer-aided instruction.

Caliber A term used to express bullet diameter in decimals of an inch or in millimeters.

Cancellous bone screw A type of bone screw with a smooth shank proximally and coarse threads distally. It is designed to be inserted into cancellous bone. The threads should not cross a fracture line.

Cannulated screw This type of orthopedic screw has the same appearance as a standard screw except that the shank is hollow, a feature that allows it to be placed over a guide pin for more exact placement.

Cantor tube A type of intestinal drainage tube with a single channel and a weighted mercury bag.

CAPD Continuous ambulatory peritoneal dialysis.

CAR Canadian Association of Radiologists.

Carey capsule A device used for small bowel biopsy.

Carpentier-Edwards valve A type of prosthetic heart valve.

Caspar plate The best known of the anterior cervical plates.

Cast gold crown Another term for a dental gold cap.

CDC Centers for Disease Control and Prevention.

CDRH Center for Devices and Radiological Health.

Celestin tube A nylon-reinforced latex tube used to bypass esophageal tumors.

Central venous catheter A type of catheter used for access to the central venous system, usually the superior vena cava or the right atrium. The catheter may be introduced surgically or percutaneously, typically into the subclavian or jugular venous system, though more peripheral access routes may be used. Central venous catheters have one to three separate lumens and are used to measure central venous pressure, withdraw blood samples, or administer medications and hyperalimentation. Drs. J.W. Broviac and R.O. Hickman and their associates independently described some of the first applications for such catheters, and their names are often used generically to refer to an indwelling central venous catheter.

Ceramics Inorganic compounds that include silicates, metallic oxides, carbides, and various refractory hydrides, sulfides, and nitrides. Ceramics have extremely low coefficients of friction, making them ideal in certain settings for articular bearing surfaces.

Cerclage wires Circumferential wires used to stabilize long bone fractures. They are often used with intramedullary fixation and work in the same manner as barrel stays.

Cerebrospinal fluid shunt Any type of shunt used to treat hydrocephalus by draining fluid out of the ventricular system of the brain into the vascular system or into a body cavity.

Cervicothoracic brace A type of cervical-spine external immobilization brace.

Charnley-Mueller hip One of the first successful hip prostheses.

Chemical shift artifacts A type of MRI artifact commonly seen at the interface of fat and soft tissue.

CHIPES Stands for *chloral hydrate, heavy metals, iodides, phenothiazines, enteric coated, solvents*; a mnemonic for remembering which classes of potentially poisonous compounds are radiopaque.

Cimino-Brescia A type of distal radial artery–to–cephalic vein fistula surgically created for reliable vascular access in patients needing chronic hemodialysis.

CLIA Clinical Laboratory Improvement Act of 1988.

Closed wound suction drains These drains offer a constant level of suction, sometimes with a choice of suction pressures.

Cloverleaf filter A type of inferior vena cava (IVC) filter.

Co-Cr alloys. Cobalt-chromium alloy used as a metallic biomaterial.

Cochlear implant A type of surgically implanted hearing aid used to treat sensorineural hearing loss.

Comet-tail (ringdown) artifact This ultrasound artifact appears as a line of intense, nearly continuous echoes trailing behind a small reflector or behind the bands of a periodic reverberative artifact. Clinically, the comet tail is seen behind gas collections, areas of cholesterolosis, metallic clips, needles, and intrauterine devices.

Composite base acrylics Biomaterials used in tooth-colored restorations and tooth veneers.

Compression plate *See* Dynamic compression plate.

Compression screw Screws that are usually used in the treatment of intertrochanteric and supracondylar femur fractures.

CON Certificate of need.

Cope loop catheter A type of catheter with a mechanism for holding the distal end of the catheter in a locked pigtail configuration to prevent accidental catheter removal.

Copper T, Copper-7, Copper T380A Types of intrauterine contraceptive devices.

Cordis sheath An access catheter manufactured by the Cordis Corporation (Miami Lakes, Florida). It is basically a thin-walled vascular sheath through which various smaller catheters can be passed. It has come to represent generically any type of sheath allowing access to the central circulation.

Cortical bone screw A type of fully threaded bone screw designed for use in cortical bone. It uses fine threads to anchor the screw on the near and far cortex of the bone.

Cotrell-Dubousset system A complex orthopedic system of rods, hooks, cross-links, and screws for the posterior fixation of the spine.

CPAP Constant positive airway pressure.

CPT American Medical Association's (AMA) *Physicians' Current Procedural Terminology,* which is published periodically.

CQI Continuous quality improvement.

CSGIT Continuous-suture, graft-inclusion technique, a technique for repair of aortic aneurysms and dissections.

CSRT Canadian Society of Radiological Technicians.

Cu-7 IUD A type of intrauterine contraceptive device.

CVAC Central venous access catheter.

CVP Central venous pressure.

Dacron Du Pont's trade name for polyethylene terephthalate polyester fiber. Dacron is a typical condensation polymer and was the first commercial polyester. Sometimes, the terms "polyester" and "Dacron" are used interchangeably.

Dalkon Shield A type of intrauterine device. It is no longer marketed because of the great number of pelvic complications associated with its use.

DCP Dynamic compression plate.

Dental amalgam An amalgam of silver, tin, and mercury used in dental applications for filling of cavities. It may also contain low concentrations of copper and zinc.

Dental restorations Another term for dental fillings.

Dental plate A plate containing artificial teeth. It is fitted to the shape of the mouth and is usually constructed from metal or acrylic materials.

Denver shunt A pleuroperitoneal shunt for use in patients with intractable pleural effusion.

Deyerle apparatus An apparatus with multiple fixation pins and a side plate. It is used for intracapsular hip fractures.

Diamond's tube A tube similar to the Abbott-Rawson tube; used for study of the small intestine.

DNR Do not resuscitate.

Dobbhoff tube A type of feeding tube developed by Drs. Dobbie and Hoffmeister. It is now a generic term for any small feeding tube.

Dome port A type of vascular access port.

Doppler phenomenon A generic term to describe the apparent change in frequency of a wave form, such as light or sound, whenever the wave source and an observer are in motion relative to each other. If the source and the observer are moving together, the observed frequency is higher than the emitted frequency. If they are moving apart, the observed frequency is lower than the emitted frequency. An important example of the latter case is the "red shift" of visible light and other electromagnetic radiation from distant galaxies, which are receding from our own galaxy, the Milky Way, because of the expansion of the universe. The Doppler phenomenon is used in many medical applications, such as color Doppler ultrasound. The phenomenon is named after Christian Doppler (1803-1853), an Austrian physicist and mathematician who first described it.

Dorsal column stimulator A type of spinal column stimulator used to reduce chronic pain or muscle spasticity.

Double-lumen endotracheal tube A tube used for differential ventilation of the two lungs to accommodate differences in compliance between them.

DRG Diagnosis-related groups.

Dual MicroPort; Dual MacroPort Types of vascular access port.

DuraPhase A type of penile prosthesis.

Dwyer/Zielke (Zielke) system A complex orthopedic fixation system used for correcting thoracolumbar scoliosis.

Dynamic compression plate (DCP) An orthopedic fracture fixation plate with oval holes designed to provide compression of the fracture as eccentrically placed screws are tightened on either side of the fracture line. They are typically used for fractures that are stable.

ECRI Emergency Care Research Institute, Plymouth Meeting, Penn.; now known as ECRI.

Eggers' plate A metallic bone plate designed for maintaining approximation of bone fragments.

EN-tube-Plus A type of feeding tube.

Endoprosthesis A term sometimes applied to a hip prosthesis that consists of a single piece—a press-fit stem with a ball that matches the diameter of the acetabulum.

Endotracheal tube A tube placed in the trachea to control respiration.

Enteroclysis A high enema (literally 'intestine wash'; accent on third syllable). Barium, methyl cellulose, and sometimes air are used in varying proportions for visualization of the entire small bowel and are instilled through a tube placed in the duodenum or proximal jejunum.

Entriflex tube A type of feeding tube.

ERCP Endoscopic retrograde cholangiopancreatogram or cholangiopancreatography.

ESKA Jonas Silicone-Silver A type of malleable penile prosthesis.

Esophageal stent A stent used in the esophagus to traverse tumors or strictures.

Ewald tube A large-bore gastric tube for the evacuation and lavage of the stomach. It is typically used in cases of poison ingestion.

F, Fr French scale (see French scale).

FACR Fellow of the American College of Radiology

FB Foreign body.

FDA The United States Food and Drug Administration.

Federal Hydrashok bullet This .45 caliber bullet often produces characteristic fragments when it deforms in body tissues. It is a hollow point bullet with a post in the center. The bullet jacket of copper forms the rim of the bullet tip.

Fine needle aspiration (FNA); fine needle aspiration cytology (FNAC); fine needle aspiration biopsy (FNAB) A popular procedure in which a small needle, typically 20 to 23 gauge, is introduced into a lesion and a few cells are aspirated for cytologic examination.

Finney Flexi-Rod (Flexirod) A type of penile prosthesis.

Fish viscera retainer A metallic device used to contain viscera inside the abdominal cavity during abdominal surgery.

Fixation screws (bone screws) Any type of screw used to approximate two pieces of bone or attach a plate or rod to a bone.

Fixation wire Any type of wire used to approximate one or more pieces of fractured bone.

Flexi-Flate A type of penile prosthesis.

Flexiflow tube A type of feeding tube.

FMC Full metal case, synonymous with full metal jacket.

Focal zone banding A sonographic artifact that results from the ultrasound beam having varying intensities along its course.

Fold-in, foldover artifact See Wraparound artifact.

Foley catheter A balloon-tipped catheter used in the urinary bladder.

Four-poster Brace A type of cervical-spine external immobilization brace.

Fr, F French scale (see below).

Frederick-Miller tube A type of intestinal feeding tube.

French scale A common scale used for denoting the size of catheters, tubes, and sounds (metal exploratory or dilating instruments). Each French unit approximates 0.33 mm in diameter; therefore 18 French is equivalent to a diameter of 6 mm.

FT Feeding tube.

Full metal case (FMC) A synonym for full metal jacket.

Full Metal Jacket A type of bullet in which a metal jacket completely covers the bullet tip (a full metal jacket, or "ball," bullet). Full metal jacket bullets typically penetrate at least 10 cm before the bullet yaws. With this type of bullet, only after significant yaw does a large temporary cavity form. Under the terms of the convention of the Hague of 1899, the jacket of a military bullet must completely cover the bullet tip.

G-tube Gastrostomy tube.

Gastrostomy Tube A tube surgically, percutaneously, or endoscopically placed into the stomach through the anterior abdominal wall and used for long-term administration of feedings.

Gauge, gage A standard of measurement, or scale by which a device is measured, such as the outside diameter of a needle. (See needle gauge chart in Appendix.)

Gehrung A type of pessary.

Gellhorn A type of pessary.

"Geometric" artifact See Linear artifact.

Glanturco-Rosch Z-stents A type of self-expanding metallic stent composed of round stainless steel. It is used in the vascular and biliary systems to keep patent areas of narrowing or obstruction by buttressing.

Gibbs artifact A frequency artifact produced by magnetic resonance imaging similar to chemical-shift and magnetic artifacts. Gibbs artifact may present as a linear area of decreased signal intensity, for example, simulating a syrinx in the cervical spinal cord. Gibbs artifact is worse on coarse matrix magnetic resonance images (such as 128×128).

Glaser Safety Slug A type of bullet consisting of hundreds of pellets of number 12 birdshot in a copper cup with a nonradiopaque fiberglass-Teflon cap.

Gore-Tex A trademark of W.L. Gore (Elkton, Maryland). It is a fluorocarbon polymer and is similar chemically to Teflon (polytetrafluoroethylene). Gore-Tex is best known for its use in sportswear, but it has also been utilized in the production of a synthetic ligament and other medical devices.

Gortex A corrupt spelling of Gore-Tex.

Gossypiboma A term used to describe the foreign-body reaction that develops around a retained surgical sponge.

Gravigards A type of intrauterine contraceptive device.

Gravity drains Surgical drains that rely on gravity and fluid-tension dynamics to drain fluids away from surgical beds and help tissue approximation and wound healing.

Greenfield filter A type of inferior vena cava (IVC) filter for use in the prevention of clot propagation to the lungs.

GSW Gunshot wound.

GT Gastrostomy tube.

Gunther filter A type of inferior vena cava filter (IVC) for use in the prevention of clot propagation to the lungs.

Hagie pin A type of orthopedic fixation pin.

Halifax clamps A type of interlaminar clamp for posterior cervical spine fixation. Halifax clamps are generally used to stabilize a single level and are used in combination with bone grafting.

Hall-Kaster valve A type of prosthetic heart valve.

Halo vest An external cervical immobilization device used for unstable fractures and dislocations. A metallic ring (the halo) is fixed to the outer table of the skull by screws. The halo is connected to a padded fiberglass or plastic thoracic cast by metal rods (the struts).

Hancock (porcine) valve A type of prosthetic heart valve manufactured from pig heart valves.

Harrington rod A device using hooks in the lamina and facet joints of the spine to support the spine in cases of fracture, infection, and tumor involvement.

Harris tube A single-lumen tube with a mercury weight. Its head is similar to the Miller-Abbott tube. It is used in study of the small intestine.

Hawkins catheter A type of self-retaining accordion catheter that assumes a Z configuration after the self-retaining device has been engaged.

HC Hickman catheter.

HCFA Health Care Financing Administration.

Hemoclips Surgical clips of various sizes used to occlude bleeding vessels.

Herbert screw A modified orthopedic screw that was originally developed for the fixation of scaphoid fractures. It is cannulated and has threads on both ends.

Heterograft A graft of tissue or an organ from one species to another species.

Hickman catheter A type of central venous catheter introduced by Dr. R.O. Hickman. It is a trade name of C.R. Bard, Inc. (Tewksbury, Massachusetts) and is often used as a generic term for any central venous catheter.

HIS Hospital information system.

HMO Health maintenance organization.

Hollow point bullet Hollow point bullets have a hole in the bullet jacket at the bullet tip. The bullet is designed to deform into a mushroom shape in tissue to maximize tissue damage.

Homograft A graft of tissue or an organ from a donor of the same species as the recipient. Sometimes considered to be synonymous with the term *allograft*.

Hulka clip A special clip designed for tubal ligations.

Hydrashok bullet *See* Federal Hydrashok bullet.

Hydroflex (AMS Hydroflex) A type of penile prosthesis.

Hydroxyapatite implant A type of implant used to supplement bone defects in the jaw and facial bones.

H₂S Chemical notation for hydrogen sulfide, a rather obnoxious gas, or pejorative term used for the Department of Health and Human Services.

IACB Intra-aortic counterpulsation balloon.

ICD Implantable cardioverter-defibrillator device, the same as an automatic implantable cardioverter defibrillator (AICD).

ID Inside diameter.

Ileo-B pouch A pouch device for collecting fluids from an ostomy site.

Ilizarov technique A technique used most often in reconstructive settings to lengthen limbs, transport bone segments, and correct angular deformities.

IMDG International Medical Device Group.

Immobilization device Any device to immobilize a patient so that a procedure may be performed. Typical examples include a head holder for cranial computed tomographic studies and a Pigg-O-Stat device to restrain a child for chest radiography.

Implant Generic term used for materials or devices placed in vivo for the treatment of medical or dental conditions.

Implantofix II A type of vascular access port.

Infusaid Model 400; Infusaid Model 600 Types of vascular access port.

Injection artifacts A type of nuclear medicine artifact that originates from the injection of radiotracer.

Interfragmentary screw An orthopedic screw that crosses a fracture line.

Intestinal tube Any type of tube used to decompress the stomach or large or small bowel, to obtain fluid samples, and to provide an access route for patient nutrition.

Intra-aortic counterpulsation balloon device (IACB) This device is used to support the circulation after cardiac surgery or acute myocardial infarction until the heart recovers adequate function of its own.

Intracranial aneurysm clip A surgical clip used to occlude an intracranial aneurysm.

Intramedullary rod An orthopedic rod inserted into the medullary space of a long bone to help with fracture fixation.

Interlocking screws Screws used with intramedullary rods to "lock" the rod in place to control fracture-fragment rotation and shortening.

Intrauterine contraceptive device (IUD) A small device placed in the uterus to prevent unwanted pregnancy. IUDs are a very popular contraceptive means in most of the world.

IOFB Intraocular or intraorbital foreign body.

Ionescu-Shiley valve A type of prosthetic heart valve.

IPA Independent practice association.

IPD Intermittent peritoneal dialysis.

IPN Intern's progress note.

IPOP Immediate postoperative period, immediate postoperative prosthesis.

IPPB Intermittent positive-pressure breathing.

IPPF Immediate postoperative prosthetic fitting.

IPPV Intermittent positive-pressure ventilation.

Iron poisoning A common type of poisoning in pediatric patients, who are highly sensitive to iron compounds. Iron poisoning is a large problem in the pediatric age group because iron-containing medications are so widely used, and adults usually do not appreciate the potential toxicity of iron tablets.

ISO International Standards Organization, an international organization formed after World War I to coordinate equipment and later software standards worldwide.

IUD Intrauterine contraceptive device.

IVC Inferior vena cava. (Avoid improper "inferior vena caval" as adjective.)

I-S Ionescu-Shiley prosthetic heart valve.

J-tube Jejunostomy tube.

Jackson-Pratt drain A flat, fenestrated, closed-wound surgical drain.

Jarvik heart A pneumatically driven biventricular device invented at the University of Utah. It completely replaces the native heart within the pericardial sac.

JCAHO Joint Commission of Healthcare Organizations.

Jejunostomy tube A tube surgically or percutaneously placed into the jejunum through the anterior abdominal wall and used for long-term administration of feedings.

Jewett nail and Jewett plate A Jewett nail is used with a plate for internal fixation of an intertrochanteric hip fracture.

Jonas Penile Prosthetic Implant A type of penile prosthesis.

JP, JP-drain, JP-tube Terms sometimes used to describe a Jackson-Pratt surgical drain.

K wire *See* Kirschner wire.

Kaneda device A spine-fixation device designed to facilitate one-stage treatment of thoracolumbar lesions.

Kimray-Greenfield (K-G) filter A type of inferior vena cava (IVC) filter used to prevent clot propagation to the lungs.

Kirschner wire A type of wire commonly used for fixation of fracture fragments during fracture reduction and skeletal traction.

Knodt rod A type of orthopedic fixation rod used for spine reconstruction.

Knowles pin A type of orthopedic fixation pin.

Kuntscher nail A type of intramedullary nail for the fixation of fractures.

Kurosaka screw A short, broad, headless orthopedic screw designed to anchor anterior cruciate grafts in the metaphysis of the tibia and femur.

LAC Left atrial catheter.

Lag screw An orthopedic screw that provides compression across a fracture line.

Lane plate A metallic bone plate used for fracture fixation.

Latex A suspension in water of particles of natural or synthetic rubber or plastic; used in rubber goods, adhesives, paints, and so on.

LCDCP Low-contact dynamic compression plate, a type of orthopedic compression plate under development. It is designed to preserve periosteal blood supply.

LeVeen shunt A peritoneal jugular shunt designed to drain ascitic fluid from the peritoneal cavity to the central venous system.

Levin tube A small-bore nasogastric tube.

LGM, Vena Tech/LGM A type of vena cava filter.

Lifeport A type of vascular access port.

Light-bulb effect A type of computed radiography artifact wherein the lower, outer portions of an image appear darkened relative to the remainder of the image because of backscattered radiation entering the photostimulable phosphor imaging plate from the patient's bed or other object.

Lillehei-Kaster Valve A type of prosthetic heart valve.

Linear artifact A type of computed tomographic artifact seen at the edges of tissues with different densities, as at the junction of the dome of the liver and the lung base.

Lippes Loop A type of intrauterine contraceptive device.

Liquid adhesives (glue) Gluelike biomaterials used to treat arteriovenous malformations, high-flow vascular fistulas, and occasionally brain tumors.

LOL Little old lady.

LOM Little old man.

Luque rods (wires) An orthopedic fixation system used for spine surgery. It provides segmental posterior stabilization of the lumbar or thoracic spine by using sublaminar wires to anchor rods.

MacroPort A type of vascular access port.

Maglinte tube An intestinal tube placed in the duodenum or jejunum for performing enteroclysis. It has an expandable balloon used to occlude the bowel lumen to prevent reflux of fluid into the stomach.

Magnetic susceptibility artifact A form of chemical-shift artifact in which artifacts may be attributable, not to the difference in the frequency precessions of fat and water, but to the magnetic susceptibilities of different materials, inhomogeneity in the static field, or the presence of magnetic materials. Magnetic artifacts are projected along the frequency-encoding axis and may have comet appearances depending on the shape of the magnetic inhomogeneity.

Malecot catheter A catheter with a bulbous tip composed of two or four wings.

Malleolar bone screw A type of cortical bone screw with a self-tapping thread.

Mammary prosthesis A breast augmentation/reconstruction implant.

Marmor hemiarthroplasty A type of hemiarthroplasty used in the knee.

McGlaughlin nail Nail designed for use with a side plate for fixation of intracapsular and intertrochanteric hip fractures.

McLean Ringer tube A type of feeding tube.

Medtronic Hall valve A type of prosthetic heart valve.

Mentor GFS A type of penile prosthetic implant.

Mentor "3-piece" A type of penile prosthetic implant.

MicroPort A type of vascular access port.

Miller Abbott tube A type of intestinal drainage and decompression tube with a weighted mercury bag and two channels.

Minnesota tube A complex, multiple balloon tube similar to a Sengstaken-Blakemore tube.

Mirror imaging artifact A type of ultrasound artifact that may be created adjacent to a highly reflective acoustic interface.

Mobin-Udin umbrella A type of inferior vena cava (IVC) filter used to prevent clot propagation to the lungs.

Modular spine-fixation system A spine-fixation system using pedicle screws designed to be used with distraction hooks, intermediate screws, and a rod *(universal rod)*.

Morscher plate An anterior cervical spine–fixation system using a plate and a hollow screw.

Moe plate A metallic bone plate used for fixation of an intertrochanteric femur fracture.

MRI port A type of vascular access port.

MRPN Medical resident progress note.

Mules (also known as **"body packers"**) People who smuggle drugs by ingesting or inserting into their rectum or vagina drug-filled packets. The packing material is typically a condom or balloon, and the packets vary in their relative radiopacities.

Multiload-250 A type of intrauterine contraceptive device.

NAD No abnormality noted or no active disease.

Napier A type of pessary.

Nasogastric tube A generic term for any rubber or plastic tube used for decompression of the stomach.

NCRP National Council on Radiation Protection and Measurement.

NDT Nondestructive testing.

NED No evidence of disease.

Needle gauge The following chart shows common needle gauges and catheter-size correlations.

NEEP Abbreviation for negative end-expiratory pressure.

Neer prosthesis A type of shoulder prosthesis.

NEFT Nasoenteric feeding tube.

NEMA National Electrical Manufacturers Association, National Eclectic Medical Association.

Nephrostomy tube A tube placed into the pelvis of the kidney for the external drainage of urine.

Neufeld nail A device designed for internal fixation of intertrochanteric femur fractures.

Neutralization plate An orthopedic fixation plate used with interfragmentary screws to protect the screw fixation by neutralizing various mechanical stresses at the fracture site. Neutralization plates are typically used in the shafts of long bones.

NEXT Nationwide Evaluation of X-ray Trends.

NG tube Nasogastric tube.

NIH National Institutes of Health.

Nissen fundoplication A surgical procedure to prevent gastroesophageal reflux.

Nissenkorn prosthesis An endourethral prosthesis used to relieve urinary retention in high-risk surgical patients.

Nitinol filter A type of inferior vena cava (IVC) filter used to prevent clot propagation to the lungs.

NMR Nuclear magnetic resonance. A synonym for magnetic resonance (MR).

No Δ Abbreviation commonly scribbled on the front of film jackets by busy radiologists. It means "*no change* from previous examination."

NOMS Not on my shift.

Norport-AC, -DL, -LS, -PT, -SP Types of vascular access ports.

Nova T IUD A type of intrauterine contraceptive device.

Novacor A type of ventricular assist device.

NPDB National Practitioner Data Bank.

Nylon The first commercial polymer made in the 1930s. Nylon is now used as a generic term for a family of polyamide polymers. These polymers are used to make fibers, fabrics, and extruded forms.

OD Outside diameter, overdose, right eye *(oculus dexter)*.

OSHA Occupational Safety and Health Administration.

Oleo plombage *See* Wax plombage

Omnicarbon valve A type of prosthetic heart valve.

OmniPhase A type of penile prosthesis.

Omniscience valve A type of prosthetic heart valve.

OOP Out of plaster.

Operations *See* Surgical procedures.

OPM Other people's money.

OREF Open reduction and external fixation.

ORIF Open reduction and internal fixation.

Orogastric tube Any tube going into the stomach through the mouth rather than through the nose (a nasogastric tube).

Orotracheal tube A tube inserted into the mouth to keep the mouth open and the teeth from biting the tongue.

Orthopod Slang term for orthopedic surgeon.

Osseointegration Chemical bonding between living bone and an implant.

OTC Over the counter. It is used in reference to drugs and medical equipment that may be bought without a prescription.

OTW Off-the-wall ('unexpected, bizarre, slightly crazy comment or behavior').

P&V Pyloroplasty and vagotomy.

PACS Picture archiving and communications system.

Palmaz endovascular stent A type of stainless steel vascular stent used to maintained the lumen in narrowed vessels and ducts. It is now also being used in other applications such as porta cava shunts.

Pantopaque An oil-based myelographic contrast agent. It is not miscible with water and is no longer used, having been replaced by low-osmolar water-soluble agents. It is very slowly absorbed and remains radiographically visible for years.

Particle reinforcement A technique used to improve the properties of bone cement. For example, inclusion of bone particles in PMMA cement somewhat improves its stiffness and considerably improves its fatigue life.

Peel-Away (Introducer, Sheath) Peel-Away is a registered trade name of Cook, Inc. (Bloomington, Indiana). It is a term often used generically for any type of introducing catheter or sheath that aids in the placement of an indwelling catheter or tube. Near the end of the procedure the Peel-Away introducer is peeled off the permanent catheter and discarded.

PEEP Positive end-expiratory pressure.

Penrose drain A traditional type of gravity drain. These drains are also convenient for use as tourniquets. Penrose drains are often made out of soft latex rubber to lessen wound irritation.

Peritoneal jugular shunt (LeVeen shunt) A shunt designed to drain fluid from the peritoneal cavity to the central venous system.

Pessary A simple mechanical device inserted in the vagina for the treatment of vaginal and uterine prolapse.

Philadelphia collar A type of cervical immobilization collar molded from plastic. It has chin and occipital supports.

PHO Physician hospital organization.

Pigtail A term used to describe the appearance of the end of a drainage catheter or angiography catheter with a curvature similar to that of a pig's tail.

Ping-Pong ball plombage A type of chest treatment used for tuberculosis in the era before antibiotics.

Platinum metals Platinum, ruthenium, rhodium, palladium, osmium, and iridium. These very expensive metals are sometimes used in alloys for surgical implants.

PMMA Poly(methyl methacrylate); often less chemically correct and thus improperly: polymethylmethacrylate.

PND Percutaneous needle drainage.

POD, pod Slang term for orthopedic surgeon.

Polycarbons (polycarbonates) High-strength polymeric thermoplastic materials that match the properties of light metals. They have a resistance to most chemicals and to water over wide temperature ranges.

Polyester (fiber) Long-chain polymeric compound produced by the combination of an ester of a dihydric alcohol (usually ethylene glycol) and terephthalic acid. Dacron was the first commercial polyester fiber, and the terms "Dacron" and "polyester" are often used interchangeably. A polyester fiber is strictly defined as a synthetic fiber containing at least 80% polyester compounds.

Polyethylene, PE A simple polymer made from ethylene $(CH_2{=}CH_2)$.

Polymers (*poly* = 'many', *mer* = 'part') Molecules linked together in long chains by the primary covalent bonding in the main backbone chain with C, N, O, Si, and so on, as side atoms.

Poly(methyl methacrylate), PMMA An acrylic polymer used in a variety of prostheses.

Polytetrafluoroethylene, polytef Chemical name for Teflon and Gore-Tex.

Porcelain veneer crown Another term for a porcelain tooth cap.

Porcine graft (valve) A biologic body part derived from a pig.

Port-A-Cath A type of vascular access port. This term has come to be used generically for any type of vascular access port with a subcutaneous reservoir for injection of medication.

Portacath, Porta Cath, PortaCath Corrupt spellings of Port-A-Cath.

Portnoy shunts A type of ventriculoperitoneal shunt.

Posterior wiring A method of providing spinal fixation with posteriorly placed stabilizing wires or plates.

Posterior cervical plates A system of plates and screws placed posteriorly for the fixation of unstable spine fractures and dislocations or to stabilize the spine after surgery.

PPE Personal protective equipment, such as gloves, mask, and gown, used for handling dangerous chemicals, blood products, and bodily fluids.

PPO Preferred provider organization.

Progestasert A type of intrauterine contraceptive device.

Prosthesis Artificial substitute for a missing body part. Sometimes the terms *prosthesis, implant,* and *medical device* are used interchangeably.

PSC Percutaneous suprapubic cystostomy.

PTBD (PTHBD) Percutaneous transhepatic biliary drain.

PTFE Polytetrafluoroethylene, the parent compound for Gore-Tex and Teflon.

Pudenz-Shultz ventricular access catheter A type of ventriculoperitoneal shunt.

QAP Quality assurance program.

Q-Port A type of vascular access port.

Radiopaque A term used to describe the ability of a substance to absorb x rays and appear opaque (white) on radiographic studies.

Rayon Any of a group of smooth textile fibers made into a filament and staple form from cellulosic material by extrusion through minute holes.

RBRVS Resource-based relative value scale.

Reconstruction breast prosthesis A breast implant (prosthesis) used to reconstruct a breast after mastectomy.

Reconstruction rod A type of orthopedic rod used to treat fractures of the femoral neck, intertrochanteric, or subtrochanteric areas. These rods have proximal locking holes oriented to allow screws to be placed into the femoral neck and head.

Reconstruction plate A type of orthopedic fixation plate that is notched between the holes, allowing it to be bent or contoured in three planes. These plates are commonly used to accommodate the complex anatomy of pelvis fractures.

Resin base acrylics Biomaterials used in dentures, removable orthodontic appliances, bite guards, temporomandibular joint orthotic appliances, temporary crowns or bridges, and denture teeth.

Retaining plate An orthodontic appliance.

Reverberation pseudomass An ultrasound artifact in which multiple reverberating echoes from a gas-filled or fluid-filled structure can simulate a mass.

Reverberation bands A type of ultrasound artifact in which bright parallel lines or bands occur at regular intervals on an ultrasound image.

Ring artifact A type of computed tomographic artifact usually caused by a faulty detector producing rings or concentric circles on CT images.

Ringdown artifact *See* Comet-tail artifact.

RIS Radiology information system.

RND Radical neck dissection.

Road rash Term used by emergency room and trauma team personnel to describe the gravel, broken glass, dirt, and other debris that gets embedded in the skin and soft tissues of motor-vehicle, bicycle, Moped, motorcycle, and pedestrian accident victims. Some of the debris, such as glass and gravel, is radiopaque and will be visible on plain film radiographs.

Round CT static artifacts A film-related artifact. Round computed tomographic film static artifacts are seen as spotlike or smudge-like low densities on film. They are created by static electric discharges at points of contact between film and cassettes.

RPG Retrograde percutaneous gastrostomy.

RPN Resident progress note. There is no standard abbreviation for "attending physician progress note," since attending physicians do not customarily write progress notes.

RSNA Radiological Society of North America.

Rubber Substance defined by American Standards for Testing and Materials (ASTM) as "a material which at room temperature can be stretched repeatedly to at least twice its original length and upon release of the stress, returns immediately with force to its approximate original length."

Rush pin A type of orthopedic fixation pin with sled-runner tip and hooked end.

s Abbreviation for 'without' (from the Latin preposition *sinö*).

Saf-T Coil A type of intrauterine contraceptive device.

SCAR Society for Computer Applications in Radiology.

SCARD Society of Chairmen of Academic Radiology Departments.

SCVIR Society of Cardiovascular and Interventional Radiology.

Scott Inflatable Prosthesis A type of penile prosthesis.

SE Starr-Edwards heart valve.

Seldinger technique A percutaneous technique for the introduction of catheters and tubes. It avoids the need for a cutdown and employs the use of a guide wire.

Shape memory alloys (SMA) Alloys that permit one to design an implant that can be changed to its desirable body form by a well-controlled heating process.

Sherman plate A type of bone-fracture fixation plate.

Side-lobe/grating-lobe artifact An artifact in which several additional sound beams may be located outside the main axis of the ultrasound beam.

Sideris patch A "patch" used to close an atrial septal defect.

Silastic rubber Trade name of Dow Corning for a condensation polymer. It is a type of soft, flexible silicone elastomer.

Silicone A generic term for organic silicon compounds polymerized for use as oils, polishes, and rubberlike materials.

Silicone rubber A trade name of Dow Corning for certain rubber polymers made from polydimethyl siloxane, which is polymerized by a condensation process. The term *silicone rubber* is also used generically for a multitude of rubberlike polymers (elastomers) derived from organic silicon compounds.

Silk tube A type of feeding tube.

Simultaneous bidirectional flow artifact A Doppler ultrasound artifact in which there is the appearance of bidirectional simultaneous flow on both sides of the zero base line.

Skeletal maturation The numbers given in these figures indicate the age of appearance of ossification centers (in ranges from the 10th to the 90th percentile). The upper range refers to males and the lower to females where two sets of numbers are given; *m* indicates age in months, *yr* indicates age in years; *AB* indicates ossification centers visible at birth. *Numbers in parentheses* indicate approximate time of fusion.

SMA Superior mesenteric artery, shape memory alloy.

Small-Carrion A type of semirigid penile prosthesis.

Smeloff-Cutter valve A type of prosthetic heart valve.

Smith-Hodges A type of pessary.

Smith-Peterson cup A type of metal cup placed on the reamed femoral head in cases of fracture or aseptic necrosis.

Smith-Petersen nail A type of flanged nail for treating fractures of the femoral neck.

Snap-Lock A type of vascular access port.

SNM Society of Nuclear Medicine.

Soft point bullet Soft point bullets have some of the lead core of the bullet exposed at the tip. Soft point bullets are designed to deform into a mushroom shape in tissue to maximize tissue damage.

Somi brace A type of cervical spine brace.

SPIE International Society for Optical Engineering.

Spinal column stimulator An electronic device with leads implanted in the epidural space, the dura, or the subarachnoid space to provide electrical signal for the relief of pain or muscle spasticity.

SR Slow-release medication, sinus rhythm, or see report. SR is often written on the front of radiographic film folders by radiologists too pressed for time to describe difficult or complex radiographic findings on a particular study.

Stainless steel A common metal alloy used as a biomaterial.

Starr-Edwards valve A type of prosthetic heart valve. Its ball-cage design was one of the first successful prosthetic valves.

STAT, stat. Abbreviation for *statim,* which means 'immediately' in Latin. It is supposed to indicate an emergency of the most extreme kind. Unfortunately, this term has been greatly abused by physicians and others who desire a radiographic study, laboratory procedure, or patient consultation done quickly for their own convenience or for the patient's convenience rather than for an emergency situation. This abuse has resulted in the term *stat* coming to have little significant meaning in many radiology, pathology, and emergency departments.

Steffee device A type of posterior spinal fixation apparatus using flat plates connected to pedicular screws.

Steinman pin A type of pin commonly used for fixation of fracture fragments during fracture reduction and skeletal traction.

Stengstaken-Blakemore tube A complex device for controlling bleeding esophageal varices. There are three lumens, one of which is used to inflate a stomach balloon for retaining the device in place and for tamponing bleeding vessels in the cardia of the stomach. A second lumen is used for inflating a long balloon positioned in the distal portion of the esophagus to compress bleeding varices. The third lumen is used for aspiration of stomach contents.

Strecker stent A flexible balloon-expandable tantalum endovascular stent.

Subdural drainage catheter Catheter commonly placed to diminish subdural hematoma reaccumulation and allow the brain to reexpand.

Sump drains A type of drainage that provides a constant low level of suction. Modern sump drains often have three lumens. One lumen allows for drainage of fluid, the second allows filtered air to be sucked into the drainage bed to provide pressure for drainage, and the third is used to irrigate the wound bed.

Suprapubic cystostomy A catheter placed through the anterior pelvic wall directly into the bladder.

Swan-Ganz catheter A registered trade name of Baxter International (now Baxter Healthcare Corp.). This term has come to represent any type of multilumen central venous catheter used for measuring hemodynamic pressures and cardiac output. The tip of the catheter is usually placed in a proximal pulmonary artery branch and may be temporarily wedged more distally for measurement of pulmonary venous or left atrial pressure.

Swanson prosthesis A type of prosthesis used in small joints, such as the fingers.

Synchromed A type of vascular access port.

Syndesmotic screw An orthopedic screw that is placed across the distal tibiofibular joint parallel to and 1 to 2 cm proximal to the ankle joint.

T-tube drain A type of traditional gravity drain configured in a T shape. T-tubes are most often used for common bile duct drainage.

Tantalum A noncorrosive, malleable metal found in some prosthetic devices. As a mesh, it was formerly used to reinforce wound closures.

TARA Total articular replacement arthroplasty.

TCu (Copper T) A type of intrauterine contraceptive device.

Teflon (polytetrafluoroethylene, polytef, PTFE) The best known of the fluorocarbon polymers, a material resulting from substituting the hydrogen atoms of polyethylene with fluorine.

TENS Transcutaneous electrical neural stimulation.

Tenckhoff catheter A peritoneal dialysis catheter.

Tension band wiring A type of orthopedic wiring used to absorb tension and apply compression to bony fragments at a fracture site.

TFE Tetrafluoroethylene, the chemical compound used to manufacture Gore-Tex, Teflon, and other fluorocarbon polymers.

THA Total hip arthroplasty.

Thoracostomy tube Another term for a chest tube. It is used to drain pleural fluid collections or reexpand the lung in cases of a pneumothorax.

Thorotrast Thorium dioxide (Thorotrast) was formerly used as a radiologic contrast agent. It was discontinued because of its carcinogenic properties. Thorium is a radioactive element and emits alpha particles.

THR Total hip replacement.

Through-transmission artifact An artifact created when tissue that lies deep to fluid-filled structures appears more echogenic than normal.

TIPS Transjugular intrahepatic portosystemic shunt or stent.

Tissue compatibility A general descriptive term describing the compatibility of a prosthesis or device for use in human tissues.

Titanium Metallic element used as an implant material because of its high corrosion resistance and relatively low density.

TKA Total knee arthroplasty.

TKR Total knee replacement.

TLD Thermoluminescent dosimeter, a device used to measure ionizing radiation.

TNM A tumor classification system that describes tumor size (T), nodal involvement (N), and metastases (M).

TNTC Too numerous to count.

TPN Total parenteral nutrition.

TQM Total quality management.

TSR Total shoulder replacement.

Tracheostomy tube A tube directly inserted into the trachea through the anterior tracheal cartilage. It bypasses the larynx and pharynx and is inserted for patients in need of long-term mechanical ventilation.

TRAM flap Transverse rectus abdominis muscle flap, a surgical procedure using a portion of the abdominal wall to construct a breast cosmetically after mastectomy.

Triflanged nail A type of fixation nail used for intracapsular hip fractures.

Twiddler's syndrome A situation in which a patient "twiddles" with his or her pacemaker pack, twisting it around in its pocket. Such an action can lead to fractured wires, pacemaker malfunction, or retraction of the pacemaker leads.

UAC Umbilical artery catheter.

UHMWPE Ultrahigh molecular weight polyethylene, a type of polyethylene popular for use as the bearing interface in total joint arthroplasty.

Umbilical catheter A type of central venous catheter used in neonates. The catheter is inserted either into the umbilical vein or into one of the umbilical arteries.

Uni-Flate 1000 A type of penile prosthesis.

Universal rod A type of spinal rod used with the modular spine-fixation system.

Ureteral stent A urinary stent placed in the ureter.

Urinary stent A generic term used for any stent employed in the urinary system to traverse benign and malignant strictures, bypass areas of dehiscence or obstructing calculi, and help with fistula healing.

Urolume stent A metallic stent used for the treatment of urethral strictures. The stent is woven in the form of a tubular mesh composed of a superalloy.

UVC Umbilical vein catheter.

V&P Vagotomy and pyloroplasty.

VAD Ventricular assist device.

van Sonnenberg catheter A sump-drainage catheter system developed for the percutaneous treatment of abscesses.

Vasport A type of vascular access port.

VBAC Vaginal birth after cesarean section.

Vena Tech filter A type of inferior vena cava (IVC) filter used to prevent clot propagation to the lungs.

Ventricular assist devices (VAD) These may be univentricular or biventricular. For example, the Novacor left ventricular assist device is an implantable electrically driven pump that takes blood through a Dacron conduit from the apex of the left ventricle and pumps it through another Dacron conduit to the aorta.

Ventriculoperitoneal shunt A shunt system designed to reduce intracranial pressure and prevent the development of hydrocephalus. Cerebrospinal fluid is shunted from the ventricular system of the brain to the peritoneal cavity.

Vitallium A trade name for a cobalt-chromium alloy used in a variety of prostheses and medical instruments.

VPMA Vice-president for medical affairs, which is often used synonymously with the term "medical director."

VP shunt Ventriculoperitoneal shunt.

Wallstent A type of self-expanding metallic stent. It is composed of a wire mesh and is used to bypass biliary and vascular obstructions.

Wax plombage (oleo plombage) Before the era of antibiotics a treatment for tuberculosis in which wax was placed in the thoracic cavity to collapse and replace the affected lung.

WHO World Health Organization.

Wiltse System An orthopedic spine-fixation system using pedicle screws connected to a rod by clamps.

WNL Within normal limits.

Wraparound (fold-in, foldover) artifact A type of magnetic resonance artifact in which a portion of the image is folded over onto some other portion of the image.

Xenograft Same as a heterograft.

XIP Perform x-ray study in plaster.

XOP Perform x-ray study out of plaster.

Yale brace A type of cervical spine brace.

Yaşargil clip A type of clip for occluding a cerebral aneurysm.

Yaw The angle between the long axis of a bullet and its path of flight.

Z-stent A generic term for a variety of metallic stents used to overcome areas of narrowing in such tubular structures as arteries, bile ducts, ureters, and the urethra.

Zickle device A system designed for the stabilization of pathologic femur fractures and subtrochanteric hip fractures. It consists of an intramedullary rod and a triflanged nail.

BIBLIOGRAPHY

Brown M, Hammond P, Johnson T. *Dictionary of medical equipment,* London, 1986, Chapman & Hall.

Churchill's illustrated medical dictionary, New York, 1989, Churchill Livingstone.

De Sola R: *Abbreviations dictionary,* ed 8, Boca Raton, Fla., 1992, CRC Press.

Dorland's illustrated medical dictionary, ed 26, Philadelphia, 1981, Saunders.

Duncan HA: *Duncan's dictionary for nurses,* ed 2, New York, 1989, Springer Publishing Co.

Gelman MI: *Radiology of orthopedic procedures, problems and complications,* Philadelphia, 1984, Saunders.

Haber K: *Common abbreviations in clinical medicine,* New York, 1988, Raven Press.

Hamilton B, Guidos B. *Medical acronyms, symbols, and abbreviations,* ed 2, New York, 1988, Neal-Schumann.

Indovina T, Lindh WQ: *The radiology word book,* Philadelphia, 1990, FA Davis.

Jablonski S: *Dictionary of medical acronyms and abbreviations,* Philadelphia, 1987, Hanley & Belfus (and St. Louis, Mosby).

Kilcoyne RF, Farrar EL: *Handbook of orthopedic terminology,* Boca Raton, Fla., 1991, CRC Press.

Logan CM, Rice MK: *Logan's medical and scientific abbreviations,* Philadelphia, 1987, Lippincott.

Medical device register 1992: The official directory of medical suppliers, vol 1 and 2, Montvale, N.J., 1992, Medical Economics.

Mosby's medical, nursing, and allied health dictionary, ed 3, St. Louis, 1990, Mosby–Year Book.

Mossman J, editor: *Acronyms, initialisms, and abbreviations dictionary,* ed 16, Detroit, 1992, Gale Research Inc.

Schmidt JE: *Medical discoveries: who and when,* Springfield, Ill, 1959, Charles C Thomas.

Segen JC, editor: *The dictionary of modern medicine,* Park Ridge, N.J., 1992, The Parthenon Publishing Group.

Stedman's medical dictionary, ed 25, Baltimore, 1990, Williams & Wilkins.

Thomas CL, editor: *Taber's cyclopedic medical dictionary,* Philadelphia, 1989, FA Davis.

Webster JG, editor-in-chief: *Encyclopedia of medical devices and instrumentation,* vol 1-4, New York, 1988, John Wiley.

Medical Device Manufacturers

· ·

The following is a list of addresses and phone numbers of manufacturers of medical devices. The products of many of these manufacturers are illustrated or discussed in this book. It is probably impossible to produce such a list without inadvertently overlooking one or more important companies. The editors apologize for any omissions.

Abbott Laboratories
14th St. & Sheridan Road
North Chicago, IL 60064
(800) 222-6883

Acromed Corporation
3303 Carnegie Ave.
Cleveland, OH 44115-2636
(800) 365-6633

Acufex Microsurgical, Inc.
130 Forbes Blvd.
Mansfield, MA 02048
(800) 343-9124

Adept-Med International, Inc.
5040 Robert J. Mathews Parkway
El Dorado Hills, CA 95630-5702
(800) 222-8445

Aesculap Inc.
1000 Gateway Blvd.
South San Francisco, CA 94080-7028
(800) 258-1946

Alcon Surgical
P.O. Box 19587
Irvine, CA 92713-9587
(714) 753-1393

Alza Corp.
950 Page Mill Rd.
Palo Alto, CA 94304-1012
(800) 227-9953

American Dental International, Coaxco, Inc.
12250 SW Myslony
Tualatin, OR 97062-8041
(800) 637-0001

American Edwards Laboratories
(Baxter Healthcare Corp., Edwards Orthop. Div.)
P.O. Box 11150
Santa Ana, CA 92711-1150
(800) 424-3278

American Medical Systems
(Pfizer Hospital Products Group, Inc.)
1101 Bren Road East
Minnetonka, MN 55343-9605
(800) 328-3881

Anchor Products Company
52 Official Road
Addison, IL 60101-4519
(800) 323-5134

Argon Medical Corporation
(A Henley International company)
P.O. Box 1970
Athens, TX 75751
(800) 927-4669

Argyle; *see* Sherwood Medical Company

Avery Laboratories, Inc.
100 Lattingtown Rd.
Glen Cove, NY 11542-1243
(516) 676-9292

Baker/Cummins
8800 NW 36th St.
Miami, FL 33178-2404
(800) 735-2315

Bard Interventional Products
C.R. Bard Inc.
200 Ames Pond Drive
Tewksbury, MA 01876
(800) 327-4227

Bard Urological
8195 Industrial Blvd.
Covington, GA 30209
(800) 526-4467

Bard Vascular System Inc.
129 Concord Road
P.O. Box M
Billerica, MA 01821
(800) 322-BARD

Baxter Healthcare Corp.
1 Baxter Parkway
Deerfield, IL 60015-4625
(708) 948-2000

Becton Dickinson
One Becton Drive
Franklin Lakes, NJ 07417
(201) 847-7100

Beiersdorf, Inc.
360 Martin Luther King Dr.
Norwalk, CT 06856-0552
(800) 233 2340

Biocontrol Technology, Inc.
300 Indian Springs Rd.
Indiana, PA 15701-9704
(412) 349-1811

Biomet Inc.
Box 587, Airport Industrial Park
Warsaw, IN 46581-0587
(219) 267 6639

Bristol-Myers/Squibb
345 Park Avenue
New York, NY 10154 0193
(212) 546-4000

Burron Medical, Inc.
824 12th Avenue
Bethlehem, PA 18018-3524
(800) 523-9695

California Medical Products
1901 Obispo Ave.
Long Beach, CA 90804-1223
(213) 494-7171

Camino Laboratories
5955 Pacific Center Blvd.
San Diego, CA 92121-4309
(619) 455-1115

Carter-Wallace
P.O. Box 1-Half Acre Rd.
Cranbury, NJ 08512
(609) 655-6000

Churchill Medical Systems
905 Sheehy Drive
Horsham, PA 19044-1241
(215) 956-0585

COBE Laboratories Inc.
1185 Oak Street
Lakewood, CO 80215-4407
(800) 525-2623

Cochlear Corp.
61 Inverness Dr. E, Ste. 200
Englewood, CO 80112-5128
(800)523-5798

Codman & Shurtleff, Inc.
(A Johnson & Johnson company)
41 Pacella Drive, Randolph Ind. Park
Randolph, MA 02368-1755
(800) 343-5966

Cook Europe A/S, William
Sandet 6, DK-4632 Bjaerskov
Denmark
3/671133

Cook Incorporated
925 S. Curry Pike
Bloomington, IN 47403-2624
(800) 457 4500

Cook Urological Inc.
1100 West Morgan Street
P.O. Box 227
Spencer, IN 47460-9426
(800) 457-4448

Coopervision; see Alcon Surgical

Coratomic, Inc.; see Biocontrol Technology, Inc.

Cordis Corporation
14201 NW 60th Ave.
Miami Lakes, FL 33014-2802
(800) 327-2490

Corpak, Inc.
100 Chaddick Dr.
Wheeling, IL 60090-6006
(800) 323-6305

Cryomedic Inc
(a Cabot Medical corporation)
2021 Cabot Blvd West
Langhorne, PA 19047
(800) 243-9886

Cutter Biological
Miles Inc.
1630 Industrial Park Street
Covina, CA 91722-3419
(818) 339-7388

Dacomed Corporation
1701 E. 79th Street
Minneapolis, MN 55420
(800) 328-1103

Davis & Geck
One Cyanamid Plaza
Wayne, NJ 07470-2012
(800) 225-5341

Davol Inc.
100 Sockanossett
P.O. Box 8500
Cranston, RI 02920-0500
(800) 556-6756

Dental Ventures of America
100 Chaparral Court #100
Anaheim, CA 92808
(714) 974-6280

Denver Splint Co., Inc.
6099 S. Quebec, Suite 200
Englewood, CO 80111-4547
(800) 888-8663

De Puy
U.S. 30 East
P.O. Box 988
Warsaw, IN 46581-0988
(800) 366-8143

DLP, Inc.
620 Watson SW
Grand Rapids, MI 49504-6393
(800) 253-1540

Dow Corning Corp., Medical Materials
2200 West Salzburg Road
Dept. C-1027
Midland, MI 48640
(517) 496-4000

(Downs Surgical, Inc., now:)
Sims Surgical, Inc.
Kit Street, P.O. Box 724
Keene, NH 03431-0724
(800) 241-0995

Du Pont Critical Care
Barley Mill Plaza
P.O. Box 80027
Wilmington, DE 19880-0027
(302) 992-5000

Du Pont Merck Pharmaceutical Co.
Barley Mill Plaza P26-2172
P.O. Box 80026
Wilmington, DE 19880-0026
(302) 992-5000

Duke Labs; see Beiersdorf, Inc.

Electromedics Inc.
7337 South Revere Parkway
Englewood, CO 80112
(800) 525-7055

ENtech, Inc.
Rt. 22E. Round Valley Industrial Park
Lebanon, NJ 08833-9622
(908) 236-6500

Ethicon Inc.
Route 22, P.O. Box 151
Somerville, NJ 08876
(908) 218-0707

Ethox Corporation
251 Seneca Street
Buffalo, NJ 14204-2088
(800) 521-1022

Flowtronics Inc.
10250 North 19th Ave., Suite B
Phoenix, AZ 85021-1945
(602) 997-1364

Fuji Medical Systems U.S.A., Inc.
90 Viaduct Road
Stamford, CT 06907-2707
(800) 431-1850

Fuji Medical Systems Co., Ltd.
7-13-8 Ginza, Chuo-ku
Tokyo 104, Japan
03/545-3311

Gish Biomedical Inc.
2350 S. Pullman Ave.
Santa Ana, CA 92705
(800) 854-0531

W.L. Gore & Associates
100 Airport Road
P.O. Box 1550
Elkton, MD 21921
(800) 528-8763

Grieshaber & Company, Inc.
3000 Cabot Blvd. West
Langhorne, PA 19047-1800
(215) 654-4872

Harbor Medical, Inc.
2489 Rice St.
St. Paul, MN 55113
(612) 483-8840

Hollister Inc.
2000 Hollister Drive
P.O. Box 250
Libertyville, IL 60048-3746
(800) 323-4060

Holter-Hausner International; see Phoenix Bioengineering, Inc.

HowMedica
359 Veterans Boulevard
Rutherford, NJ 07070-2564
(201) 507-7300

Infusaid, Inc.
1400 Providence Highway
Norwood, MA 02062-5015
(800) 451-1050

Instrument Makar, Inc.
2950 East Mt. Hope Rd.
Okemos, MI 48864-1910
(800) 248-4668

Inter-Tech Orthopedics, Inc.
(div. of Johnson & Johnson Orthopedics)
618 W. Stratford Drive
Chandler, AZ 85224
(800) 356-8834

Interventional Therapeutics Corp.
385 Oyster Point Blvd., Suite #6
South San Francisco, CA 94080-1934
(415) 952-2968

Johnson & Johnson Medical Surgikos & Patient Care
25 Arbrook Blvd, P.O. Box 130
Arlington, TX 76004
(800) 433-5170

Kirschner Medical Corp.
10 W. Aylesbury Rd.
Timonium, MD 21093-4101
(800) 638-7622

Leiras Pharmaceuticals
PL 415, 20101 Turku 10
Finland
921-62311

LifeStyle Hearing, Inc.
5470 E. Speedway Blvd., #A 104
Tucson, AZ 85712
(602) 323-0099, (800) 852-2002 (limited area)

Mallinckrodt
675 McDonnell Boulevard
P.O. Box 5840
St. Louis, MO 63134-0840
(314) 895-2000

Marquest Medical Products Inc.
11039 E. Lansing Circle
Englewood, CO 80112-5910
(800) 525-7044

McGhan Medical Corp.
700 Ward Dr.
Santa Barbara, CA 93111-2919
(800) 624-4261

Meadox Medicals, Inc.
112 Bauer Drive
Oakland, NJ 07346-3105
(800) 631-8988

Medi-Spec Div. no longer valid; see Cryomedic, Inc.

Medical Incorporated
9605 W. Jefferson Trail
Inver Grove Heights, MN 55077-4423
(800) 328-2060

Medical Action Industries, Inc.
1934 New Highway
Farmingdale, NY 11735-1204
(800) 645-7042

Medical Engineering Corp./Surgitek
3037 Mt. Pleasant Street
Racine, WI 53404-1509
(800) 558-9494

Medinvent, Inc.
163 Engle Street
Englewood, NJ 07631-2530
(800) 447-7899

Medi-tech, Inc.
480 Pleasant Street
P.O. Box 7407
Watertown, MA 02272
(800) 225-3238

Med-Tech West, Inc.
15641 Chemical Lane, Suite A
Huntington Beach, CA 92649-1506
(800) 472-8431

Medline Industries, Inc.
1 Medline Place
Mundelein, IL 60060-4486
(800) 323-5886
(800) 323-3743 (factory)

Medtronic, Inc.
7000 Central Ave. NE
Minneapolis, MN 55432-3568
(800) 328-2518

Medtronic Inc., Neurological Division
800 53rd Ave., NE
Columbia Heights, MN 55421-1241
(800) 328-0810
(800) 638-7621 (sales rep.)

Mentor Corp.
600 Pine Ave
Goleta, CA 93117-3803
(800) 235-5731

Mentor Corporation
1421 2nd Ave. NW
Stewartville, MN 55976-1615
(507) 533-4725

Micro-Aire Surgical Instruments, Inc.
24971 Avenue Stanford West
Valencia, CA 91355-1278
(800) 456-0822

Mon-A-Therm, Inc.
Mallinckrodt Medical—Anaesthesiology Dept.
675 McDonnell Blvd.
St. Louis, MO 63134-0840
(800) 833-8842

Moss Tubes, Inc.
P.O. Box 378
West Sand Lake, NY 12196
(518) 674-3109

Nellcor Inc.
25495 Whitesell Street
Hayward, CA 94545-3690
(800) 635-5267

Norfolk Medical Products, Inc.
7307 N. Ridgeway
Skokie, IL 60076-4026
(708) 674-7075

Norwich Eaton Pharmaceuticals, Inc.
17 Eaton Avenue
Norwich, NY 13815-1709
(607) 335-2111

Organon Nederland bv
Welhouder van Eschstraat 1, 5342 AV.
Oss, The Netherlands
04120-6 69 22

Organon Teknika International, N.V.
Veedijk 58, Turnhout, B-2300
Belgium
14/404-040

Ormco Corp.
1332 South Lone Hill Ave.
Glendora, CA 91740-5339
(800) 854-1741

Ortho Pharmaceutical Corp.
Route 202
Raritan, NJ 08869
(908) 218-6000

Owens & Minor, Inc.
4800 Cox Rd.
Glen Allen, VA 23060-6292
(804) 747-9794

Oxboro Medical International Inc.
13828 Lincoln St., NE
Minneapolis, MN 55304
(800) 328-7958

Pacesetter Systems
(Siemens Corporation)
12884 Bradley Avenue
Sylmar, CA 91342
(800) 423-5611

Pacific Medical Industries Inc.
3134 Bunche Avenue
San Diego, CA 92122
(619) 583-3351

Para-Gard (GynoPharma Inc.)
50 Division St.
Somerville, NJ 08876-2943
(800) 322-4966

Parkell Products, Inc.
155 Schmitt Blvd.
Farmingdale, NY 11735-1403
(800) 243-7446

Pharmacia Deltec Inc.
1265 Grey Fox Rd.
St. Paul, MN 55112-6967
(800) 433-5832

Pharmaseal Div.
(Baxter Healthcare Corp.)
27200 North Tourney Road
Valencia, CA 91355-1831
(805) 253-1300

Phoenix Bioengineering, Inc.
3rd & Mill Sts., P.O. Box 96
Bridgeport, PA 19405-1076
(215) 277-6650

PIC Design
Benson Road
Middlebury, CT 06762
(203) 758-8272

Picker International, Inc.
595 Miner Rd.
Highland Heights, OH 44143
(216) 473-3000

Professional Medical Products Inc.
P.O. Box 3288
Greenwood, SC 29648-3288
(800) 845-4560

Propper & Sons Inc.
300 Denton Avenue
New Hyde Park, NY 11040
(516) 248-0300

Pudenz-Schulte Medical ITI
P.O. Box 2090, Goleta, CA 93118;
125 B. Premona Drive
Goleta, CA 93117
(800) 826-5603

Quinton Instrument Co.
2121 Terry Ave.
Seattle, WA 98121-2791
(800) 426-0337

Research Medical
(A subsidiary of Research Industries Corp.)
6864 South 300 West
Midvale, UT 84047-1001
(800) 453-8432

Richard Wolf GmbH
Pforzheimer Strasse 24, Postfach 40
D-7134 Knittlingen, Germany
07043/350

Ross Laboratories
625 Cleveland Avenue
Columbus, OH 43215-1724
(800) 848-2607

St. Jude Medical, Inc.
1 Lillehei Plaza
St. Paul, MN 55117-1761
(800) 328-9634

Sarns Inc./3M
6200 Jackson Road
Ann Arbor, MI 48103-9300
(800) 521-2818

G.D. Searle & Company
5200 Old Orchard Rd.
Skokie, IL 60077-1034
(708) 982-7000

Sentry Medical Products
17171 Murphy Ave.
Irvine, CA 92714-5915
(800) 854-6004

Sherwood Medical Company
1915 Olive Street
St. Louis, MO 63103-1625
(800) 325-7472

Shiley
17600 Gillette Avenue
Irvine, CA 92714-5702
(800) 854-3683

Siemens Medical Instrumentation, Inc.
186 Wood Avenue South
Iselin, NJ 08830-2704
(908) 321-4500

Smith & Nephew Perry
1875 Harsh Ave., SE
Massillon, OH 44646-7123
(800) 321-9752

Smith & Nephew Richards, Inc.
1450 Brooks Road
Memphis, TN 38116-1804
(800) 821-5700

Storz Instrument Company
3365 Tree Ct. Indust. Blvd.
St. Louis, MO 63122-6615
(800) 325-9500

Strato Medical Corp.
123 Brimbal Ave.
Beverly, MA 01915-1892
(800) 637-5006

Stuart Drug & Surgical Supply Co.
1 Stuart Plaza
Donohue & Luxor Roads
Greensburg, PA 16501
(412) 837-5700

Surgicot Inc.
1 Park Patriot Dr.
P.O. Box 13956
Research Triangle Park, NC 27709
(800) 221-3410
(919) 361-0419

Synthes Ltd. (U.S.A.)
P.O. Box 1766
1690 Russell Road
Paoli, PA 19301-1222
(800) 523-0322

Target Therapeutics
130 Rio Robles
San Jose, CA 95134-1806
(800) 345-2498

Taut, Inc.
2571 Kaneville Ct.
P.O. Box 326
Geneva, IL 60134-2505
(718) 232-2507

Tecnol
7201 Industrial Park Blvd.
Fort Worth, TX 76180-6153
(800) 832-6651

3M Medical-Surgical Division
3M Center, Building 225-5S-01
St. Paul, MN 55144-1000
(800) 228-3957

Treace Medical Inc.; see Xomed-Treace

Tucson Limb & Brace
4920 E. Speedway
Tucson, AZ 85712
(602) 322-0099

Union Broach
P.O. Box 508
Emigsville, PA 17318
(800) 221-1344

United States Surgical Corporation
150 Glover Ave.
Norwalk, CT 06850-1308
(203) 866-5050

Upjohn Company
7000 Portage Road
Kalamazoo, MI 49001-0102
(800) 253-8600

Valleylab Inc.
(A Pfizer Company)
5920 Longbow Drive
Boulder, CO 80301-3202
(800) 255-8522

Weck Endoscopy
(Edward Weck & Co., Inc.)
Weck Drive, P.O. Box 12600
Research Triangle Park, NC 27709
(800) 334-9751

William Gore & Associates Inc.
Route 213 North
P.O. Box 1220
Elkton, MD 21921
(800) 528-8763

Wilson-Cook Medical Inc.
4900 Bethania Station Road
Winston-Salem, NC 27105-1203
(800) 245-4717

Xomed-Treace
6743 Southpoint Drive N.
Jacksonville, FL 32216-6218
(800) 874-5797

Young Drug Products Corp.; see Carter-Wallace

Zimmer Inc.
P.O. Box 708
Warsaw, IN 46581-0708
(800) 348-2759

ZMI Corporation
500 W. Cummings Park
Woburn, MA 01801-6506
(800) 348-9011

REFERENCE

Medical Device Register, vol 2, Medical Economics Data, 1992, a div. of Medical Economics Co., Inc., Montvale, NJ 07645.

Safe Medical Devices Act of 1990

Eve Saenz

On November 28, 1990, President Bush signed into law the "Safe Medical Devices Act of 1990," which imposes new reporting requirements on hospitals and other "device-user facilities." The act went into effect in November 1991. The act requires healthcare facilities—including hospitals, ambulatory-surgical facilities, nursing homes, and outpatient treatment facilities—to report information that "reasonably suggests" the probability that a medical device has caused or contributed to the death, serious injury, or serious illness of a patient at that facility. Such reports must, depending on the circumstances, be submitted to the Food and Drug Administration (FDA) or the device manufacturer, or both. Facilities are also required to submit FDA semiannual reports summarizing previously submitted reports.

Deaths. When the death of a patient at a device-user facility has occurred and the facility has information that reasonably suggests the probability that a device may have caused or contributed to that death, the incident must be reported to the FDA, with a copy of the report sent to the manufacturer, if known. Such reports must be sent no later than 10 working days after medical personnel (including physicians) receive or become aware of the information in the course of their duties.

Serious illness or serious injury. When a device-user facility has information that reasonably suggests the probability that a device has caused or contributed to the serious illness of a patient at the facility, the incident must be reported to the manufacturer or to the FDA if the manufacturer is not known. Such reports must be made within the same 10-working-day time frame that is required for reports of deaths.

Once a user report is received by a manufacturer, the manufacturer has the same responsibilities that it would have on receiving information from any other source to investigate and, if appropriate, to report the incident to the FDA under the existing Safe Medical Devices Act regulations.

USER REPORTING GLOSSARY

Device-user facility means a hospital, ambulatory-surgical center, nursing home, or outpatient treatment center that is not a physician's office. The FDA regulation may include an outpatient diagnostic facility that is not a physician's office.

Serious injury and serious illness mean illness or injury, respectively, that

(1) is life threatening,
(2) results in permanent impairment of a body function or permanent damage to a body structure, or
(3) necessitates immediate medical or surgical intervention to preclude permanent impairment of a body function or permanent damage to a body structure.

PLANNING AND IMPLEMENTING A USER REPORTING PROGRAM

The following are areas that each device-user facility must consider in planning and implementing a user reporting program:

1. Assign overall responsibility for program development and management.
2. Convene an ad hoc committee with representatives from areas such as Nursing, Quality Assurance/Risk Management (QA/RM), Clinical Engineering, Medicine, Safety, Material Management, and Administration. Their goal should be to review the laws and regulations of their state and community along with current practices, such as policies and procedures already in place in their institution.
3. Develop policies and procedures for internal reporting.
4. Design a reporting form.
5. Address confidentiality issues.
6. Develop a device-related investigation protocol.
7. Provide in-service education to physicians, nurses, technologists, and others who deal directly with device usage. All in-service shifts make the same information available to staff within the device-user facilities of the organization.
8. Incorporate data into risk management/quality assurance programs.
9. Develop policies and procedures for submitting agency reports.

Recall of devices. The Act grants to the FDA for the first time significant authority to recall medical devices and to issue orders to manufacturers for the immediate termination of distribution of any device where there is a reasonable probability of serious adverse health effects. In addition, the FDA requires manufacturers to notify physicians and user facilities of such orders and to instruct them to cease the use of the device. The Act also empowers the FDA to request that physicians who prescribe medical devices assist in notifying individuals of the risks associated with a recalled device.

Civil penalties. Substantial penalties can be imposed for violations in reporting device-related incidents.

SAFE MEDICAL DEVICE-TRACKING REQUIREMENTS

After the implementation of the Safe Medical Device Act in late 1991, the FDA proposed a further regulation that would include the tracking of certain devices. These regulations became effective May 28, 1992. The Safe Medical Devices Act requires that three classes of devices be tracked:

1. Permanently implantable devices, the failure of which would be reasonably likely to have serious adverse health consequences. These devices include such items as:
   • Vena cava clip
   • Cardiovascular intravascular filter
   • Vascular graft prosthesis of less than 6 mm diameter

   • Vascular graft prosthesis of 6 mm and greater diameter
   • Intracardiac patch or pledget made of polypropylene, polyethylene terephthalate, or polytetrafluoroethylene
   • Ventricular bypass (assist) device
   • Implantable pacemaker pulse generator
   • Cardiovascular permanent pacemaker electrode
   • Annuloplasty ring
   • Replacement heart valve
   • Automatic implantable cardioverter/defibrillator
   • Tracheal prosthesis
   • Intravascular occluding catheter
   • Aneurysm clip
   • Central nervous system fluid shunt and components
   • Implanted cerebellar stimulator
   • Implanted diaphragmatic/phrenic nerve stimulator
   • Artificial embolization device
   • Spinal interlaminal fixation orthosis
   • Spinal intervertebral body fixation orthosis
2. Life-sustaining or life-supporting devices to include:
   • Breathing frequency monitors (apnea monitors)
   • Pressure regulator, including mechanical oxygen regulators
   • Portable oxygen generator, including oxygen concentrators
   • Portable liquid oxygen unit
   • Tracheostomy tube and tube cuff
   • Continuous ventilator
   • Noncontinuous ventilator (IPPB)
   • DC-defibrillator (including paddles)
   • Peritoneal dialysis system and accessories, including chronic ambulatory (adult) and chronic pediatric (infant) peritoneal dialysis systems
   • Infusion pumps
3. The FDA's proposed rule also lists the following as designated devices:
   • Silicone inflatable breast prosthesis
   • Silicone gel-filled breast prosthesis
   • Silicone gel-filled testicular prosthesis
   • Silicone gel-filled chin prosthesis
   • Silicone gel-filled Angelchik antireflux valve

DATA COLLECTION AND MAINTENANCE

Manufacturers are required to track the device through distribution channels to the ultimate user (that is, a patient). Upon implantation or further distribution of a tracked device, the manufacturer must collect a wide array of product, distribution, patient, and physician information and must maintain and update that information in an effective tracking system for the life of the device. This information will be collected from device-user facilities, physicians, and other practitioners who implant or provide the tracked device to the patient. In addition, the regulation requires manufacturers to collect, if applicable, information that will terminate a manufacturer's responsibility to track a particular device, such as the date of the patient's death or the date that the device was explanted or permanently disposed of. In most institutions this tracking system will need to be newly developed in areas other than the operating room where this procedure has long been in effect. Other areas to feel the impact of this regulation will be the ambulatory care settings who routinely explant devices but have rarely been required to track the removal of the device.

Index